Subdural Hematoma

Mehmet Turgut • Ali Akhaddar
Walter A. Hall • Ahmet T. Turgut
Editors

Subdural Hematoma

Past to Present to Future Management

Springer

Editors
Mehmet Turgut
Department of Neurosurgery
Aydın Adnan Menderes University
Faculty of Medicine
Efeler, Aydın
Turkey

Department of Histology and Embryology
Aydın Adnan Menderes University Health
Sciences Institute
Efeler, Aydın
Turkey

Walter A. Hall
Department of Neurosurgery
SUNY Upstate Medical University
Syracuse, New York
USA

Ali Akhaddar
Avicenne Military Hospital of Marrakech
Department of Neurosurgery
Mohammed V University in Rabat
Rabat
Morocco

Ahmet T. Turgut
Department of Radiology
Yüksek İhtisas University Faculty of
Medicine
Balgat, Ankara
Turkey

ISBN 978-3-030-79370-8 ISBN 978-3-030-79371-5 (eBook)
https://doi.org/10.1007/978-3-030-79371-5

This Springer imprint is published by the registered company Springer Nature Switzerland AG
The registered company address is: Gewerbestrasse 11, 6330 Cham, Switzerland

Foreword

This timely book comprehensively covers one of the most frequent afflictions and yet sorely neglected issues in Neurosurgery. In particular the chronic variant of the subdural hematoma (SDH), or as Virchow coined it the "pachymeningitis hemorrhagica interna" (1857), has increased in proportion to our longevity. Additional amplifying factors as well as the diversity of clinical presentations are systematically covered in this volume.

While books about arteriovenous malformations and aneurysms are numerous, despite being relatively rare entities, a thorough analysis in one volume on SDHs is rare, despite the prevalence in real life. Also, SDHs most often represent the first surgical experience of many neurosurgeons, past, present, and future.

And most often this is good, since frequently a small operation can yield an almost instantaneous recovery. However, all of us have also seen our patients on the slippery slope of recurrent hematomas that defy your every best therapeutic effort with uncontrollable deterioration and dismal outcomes. Chronic subdural hematoma (CSDH) can provide a humbling experience.

And while few would call themselves a "CSDH" surgeon, aren't we all? And if we are, our obligation is to further our knowledge and art. Improving the lot of a patient with SDH can be easy and gratifying with a "miracle" recovery. Not being able to help a patient despite our best efforts may be fate, but it is our duty to try everything to improve the odds and it is due diligence to treat the issue with scientific rigor and sincerity.

Turgut, Akhaddar, Turgut, and Hall provide this foundation. Their book will become a standard tool for our younger colleagues, but also a reminder for all to improve our art where it matters most.

Arya Nabavi, MD, PhD, MaHM, IFAANS
Professor of Neurosurgery
Director Dept. of Neurosurgery
Nordstadt Hospital KRH
Haltenhoffstr
Hannover, Germany

Preface

Subdural hematomas (SDHs) are an interesting disease that is still widely discussed regarding its management despite it being the most common pathology in surgical practice and one of the first surgical procedures taught in residency training in neurosurgery. The incidence of this clinical entity is gradually increasing worldwide due to the extended life expectancy for adults and the common usage of antithrombotic therapy for various medical conditions. SDHs are primarily manifest in three forms, acute, subacute, and chronic, which are influenced by their etiology and the individual patient developing the malady. The pathophysiology of the development of SDHs can be described with respect to their location in the cranial vault or the spinal canal. The various histopathological changes seen in SDHs differ based on the age of the collection since its inception. There are specific predisposing medical risk factors that can lead to the occurrence of SDHs.

The clinical presentation of the SDHs is related to its intracranial location and can be different when the specific age group affected is considered. In intracranial SDHs, the anticipated modes of presentation, such as seizures, can result as can other unusual forms of presentation, such as psychiatric disorders, while spinal cord compression syndrome can occur at the spinal level of origination. The presence of neurological findings should necessitate some form on neuroimaging study in the form of computed tomography or magnetic resonance imaging to determine the underlying source of the hemorrhage. A careful clinical history can also yield a potential etiology for the SDH if a lumbar puncture or cerebrospinal fluid diversion surgery is performed, electroconvulsive therapy is administered, and an underlying hematological disorder or spontaneous intracranial hypotension is present. In some cases, specific intracranial abnormalities have been identified in association with SDHs such as arteriovenous malformations and arachnoid cysts. Not unexpectedly, head trauma and sports-related injuries can result in the development of SDHs, even with minor trauma in the elderly.

The management of SDHs is primarily surgical in nature with different anesthetic techniques being administered in order to successfully treat the hemorrhagic collection. New invasive procedures that include endoscopic drainage and middle meningeal artery embolization have been effectively employed to SDHs. Medical management in the form of corticosteroid therapy and the administration of tranexamic acid have been utilized to manage SDHs. Despite improved treatment for SDHs, postoperative complications can occur and lead to disease recurrence. Ultimately, some form of postoperative rehabilitation therapy is necessary for the elderly population that sustains a SDH, and the prognosis and clinical outcome are often influenced by a successful course of treatment. From a medicolegal point of view, it should always be kept in mind that various acts of malpractice, such as shaken baby syndrome, in addition to diagnostic and treatment errors, may complicate the management of patients with SDHs.

Aydın, Turkey — Mehmet Turgut
Marrakech, Morocco — Ali Akhaddar
Syracuse, NY, USA — Walter A. Hall
Ankara, Turkey — Ahmet T. Turgut

Contents

Chapter 1
Review of Craniospinal Acute, Subacute, and Chronic Subdural Hematomas

Ali Akhaddar

1.1 Introduction

A subdural hematoma (SDH) appears due to an accumulation of blood into the space between the dura mater and the arachnoid layer. The dura represents the pachymeninx that protects the brain within the cranial cavity and both the spinal cord and nerve roots inside the spinal canal. Most SDHs result from a rupture of bridging veins in the subdural space under certain circumstances, the most important of which is trauma in addition to some medical comorbidities and risk factors such as antiplatelet or anticoagulant agents.

SDHs represent a common and well-known entity in neurosurgical practice with various localizations, heterogeneous clinical manifestations, different neuroimaging features, as well as diverse vital and functional considerations. However, in order to simplify SDH classification, three main categories of patients must be distinguished depending on the topography and age of the hematoma:

– "Primo" Cranial acute/subacute SDH
– "Secundo" Cranial chronic SDH
– "Tertio" Spinal SDH

However, different associations are possible as discussed throughout this book.

The distinction between acute and subacute SDH on one hand and subacute and chronic SDH on the other hand is not always evident; it depends on time and neuroimaging features.

Both young and aging populations are affected by cranial SDH. Younger patients typically experience acute traumatic SDH secondary to high-energy mechanisms of injury, while older patients are more likely to present chronic SDH generally

---

A. Akhaddar (✉)
Avicenne Military Hospital of Marrakech, Department of Neurosurgery,
Mohammed V University in Rabat, Rabat, Morocco

M. Turgut et al. (eds.), *Subdural Hematoma*,
https://doi.org/10.1007/978-3-030-79371-5_1

resulting from a minor head injury with or without predisposing conditions (brain atrophy, alcoholism, coagulopathies…). Cranial acute SDHs are frequently life-threatening while chronic ones have a better prognosis if correctly managed.

Spinal localization is even more uncommon than intracranial forms of SDH with less than 260 reported cases in the literature to date [61].

A summary of cranial and spinal SDHs is given in this chapter, taking into consideration the age of hematoma and the potential association of its various forms.

1.2 Cranial Acute and Subacute Subdural Hematoma

Acute and subacute SDHs are usually associated with severe head injuries and may result from avulsed bridging veins, lacerated brain, or ruptured cortical vessels. Also, up to one third of head-injured patients with acute SDH may have a significant polytrauma [24, 40]. These hematomas can also be associated with other intracranial lesions such as contusions and intracerebral hematomas, brain swelling, diffuse axonal injuries, or epidural hematomas. Some acute/subacute SDHs may occur in patients without a history of trauma but who have bleeding disorders (receiving anticoagulant therapies or having coagulation diseases) or other unusual underlying etiologies as neoplasms or vascular malformations [13, 16, 27, 32, 41, 58]. In addition, a few cases have been described following cranial or spinal surgery [10, 12, 52, 62, 64].

Symptoms may be secondary to compression of underlying brain, injured brain parenchyma, cerebral edema, and midline shift. Frontal and temporal lobes are the most common localizations. However, some acute/subacute SDHs may be interhemispheric, along the tentorium, or in the posterior fossa [19]. A wide range of clinical presentations may occur such as altered consciousness, seizure, and neurological deficits, as well as other cardio-respiratory and systemic disorders.

In emergency situation, non-contrast computed tomography scan (CT scan) is considered the gold initial procedure in cranial injured patients because it is more accessible, faster, and less expensive. The classic intracranial SDH is an extra-axial crescentic mass with a concave inner margin that follows the surface of the brain usually with associated edema, mass effect, and midline shift. Severe presentations are accompanied by cerebral contusions, intraparenchymal hematomas, uncal herniation, effacement of basal cisterns, and dilatation of the contralateral temporal horn. Distinction between acute and subacute bleeding is occasionally confused. However, most acute forms (less than 3 days old) are hyperdense and most subacute hematomas (between 3 days and 2 weeks old) are isodense or with mixed density as compared to brain parenchyma (Figs. 1.1 and 1.2). In the same way, some forms of SDH cannot be distinguished from epidural subdural hematoma on CT scan and can even sometimes coexist [4]. When a vascular lesion is suspected, a prompt angiographic CT scan or angio-magnetic resonance (MR) (less commonly a brain angiography) can be useful to localize and diagnose the etiology [13, 18, 58]. Other

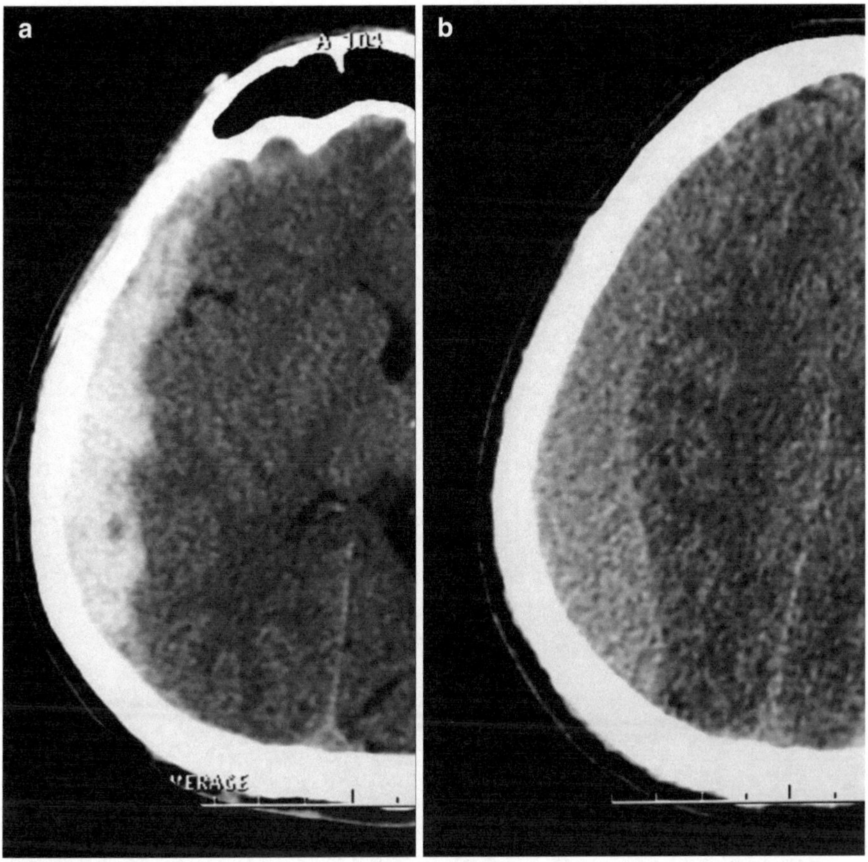

Fig. 1.1 Computed tomography appearance of acute (**a**) and subacute (**b**) subdural hematomas

testings can be useful as laboratory investigations in order to search for an occult coagulopathy or hematologic disease.

The majority of patients with acute SDH need neurocritical care [19, 36]. When surgical procedures are discussed, the neurosurgeon should always consider the underlying etiology of the bleeding, patient's general conditions and any coagulopathy that could be associated. The treatment of acute/subacute SDHs depends on the size and rate of growth of the hematoma, as well as the underlying brain damage. Some small subdural hematomas (thickness less than 10 mm in adult and less than 5 mm in children) can be managed conservatively as the blood collection may resolve spontaneously [28, 76]. Others, especially subacute and liquefied forms, can be treated by bur hole(s) and drainage. However, because of the consistency of blood clots (coagulum), large or symptomatic acute SDHs require a craniotomy for hematoma evacuation and a control of the bleeding (Fig. 1.3) [19]. Sometimes, a supplement decompressive craniectomy may be necessary [40, 60]. Postoperative complications can include high intracranial pressure, brain swelling,

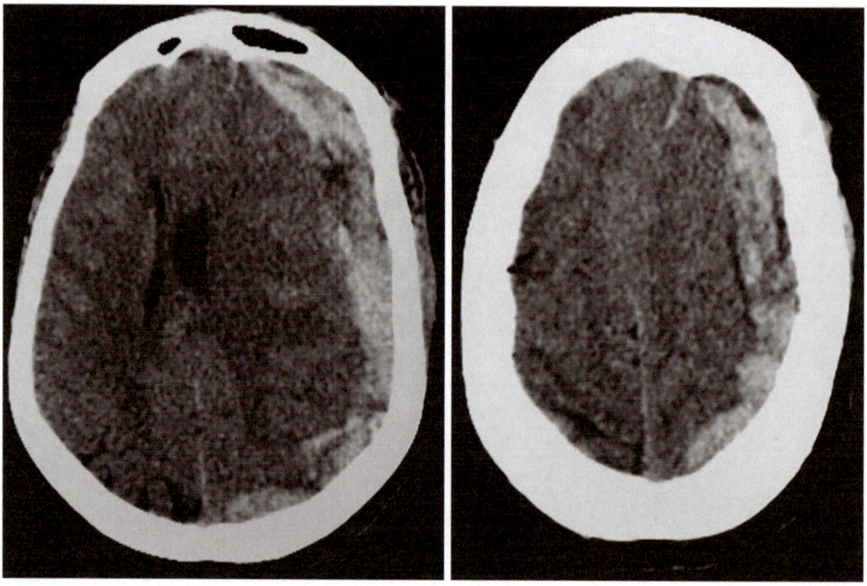

Fig. 1.2 Head axial CT scan: spontaneous (non-traumatic) left acute subdural hematoma in a patient receiving anticoagulant agent

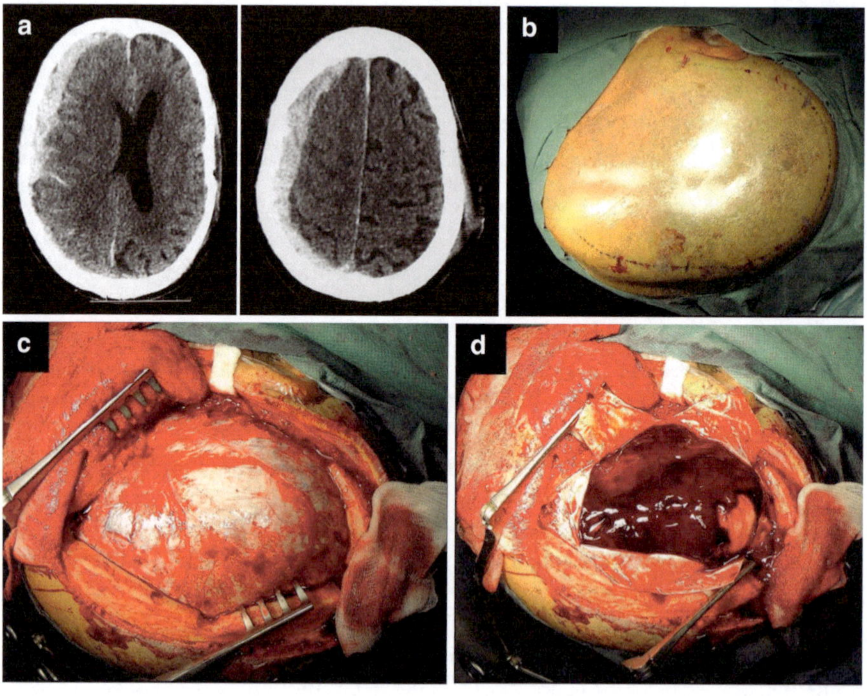

Fig. 1.3 Axial CT scan: post-traumatic acute subdural hematoma on the right side (**a**). Head position with incision mark (question-mark-shaped) on the scalp (**b**). Operative view after removing the fronto-parieto-temporal bone flap (**c**). After opening the dura in a cruciform fashion, the acute hematoma (blood clots) was revealed on the subdural space (**d**)

various forms of new intracranial bleeding, subdural recurrence, infections, seizures, and cardiopulmonary consequences. Therefore, a multidisciplinary postoperative critical care is often needed [36, 70].

The prognosis is habitually much worse than chronic SDH and epidural hematoma. The extent of primary brain lesions underlying the acute subdural hematomas seems the most significant factor affecting the outcome [22, 33, 70]. However, an aggressive medical management and a rapid surgical decompression may improve the initial neurological status [33, 40]. [For further details about cranial acute and subacute SDHs, please refer to Chap. 2 of the present book.]

1.3 Cranial Chronic Subdural Hematoma

Chronic form of SDH is a collection of old blood products (more than 3 weeks old) that have accumulated in the subdural space generally in the elderly due to brain weight diminution and subdural space expansion with age. The incidence rate of this intracranial hematoma is about 80–120 cases per 100,000 persons in aged population [11, 65]. However, this value is expected to increase considerably from 2020 to 2040 to the point that chronic SDH will become the most frequent cranial neurosurgical pathology among adults by the year 2030 in the United States of America [11, 59].

Intracranial chronic SDH had multiple potential etiologies (head injury, neoplasm, vascular malformation, intracranial hypotension,…) and risk factors (chronic alcoholism, seizure, cerebrospinal fluid shunt, cranial/spinal surgery, coagulopathies, male gender…). However, its physiopathology is not completely understood [5, 11, 34, 38, 59]. Three centuries ago, chronic SDH was recognized as a stroke [75]. One century later, it became an inflammation [63, 69, 75]. Then, a traumatic origin was accepted in the early twentieth century (traumatic tearing of the bridging veins which connect the brain cortex with the dura mater) [63, 71]. After that, various further suggestions such as osmotic pressure or effusion were advanced. Some investigators have also found that both coagulation and fibrinolysis systems were excessively activated in chronic SDH. Also, it has been proposed that more complex factors are simultaneously implicated including angiogenesis, inflammation, recurrent microbleedings, exudates, and local coagulopathy [21, 25].

Otherwise, several and various risk factors have been associated with the occurrence of this intracranial hematoma. Lately, a number of authors have assumed the role of "cranial morphology" (symmetrical or asymmetrical) on the location and development of chronic SDH (refer to Chap. 6 of the present book) [5].

Usually clinical evolution is divided into three separate stages: the initial traumatic incident (often minor and sometimes unnoticed), the latency phase, and the real clinical presentation period. Therefore, patients with chronic SDH can be asymptomatic or can have very mild symptoms such as headache, confusion, language difficulties, nausea, vomiting, vertigo, asthenia, progressive mental deterioration, gait disturbance, limb weakness, or incontinence. They may also present acute and grave symptoms with varying degrees of hemiplegia, seizures, or even coma [6, 7].

Cranial chronic SDH is usually diagnosed by CT scan. This hematoma classically appears as a concavo-convex pericerebral fluid collection along the cranial convexity. Most commonly the density of the collection is low; however, isodense and mixed or heterogeneous density lesions are also seen (Fig. 1.4a–d). Chronic SDHs are often unilateral with significant mass effect and midline shift; nevertheless, some others can be bilateral, interhemispheric, but rarely in the posterior fossa or adjacent to the skull base. Although rare, some hematomas may be organized, calcified or even ossified (Fig. 1.4e, f) [73]. In some unusual presentations, supplementary post-contrast CT scan and even better MR imaging offer important characteristics in determining the exact topography of the hematoma, its relationship with contiguous anatomic structures, and its potential underlying etiologies (e.g., tumors, vascular malformations, inflammatory lesions, infections...) (Figs. 1.5, 1.6, and 1.7) [15]. In addition, other testings can be useful as laboratory investigations in order to search for an occult coagulopathy or hematologic disease. Therefore, diagnosis of chronic SDHs can be challenging due to the variable clinical presentations of the disease and potentially subtle neuroimaging appearances (refer to Chap. 26 of the present book). For that reason, a high index of suspicion needs to be kept in mind to avoid mismanagement and possible complications of this common neurosurgical entity.

Although there is a part for nonoperative medical management strategies (Figs. 1.8 and 1.9) [Refer to Chap. 27 of the present book], surgical closed-system drainage remains the basis of current therapy in symptomatic patients. This surgical technique considerably decreases the possibility of recurrence of chronic SDH, length of hospital stay, postoperative complications, and mortality.

Formal surgical options are widely used such as burr holes (Fig. 1.10) (two, single large or trephination), twist drill craniostomy, and craniotomy (Fig. 1.11) with or without subdural closed-system drainage. Other various surgical procedures have been described worldwide but the experiences are limited and the encouraging results lack perspective [66]. Among the surgical techniques reported, we list: hollow screws, subduroperitoneal shunt, implantation of an ommaya reservoir for repetitive punctures/aspiration of subdural collections, Subdural Evacuating Port

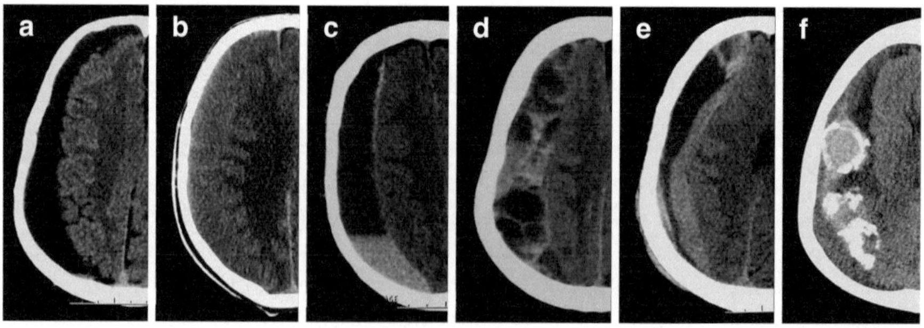

Fig. 1.4 Computed tomography appearance of various types of intracranial chronic subdural hematomas. (**a**) Low density. (**b**) Isodensity. (**c**) Acute on chronic SDH. (**d**) Mixed density with multilayer loculations. (**e**) Organized SDH. (**f**) Calcified/ossified SDH

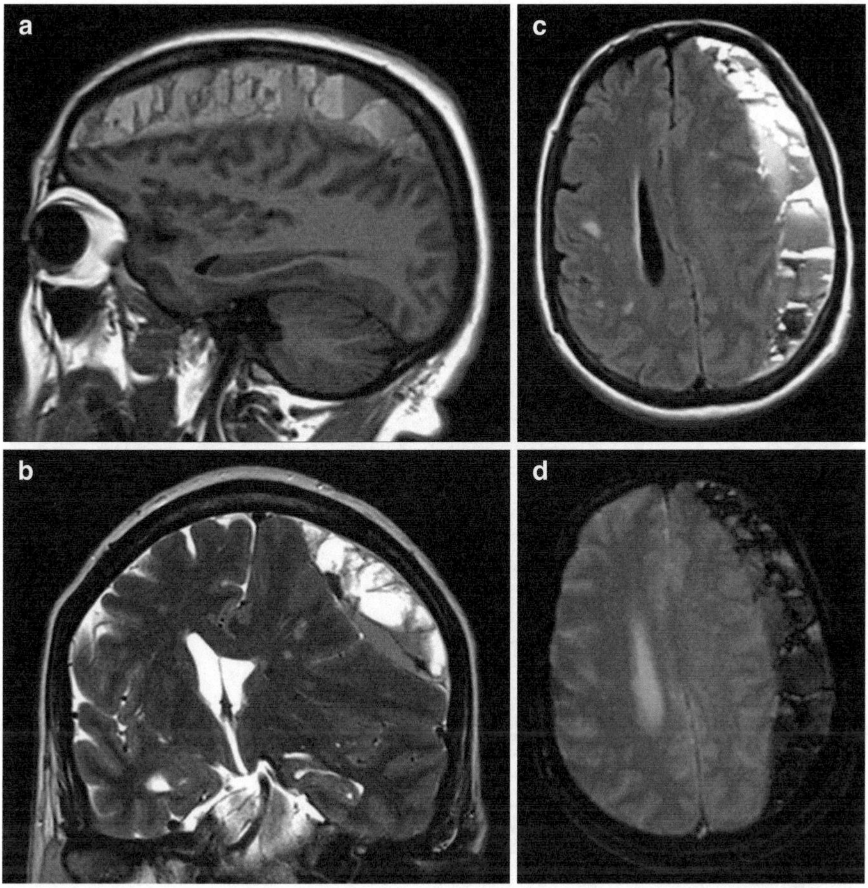

Fig. 1.5 MRI appearance of a heterogeneous mixed intracranial chronic SDH with multilayer loculations on the left side (**a**–**d**)

System (SEPS), endoscopic hematoma removal, and middle meningeal artery embolization [14, 30, 78].

Surgical evacuation of the chronic SDHs is indicated for symptomatic patients or when the hematoma had a maximum thickness superior than 10 mm with brain mass effect. Although surgery for intracranial chronic SDH is thought to be a relatively simple and safe procedure with a low complication rate, reported incidences of postoperative complications can reach 38% of operated patients [Refer to Chap. 33 of the present book]. Complications include those directly related to surgery or surgical techniques (recurrence, seizures, new intracranial bleeding, tension pneumocephalus, and infection), while others are called nonsurgical (common medical) complications. All these problems can adversely impact morbidity and mortality as well as contribute substantially to the costs of treatments and the hospital stay [65].

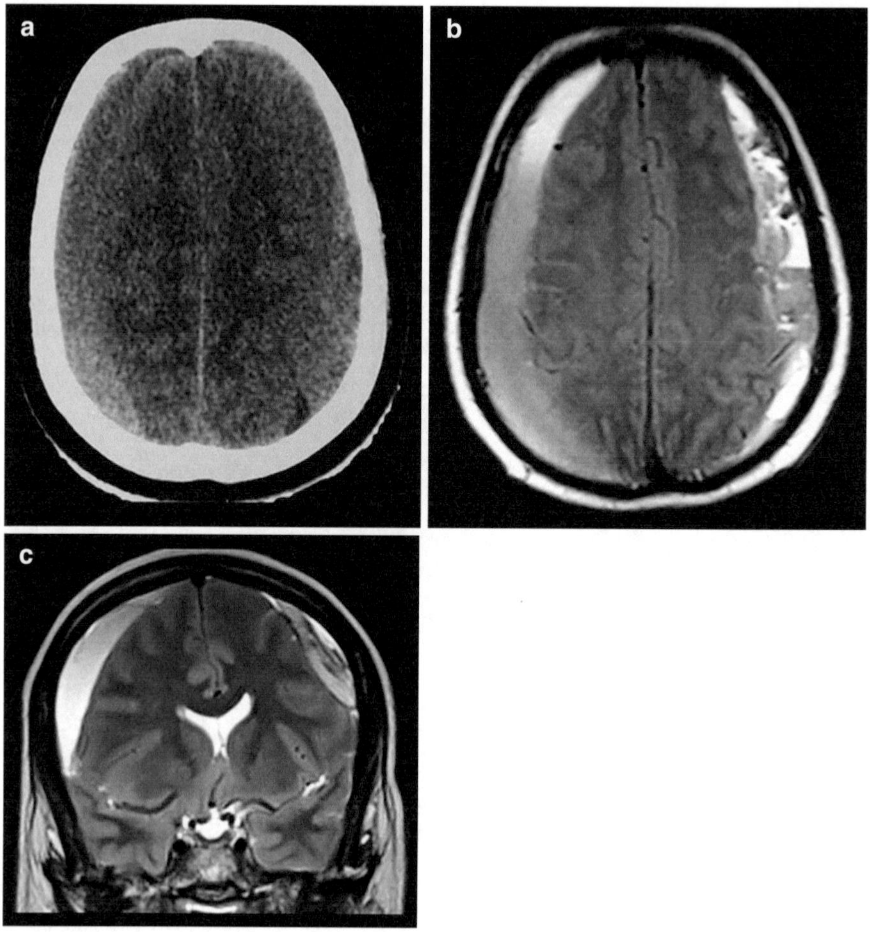

Fig. 1.6 Bilateral intracranial isodense chronic subdural hematoma on CT scan (**a**). Better distinction of the SDH on MRI: axial (**b**) and coronal (**c**) T2-weighted images

Benefit of antiepileptic agents is unclear. For some practitioners, seizure prophylaxis is used systematically. In our practice, like most neurosurgeons, antiepileptic drugs are not recommended if there are no seizures. If a late seizure occurs, a long-term therapy is required. The efficacy of corticosteroids is currently recognized [72]. They can be used as a monotherapy or as an adjunct to surgery. Coagulopathies should be corrected taking into consideration its risks/benefits.

The prognosis of chronic SDH is normally much better than the one of acute SDH. Morbidity and mortality rates of patients operated on for a chronic SDH depend mostly on the surgical technique, the patients' age and comorbidities, and the initial neurological status. The overall postoperative favorable outcome is reported to be up to 90% with younger patients usually attaining better outcomes

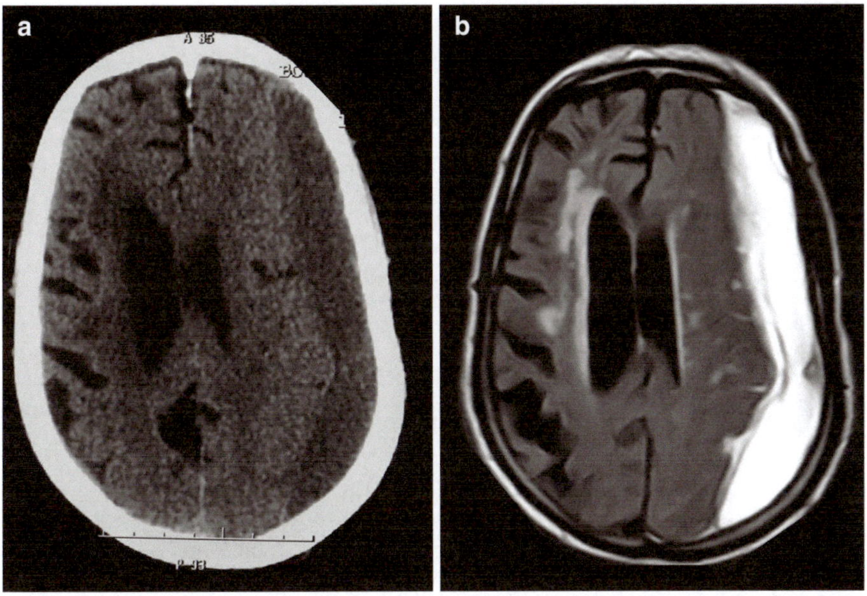

Fig. 1.7 Intracranial chronic SDH on the left side in the same patient on axial CT scan (**a**) and inversion recovery sequence (MRI) (**b**)

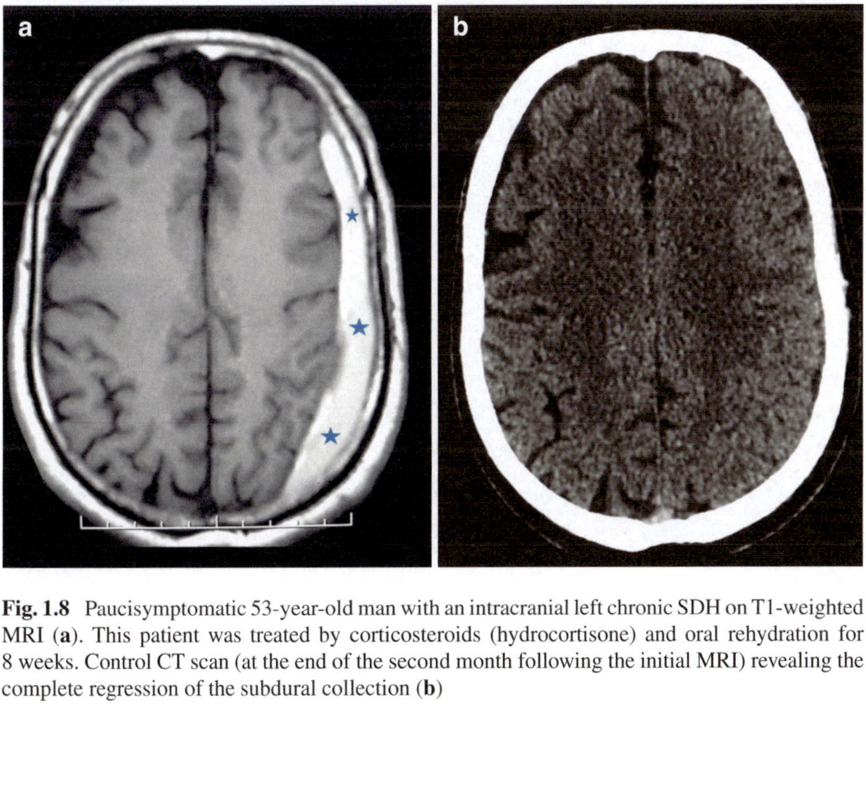

Fig. 1.8 Paucisymptomatic 53-year-old man with an intracranial left chronic SDH on T1-weighted MRI (**a**). This patient was treated by corticosteroids (hydrocortisone) and oral rehydration for 8 weeks. Control CT scan (at the end of the second month following the initial MRI) revealing the complete regression of the subdural collection (**b**)

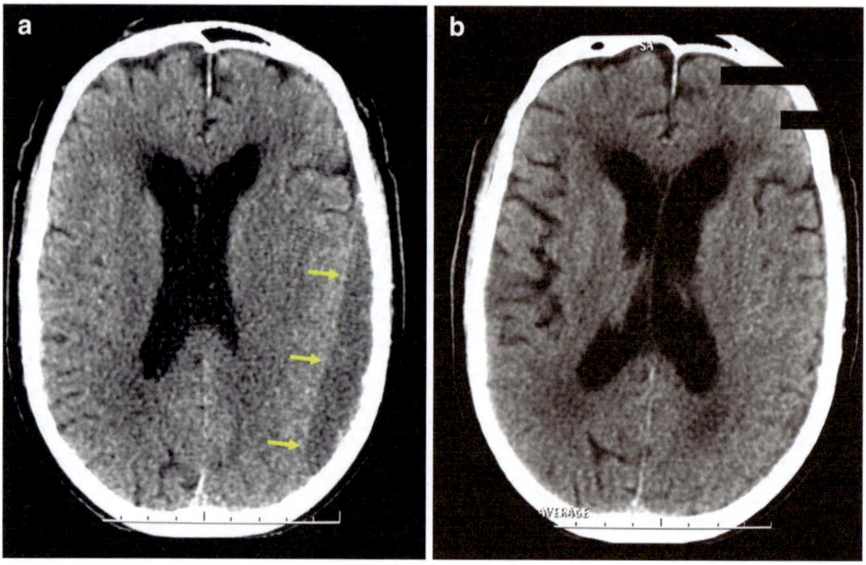

Fig. 1.9 Paucisymptomatic intracranial chronic SDH in 72-year-old man treated by corticosteroids and oral rehydration for 6 weeks. Initial CT scan (**a**) and control CT scan 2 months later showing the disappearance of the hematoma (**b**)

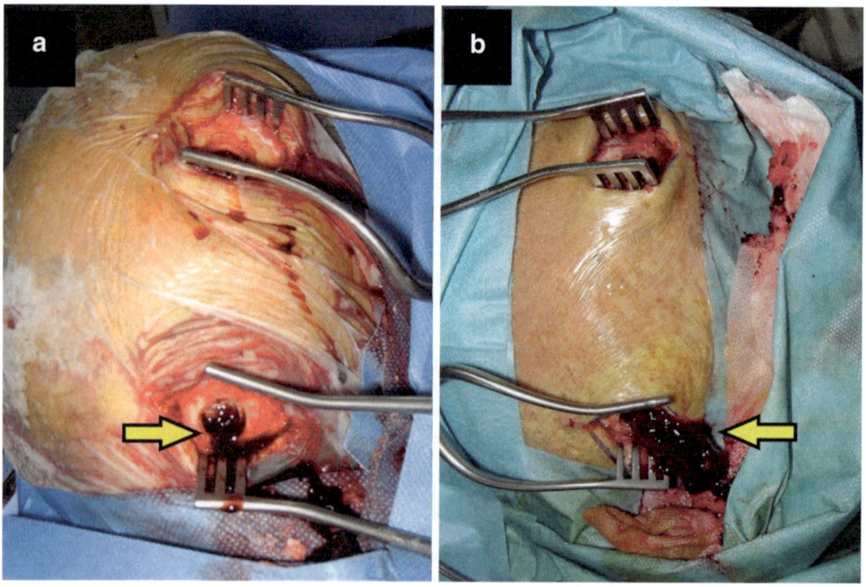

Fig. 1.10 Operative view. Surgical evacuation of chronic subdural hematomas through two burr holes. First case: evacuation of a brownish "motor oil" subdural fluid (arrow) (**a**). Another case: the chronic subdural hematoma contains darker clots (arrow) (**b**)

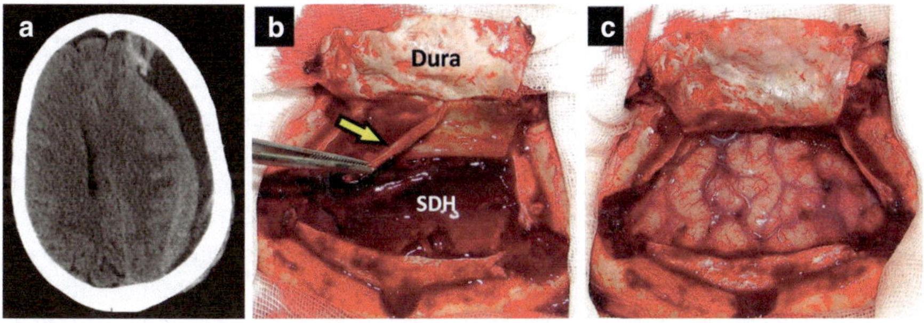

Fig. 1.11 Organized chronic/subacute subdural hematoma on axial CT scan (**a**). This patient was treated by large craniotomy and dura opening. We can see the organized SDH with its thick fibrous capsule (arrow) (**b**). Operative view of the cortical brain parenchyma following hematoma evacuation and extended membranectomy (**c**)

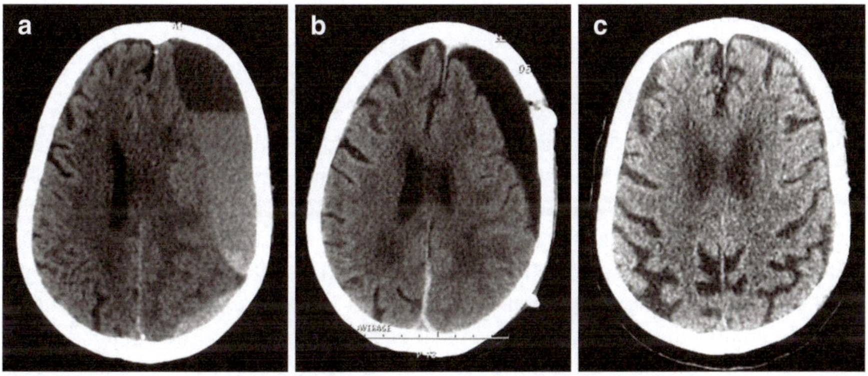

Fig. 1.12 Axial CT scan before (**a**), at third postoperative day (**b**), and 3 months after evacuation of a chronic subdural hematoma using two burr holes (**c**) with a good outcome in an 83-year-old woman

compared to the elders [66]. Also, patients with high subdural collection pressures tend to have faster cerebral expansion and better neurological improvement than cases with low pressures (Fig. 1.12).

1.4 Spinal Subdural Hematoma

The prevalence of spinal SDH is much lower than the one of cranial SDH because the intraspinal subdural space lacks important blood vessels or bridging veins which could be a cause for subdural bleeding [35, 54, 68]. Nevertheless, damage to radicular veins that cover the spinal subdural space may be the source of bleeding [61]. On the other hand, subdural hematomas are among the most uncommon types of spinal hematomas. In a systematic review of 613 patients with spinal hematomas conducted by Kreppel et al. in 2003, only 4.1% of the cases had a subdural blood collection while 75.2% (461 patients) had epidural hematomas followed by 15.7% (96 patients) with subarachnoid hematomas [46]. In a more recent review of the literature, all reported cases of spinal SDH are about 259 [35]. Chapter 40 of the present book provides an in-depth review of knowledge of the management of spinal SDH.

There are several different conditions or etiologies that can cause spinal SDH, including bleeding disorders, hematologic disease, anticoagulation therapy, traumatic injury, iatrogenic injury (lumbar puncture, epidural anesthesia, following spine or even cranial surgery), intraspinal arterio-venous malformations, and intraspinal tumors [1, 2, 8, 20, 35, 39, 48, 51, 53, 55, 61]. In some cases, the exact cause of the bleeding is not known and the SDH is then called "idiopathic" [3, 44].

Clinical symptoms of spinal SDH are not specific and vary depending on the size, level, and cause of hematomas. Apart from post-traumatic forms, most cases will present acute or subacute installation of back pain and varying degrees of neurological symptoms such as radiculopathy, leg weakness, and sphincter disturbances. Although rare, a few cases of spinal SDH also had simultaneous intracranial SDH (see below).

Long unrecognized pathology, spinal SDH has surely benefited from the contribution of MR imaging scanning that is currently the neuroimaging modality of choice [23]. MR imaging can show both the subdural hematoma, its location, and may reveal the underlying tumoral or vascular etiology. The hematoma itself has a variable T1 and T2 signal depending on the age of the bleeding (Fig. 1.13). The axial view is particularly important for differentiation between subdural and epidural hematomas. Spinal epidural hematoma has a convex lens-like form and is typically localized posteriorly to the spinal cord while subdural hematoma is usually found ventrally and laterally to and around the spinal cord in a semi-circular

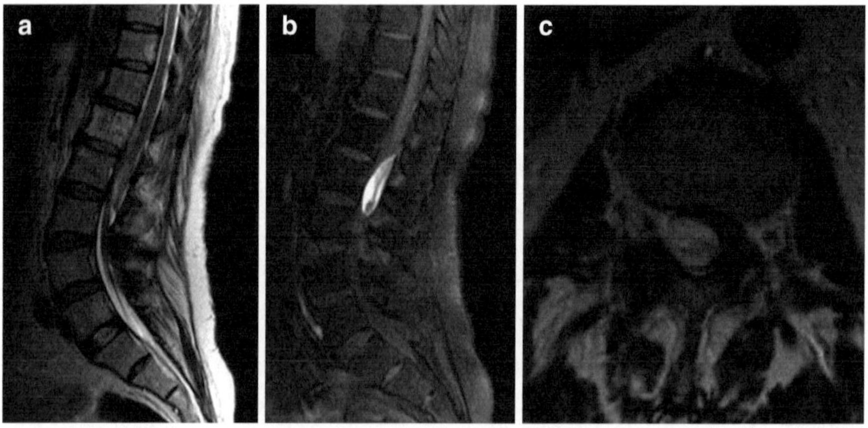

Fig. 1.13 (**a**) Preoperative images from a sagittal T2-weighted MRI, (**b**) sagittal T2-weighted FSE MRI, and (**c**) axial T2-weighted MRI revealed a spinal subdural hematoma at L2. (Reproduced from Kobayashi K et al. Eur Spine J (2017)26:2739–43; with permission) [44]

"cap sign" pattern, or in tri-radiate pattern called "inverted Mercedes Benz sign" at lumbar area [43, 47]. However, clear distinction between epidural and subdural forms of spinal hematomas before surgery can be difficult and many cases were only diagnosed intraoperatively. If a vascular malformation is suspected, a prompt spinal selective angiography should be performed or at best an angio-MR to reduce iatrogenic problems [1].

Based on many publications, treatments of spinal SDH are various [9, 49, 61]. When surgery is discussed, the neurosurgeon should always take into account the underlying etiology of the bleeding, spinal stability, patient's general conditions, and any coagulation disorders that could be associated. Generally, it appears that in patients with severe neurological symptoms, surgical decompression and evacuation have usually been achieved with good results (Fig. 1.14). However, surgical procedure should be done without delay unless the patient's conditions do not allow any anesthesia or operation. In paucisymptomatic or asymptomatic cases, both conservative and surgical treatments have allowed successful outcome. Therefore, these cases could be managed conservatively with attentive clinical follow-up. An interesting mini-invasive procedure should be mentioned: lumbar puncture for spinal SDH involving the lumbar and/or sacral column [37, 49, 56].

It is obvious that the main predictive factor of outcome will depend on neurological disorders at initial clinical presentation. Finally, patients with lumbar spinal SDH had a better outcome than those with cervical or thoracic ones.

1.5 Combination of Cranial and Spinal Subdural Hematomas

Although rare, neurosurgeons should consider the possibility of occurrence of spinal SDH in association with cranial SDH. To the best of our knowledge, less than 50 cases of craniospinal SDHs have been reported in the literature (Table 1.1) [17, 26, 29, 31, 35, 37, 42, 45, 57, 67, 68, 74, 77]. For Kokubo et al., this entity is underdiagnosed. In their prospective study, 1.19% (2 from 168) of patients surgically treated for cranial chronic SDH had concomitant lumbar SDH but these were asymptomatic [45].

This rare association can be separated into three forms as follows:

- *Type 1:* Concomitant spinal SDH and cranial SDH.
- *Type 2:* Spinal SDH developing following cranial SDH.
- *Type 3:* Cranial SDH developing following spinal SDH evacuation.

Consequently, the pathogenesis of combination of cranial and spinal SDH remains ambiguous, but a variety of hypothesis has been suggested according to the three forms:

In *type 1*, both hematomas developed as a result of trauma instead of common isolated spinal SDH, which mostly occurred owing to coagulopathy or other non-traumatic etiologies. In *type 2*, gravitational migration of the intracranial SDH

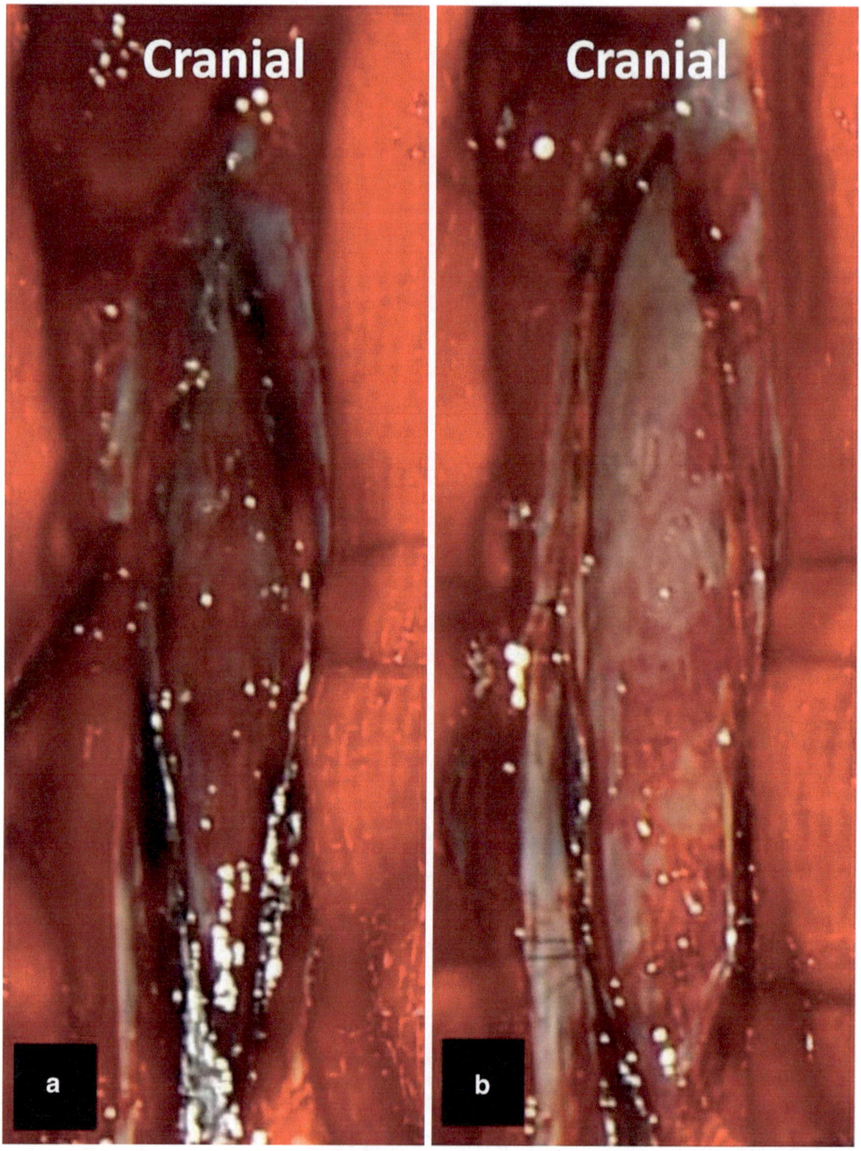

Fig. 1.14 Intraoperative photographs. (**a**) The dura and arachnoid membrane were exposed, and the spinal cord was centrally retracted to reveal a hematoma in the ventral space. This led to diagnosis of subarachnoid hematoma. (**b**) After removal of the hematoma, the spinal cord was decompressed (Reproduced from Kobayashi K et al. Eur Spine J (2017)26:2739–43; with permission) [44]

Table 1.1 Literature review of 48 patients with cranial and spinal subdural hematoma association

First author, year [reference]	Age/ sex	Predisposing event/ factors	Succession of detected lesions	Location of cranial SDH	Location of spinal SDH	Treatment of cranial SDH	Treatment of spinal SDH	Outcome
Lee, 1996 [49]	15 y/M	Trauma	Cranial	Unilateral (ASDH)	Lumbar	Conservative	Lumbar punctures	Good
Shimada, 1996 [35]	68 y/ Unk	Trauma	Cranial	Unilateral	T5-S2 (ASDH)	Conservative	Surgery	Good
Leber, 1997 [37]	54 y/M	Trauma	Cranial	Bilateral	L1-S2	Conservative	Surgery	Good
Tillich, 1999 [37]	54 y/M	Trauma	Cranial	Bilateral	T12-S2	Conservative	Surgery	Good
Kirsch, 2000 [43]	42/M	Attempting suicide	Spinal	Posterior fossa	C1-L3 (ASDH)	Conservative	Surgery	Poor
Hung, 2002 [35]	12 y/M	Trauma	Cranial	Unilateral (ASDH)	L1-L5	Conservative	Conservative	Good
Lecouvet, 2003 [68]	31 y/M	Metastatic melanosarcoma treated	Spinal	Unilateral. Posterior fossa	L1-S2	Surgery	Conservative	Improvement
Bortolotti, 2004 [35]	23 y/F	Trauma	Cranial	Unilateral	L4-S2	Conservative	Surgery	Good
Ahn, 2005 [3]	4 y/M	Trauma	Simultaneous	Unilateral. Posterior fossa	Cervico-thoracic	Conservative	Conservative	Improvement
Yamaguchi, 2005 [37]	59 y/M	Antiplatelet therapy	Simultaneous	Bilateral. Posterior fossa	T11-S1	Conservative	Conservative	Good
Jimbo, 2006 [74]	72 y/M	Anticoagulant therapy	Spinal	Multiple	L4-S2	Conservative	Surgery	Good
Sari, 2006 [67]	56 y/M	Trauma	Cranial	Interhemispheric	L1-S2	Conservative	Surgery	Good
Lee, 2007 [26]	68 y/F	No	Cranial	Unilateral	L4-S1	Surgery	Surgery	Good

(continued)

Table 1.1 (continued)

First author, year [reference]	Age/sex	Predisposing event/factors	Succession of detected lesions	Location of cranial SDH	Location of spinal SDH	Treatment of cranial SDH	Treatment of spinal SDH	Outcome
Morishige, 2007 [56]	54 y/M	No	Simultaneous	Unilateral. Posterior fossa	C1-S2	Surgery	Lumbar puncture	Good
Broc-Haro, 2008 [68]	44 y/M	No	Cranial	Unilateral (subacute SDH)	L2-L5 (ASDH)	Surgery	Conservative	Good
Gruber, 2008 [35]	4 m/M	Trauma (shaken baby)	Cranial	Unilateral (ASDH)	T10-L4	Ventricular shunt	Surgery	Improvement
Jain, 2008 [37]	12 y/M	Aplastic anemia	Simultaneous	Posterior fossa	C1-S3	Conservative	Conservative	Good
Nakajima, 2009 [37]	65 y/F	Trauma	Simultaneous	Unilateral	T12-S1	Surgery	Conservative	Good
Wong, 2009 [29]	73 y/F	Trauma	Cranial	Unilateral	T4-T10	Conservative	Conservative	Good
Yang, 2009 [37]	35 y/F	No	Simultaneous	Unilateral	L3-S1	Surgery	Surgery	Good
Hagihara, 2010 [31]	47 y/M	Trauma. Antiplatelet therapy	Cranial	Bilateral	L3-S1	Surgery	Conservative	Good
Kim K, 2010 [37]	24 y/F	Trauma	Simultaneous	Bilateral	L4-S2	Conservative	Conservative	Good
Nagashima, 2010 [37]	66 y/M	No	Spinal	Bilateral	L1-S1	Surgery	Conservative	Good
Nagashima, 2010 [37]	60 y/M	No	Cranial	Bilateral	L3-S2	Surgery	Conservative	Unk
Moscovici, 2011 [57]	88 y/M	Trauma	Cranial	Bilateral (ASDH)	L5-S1	Conservative	Surgery	Improvement
Wajima, 2012 [77]	78 y/F	Trauma Antiplatelet therapy	Cranial	Unilateral. Interhemispheric. Posterior fossa (ASDH)	S1-S2	Surgery	Conservative	Good

Wang, 2012 [37]	67 y/F	Antiplatelet therapy	Simultaneous	Unilateral	L4-S1	Surgery	Conservative	Good
Ji, 2013 [29]	47 y/F	Trauma	Simultaneous	Tentorium	L5-S2	Conservative	Conservative	Good
Jibu K, 2013 [29]	73 y/M	No	Simultaneous	Bilateral	L3-S2	Surgery	Conservative	Good
Li, 2013 [50]	26 y/M	Trauma	Cranial	Unilateral (ASDH)	T4-S1	Conservative	Conservative	Good
Moon, 2013 [37]	39 y/F	No	Spinal	Unilateral	L1-S2	Surgery	Conservative	Good
Kim, 2014 [35]	62 y/M	Trauma	Cranial	Unilateral	L2-L5	Conservative	Conservative	Good
Kokubo, 2014 [45]	83 y/M	Myelodysplastic syndrome	Cranial	Bilateral	L5-S1	Surgery	Conservative	Good
Kokubo, 2014 [45]	70 y/M	No	Cranial	Bilateral	S1	Surgery	Conservative	Good
Lin, 2014 [29]	70 y/M	No	Simultaneous	Bilateral	L4-S1	Surgery	Conservative	Good
Treister, 2014 [29]	15 y/M	Trauma	Simultaneous	Unilateral. Interhemispheric	T11-L4	Conservative	Conservative	Good
Cui, 2015 [17]	45 y/M	No	Spinal	Bilateral	L4-S3	Conservative	Surgery	Good
Kim MS, 2015 [42]	82 y/F	Trauma	Cranial	Bilateral	L3-L4	Surgery	Conservative	Good
Köksal, 2015 [35]	20 y/M	Trauma	Cranial	Unilateral (ASDH)	T10-L2	Conservative	Conservative	Improvement.
Kwon, 2015 [35]	57 y/M	Trauma	Spinal	Unilateral (ASDH)	L2-S1	Surgery	Surgery	Good
Kanamaru, 2016 [37]	67 y/M	Trauma	Cranial	Bilateral	L4-S1	Surgery	Surgery	Good
Matsumoto, 2016 [54]	58 y/M	Trauma	Cranial	Unilateral. Posterior fossa	T1-S1	Surgery	Surgery	Good

(continued)

Table 1.1 (continued)

First author, year [reference]	Age/ sex	Predisposing event/ factors	Succession of detected lesions	Location of cranial SDH	Location of spinal SDH	Treatment of cranial SDH	Treatment of spinal SDH	Outcome
Ichinose, 2018 [37]	40 y/M	Trauma	Simultaneous	Bilateral	L2-S1	Surgery	Lumbar puncture	Good
Satyarthee, 2018 [68]	14 y/M	Anaplastic anemia	Simultaneous	Posterior fossa	Thoraco-lumbar	Conservative	Conservative	Good
Uto, 2018 [74]	77 y/M	Anticoagulant and antiplatelet therapy	Spinal	Unilateral	L4-S1	Surgery	Conservative	Good
Fugita, 2019 [26]	63 y/F	Trauma	Cranial	Unilateral	L4-S1	Surgery	Conservative	Good
Golden, 2019 [29]	56 y/M	Trauma	Spinal	Bilateral (subacute)	T12-S1 (subacute)	Surgery	Surgery	Good
Hsieh, 2020 [35]	35 y/M	Trauma	Cranial	Bilateral + parafalcine (ASDH)	Thoraco-lumbar	Conservative	Conservative	Improvement

Abbreviations: *ASDH* Acute subdural hematoma, *CSDH* Chronic subdural hematoma, *m* months, *y* years, *M* male, *F* female, *C* cervical, *L* lumbar, *S* sacral, *T* thoracic, *Unk* unknown downward to form a hematoma in the spinal canal (especially the lumbosacral region) has been supposed [3, 45, 50]. It was also speculated that the newly formed spinal SDH may be caused by tearing of the bridging veins in the posterior fossa especially following surgical evacuation of the cranial SDH. Lastly, in *type 3*, intracranial hypotension caused by spinal SDH evacuation may lead to the development of the cranial hematoma. In addition, the well-known frontal cerebral atrophy in aged patients may lead to a latent space for collection of cranial SDH [29, 35, 74].

Based on our review of the literature (Table 1.1), there was no precise age of presentation. The mean age reported was 49.37 years (range, 4 months–88 years) with male predominance: there was a 35:12 male/female ratio (undetermined sex in one case). Eleven patients (22.9%) had no predisposing event or risk factors. The origin of subdural hematomas was traumatic in 28 cases (58.3%) and seven patients (14.5%) were under anticoagulant and/or antiplatelet therapy. Hematologic disease was involved in three patients (6.2%). Both SDHs were diagnosed simultaneously (*type 1*) in 14 patients (29.1%). However, cranial SDH was detected firstly (*type* 2) in 25 cases (52.2%), and spinal SDH was detected before the cranial one (*type 3*) in 9 cases (18.7%). Intracranially, most of the hematomas were supratentorial and unilateral, whereas lumbosacral area was habitually involved in the spinal SDH.

Regardless of the type of craniospinal association, the appropriate treatment of both localizations of SDH is imprecise. Previous publications described both conservative and surgical approaches with overall very good results. However, most of the cases respond very well to conservative options especially for spinal SDH. Twenty-nine patients (60.4%) with spinal SDH were managed conservatively. Sixteen patients (33.3%) underwent surgical spinal evacuation but a lumbar puncture was attempted in only three cases (6.3%) [37, 49, 56]. This last technique is simple and useful for well-liquefied spinal SDH.

In all cases, neurosurgeons should be vigilant: patients with cranial SDH who develop neurological symptoms in the lower extremities should have MRI evaluation to eliminate spinal SDH. If neurologic symptoms are severe, or patient worsening, urgent surgical evacuation should be considered.

1.6 Conclusion

Subdural hematoma is a common heterogeneous pathologic entity with various manifestations that is more complex than previously thought. It includes cranial, spinal, acute, subacute, and chronic forms with sometimes mixed combination of each type. Since the age of the population, the number of road accidents, and the need of anticoagulation therapies will rise, then an increase in incidence of SDH rate is expected in the near future especially in intracranial localizations. Although conservative medical management strategies can be applied, surgical decompression of SDH with or without drainage remains the most used therapy for many symptomatic cases. However, there is still some debate regarding the best strategy for treatment. Consequently, supplementary investigations focusing on etiopathogenesis and pathophysiology should be conducted to get a better management of SDH. When surgery is discussed, the neurosurgeon should always take into account the underlying etiology of the bleeding, clinical signs and symptoms, hematoma appearance and its localization, patient's general conditions, and any coagulation disorders that could be associated.

References

1. Abut Y, Erkalp K, Bay B. Spinal subdural hematoma: a pre-eclamptic patient with a spinal arteriovenous malformation. Anesth Analg. 2006;103:1610. https://doi.org/10.1213/01.ane.0000246274.96202.c7.
2. Abuzayed B, Oğuzoğlu SA, Dashti R, Ozyurt E. Spinal chronic subdural hematoma mimicking intradural tumor in a patient with history of Hemophilia a: case report. Turk Neurosurg. 2009;19:189–91.
3. Ahn ES, Smith ER. Acute clival and spinal subdural hematoma with spontaneous resolution: clinical and radiographic correlation in support of a proposed pathophysiological mechanism. Case report. J Neurosurg. 2005;103(2 Suppl):175–9. https://doi.org/10.3171/ped.2005.103.2.0175.
4. Akhaddar A. The yin-yang shaped image following head injury. Pan Afr Med J. 2013;16:133. https://doi.org/10.11604/pamj.2013.16.133.3555.
5. Akhaddar A, Bensghir M, Abouqal R, Boucetta M. Influence of cranial morphology on the location of chronic subdural haematoma. Acta Neurochir (Wien). 2009;151:1235–40. https://doi.org/10.1007/s00701-009-0357-7.
6. Akhaddar A, Karouache A, Boucetta M. Bilateral chronic subdural hematoma misdiagnosed as neuroleptic malignant syndrome. Emerg Med J. 2010;27:233. https://doi.org/10.1136/emj.2008.071001.
7. Akhaddar A, Boucetta M. Reversible tetraparesis due to bilateral chronic subdural haematoma. Age Ageing. 2010;39(Suppl). https://doi.org/10.1093/ageing/el_105.
8. Akiyama Y, Koyanagi I, Mikuni N. Chronic spinal subdural hematoma associated with antiplatelet therapy. World Neurosurg. 2017;105:1032.e1–5. https://doi.org/10.1016/j.wneu.2016.11.128.
9. Al B, Yildirim C, Zengin S, Genc S, Erkutlu I, Mete A. Acute spontaneous spinal subdural haematoma presenting as paraplegia and complete recovery with non-operative treatment. BMJ Case Rep. 2009;2009:bcr02.2009.1599. https://doi.org/10.1136/bcr.02.2009.1599.
10. Amagasaki K, Takusagawa Y, Kanehashi K, Abe S, Watanabe S, Shono N, et al. Supratentorial acute subdural haematoma during microvascular decompression surgery: report of three cases. J Surg Case Rep. 2017;2017(2):rjx004. https://doi.org/10.1093/jscr/rjx004.
11. Balser D, Farooq S, Mehmood T, Reyes M, Samadani U. Actual and projected incidence rates for chronic subdural hematomas in United States Veterans Administration and civilian populations. J Neurosurg. 2015;123:1209–15. https://doi.org/10.3171/2014.9.JNS141550.
12. Berger A, Constantini S, Ram Z, Roth J. Acute subdural hematomas in shunted normal-pressure hydrocephalus patients—management options and literature review: a case-based series. Surg Neurol Int. 2018;9:238. https://doi.org/10.4103/sni.sni_338_18. PMID: 30595959; PMCID: PMC6287333.
13. Caton MT Jr, Wiggins WF, Nuñez D. Non-traumatic subdural hemorrhage: beware of ruptured intracranial aneurysm. Emerg Radiol. 2019;26:567–71. https://doi.org/10.1007/s10140-019-01691-2.

14. Chari A, Kolias AG, Santarius T, Bond S, Hutchinson PJ. Twist-drill craniostomy with hollow screws for evacuation of chronic subdural hematoma. J Neurosurg. 2014;121:176–83. https://doi.org/10.3171/2014.4.JNS131212.
15. Cherif El Asri A, El Mostarchid B, Akhaddar A, Boucetta M. Chronic subdural hematoma revealing skull metastasis. Intern Med. 2011;50:791. https://doi.org/10.2169/internalmedicine.50.4654.
16. Chye CL, Lin KH, Ou CH, Sun CK, Chang IW, Liang CL. Acute spontaneous subdural hematoma caused by skull metastasis of hepatocellular carcinoma: case report. BMC Surg. 2015;15:60. https://doi.org/10.1186/s12893-015-0045-x.
17. Cui Z, Zhong Z, Wang B, Sun Q, Zhong C, Bian L. Coexistence of spontaneous spinal and undiagnosed cranial subdual hematomas. J Craniofac Surg. 2015;26:e118–9. https://doi.org/10.1097/SCS.0000000000001343.
18. de Aguiar GB, Veiga JC, Silva JM, Conti ML. Spontaneous acute subdural hematoma: a rare presentation of a dural intracranial fistula. J Clin Neurosci. 2016;25:159–60. https://doi.org/10.1016/j.jocn.2015.05.057.
19. de Amorim RL, Stiver SI, Paiva WS, Bor-Seng-Shu E, Sterman-Neto H, de Andrade AF, et al. Treatment of traumatic acute posterior fossa subdural hematoma: report of four cases with systematic review and management algorithm. Acta Neurochir (Wien). 2014;156:199–206. https://doi.org/10.1007/s00701-013-1850-6.
20. Edelson RN, Chernik NL, Posner JB. Spinal subdural hematomas complicating lumbar puncture. Arch Neurol. 1974;31:134–7. https://doi.org/10.1001/archneur.1974.00490380082011.
21. Edlmann E, Giorgi-Coll S, Whitfield PC, Carpenter KLH, Hutchinson PJ. Pathophysiology of chronic subdural haematoma: inflammation, angiogenesis and implications for pharmacotherapy. J Neuroinflammation. 2017;14:108. https://doi.org/10.1186/s12974-017-0881-y.
22. Evans LR, Jones J, Lee HQ, Gantner D, Jaison A, Matthew J, Fitzgerald MC, Rosenfeld JV, Hunn MK, Tee JW. Prognosis of acute subdural hematoma in the elderly: a systematic review. J Neurotrauma. 2019;36:517–22. https://doi.org/10.1089/neu.2018.5829.
23. Felber S, Langmaier J, Judmaier W, Dessl A, Ortler M, Birbamer G, et al. Magnetic resonance tomography in epidural and subdural spinal hematoma. Radiologe. 1994;34:656–61.
24. Fountain DM, Kolias AG, Lecky FE, Bouamra O, Lawrence T, Adams H, et al. Survival trends after surgery for acute subdural hematoma in adults over a 20-year period. Ann Surg. 2017;265:590–6. https://doi.org/10.1097/SLA.0000000000001682.
25. Fu S, Li F, Bie L. Drug therapy for chronic subdural hematoma: bench to bedside. J Clin Neurosci. 2018;56:16–20. https://doi.org/10.1016/j.jocn.2017.07.034.
26. Fujita T, Iwamoto Y, Takeuchi H, Tsujino H, Hashimoto N. Lumbar subdural hematoma detected after surgical treatment of chronic intracranial subdural hematoma. World Neurosurg. 2020;134:472–6. https://doi.org/10.1016/j.wneu.2019.11.053.
27. Gao X, Yue F, Zhang F, Sun Y, Zhang Y, Zhu X, et al. Acute non-traumatic subdural hematoma induced by intracranial aneurysm rupture: a case report and systematic review of the literature. Medicine (Baltimore). 2020;99:e21434. https://doi.org/10.1097/MD.0000000000021434.
28. Gaonkar VB, Garg K, Agrawal D, Chandra PS, Kale SS. Risk factors for progression of conservatively managed acute traumatic subdural hematoma: a systematic review and meta-analysis. World Neurosurg. 2021;146:332–41. https://doi.org/10.1016/j.wneu.2020.11.031. S1878-8750(20)32406-2.
29. Golden N, Asih MW. Traumatic subacute spinal subdural hematoma concomitant with symptomatic cranial subdural hematoma: possible mechanism. World Neurosurg. 2019;123:343–7. https://doi.org/10.1016/j.wneu.2018.12.053.
30. Golub D, Ashayeri K, Dogra S, Lewis A, Pacione D. Benefits of the subdural evacuating port system (SEPS) procedure over traditional craniotomy for subdural hematoma evacuation. Neurohospitalist. 2020;10:257–65. https://doi.org/10.1177/1941874420920520.
31. Hagihara N, Abe T, Kojima K, Watanabe M, Tabuchi K. Coexistence of cranial and spinal subdural hematomas: case report. Neurol Med Chir (Tokyo). 2010;50:333–5. https://doi.org/10.2176/nmc.50.333.

32. Hambra DV, de Danilo P, Alessandro R, Sara M, Juan GR. Meningioma associated with acute subdural hematoma: a review of the literature. Surg Neurol Int. 2014;5(Suppl 12):S469–71. https://doi.org/10.4103/2152-7806.143724.
33. Hiraizumi S, Shiomi N, Echigo T, Oka H, Hino A, Baba M, et al. Factors associated with poor outcomes in patients with mild or moderate acute subdural hematomas. Neurol Med Chir (Tokyo). 2020;60:402–10. https://doi.org/10.2176/nmc.oa.2020-0030.
34. Holl DC, Volovici V, Dirven CMF, Peul WC, van Kooten F, Jellema K, et al. Pathophysiology and nonsurgical treatment of chronic subdural hematoma: from past to present to future. World Neurosurg. 2018;116:402–11.e2. https://doi.org/10.1016/j.wneu.2018.05.037.
35. Hsieh JK, Colby S, Nichols D, Kondylis E, Liu JKC. Delayed development of spinal subdural hematoma following cranial trauma: a case report and review of the literature. World Neurosurg. 2020;141:44–51. https://doi.org/10.1016/j.wneu.2020.05.158.
36. Huang KT, Bi WL, Abd-El-Barr M, Yan SC, Tafel IJ, Dunn IF, et al. The neurocritical and neurosurgical care of subdural hematomas. Neurocrit Care. 2016;24:294–307. https://doi.org/10.1007/s12028-015-0194-x.
37. Ichinose D, Tochigi S, Tanaka T, Suzuki T, Takei J, Hatano K, et al. Concomitant intracranial and lumbar chronic subdural hematoma treated by fluoroscopic guided lumbar puncture: a case report and literature review. Neurol Med Chir (Tokyo). 2018;58:178–84. https://doi.org/10.2176/nmc.cr.2017-0177.
38. Jensen TSR, Andersen-Ranberg N, Poulsen FR, Bergholt B, Hundsholt T, Fugleholm K. The Danish Chronic Subdural Hematoma Study-comparison of hematoma age to the radiological appearance at time of diagnosis. Acta Neurochir (Wien). 2020;162:2007–13. https://doi.org/10.1007/s00701-020-04472-w.
39. Joubert C, Gazzola S, Sellier A, Dagain A. Acute idiopathic spinal subdural hematoma: what to do in an emergency? Neurochirurgie. 2019;65:93–7. https://doi.org/10.1016/j.neuchi.2018.10.009.
40. Karibe H, Kameyama M, Hayashi T, Narisawa A, Tominaga T. Acute subdural hematoma in infants with abusive head trauma: a literature review. Neurol Med Chir (Tokyo). 2016;56:264–73. https://doi.org/10.2176/nmc.ra.2015-0308.
41. Kaur G, Dakay K, Sursal T, Pisapia J, Bowers C, Hanft S, et al. Acute subdural hematomas secondary to aneurysmal subarachnoid hemorrhage confer poor prognosis: a national perspective. J Neurointerv Surg. 2021;13(5):426–9. https://doi.org/10.1136/neurintsurg-2020-016470.
42. Kim MS, Sim SY. Spinal subdural hematoma associated with intracranial subdural hematoma. J Korean Neurosurg Soc. 2015;58:397–400. https://doi.org/10.3340/jkns.2015.58.4.397.
43. Kirsch EC, Khangure MS, Holthouse D, McAuliffe W. Acute spontaneous spinal subdural haematoma: MRI features. Neuroradiology. 2000;42:586–90. https://doi.org/10.1007/s002340000331.
44. Kobayashi K, Imagama S, Ando K, Nishida Y, Ishiguro N. Acute non-traumatic idiopathic spinal subdural hematoma: radiographic findings and surgical results with a literature review. Eur Spine J. 2017;26:2739–43. https://doi.org/10.1007/s00586-017-5013-y.
45. Kokubo R, Kim K, Mishina M, Isu T, Kobayashi S, Yoshida D, et al. Prospective assessment of concomitant lumbar and chronic subdural hematoma: is migration from the intracranial space involved in their manifestation? J Neurosurg Spine. 2014;20:157–63. https://doi.org/10.3171/2013.10.SPINE13346.
46. Kreppel D, Antoniadis G, Seeling W. Spinal hematoma: a literature survey with meta-analysis of 613 patients. Neurosurg Rev. 2003;26:1–49. https://doi.org/10.1007/s10143-002-0224-y.
47. Krishnan P, Banerjee TK. Classical imaging findings in spinal subdural hematoma—“Mercedes-Benz” and “Cap” signs. Br J Neurosurg. 2016;30:99–100. https://doi.org/10.3109/02688697.2015.1071319.
48. Lee HS, Lee SH, Chung YS, Yang HJ, Son YJ, Park SB. Large spinal meningioma with hemorrhage after selective root block in the thoraco-lumbar spine. Korean J Spine. 2013;10:255–7. https://doi.org/10.14245/kjs.2013.10.4.255.

49. Lee JI, Hong SC, Shin HJ, Eoh W, Byun HS, Kim JH. Traumatic spinal subdural hematoma: rapid resolution after repeated lumbar spinal puncture and drainage. J Trauma. 1996;40:654–5. https://doi.org/10.1097/00005373-199604000-00026.
50. Li CH, Yew AY, Lu DC. Migration of traumatic intracranial subdural hematoma to lumbar spine causing radiculopathy. Surg Neurol Int. 2013;4:81. https://doi.org/10.4103/2152-7806.113647.
51. Liu J, Wu B, Feng H, You C. Spinal subdural hematoma following cranial surgery: a case report and review of the literature. Neurol India. 2011;59:281–4. https://doi.org/10.4103/0028-3886.79151.
52. Lv J, Qi X, Wang Y, Wu H, Wang K, Niu H, et al. Contralateral subdural hematoma following surgical evacuation of acute subdural hematoma: super-early intervention and clinical implications. World Neurosurg. 2019;122:24–7. https://doi.org/10.1016/j.wneu.2018.10.106.
53. Maddali P, Walker B, Fisahn C, Page J, Diaz V, Zwillman ME, et al. Subdural thoracolumbar spine hematoma after spinal anesthesia: a rare occurrence and literature review of spinal hematomas after spinal anesthesia. Cureus. 2017;9:e1032. https://doi.org/10.7759/cureus.1032.
54. Matsumoto H, Matsumoto S, Yoshida Y. Concomitant intracranial chronic subdural hematoma and spinal subdural hematoma: a case report and literature review. World Neurosurg. 2016;90:706.e1–9. https://doi.org/10.1016/j.wneu.2016.03.020.
55. Mattei TA, Rehman AA, Dinh DH. Acute spinal subdural hematoma after vertebroplasty: a case report emphasizing the possible etiologic role of venous congestion. Global Spine J. 2015;5:e52–8. https://doi.org/10.1055/s-0035-1544155.
56. Morishige M, Abe T, Ishii K, Fujiki M, Kobayashi H, Karashima A, et al. Spontaneous chronic head and spinal subdural haematoma. Acta Neurochir (Wien). 2007;149:1081–2. https://doi.org/10.1007/s00701-007-1256-4.
57. Moscovici S, Paldor I, Ramirez de-Noriega F, Itshayek E, Shoshan Y, Spektor S, et al. Do cranial subdural hematomas migrate to the lumbar spine? J Clin Neurosci. 2011;18:563–5. https://doi.org/10.1016/j.jocn.2010.07.116.
58. Mrfka M, Pistracher K, Augustin M, Kurschel-Lackner S, Mokry M. Acute subdural hematoma without subarachnoid hemorrhage or intraparenchymal hematoma caused by rupture of a posterior communicating artery aneurysm: case report and review of the literature. J Emerg Med. 2013;44:e369–73. https://doi.org/10.1016/j.jemermed.2012.11.073.
59. Neifert SN, Chaman EK, Hardigan T, Ladner TR, Feng R, Caridi JM, et al. Increases in subdural hematoma with an aging population-the future of American cerebrovascular disease. World Neurosurg. 2020;141:e166–74. https://doi.org/10.1016/j.wneu.2020.05.060.
60. Phan K, Moore JM, Griessenauer C, Dmytriw AA, Scherman DB, Sheik-Ali S, et al. Craniotomy versus decompressive craniectomy for acute subdural hematoma: systematic review and meta-analysis. World Neurosurg. 2017;101:677–85.e2. https://doi.org/10.1016/j.wneu.2017.03.024.
61. Porter ZR, Johnson MD, Horn PS, Ngwenya LB. Traumatic spinal subdural hematoma: an illustrative case and series review. Interdiscip Neurosurg. 2020;19:100570. https://doi.org/10.1016/j.inat.2019.100570.
62. Pradhan RR, Shrestha GS, Sedain G. Remote supratentorial subdural hematoma following craniectomy and evacuation of hypertensive cerebellar hematoma. Cureus. 2020;12:e6977. https://doi.org/10.7759/cureus.6977.
63. Putnam TJ, Cushing H. Chronic subdural hematoma: its pathology, its relation to pachymeningitis hemorrhagica interna and its surgical treatment. Arch Surg. 1925;11:329–39.
64. Raha A, Wadehra A, Sandhu K, Dasgupta A. Acute subdural hematoma causing neurogenic pulmonary edema following lumbar spine surgery. J Neurosurg Anesthesiol. 2017;29:63–4. https://doi.org/10.1097/ANA.0000000000000254.
65. Rauhala M, Luoto TM, Huhtala H, Iverson GL, Niskakangas T, Öhman J, et al. The incidence of chronic subdural hematomas from 1990 to 2015 in a defined Finnish population. J Neurosurg. 2019;22:1–11. https://doi.org/10.3171/2018.12.JNS183035.

66. Robinson D, Khoury JC, Kleindorfer D. Regional variation in the management of nontraumatic subdural hematomas across the United States. World Neurosurg. 2020;135:e418–23. https://doi.org/10.1016/j.wneu.2019.12.011.
67. Sari A, Sert B, Dinc H, Kuzeyli K. Subacute spinal subdural hematoma associated with intracranial subdural hematoma. J Neuroradiol. 2006;33:67–9. https://doi.org/10.1016/s0150-9861(06)77231-5.
68. Satyarthee GD, Ahmad F. Spontaneous concurrent intraspinal and intracranial subdural hematoma: management and review of literature. J Pediatr Neurosci. 2018;13:24–7. https://doi.org/10.4103/JPN.JPN_121_17.
69. Schachenmayr W, Friede RL. The origin of subdural neomembranes. Fine structure of dura-arachnoid interface in man. Am J Pathol. 1978;92:53–68.
70. Shin DS, Hwang SC. Neurocritical management of traumatic acute subdural hematomas. Korean J Neurotrauma. 2020;16:113–25. https://doi.org/10.13004/kjnt.2020.16.e43.
71. Trotter W. Chronic subdural hemorrhage of traumatic origin, and its relation to pachymeningitis hemorrhagica interna. Br J Neurosurg. 1914;2:271–91.
72. Turgut M, Akhaddar A. Dexamethasone for chronic subdural hematoma: a systematic review and meta-analysis. Acta Neurochir (Wien). 2017;159:2289–90. https://doi.org/10.1007/s00701-017-3341-7.
73. Turgut M, Akhaddar A, Turgut AT. Calcified or ossified chronic subdural hematoma: a systematic review of 114 cases reported during last century with a demonstrative case report. World Neurosurg. 2020;134:240–63. https://doi.org/10.1016/j.wneu.2019.10.153.
74. Uto T, Yonezawa N, Komine N, Tokuumi Y, Torigoe K, Koda Y, et al. A delayed-onset intracranial chronic subdural hematoma following a lumbar spinal subdural hematoma: a case report. Medicine (Baltimore). 2018;97:e12479. https://doi.org/10.1097/MD.0000000000012479.
75. Virchow R. Das haematom der dura mater. Verh Phys Med Ges Wuerzburg. 1857;7:134–42.
76. Vital RB, Hamamoto Filho PT, Oliveira VA, Romero FR, Zanini MA. Spontaneous resolution of traumatic acute subdural haematomas: a systematic review. Neurocirugia (Astur). 2016;27:129–35. https://doi.org/10.1016/j.neucir.2015.05.003.
77. Wajima D, Yokota H, Ida Y, Nakase H. Spinal subdural hematoma associated with traumatic intracranial interhemispheric subdural hematoma. Neurol Med Chir (Tokyo). 2012;52:636–9. https://doi.org/10.2176/nmc.52.636.
78. Waqas M, Vakhari K, Weimer PV, Hashmi E, Davies JM, Siddiqui AH. Safety and effectiveness of embolization for chronic subdural hematoma: systematic review and case series. World Neurosurg. 2019;126:228–36. https://doi.org/10.1016/j.wneu.2019.02.208.

Chapter 2
Cranial Acute and Subacute Subdural Hematomas

Ayhan Kanat

2.1 Introduction

Head injuries are a common mode of presentation to neurosurgical departments. Major changes in medical practice have been observed over the last decades [11]. In the 1990s, the advancements in modern diagnostic methods and medical technologies [15, 35] have intensely altered the management of patients with head trauma [14], and an improved understanding of the pathophysiologic events in cerebrovascular diseases has also occurred [6, 28, 39]. A better understanding of the pathophysiology of events after acute subdural hematoma (aSDH) has led to better patient outcomes. Currently, trauma is still a major public health problem [7] with high morbidity and mortality rates [16]. The frequency of aSDH is 11–20% in patients with head injury [31], but it occurs in about one-third of patients with severe traumatic brain injuries [3], and its mortality rate ranges between 50 and 90% [36]. There is no emergency in neurosurgical practice as worrisome as a large aSDH [36]. This review aims to assess the current knowledge of acute and subacute SDH.

2.2 Acute Subdural Hematoma

Blunt cranial traumas are commonly seen in every community and can be seen in any age group [27]. The cranium is a critical surgical region because of its content [17]. After a cranial trauma, impairments in physical, cognitive, psychological, and behavioral functioning and early complications can be seen [20] such as acute

A. Kanat (✉)
Medical Faculty, Department of Neurosurgery, Recep Tayyip Erdogan University, Rize, Turkey

M. Turgut et al. (eds.), *Subdural Hematoma*,
https://doi.org/10.1007/978-3-030-79371-5_2

subdural hemorrhage which refers to the accumulation of fresh hematoma between the dura and arachnoid membranes, usually due to tearing of the bridging cortical veins [2].

2.3 Subacute Subdural Hematoma

Delayed deterioration within 24 h after trauma may be observed in some patients with aSDH. A conversion process from aSDH to subacute subdural hematoma (sASDH) may occur [33]. Hematomas usually begin to liquefy by 2 weeks after formation [12]. In these patients, aSDH is initially absorbed and the volume is reduced, but later, there can be an increase in the mass effect of the subarachnoid hemorrhage (SAH), the density of the hematoma may decrease, and the midline shift may increase on computed tomography (CT) [33]. New neurologic deficits can be seen in patients with subacute SDH.

2.4 Pathophysiology

Atrophic brain volume and the large subdural space of elderly patients constitute the enlarged subdural space [19]. In these patients, the enlarged subdural space may compensate for the increase in hematoma volume and cerebral edema before neurological deterioration occurs [32]. The timely detection of neurological deterioration is an important issue in neurosurgical practice [5]. For that reason close neurological [23] and radiological observation should be performed in a patient with head trauma [21].

The cerebrum is one of the most important organs of the human body [8] and is located in the cranium. This structure controls all of the central nervous system [8]. The volume of the cranium cannot be changed. Inside of cranium, the sum of the volume of the brain, cerebrospinal fluid, and intracranial blood is constant [26]. This principle is known as the Monro-Kellie doctrine or hypothesis and was defined in 1783 by Monro and Kellie. In a normal cranium without an aSDH, there is an equilibrium inside of the cranium. If the volume of one of the components within the cranium changes following a SDH, an increase in intracranial pressure (ICP), the onset of coma and herniation may occur. The normal level for intracranial pressure is 5–15 mmHg. Coma may be seen at the onset of severe head injury in 25–50% of cases [2]. Coma and high rate mortality from an aSDH may depend on many factors such as the Glasgow Coma Score/Scale (GCS) at the time of presentation, the degree of mass effect of the SDH, and extent of the midline shift, and the presence of increased ICP and cerebral edema. Increased ICP (above 20 mmHg) may lead to poor neurological outcome [32]. Measurement of the midline shift and the ICP has been used in assessing the severity of the SDH. The hematoma volume is an important issue when located in the posterior fossa [38]. The blood-brain barrier is necessary for normal brain function [4, 14]. The disruption of this barrier may occur following acute and subacute SDH. Cerebral perfusion pressure (CPP) can also be altered in patients with acute SDH. CPP is important for delivery of oxygen to cerebral tissue and it is affected by cerebral blood flow which may be decreased immediately after a SDH [22].

The GCS was originally devised for patients with head trauma to evaluate impaired consciousness or coma [18]. This scale has become the worldwide standard for the assessment of the patient with a head injury. The GCS has several disadvantages such as the limited verbal reaction of intubated patients [23] with aSDH. Both parasympathetic and sympathetic nervous system disorders appear to be important factors in pupillary diameter changes [5, 29]. Pupillary changes can occur in patients with SDH from uncal herniation due to mass effect leading to compression of the oculomotor nerve and the brainstem [24]. For that reason, measuring and comparing pupil diameter by testing the reactivity to light can help diagnose oculomotor nerve injury after an aSDH, but pupillary changes can also occur due to direct orbital/ocular trauma [24].

2.5 Imaging

A non-contrast CT scan is an important radiological modality in the diagnosis of aSDH. Brain magnetic resonance imaging (MRI) can be preferred in cases with a thin aSDH, and tentorial and interhemispheric aSDH. Cerebral MRI is more sensitive than head CT for hematoma detection in these cases with a thin aSDH [2]. In an aSDH, a crescent-like or "half-moon" appearance that crosses cranial suture lines may be seen [12]. Later, delayed hematoma expansion may also be detected [32].

2.6 Management

Management of SDH is still a controversial issue because evidence-based guidelines and randomized controlled trials are lacking [31]. Decisions regarding surgery are based on SDH location, size, mass effect, midline shift, acuity, patient age, medical comorbidities, and the extent of neurological deficits [31]. Some factors such as age, comorbidities, and SDH evacuation have been identified as predictors of clinical outcome [31].

2.7 Role of Surgery

Primary or secondary brain injury may occur from an aSDH [27]. The aim of the surgical approach is to resolve the cerebral herniation in patients and to reduce secondary ischemic injury, minimally [22]. In some cases, the apparent resolution of sASDHs may be seen. Because of the mass effect on the brain of a thick clot in an aSDH, decompressive craniotomy and hematoma evacuation are useful procedures. However, in the recent decades, decompressive craniectomy has been performed as an alternative surgical procedure to decompressive craniotomy [30]. Generally, the neurologic status of the patient with an aSDH on initial presentation, the hemorrhage size and its associated midline shift, and the presence of cerebral edema on CT are important factors that influence the surgical type of procedure such as a decompressive craniotomy or craniectomy [1]. The theoretical advantage of decompressive craniectomy is the ability to have more effective control of the increased ICP, and to improve in cerebral perfusion pressure and brain partial pressure of oxygen [1]. Continuous oxygen delivery and CO_2 clearance are paramount for the maintenance of normal brain function and tissue integrity [14]. The timing of surgery has often been regarded as an important factor for the clinical outcome of the patient with aSDH [34]. Surgical indications are an aSDH with >10 mm thickness or >5 mm midline shift, a deteriorating patient with the GCS <8, unilateral or bilateral fixed dilated pupils, or evidence of elevated increased ICP >20 [9]. Out of these parameters, mass effect is a significant indication for surgical intervention regardless of patient GCS [25]. Figure 2.1a shows the CT images of a patient with an aSDH; his hematoma thickness is 12.88 mm, and the patient also has

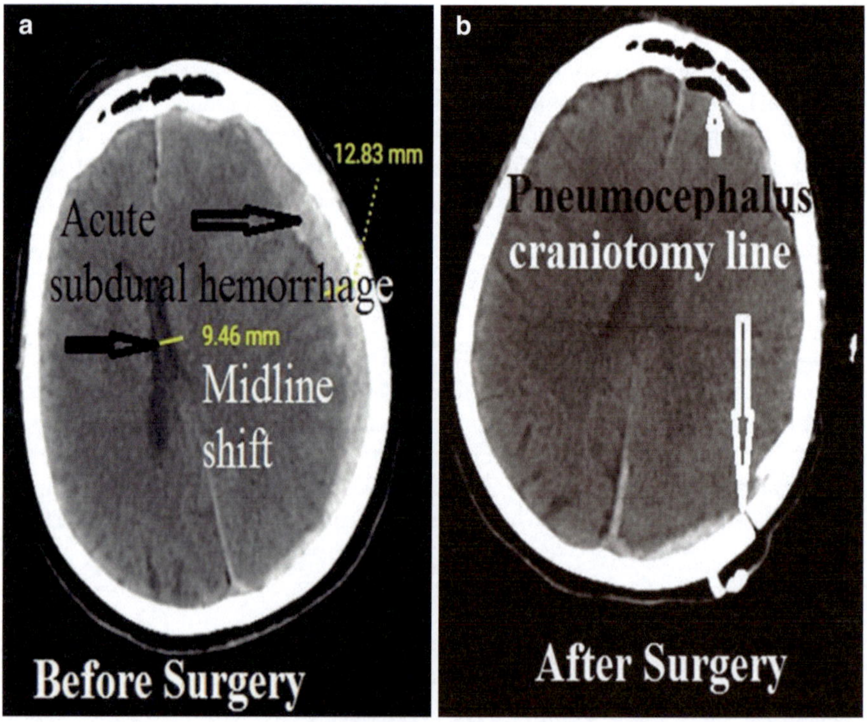

Fig. 2.1 (**a**) Shows the computed tomography images of a patient with acute subdural hematoma. His hematoma thickness is 12.88 mm, and the patient also has a 9.46 mm midline shift. (**b**) Shows the resolution of the midline shift after surgery

9.46 mm midline shift. Figure 2.1b shows the resolution of the midline shift after surgery.

Nonoperative management can be preferred in patients with thin aSDHs (clot thickness <10 mm) without significant mass effect (midline shift <5 mm) and minimal to no neurological deficits [25].

Seizures are a serious complication in patients with SDH [37]. The prevalence of seizures in SDHs is reported to be 24% in acute SDHs and 11% in chronic SDHs [37]. The use of anti-epileptic drugs for sASDH patients is a controversial issue [32].

2.8 Conclusion

The morbidity and mortality of patients following acute SDH are still high. In patients with decreased consciousness, and those with unilateral neurologic deficits (e.g., dilated pupil, motor weakness, or posturing) following a severe head injury, the presence of an acute SDH should be suspected [12]. Close clinical and radiologic follow-up is necessary to detect the rapid expansion of an aSDH. Given the important morbidity and mortality after an aSDH, it is necessary to correctly assess the damage to the human brain, which is difficult to perform on live human patients with aSDH, due to ethical issues. There are reasons to focus on experimental studies [28]. To understand the biomechanical, molecular, and cellular effects of traumatic brain injury, several injury models have been used in experimental studies [27]. The experimental studies may provide a better understanding of the effects of acute and subacute SDH than those studies of human subjects. If we consider the nervous system as a great orchestra that can express a complete range of rhythms and melodies and the most complex harmonic combinations [10], we will find it easier to understand how any traumatic acute subdural hematoma may be translated into an alteration of the rhythmic systems that synchronize the brain after disruption of the blood-brain barrier and a change in cerebral perfusion pressure. To examine the outcomes of a study, it is necessary to have testable hypotheses [13]. Outcomes are then expressed with respect to the implied goals [13]. The outcome of aSDHs has been dismal because of combined diffuse axonal injury and the accompanying increased ICP [32]. Well-orchestrated, evidenced-based, multidisciplinary studies are needed to achieve the best outcome following aSDH.

References

1. Ahmed N, Greenberg P, Shin S. Mortality outcome of emergency decompressive craniectomy and craniotomy in the management of acute subdural hematoma: a national data analysis. Am Surg. 2021;87(3):347–53. https://doi.org/10.1177/0003134820951463.
2. Al-Mufti F, Mayer SA. Neurocritical care of acute subdural hemorrhage. Neurosurg Clin N Am. 2017;28:267–78. https://doi.org/10.1016/j.nec.2016.11.009.

3. Altaf I, Shams S, Vohra AH. Role of surgical modality and timing of surgery as clinical outcome predictors following acute subdural hematoma evacuation. Pak J Med Sci. 2020;36:412–5. https://doi.org/10.12669/pjms.36.3.1771.
4. Aydin MD, Kanat A, Hacimuftuoglu A, Ozmen S, Ahiskalioglu A, Kocak MN. A new experimental evidence that olfactory bulb lesion may be a causative factor for substantia nigra degeneration; preliminary study. Int J Neurosci. 2021;131(3):220–7. https://doi.org/10.1080/00207454.2020.1737049.
5. Aydin MD, Kanat A, Yolas C, Soyalp C, Onen MR, Yilmaz I, Karaavci NC, Calik M, Baykal O, Ramazanoglu L. Spinal subarachnoid hemorrhage induced intractable miotic pupil. A reminder of ciliospinal sympathetic center ischemia based miosis: an experimental study. Turk Neurosurg. 2019;29:434–9. https://doi.org/10.5137/1019-5149.JTN.24446-18.1.
6. Celiker M, Kanat A, Aydin MDMD, Ozdemir D, Aydin N, Yolas C, Calik M, Peker HOHO. First emerging objective experimental evidence of hearing impairment following subarachnoid haemorrhage; Felix culpa, phonophobia, and elucidation of the role of trigeminal ganglion. Int J Neurosci. 2019;129:794–800. https://doi.org/10.1080/00207454.2019.1569651.
7. Celiker M, Kanat A, Ozdemir A, Celiker FB, Kazdal H, Ozdemir B, Batcik OE, Ozdemir D. Controversy about the protective role of volume in the frontal sinus after severe head trauma: larger sinus equates with higher risk of death. Br J Oral Maxillofac Surg. 2020;58:314–8. https://doi.org/10.1016/j.bjoms.2019.12.008.
8. Costa JMC, Fernandes FAO, Alves de Sousa RJ. Prediction of subdural haematoma based on a detailed numerical model of the cerebral bridging veins. J Mech Behav Biomed Mater. 2020;111:103976. https://doi.org/10.1016/j.jmbbm.2020.103976.
9. Fomchenko EI, Gilmore EJ, Matouk CC, Gerrard JL, Sheth KN. Management of subdural hematomas: part II. Surgical management of subdural hematomas. Curr Treat Options Neurol. 2018;20:34. https://doi.org/10.1007/s11940-018-0518-1.
10. Gasenzer ER, Kanat A, Neugebauer E. Neurosurgery and music; effect of Wolfgang Amadeus Mozart. World Neurosurg. 2017;102:313–9. https://doi.org/10.1016/j.wneu.2017.02.081.
11. Gasenzer ER, Kanat A, Ozdemir V, Rakici SY, Neugebauer E. Interesting different survival status of musicians with malignant cerebral tumors. Br J Neurosurg. 2020;34:264–70. https://doi.org/10.1080/02688697.2019.1701629.
12. Huang KT, Bi WL, Abd-El-Barr M, Yan SC, Tafel IJ, Dunn IF, Gormley WB. The Neurocritical and neurosurgical care of subdural hematomas. Neurocrit Care. 2016;24:294–307. https://doi.org/10.1007/s12028-015-0194-x.
13. Kanat A. Patient-evaluated outcome after surgery for basal meningiomas. Neurosurgery. 2002;51:1530–2.
14. Kanat A. Brain oxygenation and energy metabolism: part I—biological function and pathophysiology. Neurosurgery. 2003;52:1508–9.
15. Kanat A, Aydin MD, Akca N, Ozmen S: First histopathological bridging of the distance between Onuf's nucleus and substantia nigra after olfactory bulbectomy-new ideas about the urinary dysfunction in cerebral neurodegenerative disease: an experimental study Low Urin Tract Symptoms. 2021;13:383–9. https://doi.org/10.1111/luts.12371.
16. Kanat A, Aydin Y. Postcontrast magnetic resonance imaging to predict progression of traumatic epidural and subdural hematomas in the acute stage. Neurosurgery. 1999;44:685–6.
17. Kanat A, Aydin Y. Recurrent meningiomas. J Neurosurg. 1999;91:720–1.
18. Kanat A, Aydin Y. Prognostic value and determinants of ultraearly angiographic vasospasm after aneurysmal subarachnoid hemorrhage. Neurosurgery. 2000;46:505–7.
19. Kanat A, Kayaci S, Yazar U, Kazdal H, Terzi Y. Chronic subdural hematoma in adults: why does it occur more often in males than females? Influence of patient's sexual gender on occurrence. J Neurosurg Sci. 2010;54:99–103.

20. Kanat A, Romana Gasenzer E, Neugebauer E. A different aspect of the unexpected death of Mozart at the age of 35 years. CNS Spectr. 2019;24:628–31. https://doi.org/10.1017/S1092852918001736.
21. Kanat A, Yazar U, Kazdal H. Chronic subdural hygroma with thrombocythemia: first case report. J Neurosurg Sci. 2009;53:165–7.
22. Karibe H, Hayashi T, Hirano T, Kameyama M, Nakagawa A, Tominaga T. Surgical management of traumatic acute subdural hematoma in adults: a review. Neurol Med Chir (Tokyo). 2014;54:887–94. https://doi.org/10.2176/nmc.cr.2014-0204.
23. Kazdal H, Kanat A, Aydin MD, Yazar U, Guvercin AR, Calik M, Gundogdu B. Sudden death and cervical spine: a new contribution to pathogenesis for sudden death in critical care unit from subarachnoid hemorrhage; first report—an experimental study. J Craniovertebr Junction Spine. 2017;8:33.
24. Kerezoudis P, Goyal A, Puffer RC, Parney IF, Meyer FB, Bydon M. Morbidity and mortality in elderly patients undergoing evacuation of acute traumatic subdural hematoma. Neurosurg Focus. 2020;49:E22. https://doi.org/10.3171/2020.7.FOCUS20439.
25. Kvint S, Gutierrez A, Blue R, Petrov D. Surgical management of trauma-related intracranial hemorrhage—a review. Curr Neurol Neurosci Rep. 2020;20:63. https://doi.org/10.1007/s11910-020-01080-0.
26. Mokri B. The Monro-Kellie hypothesis: applications in CSF volume depletion. Neurology. 2001;56:1746–8. https://doi.org/10.1212/wnl.56.12.1746.
27. Ozdemir B, Kanat A, Kazdal H. Experimental cerebral injury models (in Turkish). Turk Norosirurji Derg. 2020;30:308–11.
28. Ozdemir B, Kanat A, Ozdemir V, Batcik OE, Yazar U, Guvercin AR. The effect of neuroscientists on the studies of autonomic nervous system dysfunction following experimental subarachnoid hemorrhage. J Craniofac Surg. 2019;30:2184–8. https://doi.org/10.1097/scs.0000000000005763.
29. Ozturk C, Ozdemir NG, Kanat A, Aydin MD, Findik H, Aydin N, Kabalar ME, Kazdal H, Yolas C, Baykal O, Calik M. How reliable is pupillary evaluation following subarachnoid hemorrhage? Effect of oculomotor nerve degeneration secondary to posterior communicating artery vasospasm: first experimental study. J Neurol Surg A Cent Eur Neurosurg. 2018;79:302–8. https://doi.org/10.1055/s-0037-1608841.
30. Rush B, Rousseau J, Sekhon MS, Griesdale DE. Craniotomy versus craniectomy for acute traumatic subdural hematoma in the United States: a national retrospective cohort analysis. World Neurosurg. 2016;88:25–31. https://doi.org/10.1016/j.wneu.2015.12.034.
31. Sharma R, Rocha E, Pasi M, Lee H, Patel A, Singhal AB. Subdural hematoma: predictors of outcome and a score to guide surgical decision-making. J Stroke Cerebrovasc Dis. 2020;29:105180. https://doi.org/10.1016/j.jstrokecerebrovasdis.2020.105180.
32. Shin D-S, Hwang S-C. Neurocritical management of traumatic acute subdural hematomas. Korean. J Neurotrauma. 2020;16:113–25. https://doi.org/10.13004/kjnt.2020.16.e43.
33. Tao Z-Q, Ding S-H, Huang J-Y, Zhu Z-G. The pathogenesis of subacute subdural hematoma: a report of 3 cases and literature review. World Neurosurg. 2018;114:e22–8. https://doi.org/10.1016/j.wneu.2018.01.147.
34. Trevisi G, Sturiale CL, Scerrati A, Rustemi O, Ricciardi L, Raneri F, Tomatis A, Piazza A, Auricchio AM, Stifano V, Romano C, De Bonis P, Mangiola A. Acute subdural hematoma in the elderly: outcome analysis in a retrospective multicentric series of 213 patients. Neurosurg Focus. 2020;49:E21. https://doi.org/10.3171/2020.7.FOCUS20437.
35. Turk O, Ozdemir NG, Demirel N, Atci IB, Kanat A, Yolas C. Nontraumatic intradiploic epidermoid cyst and older age: association or causality? J Craniofac Surg. 2018;29:e143–6. https://doi.org/10.1097/SCS.0000000000003897.
36. Vega RA, Valadka AB. Natural history of acute subdural hematoma. Neurosurg Clin N Am. 2017;28:247–55. https://doi.org/10.1016/j.nec.2016.11.007.

37. Won S-Y, Konczalla J, Dubinski D, Cattani A, Cuca C, Seifert V, Rosenow F, Strzelczyk A, Freiman TM. A systematic review of epileptic seizures in adults with subdural haematomas. Seizure. 2017;45:28–35. https://doi.org/10.1016/j.seizure.2016.11.017.
38. Yilmaz A, Musluman AM, Kanat A, Cavusoglu H, Terzi Y, Aydin Y. The correlation between hematoma volume and outcome in ruptured posterior fossa arteriovenous malformations indicates the importance of surgical evacuation of hematomas. Turk Neurosurg. 2011;21:152–9. https://doi.org/10.5137/1019-5149.JTN.3401-10.0.
39. Yolas C, Kanat A, Aydin MD, Altas E, Kanat IF, Kazdal H, Duman A, Gundogdu B, Gursan N. Unraveling of the effect of nodose ganglion degeneration on the coronary artery vasospasm after subarachnoid hemorrhage: an experimental study. World Neurosurg. 2016;86:79–87. https://doi.org/10.1016/j.wneu.2015.09.004.

Chapter 3
History of Cranial Subdural Hematoma

Nikolaos Ch. Syrmos, Vaitsa Giannouli, Sotirios Kottas, and Mehmet Turgut

3.1 Introduction

Subdural hematoma (SDH) is a collection of blood that extends into the space between the dura mater and the arachnoid meningeal layers, surrounding and protecting the human brain within the human skull. There are three types of SDH: acute, subacute, and chronic. Out of these, the chronic type develops over a 2 or 3 week period after a mild or moderate head injury coupled with chronic inflammation and with a variety of symptoms (behavioral changes, headache, focal neurological deficits, hemiparesis, seizures, etc.). The purpose of this chapter is to highlight the most important historical notes for the chronic SDH from ancient times to the modern era.

N. C. Syrmos (✉) · V. Giannouli
Medical School, Aristotle University of Thessaloniki, Thessaloniki, Macedonia, Greece

S. Kottas
Department of Neurosurgery, Papanikolaou General Hospital, Thessaloniki, Macedonia, Greece

M. Turgut
Department of Neurosurgery, Aydın Adnan Menderes University Faculty of Medicine, Efeler, Aydın, Turkey

Department of Histology and Embryology, Aydın Adnan Menderes University Health Sciences Institute, Efeler, Aydın, Turkey

M. Turgut et al. (eds.), *Subdural Hematoma*,
https://doi.org/10.1007/978-3-030-79371-5_3

3.2 Ancient History

Cranial trepanation or trephination in order to treat SDH is surely the oldest neurosurgical operation of mankind. In many parts of Africa, South America, and Melanesia, we have found documents about trepanations during the Paleolithic and Neolithic periods. Trepanation was continued from the Iron, Bronze and Stone Ages to the Hellenic Period [1, 3, 12, 22].

Hellenic Hippocrates (Ιπποκράτης) of Kos (Κώς) (460–370 BC), the first documented medical doctor and also the first neurosurgeon in the history of mankind, who together with his students and through his marvelous books, gives a detailed description of the various types of cranial trepanations used to perform accurate, and for his era, specific neurosurgical interventions (Fig. 3.1) [3, 7, 20–22].

In other parts of the world such as Central and Latin Americas, North Africa, the Mediterranean Area, and the Middle East, other important civilizations

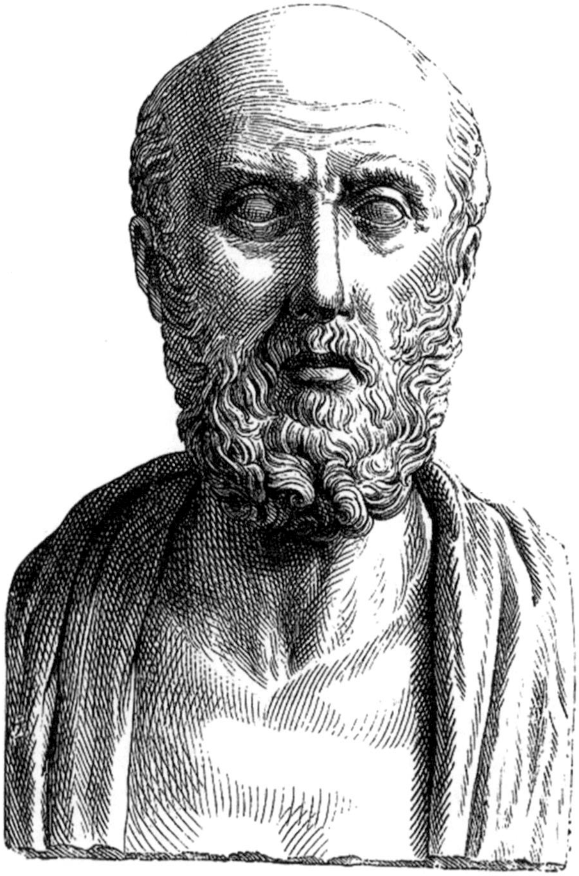

Fig. 3.1 Hippocrates (460–370 BC)

also developed (the Mayans, Incas, Aztecs, Zapotecs, Minoans, Egyptians, Babylonians, Sumerians, Assyrians, Hittites, Persians, Israelites, etc.) [3, 7, 20–22]. These civilizations developed the knowledge of cranial trepanation according to various studies and primarily through paintings and other archeological findings, that over the centuries allowed them to perform neurosurgical cranial procedures and other procedures mainly related to religious acts such as sacrifices, etc. [1, 3, 7, 12, 20, 22].

3.3 Modern History

3.3.1 Fifteenth Century

Ambroise Paré (1510–1590) was a barber surgeon from France, who served in that role for the kings Henry II, Francis II, Charles IX, and Henry III (Fig. 3.2). He was also a forensic pathologist and a pioneer anatomist of his era. Henry II was wounded in a tournament around 1559 and according to Paré had a SDH [3, 12, 17].

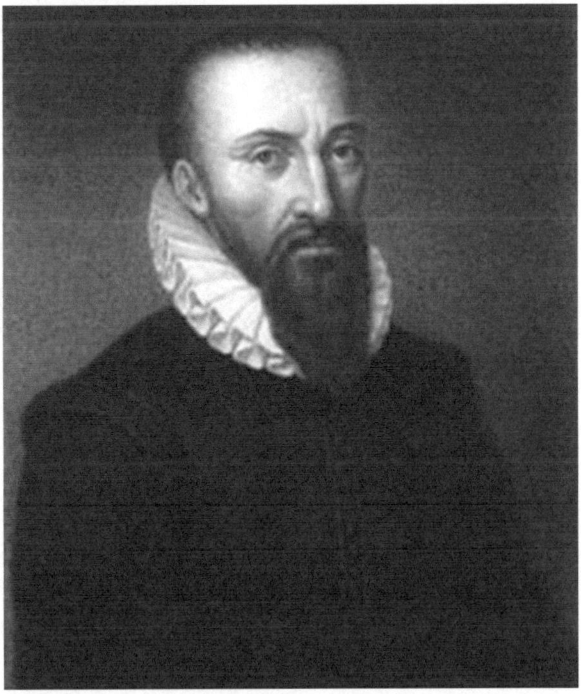

Fig. 3.2 Ambrose Paré (1510–590)

3.3.2 Sixteenth-Seventeenth Century

Johann Jakob Wepfer (December 23, 1620–January 26, 1695) was a Swiss physician from Schaffhausen. After several medical studies in his country (Basel) and abroad (Strasbourg, Padova) he returned in 1647 to his homeland [3, 4, 12]. He studied vascular brain anatomy and physiology in order to understand better cerebrovascular diseases. He performed anatomical, cadaveric, and necroscopic studies in order to describe the blood supply of the brain and the pathogenesis of the stroke. He was also a well-known scientist (pharmacologist and toxicologist) of his era [2–4, 12, 17]. According to D'Errico and German, Wepfer in 1657 was the first to describe a chronic SDH as a large cyst full of blood beneath the dura of a patient after a so-called "apoplectic stroke" attack [5, 12].

Giovanni Battista Morgagni (February 25, 1682–December 6, 1771) was an Italian anatomist (Fig. 3.3). He is considered as the father of modern anatomical pathology. He was for many years a professor of anatomy at the University of Padova in the Veneto Region, North Italy. He described, in 1857, 90 years after

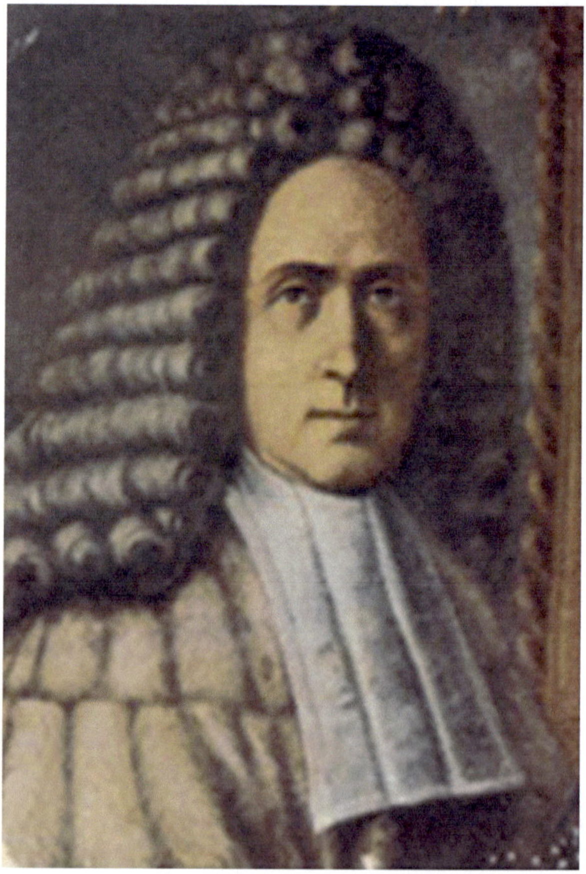

Fig. 3.3 Giovanni Battista Morgagni (1682–1771)

Johann Jakob Wepfer, a chronic SDH in a patient with a so-called "apoplectic stroke" [3, 4, 6, 12, 17].

In 1772, Hill described trephination as a method of treatment for patients with chronic SDH [3, 8, 12, 17].

3.3.3 Eighteenth-Nineteenth Century

During 1800, we have some other important pathfinder steps that allow for a better understanding of the disease:

- Bichat M, in 1800, describes in his anatomical work "*Traité des membranes en général et de diverses membranes en particulier*" extensive information about the brain meninges [3, 9, 12, 17].
- The description of Houssard in 1817 addressed the nature of the clot and of the membranes [3, 11, 12, 17].
- Thubert, in 1822, described a lesion presenting with symptoms 9 years after the initial trauma. This trauma was probably the main factor for the production of the collection of blood beneath the dura mater [3, 10, 12, 13, 17].
- The pathological, physiological, and morphological studies of Bayle, in 1826. Bayle suggested that chronic rebleeding was the main pathogenetic factor for the disease [2, 3, 12, 14, 15, 17].
- Honore de Balzac, in 1840, described a possible case of SDH, including its traumatic origin and the surgical treatment [2, 3, 12, 14, 15, 17].
- Hewit, in 1845, published an article entitled "*On extravasations of blood into the cavity of the arachnoid,*" and believed that the membrane which covered the clot was the direct result of the effusion of blood into the space and not a specific part of the arachnoid or dura [3, 12, 17].
- Heschl, in 1855, opposed the idea that hemorrhage was the primary cause for the formation of this pathologic picture but believed instead that an inflammatory membrane preceded the hemorrhage [3, 12, 16, 17].
- The etiological and histological studies of Virchow, in 1857 [3, 12, 17, 18].

Rudolf Ludwig Carl Virchow (October 13, 1821–September 5, 1902) was a polymath from Germany (Fig. 3.4). He was at the same time a physician, anthropologist, pathologist, and also an expert in other scientific fields (history and biology). He was a writer, editor, and politician [3, 12, 17, 19]. He is known worldwide as "the father of modern pathology." Virchow performed histological studies and explained the formations of the brain membranes. He recognized the occasional traumatic origin of the SDH, although he believed that the lesion was often caused by chronic inflammation called "pachymeningitis chronica hemorrhagica" of the dura mater with extravasation of blood into the subdural space and the formation of a film of fibrin over the inner surface of the dura [3, 12, 17, 23].

Kremiansky, in 1868, believed that the middle meningeal artery was always the main cause of the hemorrhage, probably due to a generalized diseased condition. He

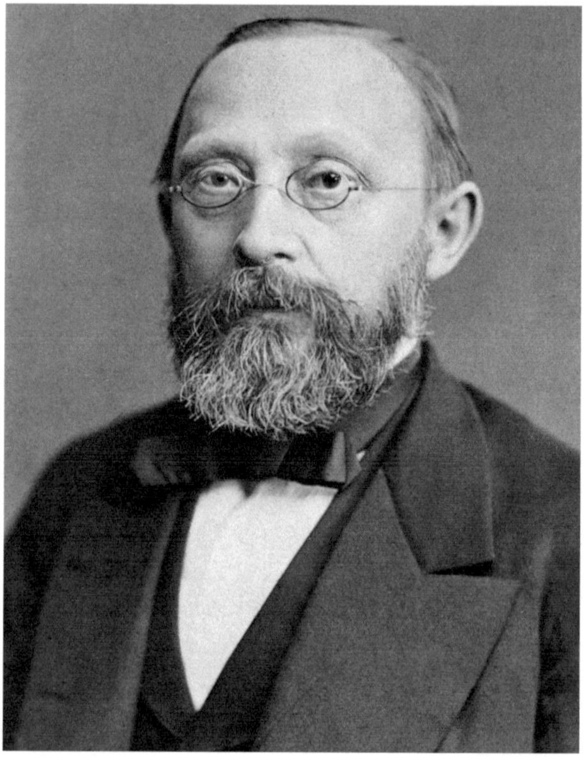

Fig. 3.4 Rudolph Virchow (1821–1902)

also recognized the possibility of local irritation playing a contributory part as well as systemic disease [3, 12, 17, 24].

In 1872, Sperling readopted the earlier view that the hemorrhage was the primary factor and that the formation of the pachymeningitic pseudomembrane was due to the organization of the extravasted material. He performed many experimental studies in dogs [3, 12, 15, 17].

Huegenin in his studies felt that brain degeneration and atrophy played a large part in the process. The same sentiments were also felt by Wigelsworth, in 1862, during his experimental work [3, 12, 15, 17].

Hulke in 1883 reported a case of a chronic SDH with successful neurosurgical treatment. However, the lesion was still regarded as an inflammatory process according to Oppenheim, in 1911 [3, 12, 15, 17].

Trauma was considered, seriously, as a possible cause of chronic SDH only from the late nineteenth century to the beginning of the twentieth century [3, 12, 15, 17, 25, 26, 28].

3.3.4 Twentieth Century

Barret in 1902 performed interesting experimental studies concerning the etiology of this SDH. He performed various studies in cats [3, 12, 15, 17, 27, 29, 30].

William Ford Robertson (1867–1923) described in detail the entire histological process involved in the formation of the membranes [12, 16, 17, 23].

Wilfrid Trotter (1872–1939) was born in England. Despite being bedridden during his childhood with serious musculoskeletal problems, he first studied medicine at London University, and then he became Professor and Chair of Surgery at the University College Hospital. He performed many surgical and oncological studies. In 1914, Trotter focused his studies on the traumatic aspect and the etiology of chronic SDH [12, 16, 17, 23].

Tracy Jackson Putnam (April 14, 1894–March 29, 1975) was an American physician. Putnam worked for the Boston City Hospital and in the New York Neurological Institute at Columbia University (Fig. 3.5) [12, 16, 17, 23].

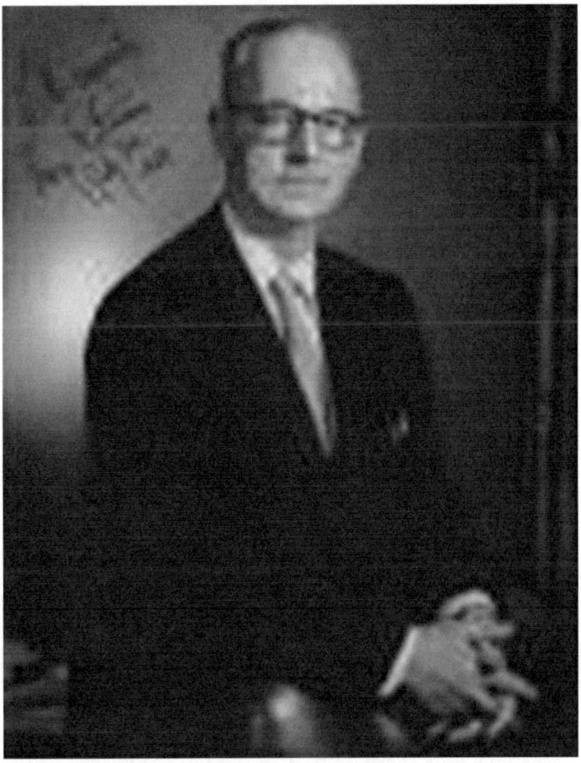

Fig. 3.5 Tracy Jackson Putnam (1894–1975)

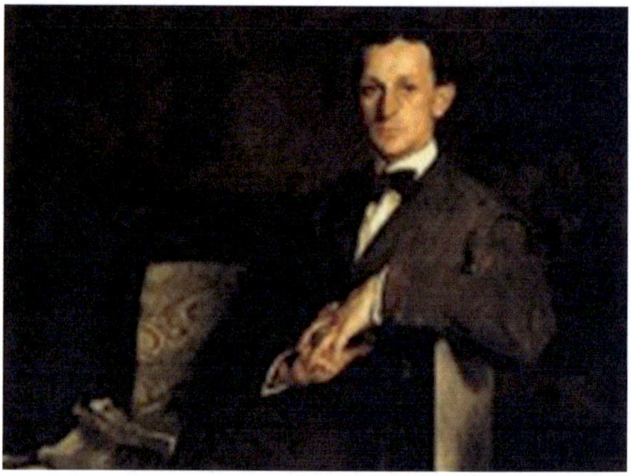

Fig. 3.6 Harvey Williams Cushing (1869–1939)

Harvey Williams Cushing (April 8, 1869–October 7, 1939) was a pioneer American neurosurgeon but also an expert in other scientific fields such as endocrinology (Fig. 3.6). He is considered the father of neurosurgery, as an autonomous medical discipline. Under him, many great neurosurgeons in the history of medicine were trained:

- Walter Dandy, the first pediatric neurosurgeon and the developer of pneumoencephalography [12, 16, 17].
- Leo M. Davidoff, founder of the Department of Neurological Surgery at the Albert Einstein College of Medicine [12, 16, 17].
- Norman Dott [12, 16, 17].
- Wilder Penfield, founder of the Montreal Neurological Institute [12, 16, 17].

Harvey Williams Cushing also described the acute SDH as an injury and also the treatment of this traumatic situation [12, 16, 17]. In September 1925, Tracy Jackson Putnam and Harvey Cushing published a paper entitled "*Chronic Subdural Hematoma. Its Pathology, Its Relation to Pachymeningitis Hemorrhagica and Its Surgical Treatment.*" In this scientific work, they described that recurrent hemorrhage caused progressive enlargement of the hematoma. Following Putnam and Cushing's studies the lesion has been called chronic SDH instead of pachymeningitis hemorrhagica interna [12, 16, 17].

Sachs, in 1920, published a review about that kind of injuries in infants. He suggested that the infants who survived may developed a chronic form of the disease [12, 17].

In 1924, Stephenson reported a case report with pachymeningitis associated with syphilis. He believed that the two conditions were associated [12, 17].

Craig, in 1928, made the statement that the mesothelial cells found lining the spaces have been classified as a part of the reticulo-endothelial system and as a result they have the power to react with the hemoglobin present. This interreaction breaks down the pigments of the blood giving it the final dark color [12, 17].

During the next several decades, diverse pathogenetic theories were proposed with the osmotic pressure theory being the generally accepted opinion for about 40 years:

- Gardner, in 1932, proposed that the expansion of the original subdural clot occurred through the osmotic attraction of cerebrospinal fluid (CSF) by blood within the semipermeable hematoma neo-membranes [12, 17].
- Zollinger, in 1934, also proposed oncotic pressure theory [30].
- Munro and Merritt, in 1936, published a series of 105 cases, studying the progression of the lesion [12, 17].
- In the same time period, Hannah and Kaump also performed studies regarding the secondary formation of the membranes inside the dura mater [12, 17].
- Giltin, in 1955, proposed an effusion theory [12].

In the 70s:

- Weir disputed the osmotic pressure theory and found no osmolarity difference between venous blood, cerebrospinal fluid, and chronic SDH fluid (1971) [25–30].
- Watanabe managed to produce a clinical form of a chronic SDH by inoculating a clot made of blood mixed and cerebrovascular fluid into the subdural space of dogs and monkeys (1972) [25–30].
- Apfelbaum failed to prove that cerebrovascular fluid was essential to produce chronic SDH (1974) [25–30].
- Sato and Suzuki reported that repeat microhemorrhage from the capillaries of the outer membrane was responsible for the enlargement of chronic SDH (1975) [25–30].
- Labadie and Glover demonstrated that injection of dexamethasone into the cerebrospinal fluid inhibits membrane formation (1976) [25–30].
- Yamada described the transformation from hygroma to hematoma (1979) [25–30].

In the 80s:

- Weir, in 1980, disagreed with the oncotic pressure theory. However, in his studies he could not explain the mechanism of hematoma enlargement [25–30].
- Markwalder, in 1981, supported the theory for rebleeding from the membrane for the formation of chronic SDH. Markwalder's review of the rebleeding theory was widely accepted [25–30].
- Asymptomatic acute SDHs were suspected as the origin of chronic SDHs (1985) [25–30].

In 90s and 20s:

- The Lee studies (1996, 1998, and 2004) uncover the relation of subdural lesions, their origin, and the natural history of chronic SDHs [10–12].

Till the end of the twentieth century:

- None of the experimental models used have managed to demonstrate a progressive enlargement of chronic SDH, except where a similar pathology of liquefied hematoma was enveloped with a neomembrane [12].
- There are still controversies regarding the origin and natural history of this lesion [12].

3.4 Conclusion

Chronic SDH remains an important neurosurgical pathological entity. From the first descriptions in ancient human history we pass into the modern era. First described during the seventeenth and eighteenth centuries it was regarded as a stroke, later considered an inflammatory disease in the nineteenth century, and finally it became a traumatic lesion in the twentieth century, thanks to the development of neurosurgery as an autonomous medical discipline. Although the cause of chronic SDH was revealed as traumatic, this lesion has still many unrevealed secrets such as: (a) how asymptomatic acute SDHs become the main source of chronic ones; and (b) why there is no clear explanation for the latent interval that exists between the initial head injury and the onset of symptoms.

References

1. Andrushko VA, Verano JW. Prehistoric trepanation in the Cuzco region of Peru: a view into an ancient Andean practice. Am J Phys Anthropol. 2008;137:4–13.
2. Apfelbaum RI, Guthkelch AN, Shulman K. Experimental production of subdural hematomas. J Neurosurg. 1974;40:336–46.
3. Castiglioni A. Storia della Medicina. Milan: A. Mondadori; 1936.
4. D'Abbondanza JA, Loch Macdonald R. Experimental models of chronic subdural hematoma. Neurol Res. 2014;36:176–88.
5. D'Errico AP, German WJ. Chronic subdural hematoma. Yale J Biol Med. 1930;3:11–20.
6. Ellis H. The Cambridge illustrated history of surgery. Cambridge: Cambridge University Press; 2009.
7. Giannouli V, Syrmos N. Information about Macedonian medicine in ancient Greece. Hell J Nucl Med. 2011;14:324–5.
8. Kaufman MH, Whitaker D, McTavish J. Differential diagnosis of holes in the calvarium: application of modern clinical data to palaeopathology. J Archaeol Sci. 1997;24:193–218.
9. Kim DJ. The appeal of holes in the head. In: Whitelaw WA, editor. The Proceedings of the 13th annual history of medicine days. Calgary: Faculty of Medicine; University of Calgary; 2004. p. 17–24.

10. Lee KS. The pathogenesis and clinical significance of traumatic subdural hygroma. Brain Inj. 1998;12:595–603.
11. Lee KS. Natural history of chronic subdural haematoma. Brain Inj. 2004;18:351–8.
12. Lee K-S. History of chronic subdural hematoma. Korean J Neurotrauma. 2015;11:27–34.
13. Marino R Jr, Gonzales-Portillo M. Preconquest Peruvian neurosurgeons: a study of Inca and pre-Columbian trephination and the art of medicine in ancient Peru. Neurosurgery. 2000;47:940–50.
14. Oka H, Motomochi M, Suzuki Y, Ando K. Subdural hygroma after head injury. A review of 26 cases. Acta Neurochir (Wien). 1972;26:265–73.
15. Oppenheim H. Textbook of nervous diseases for physicians and students. 5th ed. New York: Otto Schulze and Company; 1911.
16. Putnam TJ, Cushing H. Chronic subdural hematoma: its pathology, its relation to pachymeningitis hemorrhagica, and its surgical treatment. Arch Surg. 1925;11:329–93.
17. Richards CE. Chronic subdural hematoma with special reference to etiology, diagnosis, and treatment. MD Thesis. 1940.
18. Sato S, Suzuki J. Ultrastructural observations of the capsule of chronic subdural hematoma in various clinical stages. J Neurosurg. 1975;43:569–78.
19. Schachenmayr W, Friede RL. The origin of subdural neomembranes. I. Fine structure of the dura-arachnoid interface in man. Am J Pathol. 1978;92:53–68.
20. Syrmos N. Microcephaly in ancient Greece-the Minoan microcephalus of Zakros. Childs Nerv Syst. 2011;27:685–6.
21. Syrmos N. Historical back training in most important points of neurosurgery. Master Thesis. Aristotle University of Thessaloniki, Thessaloniki, Macedonia, Greece. 2009.
22. Syrmos N, Ampatzidis G, Fachantidou A, Mouratidis A, Syrmos C. Historical back training in most important points of neurosurgery. Ann General Psychiatry. 2010;9(Suppl 1):S89.
23. Trotter W. Chronic subdural hæmorrhage of traumatic origin, and its relation to pachymeningitis hæmorrhagica interna. Br J Surg. 1914;2:271–91.
24. Tullo E. Trepanation and Roman medicine: a comparison of osteoarchaeological remains, material culture and written texts. J R Coll Physicians Edinb. 2010;40:165–71.
25. Velasco-Suarez M, Bautista Martinez J, Garcia Oliveros R, Weinstein PR. Archaeological origins of cranial surgery: trephination in Mexico. Neurosurgery. 1992;31:313–8.
26. Watanabe S, Shimada H, Ishii S. Production of clinical form of chronic subdural hematoma in experimental animals. J Neurosurg. 1972;37:552–61.
27. Weir B. The osmolality of subdural hematoma fluid. J Neurosurg. 1971;34:528–33.
28. Weir B. Oncotic pressure of subdural fluids. J Neurosurg. 1980;53:512–5.
29. Wilberger JE. Pathophysiology of evolution and recurrence of chronic subdural hematoma. Neurosurg Clin N Am. 2000;11:435–8.
30. Zollinger R, Gross RE. Traumatic subdural hematoma: an explanation of the late onset of pressure symptoms. J Am Med Assoc. 1934;103:245–9.

Chapter 4
Understanding Chronic Subdural Hematoma: Pathophysiology

George W. Koutsouras, Sydney Colvin, and Satish Krishnamurthy

4.1 Introduction

Chronic subdural hematoma (CSDH) is a common neurological condition with an incidence ranging from 10 to 80 per 100,000 individuals, with a rising incidence among the elderly [2]. The pathophysiology of CSDH remains perplexing and appears to be multifactorial. Despite the reasonably high prevalence of CSDH, an effective initial treatment and one that lowers the recurrence rate remains to be identified [4].

The normal subdural space is maintained by dural border cells that tether the dura to the arachnoid. Chronic subdural hematoma is preceded by disruption of this gap, either spontaneously or secondary to trauma [10, 23, 28]. Once this disruption occurs, there are a constellation of events, including an inflammatory process leading to the development of neomembranes in addition to incomplete resorption of the hemorrhage that leads to CSDH formation. We describe the sequence of events that are involved in the genesis of a CSDH (Fig. 4.1).

4.2 Clinical Features

CSDHs typically cause symptoms between 4 and 7 weeks after development. Patients present with symptoms such as headache, nausea, mental status changes, weakness, seizures or even coma secondary to cortical irritation, brain compression or elevation in intracranial pressure.

G. W. Koutsouras (✉) · S. Colvin · S. Krishnamurthy
Department of Neurosurgery, Upstate University Hospital, Syracuse, NY, USA
e-mail: koutsoug@upstate.edu; sy13colv@siena.edu; krishnsa@upstate.edu

M. Turgut et al. (eds.), *Subdural Hematoma*,
https://doi.org/10.1007/978-3-030-79371-5_4

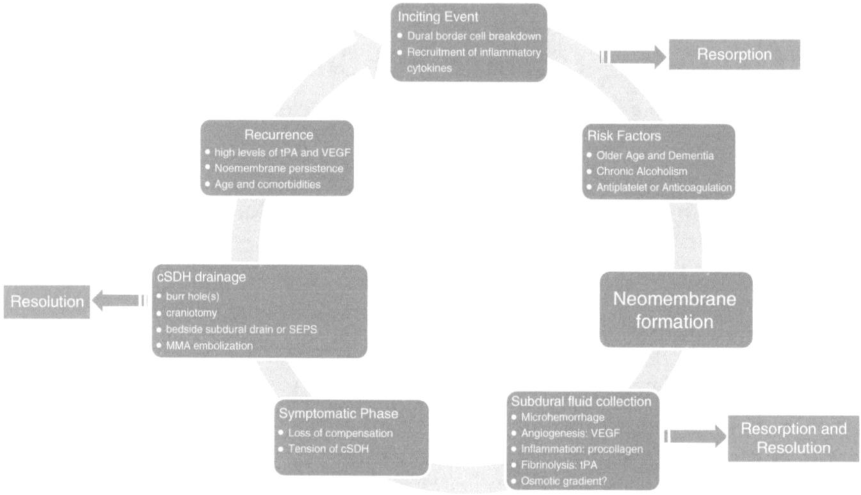

Fig. 4.1 Life cycle of chronic subdural hematoma (CSDH). The inciting event, an initial trauma with risk factors for development of CSDH, such as old age, blood thinner usage, and chronic alcoholism, lead to the neomembrane formation and subsequent seepage of red blood cells and cerebrospinal fluid into the subdural space, without an ability to resorb the fluid, leads to loss of compensatory mechanisms and symptom development. Symptom onset will herald surgical treatment of the patient. The factors that prevent recurrence include ability to remove the hematoma along with removal of the neomembrane or even reduce the CSDH vasculature via middle meningeal artery (MMA) embolization. *SEPS* subdural evacuation port system, *VEGF* Vascular Endothelial Growth Factor, *tPA* tissue plasminogen activator

In most cases, CSDH formation follows an acute subdural hematoma. However, 3–26% patients with acute SDH are found to develop CSDH [20]. This indicates that there must be other factors contributing to CSDH formation, since there is an obvious latent or asymptomatic period during which pathophysiological mechanisms lead to its development. Clotted blood undergoes liquification leaving serosanguinous fluid within the subdural space which becomes resorbed. This process is enabled by the brain parenchymal pressure which decreases the size of the subdural space. In patients with low intracranial pressure or those with cerebral atrophy, as is seen in advanced dementia or chronic alcoholics, they are more likely to accumulate this fluid within the subdural space [19]. Advancing age is a risk factor for subdural hematoma occurrence, with over 60% of patients with a CSDH are over 65 years old [2]. Subdural hematomas may also be seen in infants and children. They classically are seen in the context of nonaccidental head trauma, but could also be seen in patients with external hydrocephalus, benign enlargement of the subarachnoid spaces, idiopathic macrocephaly, and even dehydration [40]. Males are also seen to have CSDH more often than females [1]. Patients on anticoagulation or antiplatelet agents are at a higher risk of developing both acute SDH and CSDH after a trauma, than those not on blood thinners [1] (Fig. 4.2).

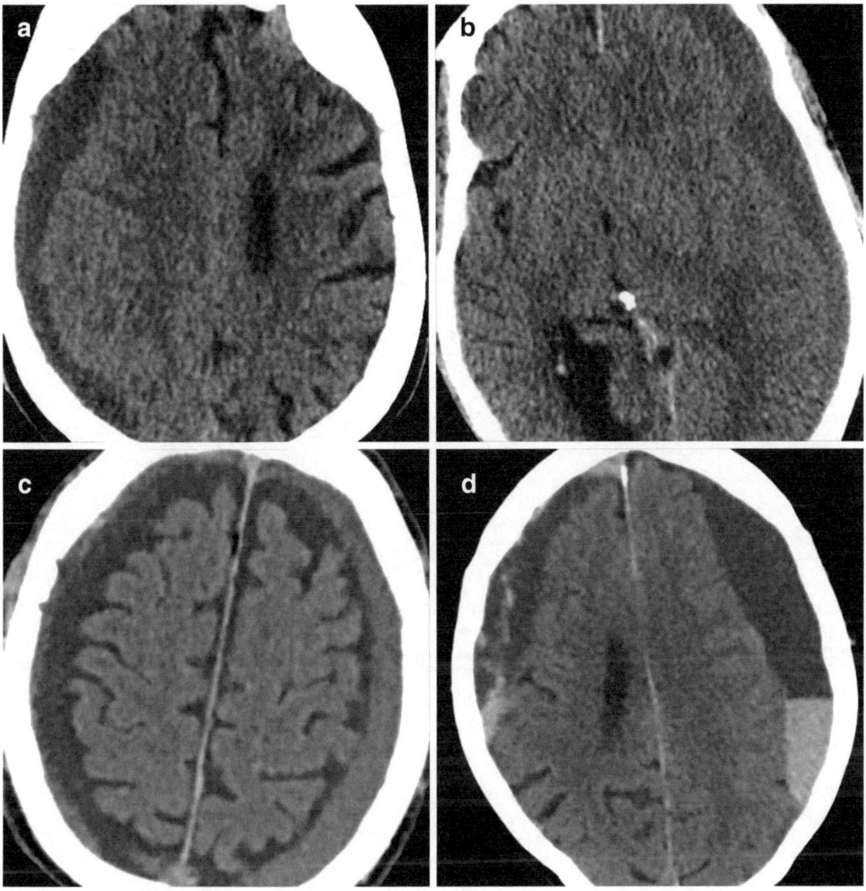

Fig. 4.2 Various hematoma densities seen on brain CT. (**a**) Low density, (**b**) iso dense, (**c**) high density (left convexity), (**d**) mixed density bilaterally, right convexity loculations

4.3 Radiographic Features

Computed tomography (CT) is the ideal diagnostic test for CSDH which is seen as an extra-axial fluid collection of different densities on CT relative to the brain parenchyma (Fig. 4.3). Isodense lesions are most commonly found. Secondary to the inflammatory process that occurs, mixed densities are also commonly seen. They are believed to be the result of continuous microbleeding and neomembrane formation. Mixed densities are also seen with acute on chronic traumatic events [10]. Magnetic resonance imaging (MRI) has been useful in differentiating various ages of CSDHs as well as from other pathologies such as subdural hygroma or in children with benign enlargement of the subarachnoid spaces [31, 48].

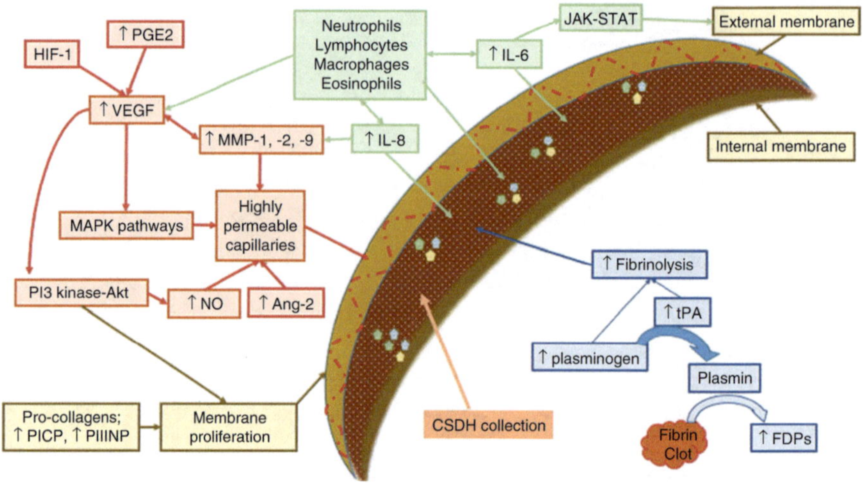

Fig. 4.3 Summary of the pathogenesis and inflammatory cascade associated with CSDH. Abbreviations: *Ang* angiopoietin, *FDPs* fibrin/fibrinogen degradation products, *HIF* hypoxia-inducible factor, *IL* interleukin, *JAK-STAT* Janus kinase-signal transducer and activator of transcription, *MAPK* mitogen-activated protein kinase, *MMP* matrix metalloproteinase, *NO* nitric oxide, *PGE* prostaglandin E, *PI3-Akt* phosphatidylinositol 3-kinase-serine/threonine kinase, *PICP* procollagen type 1, *PIIINP* procollagen type 3, *tPA* tissue plasminogen activator, *VEGF* vascular endothelial growth factor. Copyright from Edlmann et al. 2017 [5] http://creativecommons.org/licenses/by/4.0/

4.4 Pathophysiological Mechanisms

Since its first description in the early nineteenth century, the use of histopathology has identified the internal matrix of subdural hematomas and surgical advancements have highlighted a multitude of factors that influence the development and recurrence of the disease [20]. Described as early as 1875, by Virchow "pachymeningitis hemorrhagic interna," CSDH were first thought to be a product of a bacterial infection leading to chronic inflammation driving neovascularization and fibrin exudation [6]. In the early twentieth century, Schwartz, Trotter, Putnam, and Cushing all described an initial trauma that subsequently led to a chronic inflammatory process [32, 33]. In 1936, a neurosurgeon Dr. Furlow from Washington University further expanded upon the case series by Putnam and Cushing, describing two types of subdural hematomas. He classified them as reactive or traumatic type and a vascular type based on the histopathological appearance [42].

In 1946, Inglis discovered dural border cells lining the dura mater [14]. When these cells are damaged, inflammatory cells are induced and can form new membranes in the subdural space. Once these membranes form, a mixture of blood and cerebrospinal fluid (CSF) fill the subdural cavity [5]. The inflammatory cascade set in motion by the disruption of the dural border cells and the formation of a neomembrane plays a key role in the persistence of a CSDH with the accumulation of blood and CSF.

The neomembrane of CSDH consists of an external and an internal layer. Initially described in 1936, the dural cells form an external membrane after approximately 1 week. Within 3 weeks, the inner membrane develops [24]. As the CSDH develops, CSF and blood fill the subdural space which sets off a cascade of fibrin deposition with cycles of fibrinolysis primarily through the activation of tissue plasminogen activator (tPA). There is angiogenesis through the activation of vascular endothelial growth factor (VEGF), and reorganization or liquefaction of the subdural hematoma [5]. High concentrations of type 1 and 3 procollagen, fibrin, angiopoeietin-2, additional cytokines and chemokines, have been identified within CSDH fluid (Fig. 4.3).

Blood vessels and capillaries within the outer membrane are oriented towards the CSDH contents. The external membrane is found to contain fibroblasts, collagen fibrils, and migrating cells (Fig. 4.4) [7]. Blood vessels are also involved in the inflammatory response and contain permeable capillaries as well as gap junctions to allow for the migration of blood and CSF into the subdural cavity. There is some literature to suggest that as the external neomembrane develops, it can be divided into several histological subtypes that could correlate with radiographic features. For example, type II or hemorrhagic neomembrane is more often associated with rapid expansion and the greatest hematoma thickness [29]. These microcapillaries although small lead to persistent episodes of bleeding and progression of the hematoma. VEGF is a major angiogenic factor involved in the progression of CSDH. This molecule is upregulated as part of the inflammatory process, and the proteome make-up of the developing neomembrane [35, 37, 41]. VEGF creates high permeability which results in the formation of immature capillaries that cause microbleeds and thus hematoma formation. Surgical drainage is believed to reduce the amount of VEGF in the hematoma cavity and therefore alleviate the adverse effects of increased stimulation [35]. Growth factors known as angiopoietins regulate angiogenesis and vascular permeability. The proangiogenic factor angiopoietin-2 (Ang-2) may lead to adverse effects on the process of angiogenesis [12]. Overexpression of Ang-2 results in the formation of fragile vessel formation in the CSDH membrane and when combined with VEGF, which makes these vessels highly permeable, may contribute to the development of CSDH. Studies are being performed to determine the difference between normal and abnormal VEGF functions in addition to methods to mitigate the progression of CSDH. The middle meningeal artery has been observed to largely supply the microcapillaries of the neomembrane [16, 26, 36]. Enlarged middle meningeal arteries (MMA) on the same side as CSDH are the target of therapy for CSDH. MMA embolization is a technique that aims to minimize the leakage of blood products. MMA embolization results in a lower recurrence rate of 3.6% found in two case studies [16, 36]. This technique is appealing for the elderly that may have other underlying health conditions or may be on medication such as anticoagulants or antiplatelets. Several factors regarding embolization such as the choice of the embolic agent, type of anesthesia used, and the definite indications for the embolization procedure are yet to be determined.

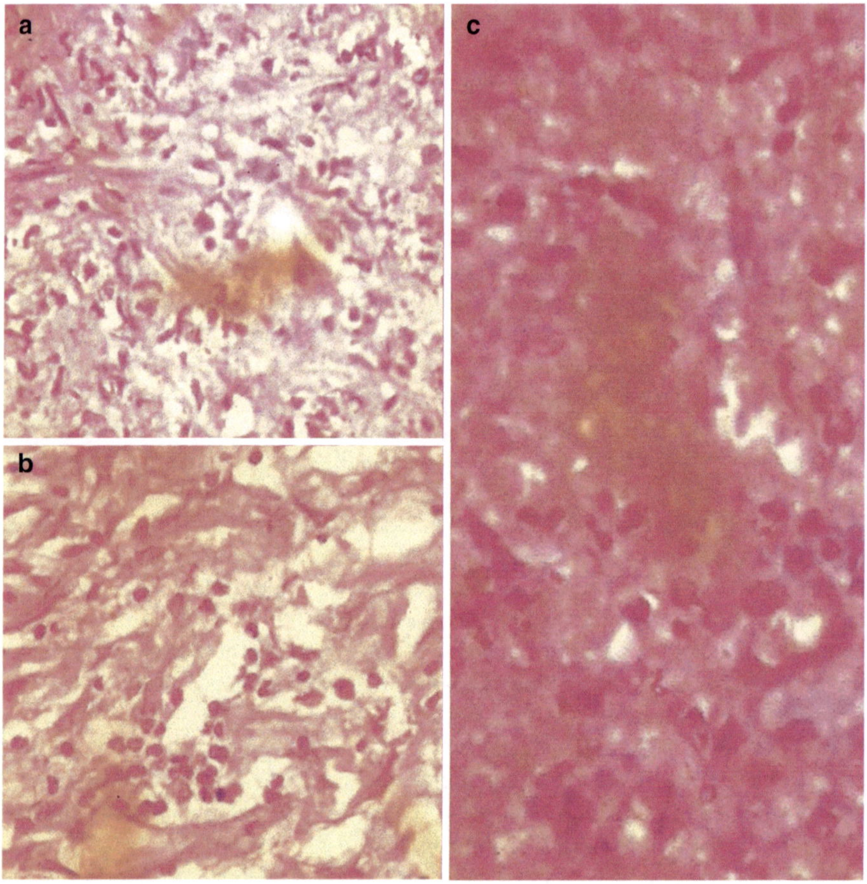

Fig. 4.4 Histological classification of outer CSDH membrane. (**a**) Type II inflammatory membrane consisting of a single layer of immature connective tissue and associated with marked vascularization and cell infiltration. (**b**) Type III hemorrhagic inflammatory membrane which consists of multiple layers associated with large diameter capillaries and marked cell infiltration with proliferation of new vessels accompanied by hemorrhage into the membrane. (**c**) Type IV scar inflammatory membrane depicting scarring with further inflammatory cell infiltration on hematoxylin and eosin. Copyright from Gandhoke et al. 2013 [7] (Copyright reprint granted)

As the subdural hematoma becomes chronic, numerous cycles of fibrin formation and fibrinolysis will occur, the development of an inner neomembrane with possible high-density septa may occur [3, 7, 27]. The inner layer of the membrane consists of four layers: the hematoma layer, intermediate layer, arachnoid surface, and the final layer. As the CSDH develops, the presence of vascular structures decreases while the number of fibrous tissues increases. The internal membrane contains mediators of CSDH that include cytokines, IL-6, and high levels of chemokines. Cytokines released in response to inflammation can be used as markers for hematoma development. IL-6 plays a role in widening gap junctions. Myofibroblasts within the internal membrane release chemokines which typically move inflammatory cells to the epicenter of the hematoma [5, 11].

CSDHs are rich in blood, cerebrospinal fluid, and protein. Given their rich protein content, mainly in the form of albumin, they are hyperosmotic to the subarachnoid CSF containing spaces. As described by Zollinger et al. in 1934, there was a belief that higher protein levels within the matrix of the hematoma led to an osmotic gradient resulting in cerebrospinal fluid seepage into the subdural space [49]. But given the presence of capillaries within the external neomembrane, it was necessary to study the gradient between CSDH and serum. Weir et al. measured the oncotic pressure differential in subdural hematoma fluid in contrast to blood oncotic pressure. He saw no convincing evidence to suggest there was an existing gradient present [43, 44]. In the authors' opinion, osmotic gradients are equalized between the compartments rapidly and it is unlikely that a gradient can be demonstrated. Higher macromolecular content of the subdural fluid increases the osmotic load and the osmotic draw of the fluid from surrounding blood vessels (especially the leaky small capillaries) can contribute to the volume of the CSDH. Thomas et al. state that osmotic gradients simultaneously exist for both CSDH growth and resorption. Despite no remarkable difference between CSDH and serum, Thomas et al. state that if the surface area of the neomembrane was greater than the surface area of the subdural hematoma, there is a mechanism of resorption that could occur. Thomas et al. proposed that the surface area of capillaries present on the neomembrane could play a role in CSDH resorption. The larger the surface area compared to the hematoma volume, the greater the chance for resorption [38].

Subdural hygromas are also a pathology seen in adults and children. In patients with a larger calvarium to brain parenchyma ratio, they may have a disproportionally large subdural space. Subdural space can accumulate cerebrospinal fluid, especially in the presence of hydrocephalus [30, 31]. In patients without expansile brain associated with craniocerebral disproportion, such as in children with macrocephaly and older patients with cerebral atrophy, hydrostatic forces play a key role in the direction of flow of fluids between subarachnoid space, subdural space, and neomembrane interface [31]. Thus, oncotic and hydrostatic pressures must be considered in the pathophysiology of CSDH. Furthermore, Nakaguchi described that secondary to traumatic tears within the arachnoid membrane, CSF can accumulate within the subdural space [8]. With subdural hygromas present, there may be an increased possibility of developing a CSDH as the pathophysiology principles of neomembrane formation and microbleeding could ultimately occur in these pathologies [18–20].

4.5 Recurrence

The possibility of recurrence of CSDH is significant and should be considered by the treating physician. Some patient-specific factors for recurrence include older age, chronic alcoholism, brain atrophy, hydrocephalus, and diabetes mellitus. Other factors include the density of the hematoma, age of hematoma, presence of bilateral CSDHs, significant postoperative residual hematoma, and even subdural air within the postsurgical cavity [15, 17, 25, 34, 39, 45, 47]. Contrary to popular belief, restarting blood thinners after CSDH drainage was not associated with high recurrence rates [9, 21, 46]. Jeong and group demonstrated a significant positive relationship between high or mixed density CSDH and the degree of recurrence [15].

There has been great attention given to the subdural neomembrane and its relationship to CSDH recurrence. As mentioned, the neomembranes are largely fed by neocapillary formation secondary to angiogenesis. Xin liu and his group in China demonstrated that removing thick inner membrane reduced the CSDH recurrence rate. They identified a significant association between a thick inner neomembrane during craniotomy and CSDH recurrence [22]. They also associated the presence of a thick inner membrane with mixed density subdural hematoma presence on CT imaging. Other studies have suggested that the increasing thickness of the membrane in combination with the tension placed on the cortex is associated with the onset of symptoms in a patient who is asymptomatic or in the latent phase [39].

Many studies have indicated a reduced recurrence rate of CSDH in patients after receiving dexamethasone in addition to surgical drainage. Dexamethasone is a synthetic corticosteroid and functions to reduce the inflammatory response that leads to CSDH. Dexamethasone reduces blood clot formation and prevents the inflammatory response resulting in a halt in neomembrane development [17]. Corticosteroids inhibit the expression of inflammatory proteins such as cytokines and chemokines involved in the development of CSDH. Researchers are still analyzing the negative side effects of the steroid especially within the elderly population. Most recently published by Hutchinson and the Dex-CSDH Trial investigators found that favorable outcomes of dexamethasone use were exceeded by negative effects in the treatment of chronic subdural hematoma [13].

4.6 Conclusion

CSDH is a fairly common neurosurgical disorder that requires treatment. Understanding the complex pathophysiological mechanisms of this disorder has paved the way for better treatment strategies to treat this condition and decrease the recurrence rate. This chapter summarizes the initiation of the hematoma formation with the disruption of the dural border cells followed by the accumulation of the blood clot resulting in a cascade of events which includes inflammation that leads to neomembrane formation. The mechanisms and timeline of outer and inner membrane formation, role of VEGF and angiopoietins in the vascularity of the membranes and osmolarity are described. Mechanisms of recurrence and factors that predict recurrence as well as the rationale underlying some of the newer modalities of treatment such as MMA embolization are discussed. Our understanding of the multifactorial process behind CSDH formation continues to pave the way for possible pharmaceutical and surgical interventions.

References

1. Baechli H, Nordmann A, Bucher HC, Gratzl O. Demographics and prevalent risk factors of chronic subdural haematoma: results of a large single-center cohort study. Neurosurg Rev. 2004;27(4):263–6.
2. Balser D, Farooq S, Mehmood T, Reyes M, Samadani U. Actual and projected incidence rates for chronic subdural hematomas in United States Veterans Administration and civilian populations. J Neurosurg. 2015;123(5):1209–15.
3. Bokka S, Trivedi A. Histopathological study of the outer membrane of the dura mater in chronic sub dural hematoma: its clinical and radiological correlation. Asian J Neurosurg. 2016;11(1):34–8.
4. Ducruet AF, Grobelny BT, Zacharia BE, Hickman ZL, DeRosa PL, Andersen KN, et al. The surgical management of chronic subdural hematoma. Neurosurg Rev. 2012;35(2):155–69.
5. Edlmann E, Giorgi-Coll S, Whitfield PC, Carpenter KLH, Hutchinson PJ. Pathophysiology of chronic subdural haematoma: inflammation, angiogenesis and implications for pharmacotherapy. J Neuroinflammation. 2017;14(1):108.
6. Feghali J, Yang W, Huang J. Updates in chronic subdural hematoma: epidemiology, etiology, pathogenesis, treatment, and outcome. World Neurosurg. 2020;141:339–45.
7. Gandhoke GS, Kaif M, Choi L, Williamson RW, Nakaji P. Histopathological features of the outer membrane of chronic subdural hematoma and correlation with clinical and radiological features. J Clin Neurosci. 2013;20(10):1398–401.
8. Gitlin D. Pathogenesis of subdural collections of fluid. Pediatrics. 1955;16(3):345–52.
9. Glover D, Labadie EL. Physiopathogenesis of subdural hematomas. Part 2: inhibition of growth of experimental hematomas with dexamethasone. J Neurosurg. 1976;45(4):393–7.
10. Haines DE, Harkey HL, al-Mefty O. The “subdural” space: a new look at an outdated concept. Neurosurgery. 1993;32(1):111–20.
11. Heula AL, Ohlmeier S, Sajanti J, Majamaa K. Characterization of chronic subdural hematoma fluid proteome. Neurosurgery. 2013;73(2):317–31.
12. Holl DC, Volovici V, Dirven CMF, Peul WC, van Kooten F, Jellema K, et al. Pathophysiology and nonsurgical treatment of chronic subdural hematoma: from past to present to future. World Neurosurg. 2018;116:402–11.e2.
13. Hutchinson PJ, Edlmann E, Bulters D, Zolnourian A, Holton P, Suttner N, et al. Trial of dexamethasone for chronic subdural hematoma. N Engl J Med. 2020;383(27):2616–27.
14. Inglis K. Subdural haemorrhage, cysts and false membranes; illustrating the influence of intrinsic factors in disease when development of the body is normal. Brain. 1946;69(3):157–94.
15. Jeong SI, Kim SO, Won YS, Kwon YJ, Choi CS. Clinical analysis of risk factors for recurrence in patients with chronic subdural hematoma undergoing Burr hole trephination. Korean J Neurotrauma. 2014;10(1):15–21.
16. Jumah F, Osama M, Islim AI, Jumah A, Patra DP, Kosty J, et al. Efficacy and safety of middle meningeal artery embolization in the management of refractory or chronic subdural hematomas: a systematic review and meta-analysis. Acta Neurochir. 2020;162(3):499–507.
17. Kamenova M, Lutz K, Schaedelin S, Fandino J, Mariani L, Soleman J. Does early resumption of low-dose aspirin after evacuation of chronic subdural hematoma with Burr-hole drainage lead to higher recurrence rates? Neurosurgery. 2016;79(5):715–21.
18. Knox B, Rorke-Adams L, Luyet F. Subdural hematoma rebleeding in relation to abusive head trauma. J Fam Violence. 2016;31(7):815–21.
19. Lee K-S. History of chronic subdural hematoma. Korean J Neurotrauma. 2015;11(2):27–34.
20. Lee KS, Bae WK, Park YT, Yun IG. The pathogenesis and fate of traumatic subdural hygroma. Br J Neurosurg. 1994;8(5):551–8.
21. Liu LX, Cao XD, Ren YM, Zhou LX, Yang CH. Risk factors for recurrence of chronic subdural hematoma: a single center experience. World Neurosurg. 2019;132:e506–e13.

22. Lutz K, Kamenova M, Schaedelin S, Guzman R, Mariani L, Fandino J, et al. Time to and possible risk factors for recurrence after Burr-hole drainage of chronic subdural hematoma: a subanalysis of the cSDH-drain randomized controlled trial. World Neurosurg. 2019;132:e283–e9.
23. Mori K, Maeda M. Surgical treatment of chronic subdural hematoma in 500 consecutive cases: clinical characteristics, surgical outcome, complications, and recurrence rate. Neurol Med Chir. 2001;41(8):371–81.
24. Munro D, Merritt HH. Surgical pathology of subdural hematoma: based on a study of one hundred and five cases. Arch Neurol Psychiatr. 1936;35(1):64–78.
25. Nagatani K, Wada K, Takeuchi S, Nawashiro H. Corticosteroid suppression of vascular endothelial growth factor and recurrence of chronic subdural hematoma. Neurosurgery. 2012;70(5):E1334; author reply E1334–6.
26. Nakagawa I, Park HS, Kotsugi M, Wada T, Takeshima Y, Matsuda R, et al. Enhanced hematoma membrane on DynaCT images during middle meningeal artery embolization for persistently recurrent chronic subdural hematoma. World Neurosurg. 2019;126:e473–e9.
27. Nakaguchi H, Tanishima T, Yoshimasu N. Factors in the natural history of chronic subdural hematomas that influence their postoperative recurrence. J Neurosurg. 2001;95(2):256–62.
28. Park H-R, Lee K-S, Shim J-J, Yoon S-M, Bae H-G, Doh J-W. Multiple densities of the chronic subdural hematoma in CT scans. J Korean Neurosurg Soc. 2013;54(1):38–41.
29. Park MH, Kim CH, Cho TG, Park JK, Moon JG, Lee HK. Clinical features according to the histological types of the outer membrane of chronic subdural hematoma. Korean J Neurotrauma. 2015;11(2):70–4.
30. Piatt JH Jr. A pitfall in the diagnosis of child abuse: external hydrocephalus, subdural hematoma, and retinal hemorrhages. Neurosurg Focus. 1999;7(4):e4.
31. Pittman T. Significance of a subdural hematoma in a child with external hydrocephalus. Pediatr Neurosurg. 2003;39(2):57–9.
32. Putnam TJ, Cushing H. Chronic subdural hematoma: its pathology, its relation to pachymeningitis hemorrhagica and its surgical treatment. Arch Surg. 1925;11(3):329–93.
33. Schwartz AB. The etiology of pachymeningitis hemorrhagica interna in infants. Am J Dis Child. 1916;XI(1):23–32.
34. Schwarz F, Loos F, Dunisch P, Sakr Y, Safatli DA, Kalff R, et al. Risk factors for reoperation after initial burr hole trephination in chronic subdural hematomas. Clin Neurol Neurosurg. 2015;138:66–71.
35. Shono T, Inamura T, Morioka T, Matsumoto K, Suzuki SO, Ikezaki K, et al. Vascular endothelial growth factor in chronic subdural haematomas. J Clin Neurosci. 2001;8(5):411–5.
36. Srivatsan A, Mohanty A, Nascimento FA, Hafeez MU, Srinivasan VM, Thomas A, et al. Middle meningeal artery embolization for chronic subdural hematoma: meta-analysis and systematic review. World Neurosurg. 2019;122:613–9.
37. Suzuki K, Takano S, Nose T, Doi M, Ohashi N. Increased concentration of vascular endothelial growth factor (VEGF) in chronic subdural hematoma. J Trauma. 1999;46(3):532–3.
38. Thomas PAW, Marshman LAG, Rudd D, Moffat C, Mitchell PS. Growth and resorption of chronic subdural hematomas: Gardner, Weir, and the osmotic hypothesis revisited. World Neurosurg. 2019;132:e202–e7.
39. Tomita Y, Yamada SM, Yamada S, Matsuno A. Subdural tension on the brain in patients with chronic subdural hematoma is related to hemiparesis but not to headache or recurrence. World Neurosurg. 2018;119:e518–e26.
40. Vinchon M, Delestret I, DeFoort-Dhellemmes S, Desurmont M, Noulé N. Subdural hematoma in infants: can it occur spontaneously? Data from a prospective series and critical review of the literature. Childs Nerv Syst. 2010;26(9):1195–205.
41. Weigel R, Hohenstein A, Schilling L. Vascular endothelial growth factor concentration in chronic subdural hematoma fluid is related to computed tomography appearance and exudation rate. J Neurotrauma. 2014;31(7):670–3.
42. Weigel R, Krauss JK, Schmiedek P. Concepts of neurosurgical management of chronic subdural haematoma: historical perspectives. Br J Neurosurg. 2004;18(1):8–18.

43. Weir B. Oncotic pressure of subdural fluids. J Neurosurg. 1980;53(4):512–5.
44. Weir B. The osmolality of subdural hematoma fluid. J Neurosurg. 1971;34(4):528–33.
45. Xu FF, Chen JH, Leung GK, Hao SY, Xu L, Hou ZG, et al. Quantitative computer tomography analysis of post-operative subdural fluid volume predicts recurrence of chronic subdural haematoma. Brain Inj. 2014;28(8):1121–6.
46. Yamamoto H, Hirashima Y, Hamada H, Hayashi N, Origasa H, Endo S. Independent predictors of recurrence of chronic subdural hematoma: results of multivariate analysis performed using a logistic regression model. J Neurosurg. 2003;98(6):1217–21.
47. You W, Zhu Y, Wang Y, Liu W, Wang H, Wen L, et al. Prevalence of and risk factors for recurrence of chronic subdural hematoma. Acta Neurochir (Wien). 2018;160(5):893–9.
48. Zahl SM, Wester K, Gabaeff S. Examining perinatal subdural haematoma as an aetiology of extra-axial hygroma and chronic subdural haematoma. Acta Paediatr (Oslo, Norway: 1992). 2020;109(4):659–66.
49. Zollinger R, Gross RE. Traumatic subdural hematoma: an explanation of the late onset of pressure symptoms. J Am Med Assoc. 1934;103(4):245–9.

Chapter 5
Experimental Models of Chronic Subdural Hematoma

Sinan Sağıroğlu, Mehmet Turgut, and R. Shane Tubbs

5.1 Introduction

Chronic subdural hematoma (CSDH) is one of the most common neurosurgical entities in clinical practice. Various complications of surgical therapy frequently develop because of the associated medical problems and advanced ages of the patients [14, 18]. Unfortunately, the ideal treatment modality of CSDH is still under debate [14, 18]. Despite numerous attempts to replicate CSDH in small animals, success in explaining its pathogenesis has been only partial [5].

In this chapter, we review the chronological development and evolution of experimental models of CSDH from their first description to the present. Experimental studies by the authors who defined the various models are given in detail.

S. Sağıroğlu (✉)
Department of Neurosurgery, Aydın Adnan Menderes University Faculty of Medicine, Efeler, Aydın, Turkey

M. Turgut
Department of Neurosurgery, Aydın Adnan Menderes University Faculty of Medicine, Efeler, Aydın, Turkey

Department of Histology and Embryology, Aydın Adnan Menderes University Health Sciences Institute, Efeler, Aydın, Turkey

R. S. Tubbs
Department of Anatomical Sciences, St. George's University School of Medicine, Grenada, WI, USA

Department of Neurosurgery, Tulane University School of Medicine, New Orleans, LA, USA

M. Turgut et al. (eds.), *Subdural Hematoma*,
https://doi.org/10.1007/978-3-030-79371-5_5

5.2 Experimental Models of Chronic Subdural Hematoma

Historically, experimental studies of subdural hematoma (SDH) were begun in 1819 by Serres, who tore the superior sagittal sinus subdurally and examined the fibrinous sac that developed adherent to the dura [16]. In 1864, Laborde injected blood into the subdural space in dogs and cats but performed no histological examination [10]. Later, Sperling and Van Vleuten experimented on rabbits in 1872 and 1898, respectively, injecting blood into the subdural space [17, 19]. Although these two studies achieved some success in producing the membrane characteristic of SDH, the histological findings were not well documented [12]. Interestingly, animal studies on the relationship of chronic alcoholism to CSDH have also been reported many times and were summarized by Saltykow [15]. However, those studies failed to produce the typical subdural membrane of CSDH.

In the following sections, the experimental CSDH models are grouped as follows: (a) subdural blood injection models, (b) subdural blood clot implantation, (c) subdural blood or clot implantation with decreased intracranial pressure (ICP), (d) subcutaneous implantation models, (e) vascular injury models, and (f) brain atrophy models. Experimental studies by the authors who defined the models in each group are then summarized in detail.

5.2.1 Subdural Blood Injection Models

A summary of six experimental studies as an example of subdural blood injection models for production of SDH are given as below in detail (Table 5.1) [4, 6, 7, 11–13]:

- *Study by Putnam and Putnam*

  Putnam & Putnam injected autologous blood into the subdural space of dogs and cats, and the animals were sacrificed after 5–50 days. Some animals produced a thin mesothelial membrane above the arachnoid, but they neither formed a liquefied hematoma cavity nor showed increased hematoma volume during the study [12]. The authors noted the similarities between their histological findings and those of traumatic SDHs [12].
- *Study by Gardner*

  Gardner suggested osmosis as the mechanism by which SDHs enlarge. He injected five dogs with autologous blood into the subdural space [6]. In seven dogs, he injected the blood into the contralateral side with a curved needle [6]. He also used semi-permeable cellophane sacs containing autologous blood, measuring the weights of the sacs pre-procedure and after 3–18 days [6]. He found a 39–103% increase in the weight and deduced that the high protein content of liquefied blood created an osmotic pressure gradient and therefore an increased hematoma volume [6]. He also noted the lack of lymphatic drainage from the

Table 5.1 Experimental subdural blood injection models

Author(s)/ ref.#	Year	Species/duration of study	Technique of study	Location	Conclusion
Putnam and Putnam [12]	1927	Dog (*n* = 3) and cat (*n* = 15)/1 day to 3 months	1–2 mL of autologous whole blood, defibrinated blood, washed fibrin injection into subdural space	1–2 cm trephine opening between longitudinal and transverse sinus angle	Lesions similar to CSDH in appearance were achieved, but progressive behavior could not be replicated
Gardner [6]	1932	Dog (*n* = 5), dog (*n* = 7), and dog (*n* = 8)	Subdural injection, subdural injection on the contralateral side, the subdural sac containing autologous whole blood	Trephine opening or burr hole at the parietal convexity	It is difficult if not impossible to reproduce the clinical picture of SDH in the dog
Christensen [4]	1944	Dog (*n* = 2), dog (*n* = 4), dog (*n* = 4), and dog (*n* = 4)/8 days to 2 months	Single and repeated subdural blood injections, with or without trauma and with or without sagittal sinus ligation	Not stated. Mostly bilateral	CSDH has a traumatic origin; superior sagittal sinus ligation contributes to cyst formation
Goodell and Mealy [7]	1963	Dog (*n* = 8)/8–72 days Dog (*n* = 4)/36 days	Subdural blood injection, IV urea administration Subdural injection of frozen and thawed blood	Parietal convexity	Subdural blood, reduced cerebral volume, tearing of bridging veins are insufficient to induce CSDH; the contribution of osmosis is unclear
Ohshima [11]	1982	Dog (*n* = 22)/30 days	Subdural autologous whole blood; blood mixed with CSF	Trephine opening and balloon expansion of the subdural space at the parietal convexity	CSF mixed with blood and low intracranial pressure (mannitol and CSF evacuation) is needed for expanding SDH
Quan et al. [13]	2015	Rat (*n* = 144)	Subdural autologous whole blood injection	Repeated subdural injection through a burr hole	Plasma levels of inflammatory markers in circulating blood parallel the organization and resolution of CSDH

Abbreviations: *CSDH* chronic subdural hematoma, *CSF* cerebrospinal fluid, *SDH* subdural hematoma, *IV* intravenous mesothelial-lined subdural space [6]. The osmotic hypothesis gained widespread acceptance after this study.

- *Study by Christensen*

  Christensen performed four types of animal experiments [4]. In the first, he used a single subdural injection of citrated blood in four dogs, which he sacrificed on the 8–11th days [4]. His results were similar to those of *Putnam and Putnam* [4]. In the second, he injected blood into two dogs each week for 3 weeks, then sacrificed the animals 1 week after the last injection [4]. He found subdural membranes with capillaries up to 50 μm diameter and a newly formed layer containing macrophages, decaying erythrocytes, and fibroblasts, as in CSDH; but there was no liquefaction of blood products [4]. In the third experiment, on four dogs, he used the same procedure as in the second but also inflicted trauma to the occipital region [4]. The findings were the same as in the foregoing, with the addition of a traumatic subarachnoid hemorrhage in the occipital region. In the fourth experiment, on four dogs, he partially ligated the superior sagittal sinus but failed to achieve any SDHs after 5 days to 2 months [4]. He ligated the superior sagittal sinus and injected subdural blood bilaterally at the same time [4]. After 11 days to 3 weeks there were lesions similar to CSDH with large cystic cavities and vascular neomembranes [4]. He acknowledged Gardner's osmotic hypothesis in his conclusion [4].

- *Study by Goodell and Mealy*

  Goodell and Mealy also conducted four experiments each on two groups, including injection of subdural blood or clot, tearing the bridging veins, using intracranial volume reducing agents, shunting, and injection of anti-inflammatory agents [7]. Some of the experiments in this study are mentioned later in this chapter. In the first experiment (group A), eight dogs were injected subdurally with fresh blood, and intravenous (IV) urea was administered to reduce the cerebral volume. The volumes of blood administered averaged 6.7 mL and the animals were sacrificed on days 8–72 after injection. No subdural collection was formed [7]. In the fourth experiment (group A), seven dogs were injected with a mixture of clot, cerebrospinal (CSF), hydrocortisone, and streptokinase-streptodornase. None of the dogs developed delayed symptoms and resolution was similar to that of previous experiments [7]. In group B, frozen and thawed blood was injected into four dogs. The two surviving dogs, sacrificed on days 24 and 36, showed resorbed hematoma and dural thickening [7]. *Goodell and Mealy* tried multiple approaches to the experimental SDH but were unable to replicate the progressive lesions or liquefaction of the hematoma [7]. They concluded that the osmotic mechanism of hematoma expansion was untenable [7].

- *Study by Ohshima*

  Ohshima experimented on 45 dogs in four groups, using a trephine opening and applying a balloon technique similar to that of *Watanabe* et al., who implanted 3–4 mL of blood or clot [11]. He also used D-mannitol on some dogs and CSF drainage to increase the subdural cavity size, as in the *Goodell and Mealy* experiments, allowing 8–10 mL injections [11]. The first group comprised nine dogs inoculated with autologous fresh blood into the subdural space [11]. Blood clot was injected into the second group (10 dogs) and blood mixed with CSF was given to the third group (13 dogs) [11]. In the fourth group, a blood-CSF mixture was inoculated, and after the seventh day of inoculation daily doses of D-mannitol 3 g/kg and heparin 200 U/kg were given [11]. The first two groups showed high-density clot at days 3–4 followed by a decrease in hematoma volume and density in follow-up computed tomography (CT) imaging. Histological examination revealed typical organization and resolution of the hematomas [11]. In the third group, low-density and iso-dense lesions were apparent, reduced in size in follow-up CT images. The lesions had mostly regressed by the 18th day CT scan. When the animals were sacrificed at 2–3 weeks, histology showed neovascular membranes and fibrous layers similar to CSDH [11]. The fourth experimental group is described in the following section.

- *Study by Quan* et al.

  Quan et al. used a model of repeated blood injection through burr holes into the frontoparietal regions of 144 rats in four groups [13]. Each rat was initially injected with 400 μL freshly drawn autologous blood, then injected with an additional 300 μL in the same area after 72 h [13]. Blood in the subdural space was confirmed with in vivo magnetic resonance imaging (MRI) evaluation [13]. The authors sacrificed the four animal groups on the 3rd, 10th, 17th, and 24th days. Each group included 12 control rats, which underwent the same procedure without blood infusions [13]. All lesions followed a typical SDH resolution pattern, with vascular neomembrane formation and inflammatory processes [13]. On MRI, all hematomas were almost completely resolved by the 24th day [13]. Enzyme-linked immunosorbent assay (ELISA) tests on peripheral blood revealed increased levels of pro-inflammatory factors such as interleukin-6 (IL-6), IL-8, and tumor necrosis factor-α, peaking at day 10 [13]. IL-10, IL-13, and other anti-inflammatory factors increased at days 17 and 24, parallel to the resolution of CSDH [13].

5.2.2 Subdural Blood Clot Implantation

A summary of four experimental studies as an example of subdural blood clot implantation models for production of SDH are given as below in detail (Table 5.2) [3, 7, 11, 20]:

- *Study by Goodell and Mealy*

  Goodell and Mealy used 21 dogs, injecting large volumes of blood clot into the subdural space in their second experimental group A. They used urea, CSF drainage, and hypothermia to reduce the cerebral volume, and up to 12.2 mL of clot was injected into the animals [7]. The surviving dogs, although initially lethargic and unsteady, improved clinically and were sacrificed between the 15th hour and day 20 [7]. Reorganization and resolution of the hematoma were documented in this group [7]. In group B, eight dogs received weekly repeated injections of blood or clot into the subdural space from 12 to 35 days. Urea, CSF

Table 5.2 Experimental subdural blood clot implantation models

Author(s)/ ref.#	Year	Species/duration of study	Technique of study	Location	Conclusion
Goodell and Mealy [7]	1963	Dog ($n = 21$)/20 days Dog ($n = 2$) Dog ($n = 7$)/35 days	Subdural clot placement and IV urea administration Subdural clot placement and repeated urea administration for 6 days Repeated subdural clot or blood placement/ injection with urea administration	Parietal convexity	Subdural blood, reduced cerebral volume, tearing of bridging veins are insufficient to induce CSDH; the contribution of osmosis is unclear
Watanabe et al. [20]	1972	Dog ($n = 14$) and monkey ($n = 5$)/7–21 days	Single subdural placement of clot formed ex vivo with or without CSF ($n = 2$)	Trephine opening and balloon expansion in the right frontotemporal region	The clot formed in the presence of CSF has a different elastic fibrinous capsule, necessary in expanding hematoma. Osmosis has no apparent effect
Apfelbaum et al. [3]	1974	Dog ($n = 2$) and cat ($n = 40$)/8–30 days	Single subdural clot placement with different preparations	Trephine opening and balloon expansion in frontotemporal convexity	CSF has no role in the expansion of lesion volume, fibrin, and subsequent membrane formation on the dural surface, and rebleeding is the key factor in progression
Ohshima [11]	1982	Dog ($n = 10$)/30 days	Subdural clot implantation	Trephine opening and balloon expansion of the subdural space at the parietal convexity	CSF mixed with blood and low intracranial pressure (mannitol and CSF evacuation) is needed for expanding SDH

Abbreviations: *CSDH* chronic subdural hematoma, *CSF* cerebrospinal fluid, *SDH* subdural hematoma, *IV* intravenous drainage, and hypothermia were again used to reduce cerebral volume [7]. Three dogs died for various reasons during follow-up and the autopsies revealed "not exceptionally large" hematomas [7]. Five dogs were sacrificed later; the resolution of the hematomas was similar to that in the first experiment [7].

- *Study by Watanabe* et al.

  Watanabe et al. studied the effects of blood clot formation in the presence of CSF and demonstrated ex vivo that the fibrin membrane of the clot was permeable and therefore highly unlikely to be implicated for the expansion of the lesion, refuting the *osmotic* hypothesis [20]. The authors used 12 dogs and five monkeys for subdural clot inoculation, and 50 dogs in six groups for subcutaneous clot inoculation [20]. Clots of 1–5 mL formed by mixing blood with CSF for 24 h at 37 °C were inoculated into the subdural space of each of the 12 dogs and five monkeys [20]. Three dogs showed progressive symptoms; nine dogs and five monkeys developed no clinical symptoms [20]. All animals were sacrificed at 7–21 days and histological findings of CSDH were demonstrated, with hematoma capsules containing reddish-brown fluid and an increased hematoma volume. The capsule adhered to the dura and tortuous, congested vascular channels were visible microscopically [20]. Two other dogs that received whole blood clots formed without CSF showed no evidence of hematoma development, but there was slight dural thickening, consistent with the results of previous studies [20].

- *Study by Apfelbaum* et al.

  Apfelbaum et al. followed similar steps to *Watanabe* et al. to reproduce the experiment [3]. Two dogs and 40 cats were used [3]. Four autologous blood samples were created for four groups of cats: 4 mL blood mixed with 1 mL of CSF, artificial CSF, or saline, or left undiluted and incubated at 37 °C for 24 h [3]. As in the study by *Watanabe* et al., the authors performed trephine opening on the skull convexity and balloon expansion, and the ex vivo coagulate was implanted into the subdural space [3]. They also made a large circular dural incision in two cats to examine the effects of dural vascularity [3]. One animal per group was sacrificed on the 8th, 10th, 13th, and 21st days. Two animals with CSF/blood were sacrificed on the 29th and 30th days, and one with saline/blood mixture was sacrificed on the 27th day [3]. Two dogs received the same treatment as the cats and were sacrificed on the 13th day [3]. All of the lesions followed the typical evolution and regression pattern of SDH. On the 21st day, only a dural thickening could be seen and the hematoma had largely resolved [3]. Ten cats were implanted with human or bovine fibrinogen mixed with human or artificial CSF, human serum, saline, or 5% glucose. Each sample was treated with thrombin and coagulated in vitro at 37 °C [3]. Human and artificial CSF samples were treated with oxalate to remove calcium ions, and calcium chloride was added to the saline and glucose solutions [3]. Two cats were implanted with a gelatin sponge, one impregnated with defibrinated blood [3]. Those animals also followed the same typical pattern of neomembrane formation and resolution [3]. Four cats had blood clots isolated from the dura by polyethylene. Three of the four animals neither developed a neomembrane nor absorbed the hematoma [3].

One cat, owing to a technical error, developed a membrane: the polyethylene barrier failed to block dural contact at the edge of the hematoma [3].

Apfelbaum et al. criticized *Watanabe* et al. because among their solutions only the CSF contained calcium ions. Only in the presence of calcium was fibrinogen converted to double-bonded fibrin [3]. They failed to obtain the same results and inferred that the key importance of a fibrin-mediated dural membrane of the hematoma; also, as the hematoma aged, neovascular channels oozed blood into the cavity, supporting the findings of *Putnam and Putnam* [3]. *Apfelbaum* et al. also commented that the absorption mechanics of the hematoma could be insufficient in large lesions owing to the disproportionate increases in surface/volume ratio as the lesion grows [3]. The authors hypothesized that reproducing human CSDH in animals is difficult because they have larger intracranial pressure differences than humans above and below the foramen of Monro [3]. The upright posture of humans is also relevant to the compartmental pressure difference [3].

- *Study by Ohshima*

  Ohshima also experimented with blood clot implantation in the second group, as mentioned in the previous section [11].

5.2.3 Subdural Blood or Clot Implantation with Decreased ICP

A summary of two experimental studies as an example of subdural blood or clot implantation with decreased ICP models for production of SDH is given below in detail (Table 5.3) [7, 11]:

- *Study by Goodell and Mealy*

  In the third experiment group A involving 15 dogs, *Goodell and Mealy* performed cisternopleural polyethylene shunts together with subdural blood clot implantation [7]. SDHs were produced in nine of the dogs. Four of those nine with shunts were also used in the second experimental group B, receiving repeated injections. Urea and hypothermia were used as additional mechanisms on five dogs [7]. In this study, all of the catheters were partially obstructed or dislocated at the time of sacrifice, so the results were inconclusive [7]. Group B consisted of two dogs that received subdural clot injections and repeated IV urea administration. Both hematomas resolved in an anticipated fashion [7].

- *Study by Ohshisima*

  In the fourth group in this study, D-mannitol and heparin were given to 13 dogs. Ten of the 13 showed no symptoms and the hematomas resolved spontaneously [11]. The lesions expanded in two dogs and hematoma progression was apparent on CT scans. At autopsy, a hemorrhagic outer neomembrane was documented [11]. In one dog, the subdural mass expanded, as seen as a low-density collection on CT, similar to a human CSDH [11]. The author concluded that the mixing of CSF with blood is an important process, together with low ICP and mechanical factors [11].

Table 5.3 Experimental subdural blood or clot implantation with decreased intracranial pressure models

Author(s)/ ref.#	Year	Species/duration of study	Technique of study	Location	Conclusion
Goodell and Mealy [7]	1963	Dog (n = 15)	Repeated subdural injection or clot implantation with cisternopleural shunt, additional IV urea, or hypothermia in some cases	Parietal convexity	Subdural blood, reduced cerebral volume, tearing of bridging veins are insufficient to form CSDH; the contribution of osmosis is unclear
Ohshima [11]	1982	Dog (n = 13)/30 days	Subdural autologous whole blood mixed with CSF injection, IV mannitol, and heparin administration	Trephine opening and balloon expansion of the subdural space at the parietal convexity	CSF mixed with blood and low intracranial pressure (mannitol and CSF evacuation) is needed for expanding SDH

Abbreviations: *CSDH* chronic subdural hematoma, *CSF* cerebrospinal fluid, *SDH* subdural hematoma, *IV* intravenous

5.2.4 Subcutaneous Implantation Models

A summary of three experimental studies as an example of subcutaneous implantation model for production of SDH is given below in detail (Table 5.4) [3, 9, 20]:

- *Study by Watanabe* et al.

  Watanabe et al. injected blood clots subcutaneously into 50 dogs, experimenting with different scenarios by inoculating the following: a clot formed in the presence of CSF; a simple blood clot; a clot formed in the presence of CSF and treated with plasmin; a fibrin clot formed in the absence of CSF; and a fibrin clot formed in the presence of CSF [20]. The authors concluded that the fibrin capsule of a hematoma that formed in the presence of CSF is more delicate than those that develop without CSF and has different characteristics. They suggested that nascent sinusoid capillaries that leak into the capsular formation could account for the expansion of the hematoma [20].
- *Study by Apfelbaum* et al.

  Apfelbaum et al. also tested subcutaneous implantation with the different compositions of blood clots mentioned in the previous section. A few of the animals showed modest enlargement of the hematoma up to twice the original size; the effect was not related to any type of clot [3].
- *Study by Labadie and Glover*

  Labadie and Glover conducted five experiments in 154 rats. They injected or surgically implanted different combinations of blood products and chemicals into dorsal subcutaneous tissue [9]. Platelet-free human plasma, autologous

Table 5.4 Experimental subcutaneous implantation models

Author(s)/ref.#	Year	Species/duration of study	Technique of study	Location	Conclusion
Watanabe et al. [20]	1972	Dog ($n = 50$)/7–21 days	The clot formed in different settings was implanted subcutaneously	Abdominal subcutaneous inoculation	The clot formed in presence of CSF has a different elastic fibrinous capsule, necessary for expanding hematoma. Osmosis has no apparent effect
Apfelbaum et al. [3]	1974	Dog ($n = 2$) and cat ($n = 40$)/8–30 days	Single subdural clot placement with different preparations	Subcutaneous abdominal incisions of four pockets	CSF has no role in the expansion of lesion volume, fibrin, and subsequent membrane formation on the dural surface, and rebleeding is the key factor for progression
Labadie and Glover [9]	1976	Rat ($n = 154$)/9 days	Injection or surgical implantation of the clot, blood, plasma, carrageenan in different combinations	Dorsal subcutaneous injection or the surgical implantation	The initial volume of the implant is the main factor in the resolution or enlargement of the lesion. CSF has no discernible effect

Abbreviations: *CSF* cerebrospinal fluid

citrated whole rat blood either hemolyzed at −20 °C or whole blood at 4 °C, human CSF, and carrageenan (extract of *Chonduru crispus*) were used in different combinations [9]. Also, in vitro controls were performed using 12 mL platelet-free, platelet-rich, hemolyzed and whole blood controls prepared and incubated at 37 °C for 100 h. All blood and plasma clots were induced by human thrombin [9]. All animals were sacrificed on day 9 after implantation. In the first experiment, the authors studied the effects of CSF on surgically implanted clots [9]. Fifty-two rats had surgically implanted in vitro coagulates, induced by human thrombin, administered immediately after forming in the dorsal subcutaneous region. Thirty-two rats received 2 mL platelet-free plasma and 1.5 mL human CSF previously filtered through a 0.22 μm millipore filter. Twenty rats received only the coagulated plasma. Comparison of the implants showed no differences with or without the presence of CSF [9]. In the second experiment, the effects of surgical incision were compared to needle injection. Thirty rats were injected with 12 mL platelet-free plasma and 2 mL human thrombin solution as soon as the two were mixed, forming in situ clots. Twenty-one rats had in vivo clots surgically implanted [9]. Surgically implanted clots were almost always recovered at autopsy and 43% of them had expanded and liquefied content. Histology showed neomembranes, fibrin clots, and neocapillaries. However, coagulated lesions injected in situ were almost always reabsorbed [9]. In the third experiment, the effects of a sterile pro-inflammatory agent, carrageenan, were tested. The authors hypothesized that stimulating inflammation contributes to neomembrane formation and lesion growth [9]. Thirteen rats were injected with carrageenan solution; nine also received 8 mL, and four 12 mL, of human plasma-thrombin mixture immediately at the same site, forming in situ clots. At autopsy, the lesions had membranes similar to those with surgical implants although with a more prominent fibroblastic reaction. Some showed evidence of central bleeding [9]. In the fourth experiment, various amounts of autologous blood frozen, thawed, and clotted in situ were injected to compare the effects of the initial volume of the lesion. Eight, 12, and 15 mL of hemolyzed blood and thrombin mixture with 1 mL of air were injected into eight, 15, and 11 rats, respectively. Rats with 12 and 15 mL injections had expanded hematomas with liquefied content [9]. In the fifth experiment, a relatively large amount of autologous blood was injected into rats. Four were injected with 16 mL of blood and thrombin solution, forming in situ clots. The results were similar to those of the fourth experiment [9].

With these experiments, *Labadie and Glover* showed an initial decrease in hematoma size to the third day but a progressive increase in size thereafter [9]. "*The larger the initial size, the more likely that subsequent enlargement will occur*" [9]. They found no relationship between CSF and lesion size. However, they noted that the anatomical location of the experimental clot could be the reason [9]. In all their samples, the albumin/globulin ratio was increased in hematoma fluids, but the osmolarity of all specimens remained constant at 289–295 mOsm/kg [9].

5.2.5 Vascular Injury Models

A summary of an experimental study as an example of vascular injury model for production of SDH is given below in detail (Table 5.5) [7]:

- *Study by Goodell and Mealy*

  In the first experiment group B, *Goodell and Mealy* sutured the bridging vein in seven dogs and tore the vein on the third day after surgery [7]. Before the venous tearing, IV urea and heparin was administered to two dogs [7]. Two heparinized dogs died acutely after the vein was torn [7]. The surviving dogs were sacrificed on days 11–72. Although there was evidence for organization and resorption of hematomas, no chronic subdural collection could be achieved [7].

Table 5.5 Experimental vascular injury models

Author(s)/ ref.#	Year	Species/ duration of study	Technique of study	Location	Conclusion
Goodell and Mealy [7]	1963	Dog (*n* = 7)/11–72 days	Tearing of the bridging veins with IV urea administration (*n* = 2 given heparin died after 2–72 h)	Parietal convexity	Subdural blood, reduced cerebral volume, tearing of bridging veins are insufficient to form CSDH; the contribution of osmosis is unclear

Abbreviations: *CSDH* chronic subdural hematoma, *IV* intravenous

Table 5.6 Experimental brain atrophy models

Author(s)/ ref.#	Year	Species/duration of study	Technique of study	Location	Conclusion
Aikawa and Suzuki [1]	1987	Mice (*n* = 48)/30 days	No injection	Intraperitoneal 6-AN administration causing hydrocephalus, later evolves into SDH	Sudden decompression of lateral ventricles and subsequent cerebral collapse causing tearing of bridging veins
Kaneko et al. [8]	1993	Dogs (*n* = 10)/7 weeks	Subdural autologous whole blood injection	Cerebral atrophy following cisternal 6-OHDA injection, followed by burr hole and blood injection	Initiation of hematoma, the formation of neomembrane, and cerebral atrophy together are the key factors in CSDH

Abbreviations: *6-AN* 6-aminonicotinamide, *6-OHDA* 6-hydroxydopamine, *CSDH* chronic subdural hematoma, *SDH* subdural hematoma

5.2.6 Brain Atrophy Models

A summary of two experimental studies as an example of brain atrophy model for production of SDH is given below in detail (Table 5.6) [1, 8]:

- *Study by Aikawa and Suzuki*

  Aikawa and Suzuki used 48 suckling mice; 38 were injected with 6-aminonicotinamide (6-AN), and 10 were controls [1]. The 6-AN was injected intraperitoneally at 25 mg/kg on the fifth postnatal day. The control group received the same treatment, but with saline [1]. Previous research by the authors had shown that 6-AN is neurotoxic and causes hydrocephalus in mice [2]. On day 9, 37 of the 38 mice developed hydrocephalus [1]. Eleven mice were sacrificed on days 20–23, eight on days 25–26, and four on days 29–30 after the injection. The authors categorized these treatment groups as early, intermediate, and late, respectively [1]. On histological and microscopic examination, the early group had a thin film of SDH covering the cerebral cortex. No inflammatory changes were seen at this stage [1]. In the intermediate group, there was a brown-colored blood clot adherent to the dura with a wide subdural cavity and neomembrane formation [1]. In the late group, a well-organized spherical hematoma was found with non-organized brownish clots. There was fresh hemorrhaging from a thick outer membrane with many blood vessels [1]. The authors proposed that the mechanism of CSDH in this model was perforation of the occipital cortex caused by a neurotoxin and subsequent abrupt decompression of the lateral ventricles causing tearing of the bridging veins [1]. Growth of the hematoma was attributed to repeated organization and bleeding from the outer membrane [1].

- *Study by Kaneko* et al.

  Kaneko et al. considered the brain atrophy model for producing CSDH. They drained 10–15 mL of CSF from the cisterna magna in 10 dogs and injected 1 mg/kg 6-hydroxydopamine (6-OHDA) dissolved in artificial CSF containing 0.01% ascorbic acid [8]. Marked ventricular enlargement was confirmed after 3–4 weeks [8]. Five dogs were examined under anesthesia and regional cerebral blood flow (rCBF) was measured by the microsphere method. The rCBFs of gray and white matter were, respectively, 49% and 47% lower than in the control group. The water contents of white and gray matter was also decreased. Therefore, the ventricular dilatation was due to brain atrophy [8]. At the third week after 6-OHDA administration, 2–3 mL of autologous blood was injected through a burr hole over the parietal convexity. The dogs developed symptoms and CT findings in the follow-up. Progressively growing hematomas developed in four dogs 2–4 weeks after the injection of blood [8]. Two dogs deteriorated clinically and CT findings showed hematoma expansion on days 7–30 and 14–28, respectively. Both animals were sacrificed and encapsulated hematomas with outer fibrous and sinusoidal neomembranes were observed [8]. The authors concluded that the *alpha* factor was the trigger or initiator of the hematoma, the *beta* factor was neomembrane formation, and the *gamma* factor was the reduction of the brain volume necessary for developing CSDH [8].

5.3 Conclusion

Although CSDH is one of the most common neurosurgical entities in clinical practice, its ideal treatment modality remains under debate. Experimental production of CSDH in small animals is very difficult and challenging. Many authors have attempted to create a verifiable model, but there is not any reproducible, well-described animal model of human CSDH in the current literature to date [5]. Studies between the early nineteenth century and the present day have demonstrated that SDH evolves into its chronic form under specific conditions. The pathophysiology of the disease is yet to be understood completely, though each experiment, thanks to advances in modern technology, brings scientists closer to the full picture. Further studies of the morphological and inflammatory processes involved in the disease are needed.

References

1. Aikawa H, Suzuki K. Experimental chronic subdural hematoma in mice. Gross morphology and light microscopic observations. J Neurosurg. 1987;67:710–6.
2. Aikawa H, Suzuki K, Ito N, Iwasaki Y, Nonaka I. 6-Aminonicotinamide-induced hydrocephalus in suckling mice. J Neuropathol Exp Neurol. 1984;43:511–21.
3. Apfelbaum RI, Guthkelch AN, Shulman K. Experimental production of subdural hematomas. J Neurosurg. 1874;40:336–46.
4. Christensen E. Studies on chronic subdural hematoma. Acta Psychiatr Neurol. 1944;19:69–148.
5. D'Abbondanza JA, Loch Macdonald R. Experimental models of chronic subdural hematoma. Neurol Res. 2014;36:176–88.
6. Gardner WJ. Traumatic subdural hematoma with particular reference to the latent interval. Arch Neurol Psychiatr. 1932;27:847–58.
7. Goodell CL, Mealey J Jr. Pathogenesis of chronic subdural hematoma. Experimental studies. Arch Neurol. 1963;8:429–37.
8. Kaneko F, Ohbayashi M, Ohshima T, Matsumoto K. An experimental chronic subdural hematoma in dogs-with a brain atrophy model. In: Nakamura N, Hashimoto T, Yasue M, editors. Recent advances in neurotraumatology. Tokyo: Springer; 1993. p. 45–8.
9. Labadie EL, Glover D. Physiopathogenesis of subdural hematomas. Part 1: histological and biochemical comparisons of subcutaneous hematoma in rats with subdural hematoma in man. J Neurosurg. 1976;45:382–92.
10. Laborde J. Contribution a l'etude des conditions pathogeniques des kystes sanguines de l'arachnoide; recherches experimentales sur les animaux. Cr Soc Biol Paris. 1864;1:70.
11. Ohshima T. Experimental study on the evolution of chronic subdural hematoma. Neurol Med Chir (Tokyo). 1982;22:696–706.
12. Putnam TJ, Putnam IK. The experimental study of pachymeningitis hemorrhagica. J Nerv Ment Dis. 1927;65:260–2.
13. Quan W, Zhang Z, Tian Q, Wen X, Yu P, Wang D, Cui W, Zhou L, Park E, Baker AJ, Zhang J, Jiang R. A rat model of chronic subdural hematoma: insight into mechanisms of revascularization and inflammation. Brain Res. 2015;1625:84–96.
14. Rovlias A, Theodoropoulos S, Papoutsakis D. Chronic subdural hematoma: surgical management and outcome in 986 cases: a classification and regression tree approach. Surg Neurol Int. 2015;6:127.
15. Saltykow. Referat, alcoholismus chronicus. Centralbl. f. allg. Path. u. path. Anat. 1911;22:849.
16. Serres A. Nouvelle division des apoplexies. Annuaire Med Chir Hop. 1819;1:246.
17. Sperling H. Ueber pachymeningitis haemorrhagica interna. Inaug.-Diss., Univ. Konigsberg. 1872.
18. Turgut M, Akhaddar A, Turgut AT. Calcified or ossified chronic subdural hematoma: a systematic review of 114 cases reported during last century with a demonstrative case report. World Neurosurg. 2020;134:240–63.
19. Van Vleuten CF. Ueber pachymeningitis haemorrhagica interna traumatica. Inaug.-Diss., Univ. Bonn. 1898.
20. Watanabe S, Shimada H, Ishii S. Production of clinical form of chronic subdural hematoma in experimental animals. J Neurosurg. 1972;37:552–61.

Chapter 6
Role of Cranial Vault Morphology on the Location of Chronic Subdural Hematoma

Ali Akhaddar

6.1 Introduction

Intracranial chronic subdural hematoma (CSDH) is a frequent and well-recognized entity in neurosurgical practice with multiple potential etiologies. However, its physiopathology is not completely understood [6, 25, 26]. Three centuries ago, CSDH was recognized as a stroke. One century later, it became an inflammation. Then, a traumatic origin was accepted in the beginning of the twentieth century [9]. After that, various further suggestions such as osmotic pressure or effusion were advanced [11, 18]. Some investigators have also found that both coagulation and fibrinolysis systems were excessively activated in CSDH [15, 26]. Furthermore, several risk factors have been associated with the occurrence of this intracranial hematoma. Lately, since the first publication of Lee KS et al. in 2001 [17], a number of authors have assumed the role of "cranial shape" (symmetrical or asymmetrical) on the localization of CSDH [2, 10, 16, 17, 22].

In this chapter, we will provide a comprehensive overview of the possible role of cranial vault morphology on the location and laterality of CSDH.

A. Akhaddar (✉)
Avicenne Military Hospital of Marrakech, Department of Neurosurgery,
Mohammed V University in Rabat, Rabat, Morocco

M. Turgut et al. (eds.), *Subdural Hematoma*,
https://doi.org/10.1007/978-3-030-79371-5_6

6.2 Methods Measuring Cranial Vault Symmetry/Asymmetry

For Lee et al., the symmetry of the cranium was checked by an easy way. The axial image of the computed tomography scan (CT scan) and/or magnetic resonance imaging (MRI) was modified to black and white. From a single point in the parieto-occipital area, three lines have been drawn: one line passing the midline and two lines touching the external cranium (outer tables) on both sides. Both angles formed by the midline and the line touching the external cranium on each side were compared. The side of the smaller angle is the cranial flat side [10, 17, 19].

In our personal experience [2], we modified the measurement method of Lee. The inner table was selected (instead of the outer table) to avoid the effect of the thickness of the skull bone both in posterior (occipital vault) and in anterior (frontal vault) regions (Fig. 6.1). The skull vault was considered symmetric if the difference between the angles of two sides of cranial convexity was less than 2° (Fig. 6.2). The side of the smaller angle was the less curved frontal or occipital bone (Fig. 6.3). All angle measurements were made at the same level of the CT-axial sections (a parallel plane approximately 6 cm above the orbito-meatal line in adults) [2]. For Khursheed, this CT scan plane was taken at 7 cm above the orbito-meatal line [16]. In another study by Oh et al., the cranial symmetry/asymmetry was measured as follows: on the best image of axial CT scan where the third ventricle is well visualized, the midline was set from anterior to posterior falx and they calculated the maximal radius on each side [22].

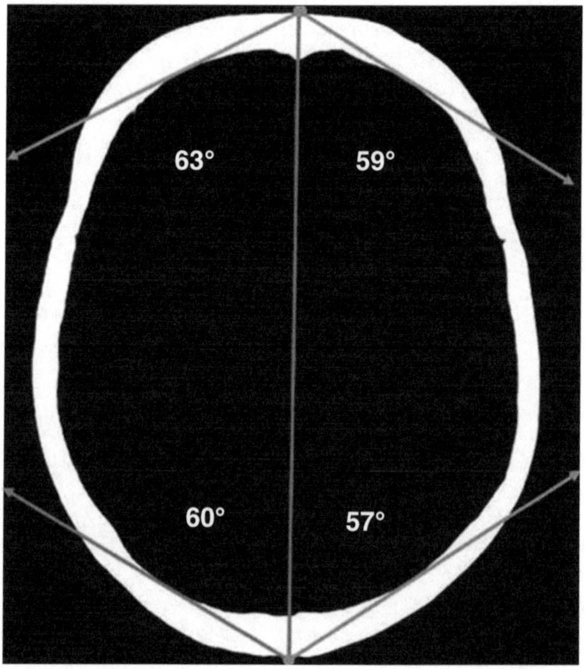

Fig. 6.1 From a single point, on the top of the cranium, three lines are drawn; one line passing the midline and two lines touching the inner table on both sides of the cranium. The side of the smaller angle is the less curved frontal convexity in an asymmetrical cranium. The same measurement was obtained for the occipital vault. (Reproduced from Akhaddar A et al. Acta Neurochir (Wien) (2009)151:1235–40; with permission)

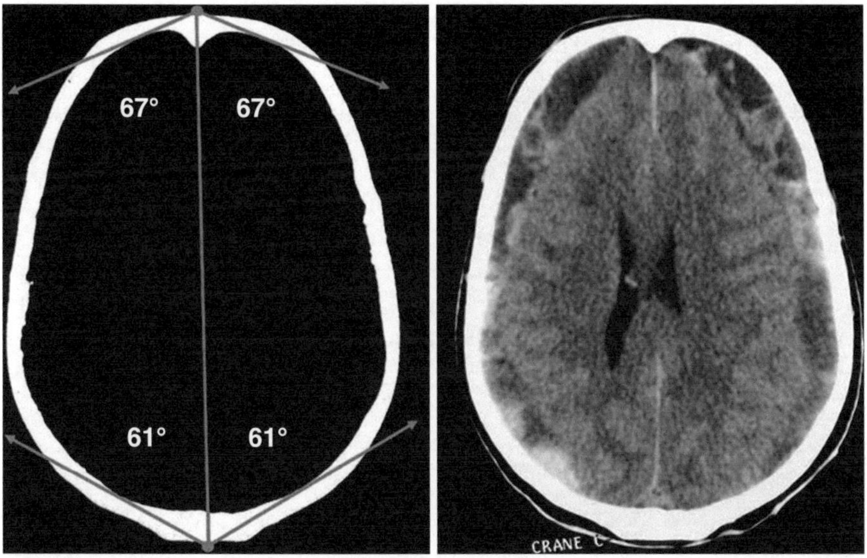

Fig. 6.2 Patient with a symmetrical frontal and occipital skull vault convexity; the CSDH is bilateral. (Reproduced from Akhaddar A et al. Acta Neurochir (Wien) (2009)151:1235–40; with permission)

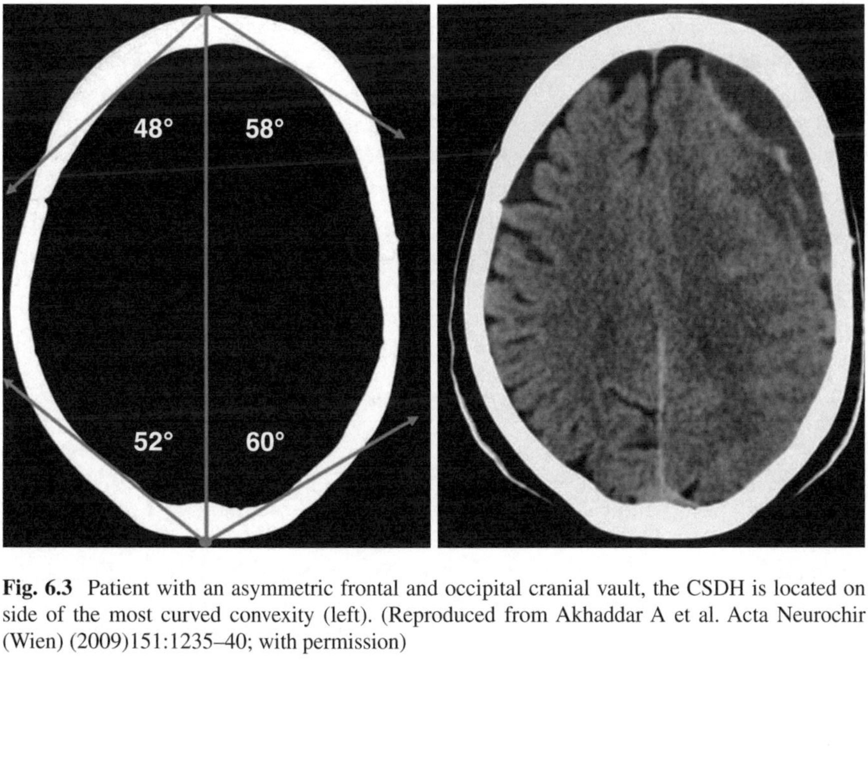

Fig. 6.3 Patient with an asymmetric frontal and occipital cranial vault, the CSDH is located on side of the most curved convexity (left). (Reproduced from Akhaddar A et al. Acta Neurochir (Wien) (2009)151:1235–40; with permission)

Recently, Hsieh and coworkers [10] used an objected semiautomated method in accordance with the concept described by Zonenshayn in 2004 for the measurement of plagiocephaly [27]. The CT images were loaded into the LabVIEW software system (National Instruments, Texas, USA). The nasion and inion, manually denoted by black spots, were considered the midline. The study was then automated, including subtraction of the cranial bone, encoding of the number of pixels, and determination of each skull region. The midline was considered as the axis, one side of the cranium could be horizontally turned over onto the other side to establish the overlapping and nonoverlapping areas. The dominant nonoverlapping side was defined as the side of the larger nonoverlapping region. The cranial index symmetry ratio was determined as twice the overlapping area divided by the total area [10].

6.3 Lateralization of Chronic Subdural Hematoma

In general human population, the shape of the cranial vault is not always symmetrical between the right and left sides [13, 14, 19, 23]. When the cranium is asymmetrical, the head has a tendency to be positioned on the flat side. If the skull is flat on the right side, the head will lie on the right side, and then the CSDH has a predisposition to develop on the left side where the cranial vault is more convex (Fig. 6.3). This hypothesis was experienced in at least four previous studies: three performed in South Korea and one in Morocco [2, 16, 17, 19].

If we consider the classic physiopathology in the development of chronic subdural hematomas [See both Chaps. 4 and 5 about Pathophysiology and Experimental models of CSDH, respectively], the authors of the four studies cited above postulated that the dura-arachnoid interface is cleaved more easily when the curved intracranial vault convexity is more prominent/curved [2, 16, 17, 19]. Additionally, the bridging veins also ruptured more easily when a significant subdural space is present. The movement of the mass parenchyma within the intracranial space makes these bridging veins more vulnerable for bleeding on the side of the more curved convexity.

6.4 Bilateral Chronic Subdural Hematoma

As shown previously, complete symmetry of the cranial vault is uncommon. The authors who were interested in this topic hypothesized that in a symmetrical curved skull convexity, the cleaved force is equal in both sides to separate the dura-arachnoid interface when direct or indirect injury occurs (Fig. 6.2). Indeed, as others, we believe that indirect head trauma seems to be more significant than direct injury in cranial CSDH [1]. This separation is probably the initiating factor that induces tissue proliferation of the dural border cell layer resulting in subsequent neo-membrane formation. In addition, the bridging veins are more likely to rupture bilaterally and therefore create equal chances of developing bilateral CSDHs on both the left and right sides. According to Lee, the symmetry must be considered on the posterior cranial vault due to the role of gravity when patients are on prone positions [18, 19]. In our opinion, both anterior (frontal) and posterior (occipital) convexities are involved in this model and this hypothesis was confirmed later [2]. These results were also reproduced in 2015 by Khursheed et al.: both symmetric frontal and occipital cranial vaults correlate with bilateral CSDH [16].

6.5 Side Prevalence of Chronic Subdural Hematoma

In literature review of a few series that mentioned the side prevalence of CSDH, it seems that the left side is more frequently involved compared to the right one (Table 6.1). MacFarlane's team had tried to explain the reason behind the increased rate of CSDH diagnosed on the left side [20].

Many studies have shown that strokes are more silent on the right side because right "non-dominant" hemispheric lesions are less frequently associated with communication difficulties (centers for language and speech and dominant hand functions are located in the left hemisphere in most left-handers) [4, 5, 7, 12, 24]. Such as ischemic strokes, other brain lesions on non-dominant brain hemisphere (most frequently on the right side) will be associated with more subtle neurologic symptoms and signs and therefore may be under-diagnosed or at least diagnosed later [3]. According to this same hypothesis, MacFarlane et al. suggested that left-sided CSDHs are more easily and more frequently recognized compared to those on the right side [20]. For MacFarlane and coworkers, CSDHs on the right side that happen but are not diagnosed may resolve or re-absorb spontaneously or patients could die if they are not diagnosed. However, the same hypothesis does not explain the prevalence of right-sided CSDH in some other series [10, 17].

Table 6.1 Four series from the literature mentioning the side prevalence of chronic subdural hematomas

Authors [reference]	Total cases	Left side location Number (%)	Right side location Number (%)
Mori et al. [21]	500	260 (52.0%)	152 (30.4%)
Gelabert-Gonzalez et al. [8]	1000	471 (47.1%)	432 (43.2%)
Akhaddar et al. [2]	110	47 (42.7%)	32 (29.1%)
MacFarlane et al. [20]	258	123 (47.6%)	92 (35.6%)

6.6 Conclusion

The concept of cranial vault symmetry/asymmetry tries to explain the side of localization and the bilaterality of CSDHs. This relative new anatomical parameter could contribute to a better understanding of the etiology and pathogenesis of CSDH. However, further prospective studies conducted by both neuroradiologists and neurosurgeons and done on larger number of patients are needed to ascertain the role of cranial morphology for the development of CSDH.

Both coronal and 3D reconstructions of the skull in addition to ethnic variations of cranial shape must be considered.

References

1. Adhiyaman V, Asghar M, Ganeshram KN, Bhowmick BK. Chronic subdural haematoma in the elderly. Postgrad Med J. 2002;78:71–5. https://doi.org/10.1136/pmj.78.916.71.
2. Akhaddar A, Bensghir M, Abouqal R, Boucetta M. Influence of cranial morphology on the location of chronic subdural haematoma. Acta Neurochir (Wien). 2009;151:1235–40. https://doi.org/10.1007/s00701-009-0357-7.
3. Baumann C, Tichy J, Schaefer JH, Steinbach JP, Mittelbronn M, Wagner M, et al. Delay in diagnosing patients with right-sided glioblastoma induced by hemispheric-specific clinical presentation. J Neurooncol. 2020;146:63–9. https://doi.org/10.1007/s11060-019-03335-4.
4. Brott T, Tomsick T, Feinberg W, Johnson C, Biller J, Broderick J, et al. Baseline silent cerebral infarction in the Asymptomatic Carotid Atherosclerosis Study. Stroke. 1994;25:1122–9. https://doi.org/10.1161/01.str.25.6.1122.
5. Dimopoulos VG, Kapsalakis IZ, Fountas KN. Skull morphology and its neurosurgical implications in the Hippocratic era. Neurosurg Focus. 2007;23:E10. https://doi.org/10.3171/foc.2007.23.1.10.
6. Drapkin AJ. Chronic subdural hematoma: pathophysiological basis for treatment. Br J Neurosurg. 1991;5:467–73. https://doi.org/10.3109/02688699108998475.
7. Foerch C, Misselwitz B, Sitzer M, Berger K, Steinmetz H, Neumann-Haefelin T, Arbeitsgruppe Schlaganfall Hessen. Difference in recognition of right and left hemispheric stroke. Lancet. 2005;366:392–3. https://doi.org/10.1016/S0140-6736(05)67024-9.
8. Gelabert-González M, Iglesias-Pais M, García-Allut A, Martínez-Rumbo R. Chronic subdural haematoma: surgical treatment and outcome in 1000 cases. Clin Neurol Neurosurg. 2005;107:223–9. https://doi.org/10.1016/j.clineuro.2004.09.015.
9. Haines DE, Harkey HL, al-Mefty O. The "subdural" space: a new look at an outdated concept. Neurosurgery. 1993;32:111–20. https://doi.org/10.1227/00006123-199301000-00017.
10. Hsieh CT, Huang CT, Chen YH, Sun JM. Association between cranial asymmetry severity and chronic subdural hematoma laterality. Neurosciences (Riyadh). 2020;25:205–9. https://doi.org/10.17712/nsj.2020.3.20190125.
11. Ito H, Yamamoto S, Saito K, Ikeda K, Hisada K. Quantitative estimation of hemorrhage in chronic subdural hematoma using the 51Cr erythrocyte labeling method. J Neurosurg. 1987;66:862–4. https://doi.org/10.3171/jns.1987.66.6.0862.
12. Ito H, Kano O, Ikeda K. Different variables between patients with left and right hemispheric ischemic stroke. J Stroke Cerebrovasc Dis. 2008;17:35–8. https://doi.org/10.1016/j.jstrokecerebrovasdis.2007.11.002.
13. Kanat A, Kayaci S, Yazar U, Kazdal H, Terzi Y. Chronic subdural hematoma in adults: why does it occur more often in males than females? Influence of patient's sexual gender on occurrence. J Neurosurg Sci. 2010;54:99–103.

14. Kanat A, Yazar U, Ozdemir B, Coskun ZO, Erdivanli O. Frontal sinus asymmetry: is it an effect of cranial asymmetry? X-ray analysis of 469 normal adult human frontal sinus. J Neurosci Rural Pract. 2015;6:511–4. https://doi.org/10.4103/0976-3147.168436.
15. Kawakami Y, Chikama M, Tamiya T, Shimamura Y. Coagulation and fibrinolysis in chronic subdural hematoma. Neurosurgery. 1989;25:25–9. https://doi.org/10.1097/00006123-198907000-00005.
16. Khursheed N, Jain A, Haneef M, Tanki H, Ramzan A, Shaheen F, et al. Skull vault morphology in subdural hematomas: a geometrical analysis. Indian J Neurotrauma. 2015;12:107–10. https://doi.org/10.1055/s-0035-1570092.
17. Kim BG, Lee KS, Shim JJ, Yoon SM, Doh JW, Bae HG. What determines the laterality of the chronic subdural hematoma? J Korean Neurosurg Soc. 2010;47:424–7. https://doi.org/10.3340/jkns.2010.47.6.424.
18. Lee KS. Chronic subdural hematoma in the aged, trauma or degeneration? J Korean Neurosurg Soc. 2016;59:1–5. https://doi.org/10.3340/jkns.2016.59.1.1.
19. Lee KS, Bae WK, Yoon SM, Doh JW, Bae HG, Yun IG. Location of the chronic subdural haematoma: role of the gravity and cranial morphology. Brain Inj. 2001;15:47–52. https://doi.org/10.1080/02699050150209129.
20. MacFarlane MR, Weerakkody Y, Kathiravel Y. Chronic subdural haematomas are more common on the left than on the right. J Clin Neurosci. 2009;16:642–4. https://doi.org/10.1016/j.jocn.2008.07.074.
21. Mori K, Maeda M. Surgical treatment of chronic subdural hematoma in 500 consecutive cases: clinical characteristics, surgical outcome, complications, and recurrence rate. Neurol Med Chir (Tokyo). 2001;41:371–81. https://doi.org/10.2176/nmc.41.371.
22. Oh JS, Shim JJ, Yoon SM, Lee KS. Influence of gender on occurrence of chronic subdural hematoma; Is it an effect of cranial asymmetry? Korean J Neurotrauma. 2014;10:82–5. https://doi.org/10.13004/kjnt.2014.10.2.82.
23. Pesce Delfino V, Potente F, Chiarelli B. Evaluation of skull vault asymmetry using methods of analytical morphometry. Boll Soc Ital Biol Sper. 1990;66:405–11.
24. Portegies ML, Selwaness M, Hofman A, Koudstaal PJ, Vernooij MW, Ikram MA. Left-sided strokes are more often recognized than right-sided strokes: the Rotterdam study. Stroke. 2015;46:252–4. https://doi.org/10.1161/STROKEAHA.114.007385.
25. Sambasivan M. An overview of chronic subdural hematoma: experience with 2300 cases. Surg Neurol. 1997;47:418–22. https://doi.org/10.1016/s0090-3019(97)00188-2.
26. Suzuki M, Kudo A, Kitakami A, Doi M, Kubo N, Kuroda K, Ogawa A. Local hypercoagulative activity precedes hyperfibrinolytic activity in the subdural space during development of chronic subdural haematoma from subdural effusion. Acta Neurochir (Wien). 1998;140:261–5. https://doi.org/10.1007/s007010050093.
27. Zonenshayn M, Kronberg E, Souweidane MM. Cranial index of symmetry: an objective semiautomated measure of plagiocephaly. Technical note. J Neurosurg. 2004;100(5 Suppl Pediatrics):537–40. https://doi.org/10.3171/ped.2004.100.5.0537.

Chapter 7
Anatomopathology and Histopathologic Changes in Chronic Subdural Hematoma

Lorenzo Gitto and Timothy E. Richardson

7.1 Introduction

Under normal physiologic conditions, the brain is suspended within the cranial cavity, cushioned and protected by cerebrospinal fluid (CSF), while the dural sinuses and other vasculature are fixed. Subdural hematomas (SDHs) commonly occur as a result of head injury, with or without direct impact. Thus, it is essential to remember that the absence of external head injuries does not necessarily exclude a traumatic etiology. For example, severe motor vehicle accidents without direct head trauma can produce rotational movements to the head, leading to vessel tearing and to SDH. This situation is particularly common in young children and in the elderly, where SDH may occur without apparent or negligible head injuries.

Generally, SDHs develop away from the point of impact. The inertia of the trauma explains this finding: since the head is freely mobile, head injury results in significant acceleration/deceleration forces that cause the skull and the brain to move asynchronously. This leads to vessel stretching and laceration with the development of SDHs. However, there are also cases of SDHs induced by cerebral

L. Gitto
Department of Pathology, State University of New York, Upstate Medical University, Syracuse, NY, USA
e-mail: GittoL@Upstate.edu

T. E. Richardson (✉)
Department of Pathology, State University of New York, Upstate Medical University, Syracuse, NY, USA

Department of Pathology and Laboratory Medicine and Glenn Biggs Institute for Alzheimer's and Neurodegenerative Diseases, University of Texas Health San Antonio, San Antonio, TX, USA
e-mail: RichardsonT2@uthscsa.edu

M. Turgut et al. (eds.), *Subdural Hematoma*,
https://doi.org/10.1007/978-3-030-79371-5_7

contusions. In such cases, the increase in cerebral pressure causes distortion and tearing of small cortical veins and the subsequent SDH.

Moreover, cortical lacerations associated with linear or depressed fractures can also cause SHDs since the sharp bone fragments can tear the intracranial vessels. In these instances, the SDH usually arises at the point of impact. Finally, spontaneous SDHs have been rarely described in the literature. Their etiology may involve arterial bleeding (e.g., due to severe hypertension) [23, 34], coagulation disorders [6], or other chronic medical conditions. Most SDHs result from indirect tearing and stretching of the parasagittal bridging veins. Thus, understanding of the anatomy and histology of these particular veins helps understand the subsequent related mechanism of injury [20].

7.2 Anatomy and Histology of the Bridging Veins and Subdural Space, and Basic Mechanism of Injury

The intracranial bridging veins allow for venous drainage of the brain. They serve as important landmarks for neurosurgeons and are implicated in many pathological conditions, particularly SDHs.

The pial veins perform the venous drainage from the cerebral hemispheres. These vessels have a circumferential smooth muscle layer and are sitting on the surface of the cortex. They receive venous blood from the subcortical veins and exit the pia mater from the parasagittal area of the brain. These vessels then course through the subarachnoid space and perforate the arachnoid membrane entering the potential subdural space. Finally, they reach and perforate the dura mater, where they converge and drain into the cerebral veins that typically drain into the nearest dural sinus. The veins located between the pia mater and the sagittal sinus are called "*bridging veins*" (Fig. 7.1) [33].

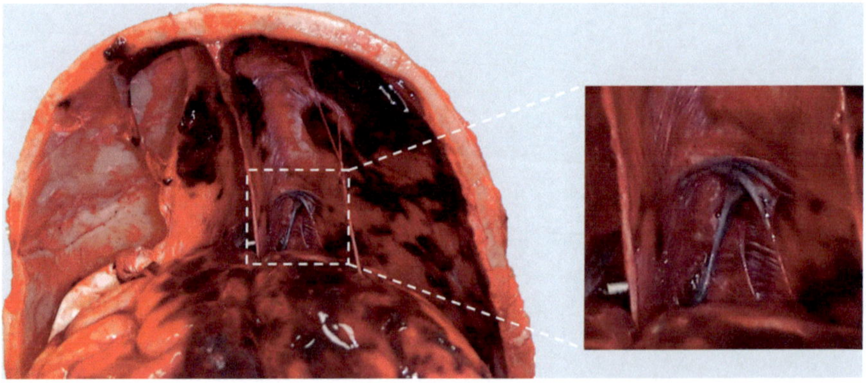

Fig. 7.1 Postmortem head examination demonstrating bridging veins between the dura and arachnoid layers

The distribution of the bridging veins is more extensive than the parasagittal convexity veins. Bridging veins are classified according to their location within the intracranial cavity.

The *posterior cranial fossa bridging veins* are located on the tentorial cerebellar surface and include the *vermian group* and the *hemispheric group*. The vermian group is located above the inferior vermis and collects blood from the terminal portions of the inferior vermian and declival veins. The hemispheric group is located on the lateral aspect of the tentorial hemispheric surface and collects blood from the terminal portions of the superior and inferior hemispheric veins [18, 19].

There are three types of hemispheric bridging veins [35]:

- *Type 1:* resulting from the union of superior and inferior hemispheric veins.
- *Type 2*: resulting from the union of superior hemispheric veins.
- *Type 3*: resulting from the union of inferior hemispheric veins.

The superior and inferior hemispheric veins have numerous collateral pathways that join the inferior portion of the suboccipital surface with the inferior vermian vein. Other bridging veins observed in the posterior cranial fossa are small veins surrounding the *jugular foramen* that collect blood from minor veins of the posterior fossa and drain in the dural sinuses.

The *temporal bridging veins* travel over the lateral aspect of the temporal lobe [9]. They are identified by their venous entry complexes, which identify a specific temporal bridging vein pattern. There is a "candelabra" type, which includes multiple venous complexes joining together into a single vein, and a "separated" type, which includes a vein entering the same area independently [29]. The temporal bridging veins are subcategorized in a mediodorsal group that drains into the sagittal sinus, and the posterior and middle cerebral groups that drain into the lateral sinus. There are three major groups of the temporal bridging veins.

- *Transverse sinus group*, located 1 cm medially to the transverse sinus and includes the posterior temporobasal vein, the middle temporal vein, and the posterior temporal vein. These veins drain into the sinus after traveling 1 cm posterior to the sinodural point (junction of the sigmoid sinus and the superior petrosal sinus).
- *Tentorial group*, located posterior to the sinodural point and drains into the tentorial sinuses [22].
- *Petrosal group*, located anterior to the sinodural point and close to the petrous ridge (which separates the middle and posterior cranial fossae). These veins collect blood from the anterior portions of the cerebellum and brainstem and drains into the superior or inferior petrosal sinus [13].

The *frontal bridging veins* are located in the anterior cranial fossa and drain the convexity, the media, and the basal sides of the brain. They are classified into two types [30].

- *Type 1* includes veins that drain into the superior sagittal sinus through a single venous trunk.

- *Type 2* includes veins that drain into the superior sagittal sinus through ≥2 venous trunks.

The direction of the blood from the bridging veins into the superior sagittal sinus is extremely variable. The direction can be anterograde, perpendicular, retrograde, hairpin shaped (changing direction shortly before entering the sinus), lacunae patterned (large venous spaces) [2, 26]. Moreover, there is great variability regarding the entrances of the bridging veins along the superior sagittal sinus. It can be divided into four segments, which receive a different number of bridging veins. These segments range from approximately 5 cm in length for segments 1 and 2, and approximately 7 cm in length for segments 3 and 4. Segments 1 and 4 receive clusters of bridging veins, while segments 2 and 3 receive only a few veins [12].

The structure of the wall of the bridging veins recalls the general architecture of the venous wall, although it can be difficult to identify histologically [8]. There are three layers, from the outer to the inner portion of the vein:

- The tunica *adventitia*, composed of dense fibrous tissue, collagen, elastin fibers that protect the vessel from overextension.
- The tunica *media*, possibly composed of smooth muscle cells [37], although there is debate concerning the presence of the tunica media [14].
- The tunica *intima*, composed of smooth endothelium covered by elastin tissue. The endothelial cells are connected by tight junctions and can be flattened or contracted cells.

The diameter of the bridging veins varies on the base of their location, ranging from 0.5 to approximately 5.0 mm. In the subarachnoid portion of the veins, their diameter is constant but increases before the outflow cuff segment, which is a narrow region at the junction of the cerebral bridging veins and superior sagittal sinus showing an ampullar bulging. At the level of this region, the diameter and length of the outflow cuff segment are smaller, and the thickness is higher than those of the cerebral bridging veins [27].

During the development of the bridging veins, their wall architecture changes. There is a variable thickness of the wall in different portions of the vein. Bridging veins have a relatively consistent wall thickness as they pass across the subarachnoid space, ranging from 50 to 200 μm, but their thickness increases as they enter the dura, where they have been found to range between 10 and 600 μm in thickness [39]. There is also a difference in the amount of collagen fibers among the different portions of the vein. The subdural portion shows a loose network of fibers compared to the tighter one that can be observed in the subarachnoid space. Moreover, the dural bridging veins show increased circumferential, as opposed to longitudinal, collagen fibers. Regardless of the portion, bridging veins are surrounded by dense fibrous tissue and loose connective tissue.

The peculiar architecture of the bridging veins makes them particularly susceptible to acceleration/deceleration forces. Angular acceleration is a quantitative expression of the change in angular velocity that a spinning object undergoes per unit time. Injury with high angular acceleration (e.g., falls with severe head impact) can result in acute SDH and diffuse axonal injury. The *more rapid* the acceleration or deceleration, and the *shorter the time* of acceleration or deceleration, the more likely one will have a subdural hematoma rather than diffuse axonal injury. Rotational and shearing forces (such as violent shaking or a blow to the face causing rotation of the head) can also cause SDH. Rotation mostly causes tearing of the bridging veins along the transverse or diagonal–frontal axis, but rotation around the vertical axis associated with translational acceleration can also occur. A rotational acceleration tolerance of approximately 10,000 rad/s^2 for pulse durations shorter than 10 ms has been estimated in human cadavers [3].

The concept of a subdural space has evolved over time, and the existence of a subdural space has been frequently questioned because of its undefined features. Haines et al. [10, 11] demonstrated that a real subdural space does not exist and there is a dural border consisting of a loose cell layer at the junction with the arachnoid. Under physiologic conditions, there is no subdural space since the dura mater is separated from the arachnoid by a thin layer of dural border cells [7]. This layer contains elongated, flattened cells lacking tight junctions with an abundant extracellular matrix and limited collagen fibers. Electron microscopy studies have demonstrated the presence of an arachnoid barrier layer loosely fused to a layer of dural border cells with no preexisting space at the interface. Therefore, there is only a "potential" or "virtual" subdural space, as the dura is normally in direct continuity with the meninges via a loose matrix of cells, but it can expand into a real space as the result of trauma, intracranial pathologies, or in the absence of cerebrospinal fluid (making it identifiable in many postmortem examinations). In the case of hemorrhage, this loose matrix of cells can easily separate, allowing the blood to collect within the layers of the dura, creating a hematoma (Fig. 7.2). Thus, a SDH results from the insinuation of hemorrhage between those layers, actually forming within the dura (intradural) [32]. As a result of this, the subdural space (or subdural cavity) is considered just a "potential" cavity, meaning a space between two adjacent structures that are typically directly apposed.

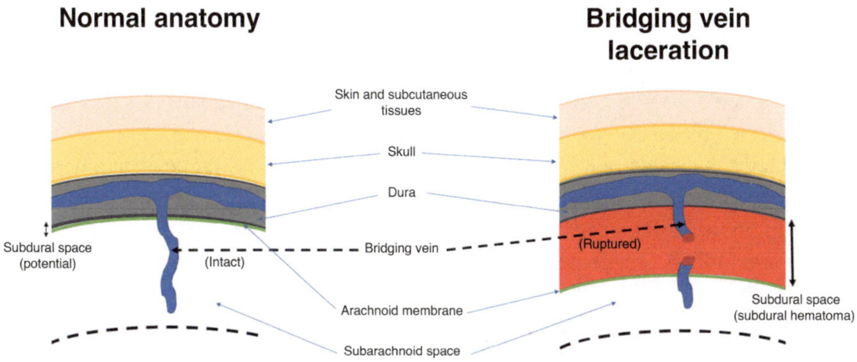

Fig. 7.2 Under physiologic conditions, there is no real subdural space as the dura is in direct continuity with the arachnoid via a loose matrix of cells. Thus, the subdural space is considered a potential space (*left*). If an injury occurs, this loose matrix of cells can be easily separated by the bleeding, allowing the blood to collect within the layers of the dura, creating a subdural hematoma (SDH) (*right*)

7.3 Anatomopathology and Histopathology

During postmortem examination, the dura mater dura is usually loosely attached to the skull cap, allowing easy detachment from the bone by pulling it backwards from the forehead. On the other hand, particularly in old age and in infancy, the dura may be very firmly adherent to the skull cap with the result that it can only be removed with considerable difficulty. It is mandatory that the dura is removed carefully, preserving the potential areas of SDHs and to avoid artifacts due to forced detachment.

On gross examination, the SDH appears as an ill-defined partially clotted blood mass, which usually covers the convexity of the cerebral hemispheres (Fig. 7.3). Three clinical stages of the subdural hematoma are described (acute, subacute, and chronic), and they can be morphologically distinguished [16, 25]. At gross examination, the following findings can be observed:

- *Acute*. Acute subdural hematomas manifest themselves clinically within 72 h of injury (Fig. 7.4). It consists of a collection of gelatinous coagulated blood or red film of liquid blood between the arachnoid and dura mater. Upon opening the cranial cavity during the postmortem examination, the dura is tense, and the blood can easily be seen underneath the dura. The clotted blood shows a variable thickness, ranging from a few millimeters to massive subdural bleeding leading to severe intracranial hypertension. After reflection of the dura, fresh coagulated blood detaches readily from the dural surface, leaving minimal to no adherent residue. Depending on the size of the hematoma, the brain can be deformed, showing accentuation of the gyral pattern on the same side as the hematoma and flattening of the gyri on the contralateral side. The subarachnoid space is often clear, and there is no extension of the hematoma into the depths of sulci. If an acute subdural hematoma evolves rapidly, it may become life-threatening and require emergent evacuation. If the bleeding is slow, there is an evolution in a subacute hematoma.
- *Subacute.* The subacute phase of SDH starts 3–7 days after acute injury, but less than 3 weeks to the appearance of clinical symptoms (Fig. 7.5). If the subdural hematoma develops slowly, a considerably larger volume of blood can be tolerated, and a subacute hematoma develops. The hematoma consists of mixed fluid and clotted blood that focally adheres to the dural surface. Organizational changes gradually take place with progressive blood autolysis and hemosiderin deposits that give a rusty-brown to golden-brown appearance to the hematoma, and lead to gelatinous adhesions usually observed on the dura (Fig. 7.6).
- *Chronic*. When the hematoma becomes clinically evident more than 3 weeks after injury, it is clinically defined as a chronic subdural hematoma (CSDH). The typical morphological feature of the CSDH is that the clot is encapsulated in fibrous membranes. If the hematoma keeps evolving from the subacute phase, the organization processes proceed both on the leptomeningeal side and on the dural side, leading to the development of tenacious fibrous tissue. The neomembranes appear to be a product of the proliferation of boundary layer cells at the upper boundary of the hematoma within the dura. The other hallmark for CSDH is liquefied hemorrhagic remnants within the neomembranes. The gross appearance of CSDHs varies with age. Recent hematomas are usually hard to distin-

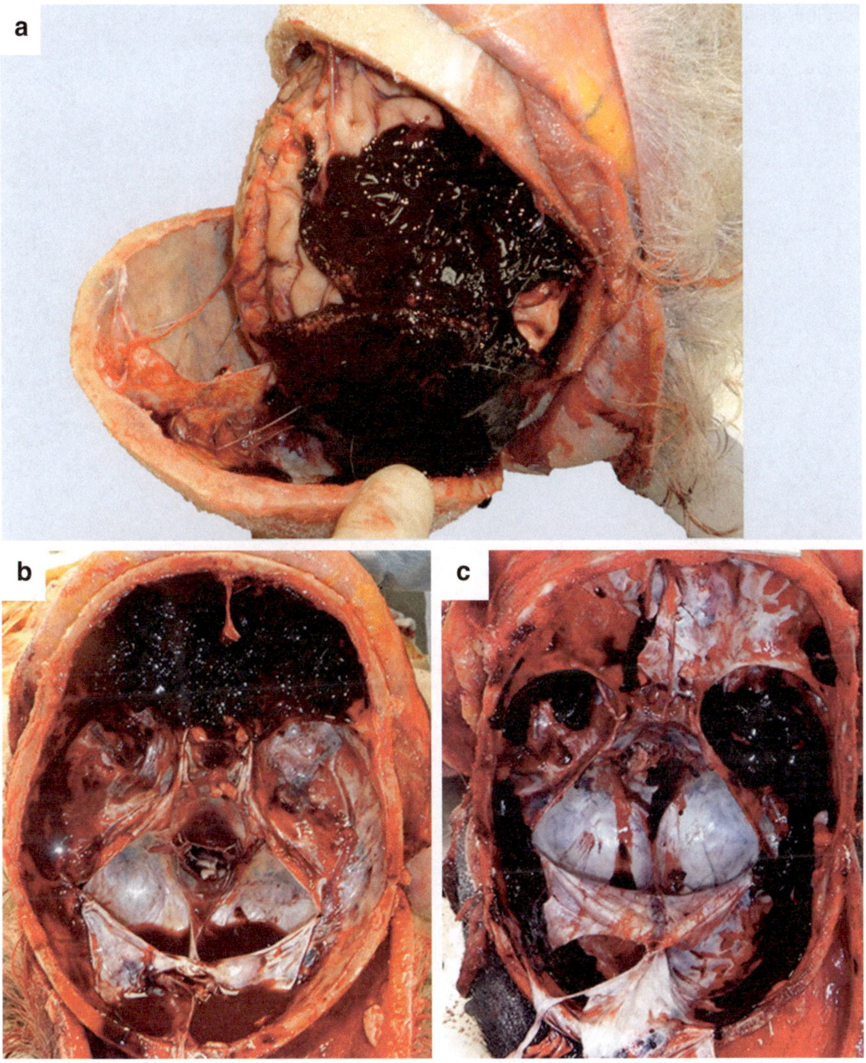

Fig. 7.3 SDHs classically develop over the brain hemisphere convexities (**a**). However, in case of severe head injury, the anterior cranial base (**b**) as well as the middle and posterior cranial bases (**c**) can be involved

guish from a subacute hematoma, being tan or red-brown with gelatinous adhesion on the dural surface, with identifiable areas of recent bleeding. Older hematomas (months to years) show thick, firm external neomembranes with a fluid content, resembling a rubber hot water bottle filled with jelly or oil. The internal liquid is frequently straw-colored (like "machinery oil"), but can be replaced by a firm, variegated tissue showing different colors due to bleeds of different ages (Figs. 7.7 and 7.8). A multiloculated appearance is frequently observed, with different amounts and colors of fluids in each locule.

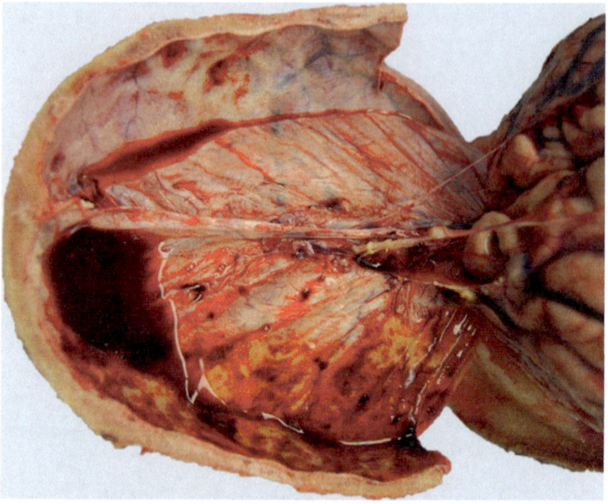

Fig. 7.4 Acute subdural hematoma, a collection of subdural liquid blood is present

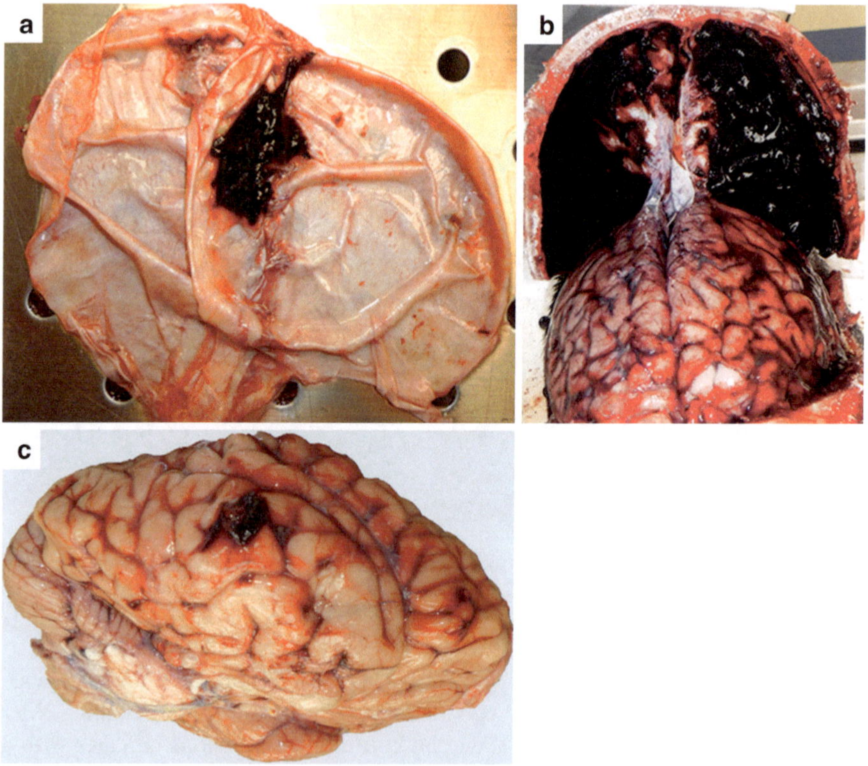

Fig. 7.5 Subacute subdural hematoma. The hematoma consists of mixed fluid and clotted blood, with early organizational changes. A typical dark-red gelatinous appearance with dural adhesions is usually observed (**a**). With the evolution of the organization changes, the hematoma becomes strongly adherent to the dural surface (**b**) and starts to adhere to the arachnoid layer. Focal residues can be observed on the brain surface, depending on the age of the hematoma (**c**)

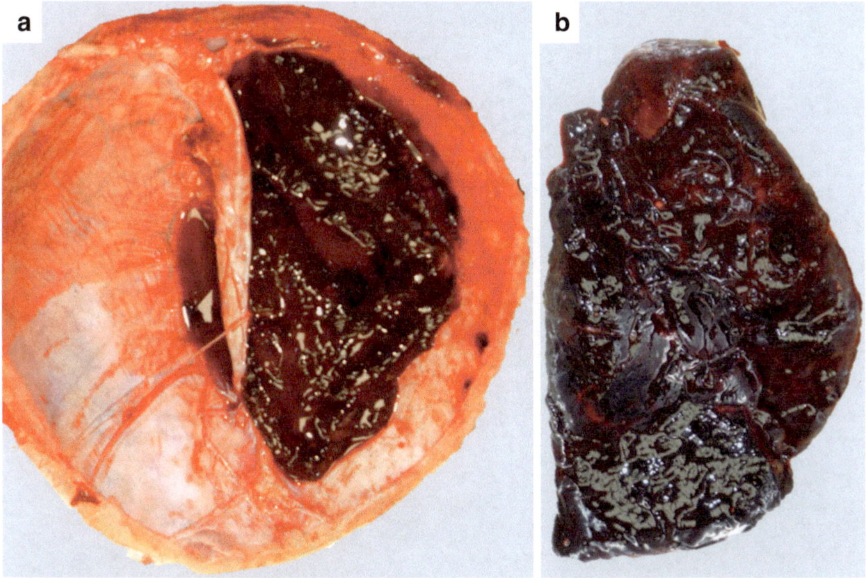

Fig. 7.6 Organizing subdural hematoma, the inferior aspect of the hematoma is shown (**a**). The superior portion was firmly attached to the dura. The superior aspect of the hematoma is shown, once it was dethatched from the dura (**b**). The outer membrane is dark-brown, irregular, and shows variegated colors due to bleeds of different ages

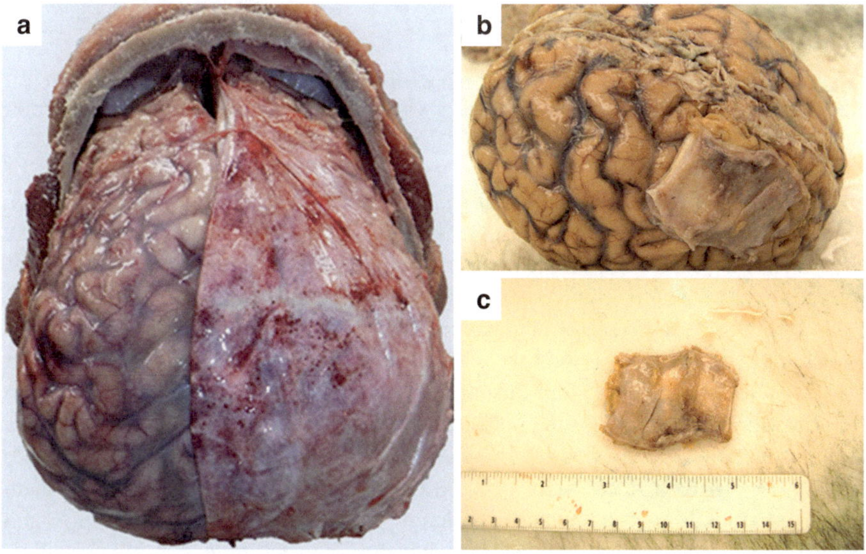

Fig. 7.7 Chronic subdural hematoma. The hematoma evolves and can slowly reabsorb (**a**), or it can rebleed, leading to fibrous tissue, thickening, and permanent discoloration of the dura with adherent fibrous neomembrane (**b**, **c**)

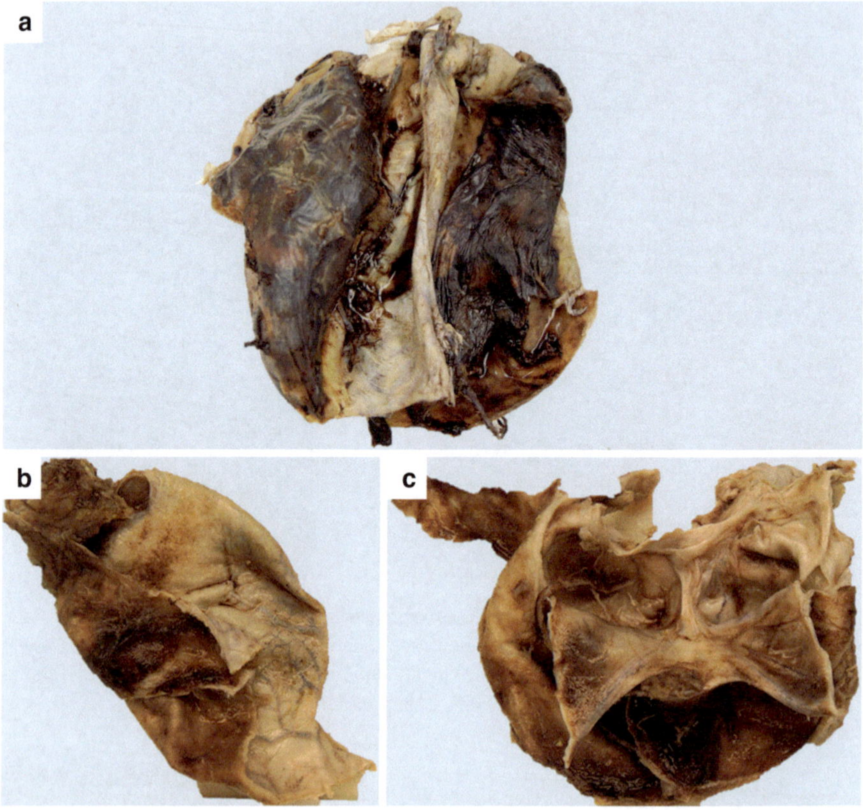

Fig. 7.8 Formalin-fixed dura with subdural hematoma. (**a**) Adherent organized hemorrhage bilaterally. (**b**, **c**) The vast majority of the dural specimen is stained brown-red with concentration over the mid falcine area

Routine histopathological examination is a relatively reliable way of dating a SDH, which can play an important role in medicolegal cases [36]. Numerous studies have been reported in the scientific literature regarding this topic. One of the first attempts to estimate the age of the subdural hematoma was made by Munro and Merritt in 1936 [21]. Since then, several subsequent papers have been published.

Nagahori et al. have studied the histological nature of the outer membrane of CSDH [24]. They proposed four different types of histological features according to the maturity and intensity of the inflammatory reaction and hemorrhage. *Type 1*, in which the membrane does not show signs of inflammation, but contains immature fibroblasts, collagen fibers, neocapillaries, and sparse cell infiltration. *Type 2*, in which inflammatory changes are prominent: there is marked cell infiltration and increased vascularization. *Type 3*, in which there are multiple fibroblastic layers associated with large capillaries on the dura surface and marked cell infiltration with small neovessels within the hematoma. *Type 4*, in which cicatricial tissue is present, with cell infiltration, neovessels, and hemorrhage [1].

The microscopic examination of SDHs allows for dating by observing specific morphological features of the hematoma (Table 7.1) [4, 5, 15, 17, 31, 38].

Table 7.1 Subdural hematoma microscopic stages

Time interval	Microscopic examination		
	Hematoma	Dural surface	Arachnoid surface
0 h	Intact red blood cells	/	/
24 h	Intact red blood cells	Thin layer of fibrin (between the dura and the clot)	Thin layer of fibrin (between the arachnoid and the clot)
36 h	Intact red blood cells	Early fibroblastic activity	Thin layer of fibrin
48–72 h	Intact red blood cells	Rare fibroblasts (spindle cells) at the interface	Thin layer of fibrin
4 days	Red blood cells breakdown (loss of sharp contour and variability of stain)	2–4 layers of fibroblasts	Thin layer of fibrin with occasional spindle cells
5 days	Red blood cells breakdown (loss of sharp contour and variability of stain)	3–6 layers of fibroblasts. Siderophages appear at the edges of the clot	Thin layer of fibrin with occasional spindle cells
7–8 days	Red blood cell lysis, early capillaries/granulation tissue, fibroblasts enter the clot, clot liquefies	12–15 layers of fibroblasts. (*The outer membrane becomes grossly identifiable*)	Layer mostly of fibrin with some fibroblasts
10–12 days	Clot is broken up in islands by capillaries, fibroblasts and a fibrin	Fibroblasts move at the edge of the clot	Siderophages appear
14–17 days	Progressive red blood cell lysis with rare elements still identifiable. Giant capillaries	Fibroblastic layer becomes approximately ½ the thickness of the dura	Fibroblastic layer appears, forming an early thin membrane. The clot can be fully encapsulated
18–28 days	Clot is liquified with areas of fresh hemorrhage and larger vessels present	Fibroblastic layer is of similar thickness of the dura. Siderophages in membrane	Well-formed membrane of similar thickness of the dura. Siderophages in membrane
29–36 days	Large capillaries	Neomembrane development	Neomembrane development
1–3 months	Enlarged capillaries with secondary fresh hemorrhages	Hyalinized membrane, increased collagen	Hyalinized membrane, increased collagen
3–6 months	Possible focal areas of rebleeding. No original red blood cells	Hyalinized membrane	Hyalinized membrane
>6 months (chronic)	At this point, estimating the age of the clot becomes difficult. No red blood cells or significant residual inflammatory cells are identifiable, the neomembrane becomes thick and calcifications may occur. Membranes can resemble the dura and may retain focal hemosiderin-laden macrophages		

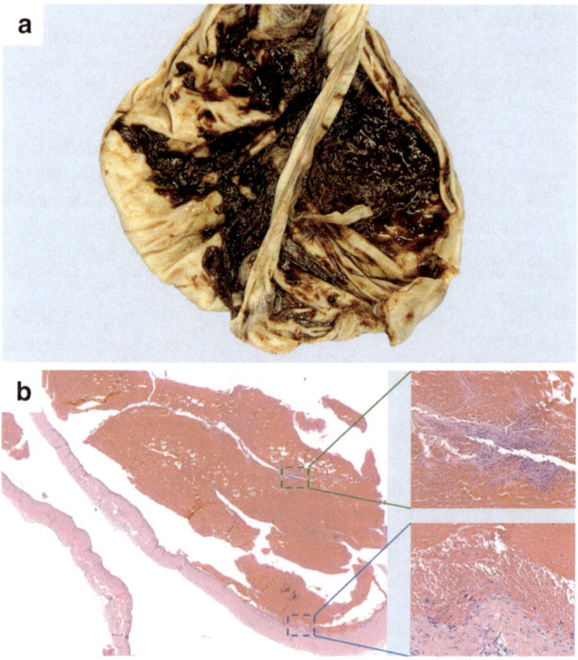

Fig. 7.9 Acute subdural hematoma. The dura (**a**) is grossly intact and contains adherent red-brown blood on the bilateral subdural surface, without evidence of neomembranes. (**b**) Microscopic examination of the dural sections demonstrates adherent blood on the subdural surface without significant fibroblast proliferation (*blue square*). A focal area of cell infiltration and fibrin is present within the hemorrhagic area (*green square*)

Following the injury, a reaction to subdural bleeding starts within a few hours. Intact red blood cells are observed within the clot (Fig. 7.9). Neutrophils that are detectable in a variable amount soon after the onset are considered to be a consequence of the injury rather than a reaction to it. Theoretically, some circulating neutrophils could spill out from the ruptured bridging veins at the time of the injury [28]. Conversely, reactive neutrophils usually appear days later, together with inflammatory changes of the vessels, forming granulation tissue as the SDH enters a histologically "organizing" phase (Fig. 7.10). There is phagocytosis and degradation of erythrocytes, as demonstrated by hemosiderin-laden macrophages. The granulation tissue comprises many capillaries, fibroblasts, collagenous fibers, and macrophages and allows the formation of the initial thin outer membrane of the hematoma. In the following days to weeks, dense network fibrin holds the hematoma together, and fibroblasts migrate from the outer layer through the hematoma to form an inner membrane lacking blood vessels. The initial outer membrane will be visible to the naked eye approximately after 1 week, while the inner layer is usually visible after 2 weeks. When the hematoma does not expand any more, the membranes become more and more fibrous, giving the typical gross appearance described above. After a period of approximately 6 months, the SDH becomes histologically "chronic." The histologic appearance of this CSDH is of a fibrous neomembrane on the subdural surface, often with scattered residual hemosiderin-laden macrophages (Fig. 7.11), but no active inflammation or erythrocytes, except in situations with secondary hemorrhage superimposed on CSDH. At this point no further age estimation is typically possible.

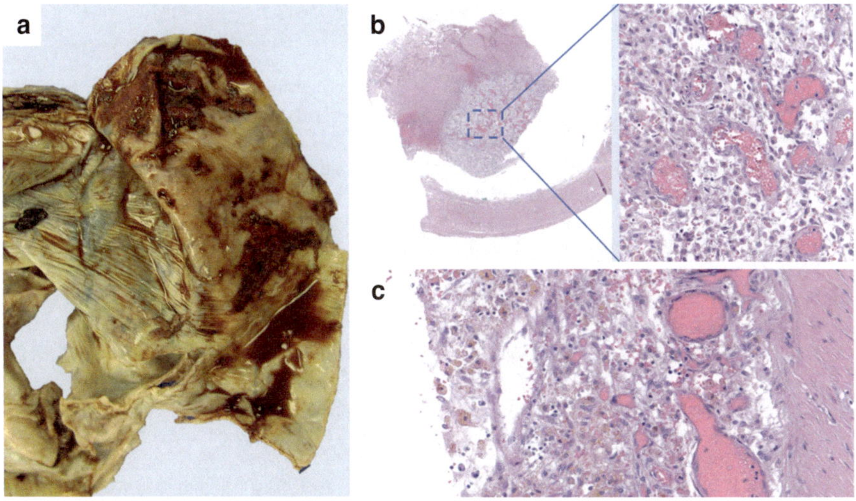

Fig. 7.10 Organizing subdural hematoma. The dura (**a**) is grossly intact with patchy areas of adherent blood bilaterally. Light microscopy of the dural sections (**b**) shows adherent red blood cells with significant fibroblast ingrowth and neovascularization, suggestive of organizing hematoma (*blue square*). Other fields show areas of more acute hemorrhage and a focal area of fibrous layers with hemosiderin deposition (**c**)

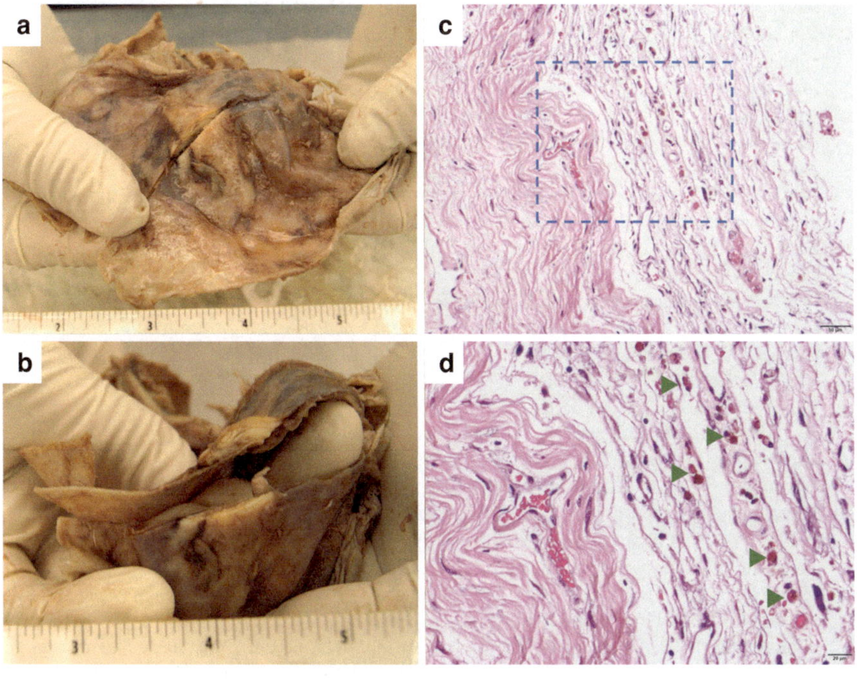

Fig. 7.11 Chronic subdural hematoma. The dura with an attached subdural neomembrane identified grossly (**a**, **b**) and (**c**) microscopic appearance of the dura (*left*) and neomembrane (*right*) with (**d**) scattered hemosiderin (*green arrow heads*)

References

1. Bokka S, Trivedi A. Histopathological study of the outer membrane of the dura mater in chronic sub dural hematoma: its clinical and radiological correlation. Asian J Neurosurg. 2016;11(1):34–8.
2. Brockmann C, Kunze S, Scharf J. Computed tomographic angiography of the superior sagittal sinus and bridging veins. Surg Radiol Anat. 2011;33(2):129–34.
3. Depreitere B, Van Lierde C, Sloten JV, Van Audekercke R, Van der Perre G, Plets C, et al. Mechanics of acute subdural hematomas resulting from bridging vein rupture. J Neurosurg. 2006;104(6):950–6.
4. Dettmeyer RB. Forensic histopathology: fundamentals and perspectives. 2nd ed. Cham: Springer International Publishing; 2018. p. 519–29.
5. DiMaio VJM, Dana MD. Handbook of forensic pathology. 2nd ed. Boca Raton: CRC Press; 2006. p. 165–9.
6. Dobran M, Iacoangeli M, Scortichini AR, Mancini F, Benigni R, Nasi D, et al. Spontaneous chronic subdural hematoma in young adult: the role of missing coagulation facto. G Chir. 2017;38(2):66–70.
7. Ducruet AF, Grobelny BT, Zacharia BE, Hickman ZL, DeRosa PL, Andersen KN, et al. The surgical management of chronic subdural hematoma. Neurosurg Rev. 2012;35(2):155–69; discussion 169.
8. Famaey N, Ying Cui Z, Umuhire Musigazi G, Ivens J, Depreitere B, Verbeken E, et al. Structural and mechanical characterisation of bridging veins: a review. J Mech Behav Biomed Mater. 2015;41:222–40.
9. Gu S-X, Yang D-L, Cui D-M, Xu Q-W, Che X-M, Wu J-S, et al. Anatomical studies on the temporal bridging veins with Dextroscope and its application in tumor surgery across the middle and posterior fossa. Clin Neurol Neurosurg. 2011;113(10):889–94.
10. Haines DE. On the question of a subdural space. Anat Rec. 1991;230(1):3–21.
11. Haines DE, Harkey HL, al-Mefty O. The "subdural" space: a new look at an outdated concept. Neurosurgery. 1993;32(1):111–20.
12. Han H, Tao W, Zhang M. The dural entrance of cerebral bridging veins into the superior sagittal sinus: an anatomical comparison between cadavers and digital subtraction angiography. Neuroradiology. 2007;49(2):169–75.
13. Harrigan MR, Deveikis JP. Handbook of cerebrovascular disease and neurointerventional technique. 3rd ed. Cham: Springer International Publishing; 2018. p. 73.
14. Kiliç T, Akakin A. Anatomy of cerebral veins and sinuses. Front Neurol Neurosci. 2008;23:4–15.
15. Leestma JE. Forensic neuropathology. 3rd ed. Boca Raton: CRC Press; 2014. p. 484–502.
16. Love S, Perry A, Ironside JW, Budka H. Greenfield's neuropathology, ninth edition—two volume set. 9th ed. London: CRC Press; 2016. p. 646–52.
17. Madea B. Handbook of forensic medicine. 1st ed. Hoboken: Wiley-Blackwell; 2014. p. 293–6.
18. Matsushima T, Rhoton AL Jr, de Oliveira E, Peace D. Microsurgical anatomy of the veins of the posterior fossa. J Neurosurg. 1983;59(1):63–105.
19. Matsushima T, Suzuki SO, Fukui M, Rhoton AL Jr, de Oliveira E, Ono M. Microsurgical anatomy of the tentorial sinuses. J Neurosurg. 1989;71(6):923–8.
20. Mortazavi MM, Denning M, Yalcin B, Shoja MM, Loukas M, Tubbs RS. The intracranial bridging veins: a comprehensive review of their history, anatomy, histology, pathology, and neurosurgical implications. Childs Nerv Syst. 2013;29(7):1073–8.
21. Munro D. Surgical pathology of subdural hematoma: based on a study of one hundred and five cases. Arch Neurol Psychiatr. 1936;35(1):64.
22. Muthukumar N, Palaniappan P. Tentorial venous sinuses: an anatomic study. Neurosurgery. 1998;42(2):363–71.

23. Naama O, Belhachmi A, Ziadi T, Boulahroud O, Abad Elasri C, Elmostarchid B, et al. Acute spontaneous subdural hematoma: an unusual form of cerebrovacular accident. J Neurosurg Sci. 2009;53(4):157–9.
24. Nagahori T, Nishijima M, Takaku A. Histological study of the outer membrane of chronic subdural hematoma: possible mechanism for expansion of hematoma cavity. No Shinkei Geka. 1993;21(8):697–701.
25. Oehmichen M, Auer RN, König HG. Forensic neuropathology and associated neurology. Berlin: Springer; 2006. p. 126–38.
26. Oka K, Rhoton AL Jr, Barry M, Rodriguez R. Microsurgical anatomy of the superficial veins of the cerebrum. Neurosurgery. 1985;17(5):711–48.
27. Pang Q, Wang C, Hu Y, Xu G, Zhang L, Hao X, et al. Experimental study of the morphology of cerebral bridging vein. Chin Med Sci J. 2001;16(1):19–22.
28. Rao MG, Singh D, Vashista RK, Sharma SK. Dating of acute and subacute subdural haemorrhage: a histo-pathological study. J Clin Diagn Res. 2016;10(7):HC01–7.
29. Sakata K, Al-Mefty O, Yamamoto I. Venous consideration in petrosal approach: microsurgical anatomy of the temporal bridging vein. Neurosurgery. 2000;47(1):153–61.
30. Sampei T, Yasui N, Okudera T, Fukasawa H. Anatomic study of anterior frontal cortical bridging veins with special reference to the frontopolar vein. Neurosurgery. 1996;38(5):971–5.
31. Saukko PJ, Knight B. Knight's forensic pathology. 4th ed. London: Hodder Arnold; 2015. p. 185–8.
32. Schachenmayr W, Friede RL. The origin of subdural neomembranes. I. Fine structure of the dura-arachnoid interface in man. Am J Pathol. 1978;92(1):53–68.
33. Schaller B. Physiology of cerebral venous blood flow: from experimental data in animals to normal function in humans. Brain Res Brain Res Rev. 2004;46(3):243–60.
34. Sung SK, Kim SH, Son DW, Lee SW. Acute spontaneous subdural hematoma of arterial origin. J Korean Neurosurg Soc. 2012;51(2):91–3.
35. Ueyama T, Al-Mefty O, Tamaki N. Bridging veins on the tentorial surface of the cerebellum: a microsurgical anatomic study and operative considerations. Neurosurgery. 1998;43(5):1137–45.
36. van den Bos D, Zomer S, Kubat B. Dare to date: age estimation of subdural hematomas, literature, and case analysis. Int J Legal Med. 2014;128(4):631–40.
37. Vignes J-R, Dagain A, Guérin J, Liguoro D. A hypothesis of cerebral venous system regulation based on a study of the junction between the cortical bridging veins and the superior sagittal sinus: laboratory investigation. J Neurosurg. 2007;107(6):1205–10.
38. Whitwell HL, editor. Forensic neuropathology. London: Hodder Arnold; 2005.
39. Yamashima T, Friede RL. Why do bridging veins rupture into the virtual subdural space? J Neurol Neurosurg Psychiatry. 1984;47(2):121–7.

Chapter 8
Epidemiology and Predisposing Factors of Chronic Subdural Hematoma

Abad Cherif El Asri, Ali Akhaddar, and Miloudi Gazzaz

8.1 Introduction

Chronic subdural hematoma (CSDH), which remains one of the most frequent diagnoses in neurosurgical practice, is characterized by a pathological collection of blood in the subdural space with an insidious onset and progression [11, 35, 50]. Given an increased occurrence in the elderly, the incidence rates have been rising with the demographic shift towards an aging population and it is expected to double by the year 2030 [40, 47]. This increase in incidence has previously been attributed to an aging population in the Occident [25, 40, 42, 47]. However, other factors such as improvement in diagnostic ability due to physicians' evolving index of suspicion and the availability of more computed tomography (CT) scanners cannot be excluded [27, 44]. In approximately 20–25% of the cases, CSDHs are bilateral [27]. Many risk factors for the development of CSDH have been described in the literature. In fact, more than one of the contributing factors can be present, and they can have a cumulative effect [20, 40, 50]. These factors include old age, direct or indirect head trauma, coagulopathy, and treatment with antiplatelet agents and anticoagulants. Among them, a history of head trauma is commonly considered as the most important risk factor [22, 24, 32]. Other significant risk factors are bleeding tendency, kidney disease, hemodialysis, liver dysfunction, epilepsy, previous shunt surgery, chemotherapeutic agent administration, and arachnoid cysts [22, 32].

A. C. El Asri (✉) · M. Gazzaz
Department of Neurosurgery, Mohamed V Military Hospital, Mohamed V, University Mohammed V of Rabat, Rabat, Morocco

A. Akhaddar
Avicenne Military Hospital of Marrakech, Department of Neurosurgery, Mohammed V University in Rabat, Rabat, Morocco

M. Turgut et al. (eds.), *Subdural Hematoma*,
https://doi.org/10.1007/978-3-030-79371-5_8

Recently, because of the improvement in life expectancy leading to an aging population, many receiving anticoagulant and antiplatelet treatment, the incidence of CSDH has been increasing over the years.

8.1.1 Incidence

The incidence of chronic subdural hematoma has been on the rise around the world. In a Finnish study conducted by Foelholm and Waltimo in 1967, 64 residents of the city of Helsinki diagnosed with CSDH were included over a 7-year period, rendering an overall incidence of 1.72 per 100,000 persons per year [13]. While in 2015, Rauhala et al. indicated that the incidence of CSDH had doubled from 8.2 to 17.6/100,000/year in the general population of Finland [37]. Additionally, in a recent study by Balser and colleagues focusing on the veteran population in United States, an overall incidence rate of 79.4 per 100,000 persons per year was observed [47].

In Asia, especially in Japan, the findings were no different. The elderly population of Japan outnumbers the elderly population of any other country worldwide. Hence, the incidence of CSDH in Japan has also been on the rise. In 1992, Kudo et al. reported that the incidence of CSDH in the local area of Awagishima Japan was 13.1/100,000/year [27]. Furthermore, another Japanese study examining the incidence of CSDH between 2005 and 2007 used data from a national registry. The authors reported an increased incidence of CSDH of 20.6 per 100,000 persons per year, with 76.5 in the 70–79-year-old age group and 127.1 in the 80-year-old age group [23]. Consequently, the annual incidence of CSDH in Japan (number of newly diagnosed cases) has been estimated to be 24,000 based on the current Japanese population which is around 120 million [44].

In Africa, the exact incidence cannot be determined because there are no specific studies that indicate the incidence of CSDH in African countries. All the studies quote western literature as a reference to the incidence of CSDH.

8.1.2 Age

Epidemiologic studies have reported a significant increase in the incidence of CSDH in the elderly compared with other age cohorts. In addition, most CSDH case series also reported their cohort to be composed of patients with advanced age with a mean age of 55–60 years, with some greater than 70 years of age [3, 10, 11, 14]. The mean age of CSDH patients has been reported to be 60 years in India [34], 64.3 years in Brazil [43], 68.9 years in Switzerland [31], 69.0 years in Korea [38], 69.3 years in Canada [19], 71.4 years in Germany [41], 72.7 years in Spain [15], and 62 years in Morocco [8]. As the population continues to mature, the incidence is expected to double by the year 2030 [11, 27, 50]. A large demographic study found the prevalence of CSDH in patients older than 65 years to be significantly higher (69% vs. 31%) [4]. Another study based in North Wales reported a lower incidence of 8.2 per 100,000 persons per year in elderly patients above 65 years over a 3-year period between 1996 and 1999 [1]. In comparison, a more recent analysis from 2005 to 2007 using a national registry in Japan revealed a relatively higher incidence rate of 20.6 per 100,000 persons per year (76.5 in population aged 70–79 years) [23].

The underlying reason for the greater prevalence of CSDH among the elderly is not completely understood, but may be attributed to a higher risk of falls in this population.

8.1.3 Sex

Men are more frequently affected by CSDH than women. The Finnish epidemiologic study on the incidence of CSDH demonstrated an overall higher incidence for men than for women. This trend was unchanged in the same cohort after stratification by age [13]. Similarly, a male gender predominance for the incidence and prevalence of the disease was also observed in other CSDH studies [10, 33]. The male/female ratio was reported as 4.8:1 in Brazil [43], 4.2:1 in Canada [19], 3.4:1 in India [34], 2.6:1 in Korea [38], 2.4:1 in Germany [41], 1.9:1 in Switzerland [31], 1.7:1 in Spain [15], and 5.3:1 in Morocco [8]. The percentage of female CSDH patients has demonstrated a tendency to increase over time in Japan, while the percentage of male CSDH patients has thus shown a corresponding decrease. The percentage of female CSDH patients reportedly tends also to increase with the aging of society when the male gender has been recognized to be a potential risk factor for CSDH [35].

8.1.4 Risk Factors for Chronic Subdural Hematoma

It is evident in the literature that CSDH is not a static disease, and that the risk of development, progression, and recurrence of CSDH may be influenced significantly by several risk factors [11, 40, 50].

8.1.4.1 Head Trauma

In the literature, head trauma is considered as the main precipitating factors for the development of CSDH, and it can be identified in about 50–70% of the patients suffering from CSDH [5, 20, 22, 24]. Although previous minor head injuries could sometimes be unrecognized, the traumatic events usually preceded the CSDH development [5, 22, 30, 35]. According to a nationwide, population-based study in Finland examining the total traumatic brain injury from 1991 to 2005, the overall incidence was 101 per 100,000 persons per year, significantly lower than that reported in other countries, including the Netherlands, Estonia, and New Zealand [12, 26, 46]. In the veteran study where traumatic brain injury within the included population is considered highly prevalent, the projected incidence rate of CSDH was reported to be 121.4, which is significantly higher than that of the general population in other studies; conversely, in the same study, the predicted incidence of CSDH was only 17.4 in civilian based models [4]. However, the exact vascular source of bleeding following trauma was reported to be the bridging veins that extended from the cerebral cortex to the dural venous sinuses that are often stretched and fragile in elderly patients with brain atrophy [36, 44]. This belief has been disputed based on the long delay (mean of 4–7 weeks) between the trauma and the development of actual symptoms, whereby even a slow venous bleed would be expected to form a symptomatic collection within a few days. This event is followed by the ingrowth of neo-capillaries, enzymatic fibrinolysis, and liquefaction of the blood clot. Fibrin degradation products are re-incorporated into new blood clots and further inhibit hemostasis [7, 44].

8.1.4.2 Advanced Age

As confirmed in previous studies, CSDH is a common disease in the elderly patients. Older people have a higher tendency to have CSDH, because of brain atrophy [20, 22, 28, 29]. The degree of brain atrophy was an independent predictive factor for developing CSDH which tends to occur in elderly people. Since brain atrophy causes enlargement of the subarachnoid space and stretching of the bridging veins, these developments provoke tearing of the bridging veins and bleeding into the cerebrospinal fluid in the subdural space after mild head injury [4, 11, 25, 47]. The degree of brain atrophy is classified into four stages according to the visual rating of brain atrophy scale [11, 33, 47]. The severity of atrophy correlates with the delay in diagnosis.

In addition, older people tend to fall more often than do the young and suffer minor head traumas. Lastly, with increasing age, the incidence of blood thinner administration rises, leading to increased risk for hemorrhage. The reported peak age for CSDH was the seventh decade of life [11, 20, 22, 24, 32]. The importance of the advanced age as a risk factor of CSDH will increase with the evolution of an aging society.

A temporal analysis of a defined Finnish population extending from 1990 to 2015 confirmed this trend by reporting an overall doubling of the incidence over that time period from 8.2 to 17.6 per 100,000 persons per year with most of the increase occurring among the population aged 80 years or more [37]. In addition to the shift towards aging populations, the increased use of anticoagulation and antiplatelet medications partly accounts for the temporal trend as well [2, 39]. As demonstrated by Toi et al., the age peak for CSDH has also been rising over time. In Japan, most CSDH reported in a 1972 study occurred in the population aged 50–59 years, while most cases occurred in the population aged 80–89 years in Toi et al.'s analysis of 63,358 cases from 2010 to 2013 [44].

8.1.4.3 Chronic Alcoholism

Alcoholism is well known to be associated with CSDH. The reason for the greater propensity of patients with chronic alcohol addiction for hematoma formation is unknown. However, it was proposed by some authors that persistent alcohol intake induces brain atrophy and coagulation dysfunction (secondary to liver malfunction) [11, 20, 24, 42]. Chronic alcoholism also leads to a higher chance of unrecognized head trauma, which might definitely play a major role in CSDH development in these patients with reported rates of CSDH with chronic alcoholism ranging from 6 to 35% [24, 30, 42].

8.1.4.4 Male Gender

Men, from all age groups, suffer disproportionally higher rates of CSDH than women [11, 42, 45, 50]. Though specific reasons could not be proved, suggested theories include trauma, morphological causes, and hormonal factors. The difference in gender distribution of CSDH might not be related to falls; in one study, the risk of a fall was reported to be similar between the two gender groups. However, the authors also noted that male gender may have been more likely to be exposed to injuries or other CSDH-related factors in general [3]. Giuffrè et al. observed a higher incidence of estrogen receptors and progesterone receptors in men rather than in women in their study on the hematoma external membrane [16]. Other factors that may explain the known male predisposition for CSDH might be related to alcohol use and epilepsy [40].

8.1.4.5 Coagulopathy

Aside from demographic risk factors, coagulopathies, including therapeutic anticoagulation (AC) and antiplatelet (AP) therapy, are known contributors to the pathogenesis of cSDH. Medical conditions include sepsis, hepatic failure, all forms of hemophilia, disseminated intravascular coagulation, and renal dialysis [11, 42, 50]. Because most patients with CSDH were elderly, an increased proportion of patients on anticoagulant agents for the prevention or treatment of systemic diseases is superimposed. It has been reported that more than a third of the cases with CSDH are treated with oral anticoagulation or antiplatelet therapy at the time of diagnosis [11, 40, 42, 50]. Lindvall and Koskinen reported a similar finding that 71% in the non-trauma group were treated with ACs/APs compared to 18% in the trauma group [30]. However, based on its unique cost-effectiveness and widespread availability for prevention of cardio-cerebrovascular events, the utilization of AC and AP treatments has changed the incidence of intracerebral hemorrhage and subdural hematomas [39]. However, Rust et al. reported that there is a 42.5 times higher possibility of developing a CSDH when taking warfarin compared to cases where no medication was taken [2, 18, 19, 30, 39]. These findings suggest that there is a causative role of the ACs/APs in the development of CSDH unrelated to head trauma or alcoholism. Besides the occurrence of CSDH, both anticoagulant and antiplatelet agents were also proposed potentially to be associated with the expansion of the hematoma [45]. The association of both medications with recurrence of CSDH was less clear and has been reported to be irrelevant in many studies [17, 40, 45].

Despite the well-recognized benefits of these drugs, concerns have been raised recently about their main side effect, hemorrhagic complications and more specifically in hemorrhagic stroke. This phenomenon will probably be more frequent in the future with the widespread use of ACs/APs [2, 5, 11, 45, 49, 50].

8.1.4.6 Intracranial Hypotension

Intracranial hypotension is mainly caused by a CSF leak related to traumatic or postoperative CSF fistulas, lumbar puncture or drainage, overshunting after placement of a ventriculoperitoneal shunt, iatrogenic or disease-induced dehydration or spontaneous events [21, 42, 48]. Subdural hematomas may result in up to 8% of the patients shunted for normal-pressure hydrocephalus. There can be an increased traction on the bridging veins, leading to a higher likelihood of hematoma formation [6, 21, 48]. Although the introduction of adjustable-pressure valves has decreased the rate of this hemorrhagic complication, intracranial hypotension resulting from overshunting is still a significant problem despite the use of this device and the management is still a challenge [21].

8.1.4.7 Other Causes

Other rare causes of spontaneous subdural hematomas have been described: vascular malformation (e.g., cerebral aneurysms and arteriovenous malformations) [11, 42, 50], benign (e.g., convexity meningiomas) and malignant tumors, carcinomatosis/sarcomatosis meningitis, and infections (e.g., bacterial and tuberculous meningitis) [9].

8.2 Conclusions

The incidence of CSDH is gradually increasing worldwide. Many authors consider it as a result of underlying disease and advanced frailty rather than a primary event in older patients [33]. They compared this neurosurgical condition to hip fractures which carries high short- and long-term mortality. The explanations for the high incidence include an aging population, a low threshold for imaging patients with recurrent falls and confusion and the increasing use of anti-thrombotic agents. Patients with high risks for developing a CSDH have to be identified and consequently the diagnosis must be suspected even with mild symptoms. The prognosis will depend on the early diagnosis and the administration of prompt appropriate treatment.

References

1. Asghar M, Adhiyaman V, Greenway MW, Bhowmick BK, Bates A. Chronic subdural haematoma in the elderly—a North Wales experience. J R Soc Med. 2002;95(6):290–2.
2. Aspegren O, Åstrand R, Lundgren MI, Romner B. Anticoagulation therapy a risk factor 323 for the development of chronic subdural hematoma. Clin Neurol Neurosurg. 2013;115(7):981–4.
3. Baechli H, Nordmann A, Bucher HC, Gratzl O. Demographics and prevalent risk factors of chronic subdural haematoma: results of a large single-center cohort study. Neurosurg Rev. 2004;27:263–6.
4. Balser D, Farooq S, Mehmood T, et al. Actual and projected incidence rates for chronic subdural hematomas in United States veterans administration and civilian populations. J Neurosurg. 2015;123(5):1209–15.
5. Choi WW, Kim KH. Prognostic factors of chronic subdural hematoma. J Korean Neurosurg Soc. 2002;32:18–22.
6. Dietrich U, Lumenta C, Sprick C. Subdural hematoma in a case of hydrocephalus and macrocrania. Experience with a pressure-adjustable valve. Childs Nerv Syst. 1987;3(4):242–4.
7. Edlmann E, Giorgi-Coll S, Whitfield PC, Carpenter KLH, Hutchinson PJ. Pathophysiology of chronic subdural haematoma: inflammation, angiogenesis and implications for pharmacotherapy. J Neuroinflammation. 2017;14(1):108.
8. El Asri AC, Benzagmout M, Chakour K, Chaoui MF, Laaguili J, Gazzaz M, Baallal H, El Mostarchid B. Variation of ventricular size after surgical treatment of chronic subdural hematoma. Asian J Neurosurg. 2019;14(1):122–5.
9. El Asri AC, El Mostarchid B, Akhaddar A, Boucetta M. Chronic subdural hematoma revealing skull metastasis. Intern Med. 2011;50(7):791.
10. Farhat Neto J, Araujo JLV, Ferraz VR, et al. Chronic subdural hematoma: epidemiological and prognostic analysis of 176 cases. Rev Col Bras Cir. 2015;42(5):283–7.
11. Feghali J, Yang W, Huang J. Updates in chronic subdural hematoma: epidemiology, etiology, pathogenesis, treatment and outcome. World Neurosurg. 2020;141:339–45.
12. Feigin VL, Theadom A, Barker-Collo S, et al. Incidence of traumatic brain injury in New Zealand: a population-based study. Lancet Neurol. 2013;12(1):53–64.
13. Foelholm R, Waltimo O. Epidemiology of chronic subdural haematoma. Acta Neurochir (Wien). 1975;32(3–4):247–50.
14. Fujioka S, Matsukado Y, Kaku M, Sakurama N, Nonaka N, Miura G. CT analysis of 100 cases with chronic subdural hematoma with respect to clinical manifestation and the enlarging process of the hematoma (author's transl). Neurol Med Chir (Tokyo). 1981;21:1153–60.
15. Gelabert-González M, Iglesias-Pais M, García-Allut A, Martínez-Rumbo R. Chronic subdural haematoma: surgical treatment and outcome in 1000 cases. Clin Neurol Neurosurg. 2005;107:223–9.
16. Giuffrè R, Palma E, Liccardo G, Sciarra F, Pastore FS, Concolino G. Sex steroid hormones in the pathogenesis of chronic subdural haematoma. Neurochirurgia (Stuttg). 1992;35:103–7.
17. Gonugunta V, Buxton N. Warfarin and chronic subdural haematomas. Br J Neurosurg. 2001;15(6):514–7.
18. Hirakawa K, Hashizume K, Fuchinoue T, Takahashi H, Nomura K. Statistical analysis of chronic subdural hematoma in 309 adult cases. Neurol Med Chir (Tokyo). 1972;12:71–83.
19. Jack A, O'Kelly C, McDougall C, Findlay JM. Predicting recurrence after chronic subdural haematoma drainage. Can J Neurol Sci. 2015;42:34–9.
20. Jeong JE, Kim GK, Park JT, Lim YJ, Kim TS, Rhee BA, et al. A clinical analysis of chronic subdural hematoma according to age factor. J Korean Neurosurg Soc. 2000;29:748–53.
21. Kamano S, Nakano Y, Imanishi T. Management with a programmable pressure valve of subdural hematomas caused by ventriculoperitoneal shunt: case report. Surg Neurol. 1991;35:381–3.
22. Kang HL, Shin HS, Kim TH, Hwang YS, Park SK. Clinical analysis of recurrent chronic subdural hematoma. J Korean Neurosurg Soc. 2006;40:262–6.
23. Karibe H, Kameyama M, Kawase M, et al. Epidemiology of chronic subdural hematomas. No Shinkei Geka. 2011;39(12):1149–53.

24. Ko BS, Lee JK, Seo BR, Moon SJ, Kim JH, Kim SH. Clinical analysis of risk factors related to recurrent chronic subdural hematoma. J Korean Neurosurg Soc. 2008;43:11–5.
25. Kolias AG, Chari A, Santarius T, Hutchinson PJ. Chronic subdural haematoma: modern management and emerging therapies. Nat Rev Neurol. 2014;10(10):570–8.
26. Koskinen S, Alaranta H. Traumatic brain injury in Finland 1991-2005: a nationwide register study of hospitalized and fatal TBI. Brain Inj. 2008;22(3):205–14.
27. Kudo H, Kuwamura K, Izawa I, Sawa H, Tamaki N. Chronic subdural hematoma in elderly people: present status on Awaji Island and epidemiological prospect. Neurol Med Chir. 1992;32(4):207–9.
28. Kwon HJ, Youm JY, Kim SH, Koh HS, Song SH, Kim Y. Postoperative radiological changes in chronic subdural hematoma and its relation to recurrence. J Korean Neurosurg Soc. 2004;35:410–4.
29. Lee JK, Choi JH, Kim CH, Lee HK, Moon JG. Chronic subdural hematomas: a comparative study of three types of operative procedures. J Korean Neurosurg Soc. 2009;46:210–4.
30. Lindvall P, Koskinen LO. Anticoagulants and antiplatelet agents and the risk of development and recurrence of chronic subdural haematomas. J Clin Neurosci. 2009;16:1287–90.
31. MacFarlane MR, Weerakkody Y, Kathiravel Y. Chronic subdural haematomas are more common on the left than on the right. J Clin Neurosci. 2009;16:642–4.
32. Markwalder TM. Chronic subdural hematomas: a review. J Neurosurg. 1981;54:637–45.
33. Miranda LB, Braxton E, Hobbs J, Quigley MR. Chronic subdural hematoma in the elderly: not a benign disease. J Neurosurg. 2011;114(1):72–6.
34. Nayil K, Ramzan A, Sajad A, Zahoor S, Wani A, Nizami F, et al. Subdural hematomas: an analysis of 1181 Kashmiri patients. World Neurosurg. 2012;77:103–10.
35. Nioka H, Matsuda M, Handa J. [A review of cases of a chronic subdural hematoma: an analysis of findings in two age groups]. Jpn J Neurosurg (Tokyo). 1995;4:359–63.
36. Ommaya AK, Yarnell P. Subdural haematoma after whiplash injury. Lancet (London, England). 1969;2(7614):237–9.
37. Rauhala M, Luoto TM, Huhtala H, et al. The incidence of chronic subdural hematomas from 1990 to 2015 in a defined Finnish population. J Neurosurg. 2019;132(4):1147–57.
38. Ro HW, Park SK, Jang DK, Yoon WS, Jang KS, Han YM. Preoperative predictive factors for surgical and functional outcomes in chronic subdural hematoma. Acta Neurochir (Wien). 2016;158:135–9.
39. Rust T, Kiemer N, Erasmus A. Chronic subdural haematomas and anticoagulation or antithrombotic therapy. J Clin Neurosci. 2006;13(8):823–7.
40. Santarius T, Kirkpatrick PJ, Kolias AG, Hutchinson PJ. Working toward rational and evidence based treatment of chronic subdural hematoma. Clin Neurosurg. 2010;57:112–22.
41. Schwarz F, Loos F, Dünisch P, Sakr Y, Safatli DA, Kalff R, et al. Risk factors for reoperation after initial burr hole trephination in chronic subdural hematomas. Clin Neurol Neurosurg. 2015;138:66–71.
42. Sim YW, Min KS, Lee MS, Kim YG, Kim DH. Recent changes in risk factors of chronic subdural hematoma. J Korean Neurosurg Soc. 2012;52:234–9.
43. Sousa EB, Brandão LFS, Tavares CB, Borges IBC, Freire Neto NG, Kessler IM. Epidemiological characteristics of patients who underwent surgical drainage of chronic subdural hematomas in Brasília, Brazil. BMC Surg. 2013;13:5.
44. Toi H, Kinoshita K, Hirai S, et al. Present epidemiology of chronic subdural hematoma in Japan: analysis of 63,358 cases recorded in a national administrative database. J Neurosurg. 2018;128(1):222–8.
45. Torihashi K, Sadamasa N, Yoshida K, et al. Independent predictors for recurrence of chronic subdural hematoma: a review of 343 consecutive surgical cases. Neurosurgery. 2008;63(6):1125–9; discussion: 1129.
46. Ventsel G, Kolk A, Talvik I, et al. The incidence of childhood traumatic brain injury in Tartu and Tartu County in Estonia. Neuroepidemiology. 2008;30(1):20–4.

47. Welling LC, Welling MS, Teixeira MJ, Figueiredo EG. Chronic subdural hematoma: so common and so neglected. World Neurosurg. 2018;111:393–4.
48. Weiner HLCS, Cohen H. Current treatment of normal-pressure hydrocephalus: comparison of flow-regulated and differential-pressure shunt valves. Neurosurgery. 1995;37:877–84.
49. Wintzen AR, Tijssen JG. Subdural hematoma and oral anticoagulant therapy. Arch Neurol. 1982;39:69–72.
50. Yang W, Huang J. Chronic subdural hematoma epidemiology and natural history. Neurosurg Clin N Am. 2017;28:205–10.

Chapter 9
Main Clinical Presentations of Chronic Subdural Hematomas

Michelle E. De Witt and Walter A. Hall

9.1 Introduction

Chronic subdural hematomas (CSDHs) are a commonly encountered neurosurgical condition with significant associated morbidity and mortality [44, 50], with an increasing incidence in the global population [3, 69]. Anatomically, they are located between the arachnoid mater and the dura mater, within the dural border cell layer [40, 56]. On imaging, they are seen as concave or crescent-shaped extra-axial lesions, which may cross suture lines and appear hypo- or iso-dense/intense relative to the brain parenchyma [44, 57]. Headaches, gait disturbance, confusion, and/or behavioral changes are the most common symptoms that trigger patient presentation to the office, emergency department, or urgent care center. On examination, motor weakness, disorientation, and/or confusion are frequently noted [21, 46, 58]. However, patient presentation with CSDHs can be quite variable. The non-specificity and variability of symptoms of presentation combined with a high frequency of comorbidities in the presenting population can be diagnostically challenging [40, 58]. There is a multifold importance in the recognition of the patient presenting with a CSDH. Patients who are symptomatic from an underlying CSDH benefit from timely surgical intervention to improve morbidity and mortality rates. Additionally, the diagnosis of a CSDH may have some prognostic value as a "fragility" marker [44]. In multiple studies, patients who have had CSDHs have increased mortality rates compared to the general population [44, 50].

M. E. De Witt (✉)
Department of Neurosurgery, SUNY Upstate University Hospital, Syracuse, NY, USA
e-mail: Dewittm@upstate.edu

W. A. Hall
Department of Neurosurgery, SUNY Upstate Medical University,
Syracuse, New York, USA
e-mail: Hallw@upstate.edu

M. Turgut et al. (eds.), *Subdural Hematoma*,
https://doi.org/10.1007/978-3-030-79371-5_9

9.2 Signs and Symptoms

A multitude of clinical signs and symptoms can be associated with a CSDH. In broad terms, most signs and symptoms described can be considered to stem from either mass effect of the hematoma or from increased intracranial pressure [58]. Reported symptoms can include weakness, gait unsteadiness, lightheadness, difficulty writing, speech changes, increased fatigue, irritability, personality changes, headache, delirium, memory loss, confusion, decreased appetite, diminished activity, sensory changes, nausea/vomiting, urinary incontinence, behavioral changes, tinnitus or another hearing disturbance, syncope, vertigo, and blurred vision. Signs include motor weakness, sensory loss, seizures, anisocoria, papilledema, diplopia, other focal neurological deficits, parkinsonism, lethargy, and coma [3, 7, 13, 16, 21, 28, 31, 42, 44, 56, 58, 59, 66]. Age-related differences in clinical signs and symptoms may be seen (Table 9.1). Significant heterogeneity in presenting complaints, as well as in the reporting of additional signs or symptoms, stymies a detailed cross-study assessment of the clinical presentation of these patients [8]. Despite this, careful review of the literature still reveals commonalities in the presentation of these patients which are described below.

9.2.1 *Headache*

Headache is one of the most common presenting symptoms of patients with CSDHs. In most studies, headaches are noted as occurring in anywhere from 25 to 90% of patients [7, 28, 31, 42, 46, 58]. However, Adhiyaman's study from North Wales in 2017 reports no headaches in his group of 66 patients [3].

The etiology of headache in this population may vary. A commonly cited etiology is elevated intracranial pressure [36, 39, 58]. Induced stretch of the meningeal arteries and veins has also been suggested as an etiology for headaches in these patients [66]. Lastly, although less common, orthostatic headaches in the setting of intracranial hypotension have been clearly described [48, 59, 66], and a thorough history and examination will elucidate these headaches.

Yamada et al. retrospectively assessed 1080 patients with CSDHs who had been treated surgically. Headache was present in 22.6%. Notably, headache in this series

Table 9.1 Age-related differences in the clinical presentation of chronic subdural hematomas

Younger patients	Elderly patients
Common symptoms: Headache, nausea, vomiting	Common symptoms: Confusion, cognitive changes, motor deficits
Lower frequency of bilateral cSDH	Higher frequency of bilateral cSDH
Decreased thickness of cSDH	Increased thickness of cSDH
Increased male:female ratio	Decreased male:female ratio

cSDH chronic subdural hematoma

was found to be significantly associated with younger age at presentation [66], which had been previously noted in other studies [16, 21, 36, 42, 46]. They additionally found that the ratio of midline shift to hematoma thickness was the most influential factor for the presence of headache. Manometry was used to measure intra-hematoma pressure in a subset of these patients and was not found to be associated with headache [66]. These findings may support the rationale that headache in chronic subdural patients is due to stretch of pain-sensitive vasculature; however, the intra-hematoma pressure may not be reflective of the overall intracranial pressure.

9.2.2 *Gait Disturbance*

Altered gait is a frequent complaint in the patient presenting with a CSDH. This may also be associated with a history of recurrent falls. Several studies have reported that a history of falls may be a presenting complaint in up to 2/3 of patients [3, 46]. Other studies have reported similar percentages in patients for whom a fall was determined to be the etiology of a CSDH. However, it may be that these falls reported in the literature were instead the manifestation of an already present hematoma [3]. Gait disturbance may also be correlated with the presence of motor deficits on examination.

9.2.3 *Nausea/Vomiting*

Nausea or vomiting is another symptom that patients with CSDHs may describe. In these patients, the presence of nausea and vomiting is concerning for elevated intracranial pressure. In several large series, increased intracranial pressure was noted to be present in approximately 3.0–12.5% of patients [42, 46, 64, 66]. Nausea and vomiting are more likely to be seen in younger patients. These findings, combined with the propensity of younger patients to present with headaches, suggest that younger patients are more likely to present with symptoms of elevated intracranial pressure [36, 39].

9.2.4 *Behavioral Disturbance*

Behavioral changes, which may include increased irritability, increased fatigue, personality or intellectual changes, have been noted in 24.8–35% of patients [7, 42, 58]. Gelabert et al. in a review of 1000 patients found that behavioral changes were the most frequent complaint in the elderly population, defined in that study as >70 years old [21].

9.2.5 *Altered Consciousness*

Confusion, disorientation, and worsening dementia are all frequently seen in patients presenting with CSDHs. Rates in the literature range from 17 to 70% of patients and are more commonly seen in elderly patients [3, 28, 31, 46, 66].

Less commonly seen than mild alterations in mental status, a depressed level of consciousness, which includes patients comatose on presentation, can be seen. Rates of depressed consciousness on presentation range from 10.9 to 28.8% [7, 28, 42, 46, 66]. However, in part, this range reflects the imprecision in the terminology used in the literature with some studies reporting depressed consciousness without further definition. Rates of coma, when reported, range from 2.5 to 12.6% across multiple cases series [19, 21, 31, 42, 46].

Unsurprisingly, mental status on admission has been found to be an important predictor of outcome, with decreased mental status being associated with poor outcomes [21, 44, 52]. This has also been found to be associated with long-term excess mortality rates in this population [50].

9.2.6 *Motor Deficits*

One of the predominant clinical signs noted in patients with CSDHs is the presence of motor weakness on examination. As a symptom, patients may describe weakness, clumsiness, and/or imbalance which may all correlate with this physical finding. The presence of a contralateral motor deficit is quite common in these patients and has been reported in anywhere from 40.3 to 60.6% of patients upon presentation [5, 28, 42, 46, 66]. In most patients, a contralateral hemiparesis with the contralateral arm and leg both being affected is seen. However, a motor deficit where leg paresis is significantly greater than the arm weakness or contralateral lower extremity weakness in the absence of an upper extremity weakness may also be seen. This is particularly true in patients presenting with interhemispheric CSDHs due to the proximity of the hematoma to the paracentral lobule [17, 55]. Contralateral upper extremity monoparesis may be seen. Furthermore, case reports exist of CSDHs presenting with motor weakness localized to the contralateral hand or foot only which may be confused with a peripheral neuropathy on initial presentation [30, 63]. Rarely, patients may present with paraparesis or quadriparesis as well [24, 28, 33, 35].

9.2.7 *Seizures*

Acute seizures are a less common, but serious, clinical event associated with CSDH. In several case series of clinical presentations of CSDHs, the reported incidence of seizures is markedly variable, ranging from 0.4 to 42% [12, 21, 31, 32, 42, 46, 53, 58, 64, 66]. In part, the variability of the described incidence may be due to underdiagnosis. In many studies, electroencephalogram (EEG) studies were not done routinely for CSDH patients and instead were ordered based on the clinicians' index of suspicion. In up to 2% of cases, patients may present in status epilepticus. In a recent case series of 375 patients by Won et al., both a Glasgow coma score (GCS) of ≤13 and a history of a remote stroke were found to be independent predictors of acute seizures in these patients [64].

9.3 Patient Demographics

9.3.1 Gender

CSDHs are more commonly seen in the male population. This observed gender predilection has been noted across numerous studies worldwide with the ratio of males to females diagnosed with CSDHs ranging from 1.7 to 4.4 depending on the case series [6, 9, 14–16, 19, 21, 28, 31, 38, 42, 46, 47, 51, 58, 66]. A male preponderance has been also noted in low and lower-middle income countries (LMICs) [31, 43]. Some studies have further analyzed gender predilection as a function of age. These studies suggest that the ratio of male to female patients decreases with increasing age [16, 28, 38, 62, 66]. Indeed, in a cases series of 1080 patients, the cohort of patients >90 years old showed that the number of female patients exceeded the number of male patients [66]. It has been suggested that part of the change in the observed male:female ratio stems from the etiology of the CSDH; younger patients (<65 years old) are more likely to develop a CSDH as a result of trauma and males are also more likely to have a reported history of trauma [31, 58]. However, in the elderly population, the index trauma is often a minor trauma, typically a fall [31, 42, 44], and in approximately 1/3 of cases, no inciting event or underlying etiology is noted [44]. Therefore, this is unlikely to fully account for the observed increase of the proportion of females with cSDH by increasing decade in the elderly population. Instead, it has been suggested that this reflects the known higher life expectancy of females [20, 21].

9.3.2 Age

While CSDHs can occur in all ages from neonates [18, 37, 49] to the very elderly [22, 66], the overwhelming majority of patients who present with CSDHs are elderly. The age at presentation varies globally with higher average ages at presentation reported in data from upper-middle income or upper income countries. Indeed, some studies from these regions have estimated that the elderly represent upwards of 90% of all patients with CSDH, with an average age of onset ranging from 62.9 to 83.8 years old [19, 21, 26, 42, 62]. Data from LMICs, countries whose economies with ≤$4045 gross national income per capita per The World Bank Group [23], have shown a younger average age of presentation [1, 13, 31]. However, as the average age of the population increases in these countries, the overall age at presentation is also increasing [43], mimicking the pattern already noted in more developed countries [62].

The association of age with CSDHs is multifactorial. First, as the cerebral parenchyma atrophies with age, the dural cell border layer and the bridging veins traversing it are put under stretch. In this setting, the stretched bridging veins are highly susceptible to minor trauma which may create venous tears [2, 9, 34, 54, 56, 67]. This leads to acute bleeding in this layer—the now actualized subdural space—which may over time become a chronic subdural hematoma. Supporting this, volumetric analyses of computed tomography (CT) brain scans of patients with cSDHs compared to age-matched controls have shown positive association between cerebral atrophy and presentation with CSDHs [27, 68], although Ju et al. suggest that this is an indirect marker of the subdural volume which is more predictive [27]. Secondly, the incidence of falls and minor head traumas increase with increasing age [52, 57, 58]. Thirdly, increasing age is also associated with an increasing use of anti-platelet agents or anti-coagulants, thus increasing this population's risk for hemorrhage [52, 57].

9.4 Imaging

CSDHs are extra-axial fluid collections, located between the arachnoid mater and the dura mater, which may be enclosed in a hematoma capsule [40]. They are most commonly diagnosed via non-contrasted CT images of the brain. On CT scans, cSDHs are typically seen as a concave or crescent-shaped extra-axial lesion, which may cross suture lines [57, 65]; rarely, they may be convex in appearance, mimicking an epidural hematoma [4, 65]. The CSDH will appear hypo- or isodense relative to the brain parenchyma [44, 57, 65]. Rarely, calcified CSDHs may be seen [61]. Although an uncommon cause of chronic subdural hematomas, contrasted CT imaging may help detect primary or metastatic dural-based neoplasms [10, 65].

Magnetic resonance imaging of the brain is less commonly indicated in these patients. When performed, CSDHs are seen as extra-axial areas of iso- or hyperintensity on T1-weighted or fluid-attenuated inversion recovery (FLAIR) images. MRI imaging may be useful in the detection of subdural membranes and intrahematoma loculations, and more sensitive at detecting small bilateral iso-dense hematomas or small amounts of acute hemorrhage [56, 65]. Contrasted MRI sequences may be useful in the evaluation of suspected intracranial hypotension to assess for pachymeningeal enhancement [11, 59] or to evaluate for primary or metastatic dural-based neoplasms. Both contrasted MRI sequences and diffusion weighted images (DWI) may be useful in the diagnosis of infected subdural hematomas [65].

9.4.1 Localization

The vast majority of CSDHs are located along the convexity of the cerebral hemispheres, although a myriad of other locations have also been described including falcine [17, 55], spinal [25, 41], and posterior fossa [45, 60]. The convexity CSDHs can be unilateral (left or right) or bilateral. There is a tendency towards presentation with a left-sided CSDH in the literature which has been noted in several case series [14, 39, 42, 46, 66]. There have been a few theories proposed to explain this observation. One hypothesis is that right-sided CSDHs are diagnosed less frequently than left, but the true incidence is likely equal [39]. Others have suggested that this tendency is due to asymmetries in cranial morphology [29, 34].

Bilateral CSDHs also occur but are less common than unilateral CSDHs. Anywhere from 9.7 to 34.8% of patients presenting with CSDHs have been found to have bilateral hematomas [7, 14, 42, 46, 62, 66]. Several studies have found that bilateral subdural hematomas are more likely to be seen in elderly patients [6, 46, 62]. This is thought to be due to the presence of cerebral atrophy which causes increased traction on the bridging veins over both hemispheres.

9.4.2 Size

The thickness of CSDHs on imaging studies has been shown to be associated with both increasing age [16, 36, 66] and the presence of bilateral subdural hematomas [46]. It is likely that this association is reflective of the underlying cerebral atrophy of the brain parenchyma. As noted previously, cerebral atrophy is directly associated with age and has itself been linked with the presence of bilateral CSDHs. If then, there is underlying cerebral atrophy, it may take a larger hematoma to cause enough mass effect to produce symptoms triggering a patient's presentation.

9.5 Conclusion

The incidence of CSDHs has been progressively climbing worldwide; thus an awareness of the clinical presentation of CSDHs is of increasing importance. Younger patients are more likely to present with signs and symptoms of elevated intracranial pressure. Older patients typically display cognitive changes and focal deficits, predominantly motor weakness, on presentation. Most patients with CSDHs are elderly, and the development of CSDHs in this population is associated with cerebral atrophy, as are hematoma size and the presence of bilateral hematomas. Clinician familiarity with the presentation of CSDHs is essential to ensure timely diagnosis and management of these lesions to mitigate the morbidity and mortality rates in these patients.

References

1. Adeolu AA, Rabiu TB, Adeleye AO. Post-operative day two versus day seven mobilization after burr-hole drainage of subacute and chronic subdural haematoma in Nigerians. Br J Neurosurg. 2012;26:743–6.
2. Adhiyaman V, Chatterjee I. Increasing incidence of chronic subdural haematoma in the elderly. QJM. 2017;110:775.
3. Adhiyaman V, Chattopadhyay I, Irshad F, Curran D, Abraham S. Increasing incidence of chronic subdural haematoma in the elderly. QJM. 2017;110:375–8.
4. Agrawal A. Bilateral biconvex frontal chronic subdural hematoma mimicking extradural hematoma. J Surg Tech Case Rep. 2010;2:90–1.
5. Akakin A, Yilmaz B, Ekşi M, Özcan-Ekşi EE, Demir MK, Toktaş ZO, Konya D. Recurrent cranial chronic subdural hematoma due to cervical cerebrospinal fluid fistula: repair of both entities in the same session. J Craniofac Surg. 2016;27:e578–80.
6. Baechli H, Nordmann A, Bucher HC, Gratzl O. Demographics and prevalent risk factors of chronic subdural haematoma: results of a large single-center cohort study. Neurosurg Rev. 2004;27:263–6.
7. Cameron MM. Chronic subdural haematoma: a review of 114 cases. J Neurol Neurosurg Psychiatry. 1978;41:834–9.
8. Chari A, Hocking KC, Edlmann E, Turner C, Santarius T, Hutchinson PJ, Kolias AG. Core outcomes and common data elements in chronic subdural hematoma: a systematic review of the literature focusing on baseline and peri-operative care data elements. J Neurotrauma. 2016;33:1569–75.
9. Chen JC, Levy ML. Causes, epidemiology, and risk factors of chronic subdural hematoma. Neurosurg Clin N Am. 2000;11:399–406.
10. Cheng YK, Wang TC, Yang JT, Lee MH, Su CH. Dural metastasis from prostatic adenocarcinoma mimicking chronic subdural hematoma. J Clin Neurosci. 2009;16:1084–6.
11. Chung SJ, Kim JS, Lee MC. Syndrome of cerebral spinal fluid hypovolemia: clinical and imaging features and outcome. Neurology. 2000;55:1321–7.
12. Cole M, Spatz E. Seizures in chronic subdural hematoma. N Engl J Med. 1961;265:628–31.
13. Dakurah TK, Iddrissu M, Wepeba G, Nuamah I. Chronic subdural haematoma: review of 96 cases attending the Korle Bu Teaching Hospital, Accra. West Afr J Med. 2005;24:283–6.
14. de Araújo Silva DO, Matis GK, Costa LF, Kitamura MA, de Carvalho Junior EV, de Moura Silva M, Barbosa BJ, Pereira CU, da Silva JC, Birbilis TA, de Azevedo Filho HR. Chronic subdural hematomas and the elderly: surgical results from a series of 125 cases: old "horses" are not to be shot! Surg Neurol Int. 2012;3:150.
15. Ernestus RI, Beldzinski P, Lanfermann H, Klug N. Chronic subdural hematoma: surgical treatment and outcome in 104 patients. Surg Neurol. 1997;48:220–5.
16. Fogelholm R, Heiskanen O, Waltimo O. Chronic subdural hematoma in adults. Influence of patient's age on symptoms, signs, and thickness of hematoma. J Neurosurg. 1975;42:43–6.
17. Fruin AH, Juhl GL, Taylon C. Interhemispheric subdural hematoma. Case report. J Neurosurg. 1984;60:1300–2.
18. Gabaeff SC. Investigating the possibility and probability of perinatal subdural hematoma progressing to chronic subdural hematoma, with and without complications, in neonates, and its potential relationship to the misdiagnosis of abusive head trauma. Leg Med (Tokyo). 2013;15:177–92.
19. Gastone P, Fabrizia C, Homere M, Cacciola F, Alberto M, Nicola DL. Chronic subdural hematoma: results of a homogeneous series of 159 patients operated on by residents. Neurol India. 2004;52:475–7.
20. Gelabert-González M, Fernández-Villa JM, López-García E, García-Allut A. [Chronic subdural hematoma in patients over 80 years of age]. Neurocirugia (Astur). 2001;12:325–30.

21. Gelabert-González M, Iglesias-Pais M, García-Allut A, Martínez-Rumbo R. Chronic subdural haematoma: surgical treatment and outcome in 1000 cases. Clin Neurol Neurosurg. 2005;107:223–9.
22. Gelabert-González M, Román-Pena P, Arán-Echabe E. Chronic subdural hematoma in the oldest-old population. Neurosurg Rev. 2018;41:983–4.
23. Group TWB. World Bank Country and Lending Groups. 2020. Accessed 28 Dec 2020.
24. Herath H, Matthias AT, Kulatunga A. Acute on chronic bilateral subdural hematoma presenting with acute complete flaccid paraplegia and urinary retention mimicking an acute spinal cord injury: a case report. BMC Res Notes. 2017;10:627.
25. Ichinose D, Tochigi S, Tanaka T, Suzuki T, Takei J, Hatano K, Kajiwara I, Maruyama F, Sakamoto H, Hasegawa Y, Tani S, Murayama Y. Concomitant intracranial and lumbar chronic subdural hematoma treated by fluoroscopic guided lumbar puncture: a case report and literature review. Neurol Med Chir (Tokyo). 2018;58:178–84.
26. Jones S, Kafetz K. A prospective study of chronic subdural haematomas in elderly patients. Age Ageing. 1999;28:519–21.
27. Ju MW, Kim SH, Kwon HJ, Choi SW, Koh HS, Youm JY, Song SH. Comparison between brain atrophy and subdural volume to predict chronic subdural hematoma: volumetric CT imaging analysis. Korean J Neurotrauma. 2015;11:87–92.
28. Kak VK, Gleadhill CA. Chronic subdural haematoma (a review of 66 cases). Ulster Med J. 1971;40:163–8.
29. Kim BG, Lee KS, Shim JJ, Yoon SM, Doh JW, Bae HG. What determines the laterality of the chronic subdural hematoma? J Korean Neurosurg Soc. 2010;47:424–7.
30. Kim HI, Oh YJ, Cho YN, Choi YC. Subdural hemorrhage mimicking peripheral neuropathy. J Korean Neurosurg Soc. 2014;56:166–7.
31. Kitya D, Punchak M, Abdelgadir J, Obiga O, Harborne D, Haglund MM. Causes, clinical presentation, management, and outcomes of chronic subdural hematoma at Mbarara Regional Referral Hospital. Neurosurg Focus. 2018;45:E7.
32. Kotwica Z, Brzeiński J. Epilepsy in chronic subdural haematoma. Acta Neurochir (Wien). 1991;113:118–20.
33. Kumar AS, Alugolu R. Chronic subdural hematoma presenting as diplegia—a rare presentation. J Neurosci Rural Pract. 2014;5:445–6.
34. Lee KS. Chronic subdural hematoma in the aged, trauma or degeneration? J Korean Neurosurg Soc. 2016;59:1–5.
35. Lesoin F, Destee A, Jomin M, Warot P, Wilson SG. Quadriparesis as an unusual manifestation of chronic subdural haematoma. J Neurol Neurosurg Psychiatry. 1983;46:783–5.
36. Liliang PC, Tsai YD, Liang CL, Lee TC, Chen HJ. Chronic subdural haematoma in young and extremely aged adults: a comparative study of two age groups. Injury. 2002;33:345–8.
37. Lin CL, Hwang SL, Su YF, Tsai LC, Kwan AL, Howng SL, Loh JK. External subdural drainage in the treatment of infantile chronic subdural hematoma. J Trauma. 2004;57:104–7.
38. Luxon LM, Harrison MJ. Chronic subdural haematoma. Q J Med. 1979;48:43–53.
39. MacFarlane MR, Weerakkody Y, Kathiravel Y. Chronic subdural haematomas are more common on the left than on the right. J Clin Neurosci. 2009;16:642–4.
40. Markwalder TM. Chronic subdural hematomas: a review. J Neurosurg. 1981;54:637–45.
41. Matsumoto H, Matsumoto S, Yoshida Y. Concomitant intracranial chronic subdural hematoma and spinal subdural hematoma: a case report and literature review. World Neurosurg. 2016;90:706.e1–9.
42. Mekaj AY, Morina AA, Mekaj YH, Manxhuka-Kerliu S, Miftari EI, Duci SB, Hamza AR, Gashi MM, Xhelaj MR, Kelmendi FM, Morina Q. Surgical treatment of 137 cases with chronic subdural hematoma at the university clinical center of Kosovo during the period 2008-2012. J Neurosci Rural Pract. 2015;6:186–90.
43. Mezue WC, Ohaebgulam SC, Chikani MC, Erechukwu AU. Changing trends in chronic subdural haematoma in Nigeria. Afr J Med Med Sci. 2011;40:373–6.

44. Miranda LB, Braxton E, Hobbs J, Quigley MR. Chronic subdural hematoma in the elderly: not a benign disease. J Neurosurg. 2011;114:72–6.
45. Mochizuki Y, Kobayashi T, Kawashima A, Funatsu T, Kawamata T. Chronic subdural hematoma of the posterior fossa treated by suboccipital craniotomy. Surg Neurol Int. 2018;9:20.
46. Mori K, Maeda M. Surgical treatment of chronic subdural hematoma in 500 consecutive cases: clinical characteristics, surgical outcome, complications, and recurrence rate. Neurol Med Chir (Tokyo). 2001;41:371–81.
47. Nakaguchi H, Tanishima T, Yoshimasu N. Factors in the natural history of chronic subdural hematomas that influence their postoperative recurrence. J Neurosurg. 2001;95:256–62.
48. Osada Y, Shibahara I, Nakagawa A, Sakata H, Niizuma K, Saito R, Kanamori M, Fujimura M, Suzuki S, Tominaga T. Unilateral chronic subdural hematoma due to spontaneous intracranial hypotension: a report of four cases. Br J Neurosurg. 2020;34:632–7.
49. Powers CJ, Fuchs HE, George TM. Chronic subdural hematoma of the neonate: report of two cases and literature review. Pediatr Neurosurg. 2007;43:25–8.
50. Rauhala M, Helén P, Seppä K, Huhtala H, Iverson GL, Niskakangas T, Öhman J, Luoto TM. Long-term excess mortality after chronic subdural hematoma. Acta Neurochir (Wien). 2020;162:1467–78.
51. Robinson RG. Chronic subdural hematoma: surgical management in 133 patients. J Neurosurg. 1984;61:263–8.
52. Rozzelle CJ, Wofford JL, Branch CL. Predictors of hospital mortality in older patients with subdural hematoma. J Am Geriatr Soc. 1995;43:240–4.
53. Rubin G, Rappaport ZH. Epilepsy in chronic subdural haematoma. Acta Neurochir (Wien). 1993;123:39–42.
54. Santarius T, Kirkpatrick PJ, Kolias AG, Hutchinson PJ. Working toward rational and evidence-based treatment of chronic subdural hematoma. Clin Neurosurg. 2010;57:112–22.
55. Schilder JC, Weisfelt M. Ataxia associated with an interhemispheric subdural hematoma: a case report. Cases J. 2009;2:8876.
56. Soleman J, Nocera F, Mariani L. The conservative and pharmacological management of chronic subdural haematoma. Swiss Med Wkly. 2017;147:w14398.
57. Soleman J, Taussky P, Fandino J, Muroi C. Evidence based treatment of chronic subdural hematoma. In: Sadaka DF, editor. Traumatic brain injury. InTechOpen; 2014.
58. Sousa EB, Brandão LF, Tavares CB, Borges IB, Neto NG, Kessler IM. Epidemiological characteristics of 778 patients who underwent surgical drainage of chronic subdural hematomas in Brasília, Brazil. BMC Surg. 2013;13:5.
59. Takahashi K, Mima T, Akiba Y. Chronic subdural hematoma associated with spontaneous intracranial hypotension: therapeutic strategies and outcomes of 55 cases. Neurol Med Chir (Tokyo). 2016;56:69–76.
60. Takemoto Y, Matsumoto J, Ohta K, Hasegawa S, Miura M, Kuratsu J. Bilateral posterior fossa chronic subdural hematoma treated with craniectomy: case report and review of the literature. Surg Neurol Int. 2016;7:S255–8.
61. Turgut M, Akhaddar A, Turgut AT. Calcified or ossified chronic subdural hematoma: a systematic review of 114 cases reported during last century with a demonstrative case report. World Neurosurg. 2020;134:240–63.
62. Uno M, Toi H, Hirai S. Chronic subdural hematoma in elderly patients: is this disease benign? Neurol Med Chir (Tokyo). 2017;57:402–9.
63. Weisberg SD, Houten JK. An unusual presentation of chronic subdural hematoma with isolated footdrop. World Neurosurg. 2019;121:166–8.
64. Won SY, Dubinski D, Sautter L, Hattingen E, Seifert V, Rosenow F, Freiman T, Strzelczyk A, Konczalla J. Seizure and status epilepticus in chronic subdural hematoma. Acta Neurol Scand. 2019;140:194–203.
65. Yadav YR, Parihar V, Namdev H, Bajaj J. Chronic subdural hematoma. Asian J Neurosurg. 2016;11:330–42.

66. Yamada SM, Tomita Y, Murakami H, Nakane M, Yamada S, Murakami M, Hoya K, Nakagomi T, Tamura A, Matsuno A. Headache in patients with chronic subdural hematoma: analysis in 1080 patients. Neurosurg Rev. 2018;41:549–56.
67. Yamashima T, Friede RL. Why do bridging veins rupture into the virtual subdural space? J Neurol Neurosurg Psychiatry. 1984;47:121–7.
68. Yang AI, Balser DS, Mikheev A, Offen S, Huang JH, Babb J, Rusinek H, Samadani U. Cerebral atrophy is associated with development of chronic subdural haematoma. Brain Inj. 2012;26:1731–6.
69. Yang W, Huang J. Chronic subdural hematoma: epidemiology and natural history. Neurosurg Clin N Am. 2017;28:205–10.

Chapter 10
Seizures in Chronic Subdural Hematoma

Amal Satté and Jamal Mounach

10.1 Introduction

Even though seizures are a known complication of chronic subdural hematoma (CSDH), several aspects of this condition remain a matter of debate, beginning with the definition, classification, and pathophysiology, and including the diagnostic criteria and management. The first classification of seizure and epilepsy types was proposed by Gatsaut in 1969. Over the years, the definitions of seizures and epilepsy and their classifications have evolved. Multiple revisions have been made by the International League against Epilepsy (ILAE), taking into account the clinical, electroencephalography (EEG), imaging, and genetic findings. An epileptic seizure is defined as a transient occurrence of signs and/or symptoms due to abnormal excessive or synchronous neuronal activity in the brain [13].

Previously, epilepsy was defined as a disorder characterized by the occurrence of at least two unprovoked seizures, more than 24 h apart [13]. The ILAE and the International Bureau for Epilepsy (IBE) have recently agreed that epilepsy is best considered to be a disease rather than a disorder. The revised practical definition implies that the epilepsy can be diagnosed in the following conditions: (1) at least two unprovoked or reflex seizures occurring >24 h apart; (2) one unprovoked or reflex seizure with a probability of at least 60% of having another seizure within the next 10 years; and (3) diagnosis of an epilepsy syndrome.

Provoked seizures are caused by a transient factor acting on a normal brain to temporarily lower the seizure threshold. Examples of this are hypoglycemia, hyperglycemia, and alcohol or drug abuse.

A. Satté (✉) · J. Mounach
Department of Neurophysiology, Mohammed V Teaching Military Hospital, Mohammed V University in Rabat, Rabat, Morocco

M. Turgut et al. (eds.), *Subdural Hematoma*,
https://doi.org/10.1007/978-3-030-79371-5_10

The term "unprovoked" means the absence of a transient provocative factor producing a seizure at that point of time [11, 12].

Acute symptomatic seizures result from acute brain processes like trauma, encephalitis, and stroke. Some authors group acute symptomatic seizures with provoked seizures as they both have a low risk of subsequent seizures. However, unlike provoked seizures, acute symptomatic seizures can cause cerebral changes which can lead to remote symptomatic seizures [7, 16].

In the setting of CSDH, seizures should be classified as either acute or remote symptomatic seizures. Acute symptomatic seizures are defined as a clinical seizure occurring at the time of a systemic insult or in close temporal association with a documented brain insult. Seizures are considered acute symptomatic if they occur within the first 7 days of an insult [5, 6, 25]. In CSDH, close temporal relationship was defined as within 1 week of the initial clinical diagnosis of CSDH or recurrence of the hematoma [48]. Remote symptomatic seizures occur in the absence of an acute precipitating factor (i.e., they are unprovoked seizures) but with evidence of a past static injury [25]. In CSDH, they are defined after 1 week of the clinical diagnosis of CSDH without an associated hematoma recurrence or any other acute brain injury [48].

It is important to note that most of the studies dealing with CSDH did not distinguish between early and remote or late symptomatic seizures [49]. Larger studies differentiating the two types of seizures are required to better understand risk factors, clinical features, and prognosis.

10.2 Epidemiology of Seizures in Chronic Subdural Hematoma

The incidence of acute symptomatic seizures in CSDH ranges between 2 and 42%. This incidence is overall lower than that in acute subdural hematoma (SDH) [26, 49]. Clinical risk factors for posttraumatic seizures include alcohol abuse, previous stroke, change in mental status, low Glasgow Coma Scale at presentation, and mean Glasgow outcome scale by discharge. Radiological risk factors include brain atrophy and mixed density SDH. Patients treated with open craniotomy were also more at risk for developing seizures, especially late symptomatic seizures. Older age, the degree of midline shift, and hematoma size were not predictors of seizures [17, 39, 49].

10.3 Pathophysiology

There are several mechanisms underlying CSDH symptomatic seizures. One of the mechanisms proposed is the direct cortical irritation caused by mass effect, which could also reduce the regional blood flow [21, 39]. On the other hand, fibrinogen degradation products result in membrane formation and irritation of the cortex [49].

However, patients who underwent capsulotomy were more prone to present with seizures than those who underwent burr-hole drainage. This suggests a possible role for gliosis caused either by the SDH or the surgical technique. Mixed density subdural hematoma could be associated to more mass effect and increasing fibrinogen degradation products, which consequently contribute to cortical irritation and hyperexcitability [39, 49]. Finally, associated brain lesions could probably play an important role. These can be either coexisting brain injuries such as cerebral contusions or preexisting lesions caused by stroke, alcohol abuse, or brain atrophy [39, 49].

10.4 Seizure Types

The 2017 ILAE classification of seizures differentiates between focal, generalized, and undetermined onset of seizures [12]. Unfortunately, most of the studies dealing with cSDH did not describe the types of seizures. As CSDH is responsible for regional irritation, it is expected to cause focal rather than generalized seizures. The limited data describing clinical features show that only 20–40% of seizures are focal and 60–80% are generalized [8, 17]. However these studies did not specify whether seizures were really generalized or focal with impaired awareness (formally called secondary generalized) [39]. Focal seizures reported are either Jacksonian march motor or sensory seizures. Ictal speech disorders like aphasia, paraphasia, or word finding difficulty remain rare in CSDH [2]. Levin reported a case of a patient with chronic bilateral subdural hematomas that presented with ictal automatisms that was originally misdiagnosed with a functional neurological disorder [40]. Status epilepticus (SE) is less frequent but is consistently associated with a poor outcome [38, 48]. In a study over 23 years of more than 1,583,255 admissions with a diagnosis of SDH, the prevalence of SE was 0.5%. Seifi showed in this study that the mortality was higher among older patients, blacks, and in those with respiratory, metabolic, hematological, and renal system dysfunction [38]. Nonconvulsive status epilepticus revealed by a decreased level of consciousness or focal deficits were also reported [10]. Symptoms are typically out of proportion to imaging findings, and may go underdiagnosed, which highlights the important role of electroencephalography.

10.5 EEG Findings in cSDH

Very few studies describe the EEG findings in CSDH. With the advent and development of imaging techniques, EEG lost its place for establishing a positive diagnosis of CSDH. However, it remains an important tool that provides valuable information for the management of patients with cSDH. SDHs lead to an increase in the distance between the cortex and the recording electrode, resulting in reduced amplitude as compared with the opposite hemisphere. On the other hand, SDHs act like a filter for fast activities which results in slowing and disruption or disappearance of posterior dominant rhythm. Bilateral diffuse slowing is the most often encountered EEG abnormality in CSDH and is typically more prominent in the hemisphere involved with the hematoma [19]. Slowing and attenuation are classical but not specific signs of SDHs. They can also result from scalp edema, meningiomas, infarcts, hygromas, and postictal effect [23] (Figs. 10.1 and 10.2).

Periodic Lateralized Epileptiform Discharges (PLEDs) or Lateralized Periodic Discharges (LPDs) have also been reported in CSDH and can be observed either before or after evacuation of the hematoma [35, 44]. This pattern consists of periodic or quasiperiodic spikes or sharp waves that occur at 1- to 3-s intervals. The mechanisms for production of PLEDs are not fully understood. Most of the studies suggest that they are caused by partial functional or anatomic isolation, or deafferentation of the cerebral cortex [44]. They are not always associated with seizures. Therefore, their interpretation can be difficult, but it is vital to distinguish between ictal and non-ictal origin so as to better adjust the treatment. Periodic lateralized discharges are subdivided into PLEDs plus and PLEDs proper. Periodic LEDs plus are characterized by fast rhythms, spikes or polyspikes inside the rhythm and are more often associated with seizures (preictal/ictal) especially if the periodicity is short (1 Hz or more), the amplitude is high, there is fluctuation of the frequency and morphology, and periods of flattening occur. Periodic LEDs proper are less often associated with seizures (6%, versus 74% in PLEDs plus), especially when they are monomorphic, with a long periodicity (0.5 Hz or less), and a low amplitude [14, 31]. Figure 10.3a, b illustrates the reasoning in such situations.

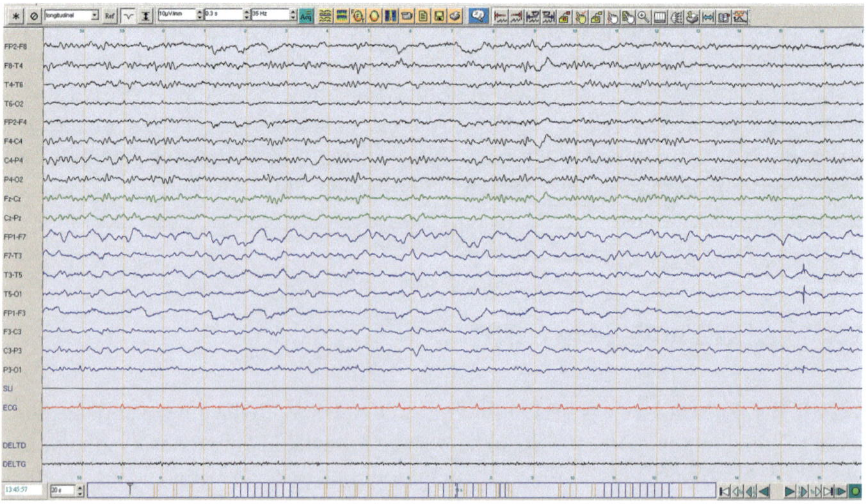

Fig. 10.1 Left hemispheric slowing related to a left cSDH in a 64-year-old woman

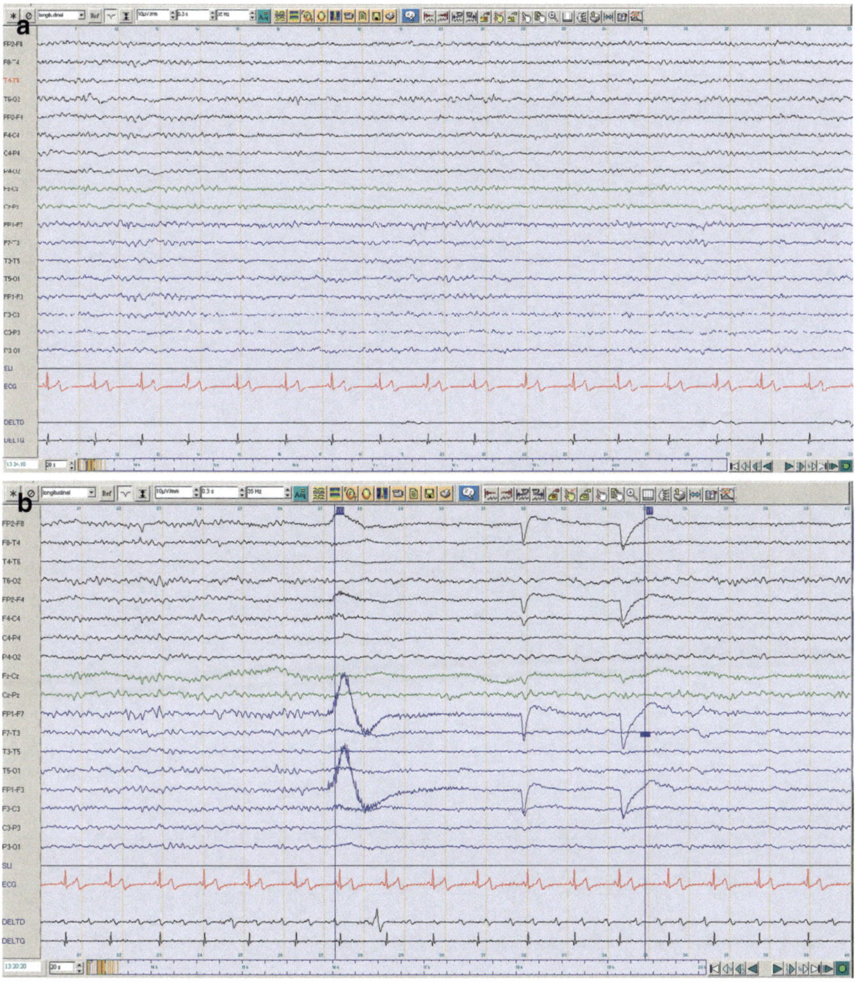

Fig. 10.2 (**a**, **b**) A 58-year-old man with bilateral subdural hematomas who presented with confusion. The EEG shows bilateral diffuse slowing

In patients with PLEDs, longer periods of monitoring provide significant information and may detect subclinical seizures (Fig. 10.4).

Epileptiform discharges are common. They can be lateralized to the side of the SDH or are bilateral. Midline epileptiform discharges can be a sign of midline shift. Contralateral discharges were also reported and can be related to either mass effect, an associated injury, or a prior brain disease [34, 39] (Fig. 10.4).

Focal intermittent rhythmic delta activity (FIRDAs) can be seen with focal potential epileptogenicity [39] (Fig. 10.4).

Status epilepticus is typically characterized by continuous rhythmic activity. However, in some nonconvulsive status epilepticus and subclinical seizures

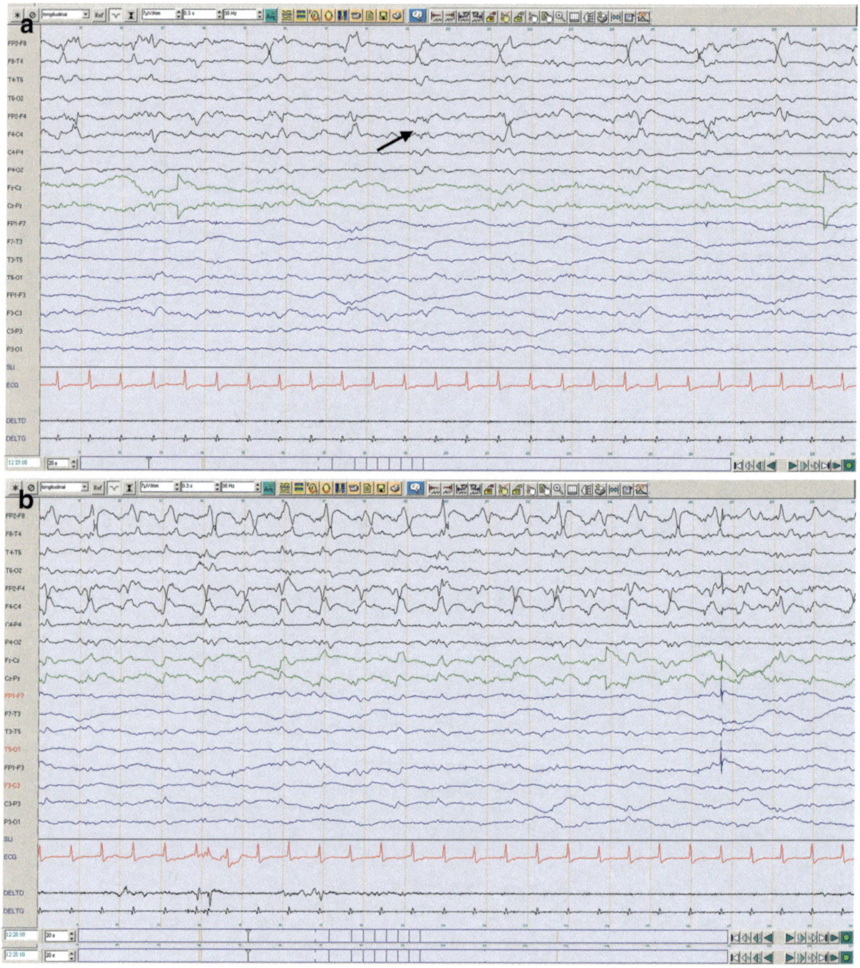

Fig. 10.3 (**a**, **b**) Postoperative prolonged EEG in a 65-year-old patient operated on for a right cSDH who presented with a single brief episode of left-sided clonic movements followed by impaired consciousness. The EEG shows right Periodic Lateralized Epileptiform Discharges that can be classified as PLEDs plus because they are sometimes associated with a fast rhythm inside the complexes (arrow). The periodicity in Fig. 10.3b is 1 Hz, the amplitude is high, there is an obvious fluctuation of the frequency and the morphology between Fig. 10.1a and b. On the other hand, the patient had a seizure. All these features support a pre-ictal/ictal origin that requires urgent treatment to avoid developing status epilepticus

standard EEG may not be suggestive of seizures. In the setting of SDH, especially in comatose patients, it is strongly recommended to incorporate long-term EEG monitoring which allows one to better explore for PLEDs and identify proper seizure activities [3, 10, 19, 38].

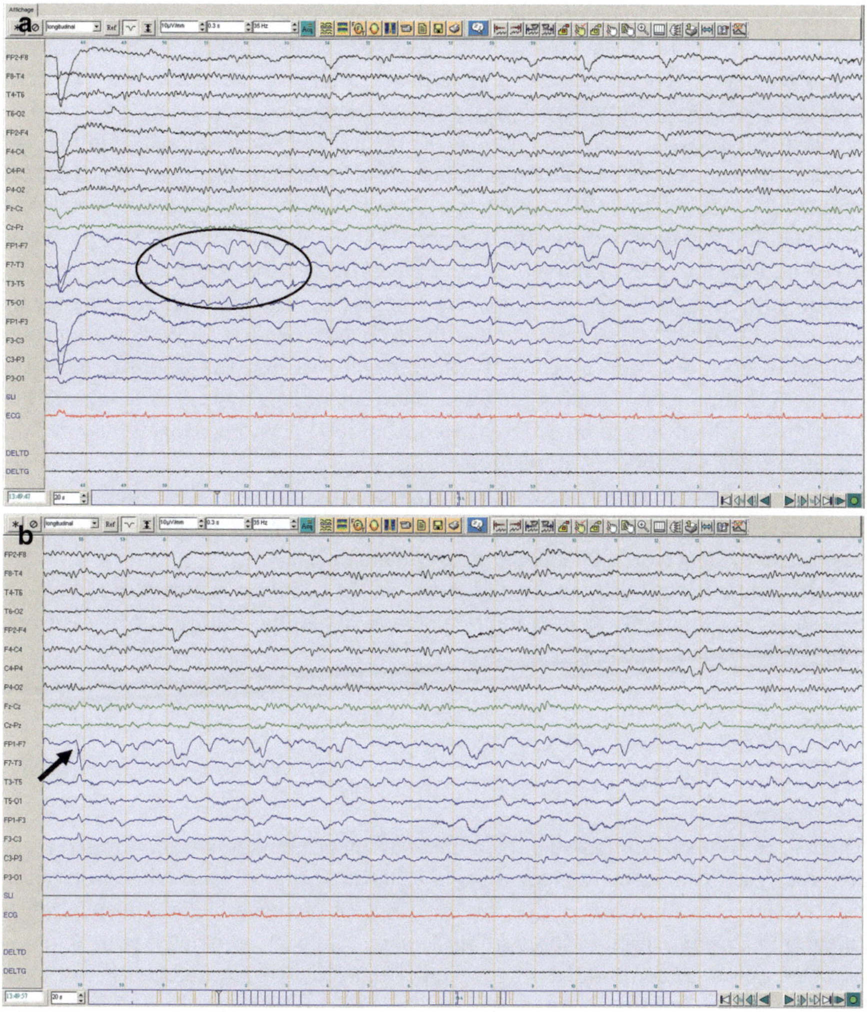

Fig. 10.4 (**a**, **b**) A 48-year-old man who presented with a generalized tonic-clonic seizure and had a left chronic subdural hematoma. The EEG shows left frontal intermittent rhythmic delta activity FIRDA (oval) and spikes on F7 (arrows)

10.6 Differential Diagnosis of Seizures in cSDH

Differential diagnosis of seizures in the setting of CSDH includes all the conditions that may cause transient or fluctuating neurological symptoms. Determining the underlying mechanism of such events can be challenging but is important because many patients will be diagnosed as epileptic despite a negative workup.

Brain injury after SDH may be caused by many factors such as hematoma volume, increased intracranial pressure (ICP), or blood constituents.

Cortical spreading depolarization is a propagating depolarization wave of neurons and glial cells in the cerebral gray matter, followed by the transient suppression of electrical activity [43]. Recently, in a prospective observational study of 40 patients who underwent CSDH evacuation, Mohammad et al. found that cortical spreading depolarization (SD) was detected in 6 patients (15%) and was associated with neurological deterioration after surgery [24]. In another study, Levesque compared clinical and EEG findings in 59 patients with SDH. He found that clonic movements, impaired awareness, positive symptoms, response to antiseizure medication, and mortality were associated with EEG abnormalities while dysphasia and prolonged episodes were associated with a negative EEG. He proposed the term NESIS (NonEpileptic, Stereotypical and Intermittent Symptoms) to designate the latter group which should be differentiated from ictal phenomena as it has specific prognostic and therapeutic implications [22].

Transient ischemia may occur after CSDH and may also cause fluctuating symptoms. EEG monitoring and transcranial doppler sonography can provide additional supportive evidence of a hemodynamic mechanism [1].

Lastly, conditions linked to the disposition of the patient may also cause transient neurological symptoms such as hypoglycemia, hyperglycemia, abrupt alcohol or drug withdrawal during hospitalization.

10.7 Treatment

There is currently no consensual recommendation, nor randomized controlled trials for prophylactic antiseizure medication in CSDH. Arguments for using prophylactic antiseizure medication are that the incidence of preoperative and postoperative seizures in CSDH is high in some studies and that they are associated with an unfavorable clinical outcome and a high mortality rate [15, 46]. Arguments against their use are that the impact of antiseizure medications did not affect the outcome at discharge [42, 47, 48]; in many patients, seizures were well controlled after hematoma removal without the need to give antiseizure medication [33, 50]. On the other hand, using antiseizure medication is not without consequences as most of them have many side effects and drug interactions. A Cochrane review studied the use of prophylactic medication in CSDH. The authors found that no conclusions can be reached from the currently available information. And that randomized controlled trials are required [30]. Until a consensus has been reached, medications should be weighed against the risks associated with these therapies. Clinician must assess each situation, taking into account the risks factors for developing seizures and the patient clinical history and physical examination. Moreover, given the valuable information provided by EEG, we believe that EEG (including preoperative EEG, postoperative EEG and long-term EEG monitoring whenever possible) should be an integral part of the evaluation criteria to decide whether to start treatment or not.

In cases of CSDH, because of the lack of evidence on which antiseizure drug to use and the dosing and duration of the treatment, choices are usually driven by habit or training, rather than by evidence. Currently, phenytoin is widely used for seizure prophylaxis. However, new antiepileptic drugs with less side effects can be used. Several studies have shown that levetiracetam is as effective as phenytoin in patients with TBI and in CSDH [20, 29, 32]. Moreover, unlike levetiracetam, phenytoin requires close monitoring because it has more side effects and causes drug interactions.

In status epilepticus, first-line treatment consists of benzodiazepines while second line antiseizure drugs include intravenous phenytoin, fosphenytoin, valproic acid, phenobarbital, levetiracetam, and lacosamide. Convention in the United States and many other countries leans toward the use of phenytoin or fosphenytoin [27]. However, a recent meta-analysis and cost effectiveness study showed that the available evidence does not support the preeminence of phenytoin, either in terms of effectiveness or in terms of cost-effectiveness. According to the same study, valproates and phenobarbital were more effective and phenobarbital were more effective than phenytoin for status epilepticus [37].

In the elderly, the choice of a drug should be a thoughtful decision that considers not only the diagnosis but also the patient's medical history and the propensity of the drugs for adverse effects and their drug-drug interactions. In a patient with hepatic disease, drugs that are not metabolized in the liver, such as levetiracetam, are preferred. Conversely, in the case of renal failure, carbamazepine or valproates are given. Some new drugs (gabapentin, pregabalin, levetiracetam) do not interact with other medications, hepatic enzymes, and plasma proteins which make them more suitable for patients in this age group [18].

Prophylactic antiseizure treatment duration remains a matter of debate, ranging from 3 months to 2 years unless seizures occur [17, 26, 39, 41, 48]. To clarify these ambiguities controlled clinical studies in these areas are necessary.

Lastly, data regarding the long-term outcome of patients with CSDH acute symptomatic seizures are lacking. For patients who experience seizures several months following the CSDH occurrence, the treatment is similar to that for other forms of symptomatic epilepsy [39].

10.8 Prognosis

Several studies agree that patients with seizures after CSDH have a worse outcome after discharge compared to those without seizures [4, 17, 28, 48, 50]. Seizures are an independent predictor for unfavorable outcome regarding physical, cognitive, and psychosocial reintegration [48]. Though seizures worsen early functional outcome, delayed favorable recovery is possible [17, 28]. Mortality rates are higher in patients with CSDH associated seizures [4, 36].

Specific data regarding long-term seizure control and outcome of patients with SDH are lacking [39]. Patients with acute symptomatic seizures may have delayed ictal manifestations with a trend toward developing epilepsy [17].

Seizures are among the risk factors for recurrence in CSDH with an odds ratio of 2.5 according to Won et al. [9, 45].

EEG findings can be very helpful in predicting functional outcome. Patients with epileptiform discharges on EEG had a poor functional outcome at the time of hospital discharge and at 6 months follow-up [28, 35, 39].

References

1. Alkhachroum AM, Fernandez-Baca Vaca G, Sundararajan S, Degeorgia M. Post-subdural hematoma transient ischemic attacks: hypoperfusion mechanism supported by quantitative electroencephalography and transcranial Doppler sonography. Stroke. 2017;48(3):e87–90.
2. Alliez J-R, Balan C, Kaya J-M, Leone M, Reynier Y, Alliez B. Hématome sous-dural chronique de l'adulte. EMC—Neurol. 2007;4(4):1–9.
3. Banoczi W. ICU-cEEG monitoring. Neurodiagn J. 2020;60(4):231–71.
4. Battaglia F, Lubrano V, Ribeiro-Filho T, Pradel V, Roche PH. Incidence et impact clinique des crises comitiales périopératoires pour les hématomes sous-duraux chroniques. Neurochirurgie. 2012;58(4):230–4.
5. Beghi E, Carpio A, Forsgren L, Hesdorffer DC, Malmgren K, et al. Recommendation for a definition of acute symptomatic seizure. Epilepsia. 2010;51(4):671–5.
6. Beleza P. Acute symptomatic seizures: a clinically oriented review. Neurologist. 2012;18(3):109–19.
7. Bergey GK. Management of a first seizure. Contin Lifelong Learn Neurol. 2016;22:38–50.
8. Chen CW, Kuo JR, Lin HJ, Yeh CH, Wong BS, et al. Early post-operative seizures after burr-hole drainage for chronic subdural hematoma: correlation with brain CT findings. J Clin Neurosci. 2004;11(7):706–9.
9. Chon KH, Lee JM, Koh EJ, Choi HY. Independent predictors for recurrence of chronic subdural hematoma. Acta Neurochir (Wien). 2012;154(9):1541–8.
10. Driver J, DiRisio AC, Mitchell H, Threlkeld ZD, Gormley WB. Non-electrographic seizures due to subdural hematoma: a case series and review of the literature. Neurocrit Care. 2019;30(1):16–21.
11. Fisher RS, Acevedo C, Arzimanoglou A, Bogacz A, Cross JH, et al. ILAE Official Report: a practical clinical definition of epilepsy. Epilepsia. 2014;55(4):475–82.
12. Fisher RS, Cross JH, French JA, Higurashi N, Hirsch E, et al. Operational classification of seizure types by the International League Against Epilepsy: position paper of the ILAE Commission for Classification and Terminology. Epilepsia. 2017;58(4):522–30.
13. Fisher RS, Van Emde Boas W, Blume W, Elger C, Genton P, et al. Response: definitions proposed by the International League Against Epilepsy (ILAE) and the International Bureau for Epilepsy (IBE) [4]. Epilepsia. 2005;46(10):1701–2.
14. Gelisse P, Crespel A, Genton P. Atlas of electroencephalography. In: Neurology and critical care. Montrouge: John Libbey Eurotext; 2019. p. 3346.
15. Grobelny BT, Ducruet AF, Zacharia BE, Hickman ZL, Andersen KN, et al. Preoperative antiepileptic drug administration and the incidence of postoperative seizures following bur hole-treated chronic subdural hematoma: clinical article. J Neurosurg. 2009;111(6):1257–62.
16. Hesdorffer DC, Benn EKT, Cascino GD, Hauser WA. Is a first acute symptomatic seizure epilepsy? Mortality and risk for recurrent seizure. Epilepsia. 2009;50(5):1102–8.
17. Huang YH, Yang TM, Lin YJ, Tsai NW, Lin WC, et al. Risk factors and outcome of seizures after chronic subdural hematoma. Neurocrit Care. 2011;14(2):253–9.
18. Jankovic SM, Dostic M. Choice of antiepileptic drugs for the elderly: possible drug interactions and adverse effects. Expert Opin Metab Toxicol. 2012;8(1):81–91.

19. Kaminski HJ, Hlavin ML, Likavec MJ, Schmidley JW. Transient neurologic deficit caused by chronic subdural hematoma. Am J Med. 1992;92(6):698–700.
20. Khan NR, Vanlandingham MA, Fierst TM, Hymel C, Hoes K, et al. Should levetiracetam or phenytoin be used for posttraumatic seizure prophylaxis? A systematic review of the literature and meta-analysis. Neurosurgery. 2016;79(6):775–81.
21. Kwon TH, Park YK, Lim DJ, Cho TH, Chung YG, et al. Chronic subdural hematoma: evaluation of the clinical significance of postoperative drainage volume. J Neurosurg. 2000;93(5):796–9.
22. Levesque M, Iorio-Morin C, Bocti C, Vézina C, Deacon C. Nonepileptic, stereotypical, and intermittent symptoms (NESIS) in patients with subdural hematoma: proposal for a new clinical entity with therapeutic and prognostic implications. Neurosurgery. 2020;87(1):96–103.
23. Marcuse LV, Fields MC, Yoo J, Rowan AJ. Rowan's primer of EEG. 2nd ed. Elsevier; 2016. p. 87–9.
24. Mohammad LM, Abbas M, Shuttleworth CW, Ahmadian R, Bhat A, et al. Spreading depolarization may represent a novel mechanism for delayed fluctuating neurological deficit after chronic subdural hematoma evacuation. J Neurosurg. 2020;134(3):1294–302.
25. Nowacki TA, Jirsch JD. Evaluation of the first seizure patient: key points in the history and physical examination. Seizure. 2017;49:54–63.
26. Ohno K, Maehara T, Ichimura K, Suzuki R, Hirakawa K, Monma S. Low incidence of seizures in patients with chronic subdural haematoma. J Neurol Neurosurg Psychiatry. 1993;56(11):1231–3.
27. Pichler M, Hocker S. Management of status epilepticus, vol. 140. 1st ed. Elsevier B.V.; 2017. p. 131–51.
28. Rabinstein AA, Chung SY, Rudzinski LA, Lanzino G. Seizures after evacuation of subdural hematomas: incidence, risk factors, and functional impact: clinical article. J Neurosurg. 2010;112(2):455–60.
29. Radic JAE, Chou SHY, Du R, Lee JW. Levetiracetam versus phenytoin: a comparison of efficacy of seizure prophylaxis and adverse event risk following acute or subacute subdural hematoma diagnosis. Neurocrit Care. 2014;21(2):228–37.
30. Ratilal BO, Pappamikail L, Costa J, Sampaio C. Anticonvulsants for preventing seizures in patients with chronic subdural haematoma. Cochrane Database Syst Rev. 2013;2013(6):CD004893.
31. Reiher J, Rivest J, Maison FG, Leduc CP. Periodic lateralized epileptiform discharges with transitional rhythmic discharges: association with seizures. Electroencephalogr Clin Neurophysiol. 1991;78(1):12–7.
32. Rowe AS, Goodwin H, Brophy GM, Bushwitz J, Castle A, et al. Seizure prophylaxis in neurocritical care: a review of evidence-based support. Pharmacotherapy. 2014;34(4):396–409.
33. Rubin G, Rappaport ZH. Epilepsy in chronic subdural haematoma. Acta Neurochir (Wien). 1993;123:39–42.
34. Rudzinski LA, Rabinstein AA. Response to "epileptiform discharges in acute subdural hematoma: to treat or not to treat". J Clin Neurophysiol. 2012;29(3):287.
35. Rudzinski LA, Rabinstein AA, Chung SY, Wong-Kisiel LC, Burrus TM, et al. Electroencephalographic findings in acute subdural hematoma. J Clin Neurophysiol. 2011;28(6):633–41.
36. Sabo RA, Hanigan WC, Aldag JC. Chronic subdural hematomas and seizures: the role of prophylactic anticonvulsive medication. Surg Neurol. 1995;43(6):579–82.
37. Sánchez Fernández I, Gaínza-Lein M, Lamb N, Loddenkemper T. Meta-analysis and cost-effectiveness of second-line antiepileptic drugs for status epilepticus. Neurology. 2019;92(20):E2339–48.
38. Seifi A, Asadi-Pooya AA, Carr K, Maltenfort M, Emami M, et al. The epidemiology, risk factors, and impact on hospital mortality of status epilepticus after subdural hematoma in the United States. Springerplus. 2014;3(1):1–10.

39. Shihabuddin B, Hinduja A, Yaghi S. Seizures in cerebrovascular disorders. In: Koubeissi MZ et al., editors. Seizures in subdural hematoma. Springer science+business media; 2015. p. 55–69.
40. Levin S. Psychomotor epilepsy as a manifestation of subdural hematoma. Am J Psychiatry. 1951;107(7):501–2.
41. Song Y, Cao C, Xu Q, Gu S, Wang F, et al. Piperine attenuates TBI-induced seizures via inhibiting cytokine-activated reactive astrogliosis. Front Neurol. 2020;11:431.
42. Spoelhof B, Sanchez-Bautista J, Zorrilla-Vaca A, Kaplan PW, Farrokh S, et al. Impact of antiepileptic drugs for seizure prophylaxis on short and long-term functional outcomes in patients with acute intracerebral hemorrhage: a meta-analysis and systematic review. Seizure. 2019;69:140–6.
43. Taş YÇ, Solaroğlu İ, Gürsoy-Özdemir Y. Spreading depolarization waves in neurological diseases: a short review about its pathophysiology and clinical relevance. Curr Neuropharmacol. 2018;17(2):151–64.
44. Westmoreland BF. Periodic lateralized epileptiform discharges after evacuation of subdural hematomas. J Clin Neurophysiol. 2001;18(1):20–4.
45. Won SY, Dubinski D, Eibach M, Gessler F, Herrmann E, et al. External validation and modification of the Oslo grading system for prediction of postoperative recurrence of chronic subdural hematoma. Neurosurg Rev. 2021;44(2):961–70.
46. Won SY, Dubinski D, Freiman T, Seifert V, Gessler F, et al. Acute-on-chronic subdural hematoma: a new entity for prophylactic anti-epileptic treatment? Eur J Trauma Emerg Surg. 2020. https://doi.org/10.1007/s00068-020-01508-9.
47. Won SY, Dubinski D, Herrmann E, Cuca C, Strzelczyk A, et al. Epileptic seizures in patients following surgical treatment of acute subdural hematoma—incidence, risk factors, patient outcome, and development of new scoring system for prophylactic antiepileptic treatment (GATE-24 score). World Neurosurg. 2017;101:416–24.
48. Won SY, Dubinski D, Sautter L, Hattingen E, Seifert V, et al. Seizure and status epilepticus in chronic subdural hematoma. Acta Neurol Scand. 2019;140(3):194–203.
49. Won SY, Konczalla J, Dubinski D, Cattani A, Cuca C, et al. A systematic review of epileptic seizures in adults with subdural haematomas. Seizure. 2017;45:28–35.
50. Yamada T. Evaluation of seizures in patients with chronic subdural hematoma treated by Burr-hole surgery and risk factors for seizures. Int J Brain Disord Treat. 2017;3(1):1–8.

Chapter 11
Chronic Subdural Hematoma with Psychiatric Disorders

Umut Kirli, Öykü Özçelik, and Osman Vırıt

11.1 Etiology of Chronic Subdural Hematoma Related to Mental Disorders

The association between alcohol and chronic subdural hematoma (CSDH) has been well documented. Alcohol use disorders are one of the most common risk factors for development of CSDH. A study presenting the etiological factors of patients with subacute or chronic subdural hematomas in the absence of head trauma showed that alcohol use disorders were of the most common precipitating factors along with epilepsy [8]. Furthermore, a case series of CSDH with a relative large sample (n = 1000) demonstrated that excessive alcohol use was the third most common concomitant diagnosis (n = 132, 13.2%) following hypertension and diabetes mellitus [19]. Alcohol use disorders were also associated with a poorer prognosis for CSDH [39]. Several mechanisms linking the excessive alcohol use and CSDH were proposed. Alcohol use leads to increased risk of falls and head trauma, particularly in the elderly [30]. Excessive alcohol use may also mediate other risk factors for CSDH, such as cerebral atrophy [38], hypertension [23], diabetes [49], and altered coagulation and functioning of platelets [2].

Substance use, particularly stimulant drugs (i.e., amphetamine, methamphetamine, ecstasy, khat, and cocaine), was associated with intracranial hemorrhage risk. Hypertensive bursts have been proposed as a plausible mechanism. Furthermore, the association between substance use and intracranial hemorrhage may partly be mediated by alcohol use [3, 7, 34, 36, 40, 43, 52]. However, the association between

U. Kirli
Institute on Drug Abuse, Toxicology and Pharmaceutical Science, Ege University, Izmir, Turkey

Ö. Özçelik · O. Vırıt (✉)
Department of Psychiatry, Muğla Sıtkı Koçman University School of Medicine, Muğla, Turkey

M. Turgut et al. (eds.), *Subdural Hematoma*,
https://doi.org/10.1007/978-3-030-79371-5_11

substance use and CSDH has not been as well described as the association with alcohol use disorders. As far as we are aware, no studies have yet directly linked CSDH with substance use. However, there are two case reports in the literature describing cases with cocaine abuse and a combination of widespread cerebral infarction and subdural hematoma, and with amphetamine-induced vasculitis and a combination of subdural and subarachnoid hemorrhage [10, 37]. Furthermore, some indirect associations through trauma caused by falls, accidents, and homicides have been documented [22]. Further studies are needed to draw precise conclusions on this issue. However, clinicians should be aware of the potential association of CSDH with substance use.

The use of selective serotonin reuptake inhibitors (SSRIs) may lead to prolongation of the bleeding time, as a function of altered platelet aggregability and activity due to inhibition of serotonin reuptake into platelets [4, 21]. These findings raised the question of whether the use of these medications may be associated with the risk of intracranial hemorrhage, especially in the elderly [14]. Meta-analysis showed an elevated risk of intracranial hemorrhage associated with SSRIs. However, the absolute risk on hemorrhage was very low [20, 32]. New onset depression itself might also be associated with an intracranial hemorrhage risk, suggesting a possibility of indication bias [12]. However, compared with the use of tricyclic antidepressants, the risk of intracranial hemorrhage was reported to be higher with the use of SSRIs. This result demonstrates an individual risk associated with the use of SSRI's, plausibly mediated by altered platelet functioning. The current use of antidepressants with a stronger affinity for the serotonin transporter (paroxetine, sertraline, fluoxetine, duloxetine, and clomipramine) had a higher risk than antidepressants with weak serotonin reuptake inhibition (agomelatine, amoxapine, desipramine, dosulepin, doxepin, isocarboxazide, iprindole, lofepramine, maprotiline, mianserin, mirtazapine, moclobemide, nefazodone, nortriptyline, reboxetine, phenelzine, protriptyline, tranylcypromine, trimipramine, viloxazine) [41]. Furthermore, the risk of intracranial hemorrhage was relatively higher during the first 30 days following the initiation of use and with the combination with the anticoagulants. There is also some evidence, despite contradictory, indicating increased risk for the combinations of SSRIs with antiplatelets [9, 20, 28, 32, 41].

Although a slightly increased risk of intracranial hemorrhage associated with SSRIs has been shown, especially in the first month of their use, these studies have not presented specific data with the risk of subdural hemorrhage. The etiology of CSDH may differ from other types of intracranial hemorrhage in some respects [29]. A recent study with a large sample showed an increased risk of subdural hemorrhage with the use of antidepressants. The increase in the risk was highest in the first month of use, and was close to zero after the third year. The risk was slightly higher with the use of SSRIs in comparison with non-SSRIs. Furthermore, the risk was increased with the use of drug combinations including anticoagulants and to a lesser degree antiplatelets/nonsteroidal anti-inflammatory drugs (NSAIDs). However, the absolute risk was remarkably low [18].The choice of never using antidepressants also gives rise to some other risks. Therefore, the risk-benefit balance should be considered while using the antidepressants in the elderly.

Some antidepressants, particularly tricyclic antidepressants but also SSRIs, have been associated with the risk of falls [46], suggesting that the association between antidepressants and subdural hematoma may not be solely attributed to the effects on platelet functioning. Furthermore, antipsychotics, anxiolytics, hypnotics, and sedatives, especially benzodiazepines with a long elimination half-life, have also been associated with the risk of falls, especially in the elderly [30, 31, 50]. Therefore, these mediations may also be associated with the risk of CSDH via increasing the risk of falls. Particularly in the elderly, these medications should be used with caution, and in the lowest doses as possible.

Electroconvulsive therapy (ECT) is a commonly used and a relatively safe treatment option for mental disorders. However, ECT has been shown to increase the metabolic demand of the brain and intracranial pressure [44]. Therefore, ECT may have an association with subdural hematoma, particularly in the presence of other risk factors such as a history of subdural hematoma, cerebral atrophy, excessive use of alcohol and antiplatelet or anticoagulant medication use [13]. Rare cases of subdural hematoma associated with ECT have been presented in the literature (five cases), one of whom died [13, 42]. On the other hand, there are reports proposing that ECT may be successfully used even in patients with subdural hematoma without mass effect [51]. Results from well-designed controlled studies are needed before drawing precise conclusions on this issue. However, brain imaging is inevitable prior to starting ECT sessions, and benefit-risk balance should be considered according to the characteristics of each individual case. Delirium, focal neurological deficit or altered consciousness following ECT should alert clinicians for a possible subdural hematoma.

Patients with intellectual disabilities and dementia are considered to be at high risk for CSDH [1, 15]. Furthermore, the prognosis for subdural hematoma may be worse in patients with dementia [1]. Conversely, the progressive mental manifestations of CSDH may mimic a dementia, which has been detailed below. Therefore, clinicians should consider the possibility of a CSDH in certain cases diagnosed with "atypical" dementia, where the symptoms may be reversible after appropriate treatment.

11.2 Mental Manifestations of Chronic Subdural Hematoma

In the case of chronic subdural hematoma (CSDH), there is a time frame between the initial injury and the clear manifestations of the index pathology. A retrospective study evaluating the medical records of 1000 CSDH cases found that the mean interval was 49.1 days [19]. Furthermore, mental symptoms were reported to be the first clinical manifestation of CSDH in about half of the patients [24]. Therefore, it is very common that patients with CSDH are referred to psychiatry clinics due to their preceding mental symptoms. Following this reasoning, it is crucial to define the mental symptoms associated with CSDH. However, the literature on the mental manifestations of the CSDH is insufficient and incomplete.

A study retrospectively investigating the clinical manifestations of 79 patients with subacute or chronic subdural hematomas demonstrated that 58% of patients had mental disturbances according to DSM-III criteria on admission. Remarkably, in one-fifth of these patients, mental disorders were the initial manifestations. Delirium was the most common diagnosis, followed by dementia and organic affective syndromes [5]. Similarly, a study presenting the clinical manifestations of 70 CSDH patients demonstrated that personality or intellectual changes were the most common clinical findings along with hemiparesis [8].

Changes in cognitive processes due to CSDH vary from subtle alterations in attention, concentration, language, memory, judgment to confusion, dementia, and delirium. Changes in personality and behavior are usually noted by family members. These changes are present as sleep disturbances, altered circadian rhythm, decreased self-care and fatigue to impulsivity, increased talkativeness, emotional bursts, and psychotic symptoms [35].

Progressive mental symptoms are more common in elderly than younger patients [47, 48]. On the other hand, younger patients are more prone to develop acute presentations. This difference in relation to age group is explained in accordance with the larger brain volume of younger patients limiting the free space in which the hematoma can develop [35]. Cases with CSDH presenting with positive psychotic symptoms (delusions and hallucinations) were reported predominantly in individuals older than 70 years of age [6, 17, 26]. However, there are exceptional cases in younger age groups presenting with negative psychotic and disorganized symptoms [27]. Mental symptoms often resolve following the resorption of the hematoma. It was proposed that mental symptoms in younger patients which had never occurred before the onset of CSDH have a greater chance to remit [24].

For the treatment of mental symptoms in the presence of CSDH, appropriate psychotropic medications may be used when needed. However, it should be kept in mind that the risk of side effects (i.e., hyponatremia, extrapyramidal side effects) may be greater in these patients [27, 33, 45]. There is a case report presenting neuroleptic malignant syndrome with the use of clozapine (an antipsychotic with a very low affinity for D_2 receptors) in a patient with CSDH [16].

The diagnosis of CSDH may be missed in psychiatry clinics. A classical study based on necropsies of 200 patients who were deceased in a mental hospital showed that 14 patients (7%) had a subdural hematoma, eight of which were chronic or subacute subdural hematomas. However, only one of these patients had an antemortem diagnosis with a computed tomography (CT) scan [11]. The most common misdiagnoses include dementia (Alzheimer's or vascular) and affective and psychotic syndromes. In most cases, dementia is not considered to be reversible. However, cognitive and affective disturbances due to CSDH may resolve if accurately treated [25]. Therefore, it is crucial to diagnose CSDH as early as possible. Some features may help determine the differential diagnosis between Alzheimer's dementia and CSDH. Patients with Alzheimer's have problems in encoding new information in first priority. However, patients with CSDH have more considerable deficits in retrieving the earlier encoded information. Furthermore, the history of memory deficits in Alzheimer's dementia is commonly expressed as in months to years, whereas in CSDH the history of memory deficits is commonly expressed as in weeks [35].

11.3 Conclusions

Clinicians should keep in mind that CSDH may manifest itself as a series of mental disorders without neurological symptoms [5]. Therefore, in psychiatric practice, particularly in the elderly and in patients with alcohol use disorders, epilepsy, and dementia, the possibility of CSDH should be carefully evaluated. In cases listed below, neuroimaging should be considered:

1. Presence of neurological symptoms co-occurring with mental disorders or a history of head trauma
2. Cognitive changes such as altered consciousness, cooperation, attention, orientation; progressive intellectual impairment or personality changes
3. Unusual psychiatric symptoms and limited response to these symptoms despite appropriate treatment
4. Unexpected side effects (i.e., occurrence of extrapyramidal side effects as a response to low potency D_2 blockade or in low doses)

References

1. Arca R, Ricchi V, Murgia D, Melis M, Floris F, Mereu A, Contu P, Marrosu F, Cossu G. Parkinsonism and dementia are negative prognostic factors for the outcome of subdural hematoma. Neurol Sci. 2016;37(8):1299–303.
2. Ballard HS. The hematological complications of alcoholism. Alcohol Health Res World. 1997;21(1):42–52.
3. Bede P, El-Kininy N, O'Hara F, Menon P, Finegan E, Healy D. 'Khatatonia'—cathinone-induced hypertensive encephalopathy. Neth J Med. 2017;75(10):448–50.
4. Bismuth-Evenzal Y, Gonopolsky Y, Gurwitz D, Iancu I, Weizman A, Rehavi M. Decreased serotonin content and reduced agonist-induced aggregation in platelets of patients chronically medicated with SSRI drugs. J Affect Disord. 2012;136(1–2):99–103.
5. Black DW. Mental changes resulting from subdural haematoma. Br J Psychiatry. 1984;145:200–3.
6. Brunekreeft JA, Peerdeman SM, Rhebergen D. Subdural hematoma and depression (in German). Tijdschr Psychiatr. 2008;50(5):295–9.
7. Bruno A. Cerebrovascular complications of alcohol and sympathomimetic drug abuse. Curr Neurol Neurosci Rep. 2003;3(1):40–5.
8. Cameron MM. Chronic subdural haematoma: a review of 114 cases. J Neurol Neurosurg Psychiatry. 1978;41(9):834–9.
9. Castro VM, Gallagher PJ, Clements CC, Murphy SN, Gainer VS, Fava M, Weilburg JB, Churchill SE, Kohane IS, Iosifescu DV, Smoller JW, Perlis RH. Incident user cohort study of risk for gastrointestinal bleed and stroke in individuals with major depressive disorder treated with antidepressants. BMJ Open. 2012;2(2):e000544.

10. Chaudhary SC, Sawlani KK, Malhotra HS, Apurva, Nanda S, Rao PK. Cocaine abuse: an unusual association. J Assoc Physicians India. 2016;64(11):77–9.
11. Cole G. Intracranial space-occupying masses in mental hospital patients: necropsy study. J Neurol Neurosurg Psychiatry. 1978;41(8):730–6.
12. Daskalopoulou M, George J, Walters K, Osborn DP, Batty GD, Stogiannis D, Rapsomaniki E, Pujades-Rodriguez M, Denaxas S, Udumyan R, Kivimaki M, Hemingway H. Depression as a risk factor for the initial presentation of twelve cardiac, cerebrovascular, and peripheral arterial diseases: data linkage study of 1.9 million women and men. PLoS One. 2016;11(4):e0153838.
13. Dauleac C, Vinckier F, Bourdillon P. Subdural hematoma and electroconvulsive therapy: a case report and review of the literature. Neurochirurgie. 2019;65(1):40–2.
14. de Abajo FJ. Effects of selective serotonin reuptake inhibitors on platelet function: mechanisms, clinical outcomes and implications for use in elderly patients. Drugs Aging. 2011;28(5):345–67.
15. de Las Heras J, Aldamiz-Echevarria L, Cabrera A. Frontoparietal subdural hematoma in a child with mental regression. JAMA Neurol. 2018;75(6):759–60.
16. Duggal HS. Clozapine-induced neuroleptic malignant syndrome and subdural hematoma. J Neuropsychiatry Clin Neurosci. 2004;16(1):118–9.
17. Feki I, Abida I, Baati I, Masmoudi J, Jaoua A. Chronic subdural hematoma and neuropsychiatric disorders: report of a case. Eur Psychiatry. 2015;30:1271.
18. Gaist D, Garcia Rodriguez LA, Hald SM, Hellfritzsch M, Poulsen FR, Halle B, Hallas J, Pottegard A. Antidepressant drug use and subdural hematoma risk. J Thromb Haemost. 2020;18(2):318–27.
19. Gelabert-Gonzalez M, Iglesias-Pais M, Garcia-Allut A, Martinez-Rumbo R. Chronic subdural haematoma: surgical treatment and outcome in 1000 cases. Clin Neurol Neurosurg. 2005;107(3):223–9.
20. Hackam DG, Mrkobrada M. Selective serotonin reuptake inhibitors and brain hemorrhage: a meta-analysis. Neurology. 2012;79(18):1862–5.
21. Halperin D, Reber G. Influence of antidepressants on hemostasis. Dialogues Clin Neurosci. 2007;9(1):47–59.
22. Heninger M. Subdural hematoma occurrence. Am J Forensic Med Pathol. 2013;34(3):237–41.
23. Husain K, Ansari RA, Ferder L. Alcohol-induced hypertension: mechanism and prevention. World J Cardiol. 2014;6(5):245–52.
24. Iliescu IA, Constantinescu AI. Clinical evolutional aspects of chronic subdural haematomas—literature review. J Med Life. 2015;8(Spec Issue):26–33.
25. Ishikawa E, Yanaka K, Sugimoto K, Ayuzawa S, Nose T. Reversible dementia in patients with chronic subdural hematomas. J Neurosurg. 2002;96(4):680–3.
26. Jomli R, Zgueb Y, Nacef F, Douki S. Chronic subdural hematoma and psychotic decompensation (in France). Encéphale. 2012;38(4):356–9.
27. Kar SK, Kumar D, Singh P, Upadhyay PK. Psychiatric manifestation of chronic subdural hematoma: the unfolding of mystery in a homeless patient. Indian J Psychol Med. 2015;37(2):239–42.
28. Kharofa J, Sekar P, Haverbusch M, Moomaw C, Flaherty M, Kissela B, Broderick J, Woo D. Selective serotonin reuptake inhibitors and risk of hemorrhagic stroke. Stroke. 2007;38(11):3049–51.
29. Kolias AG, Chari A, Santarius T, Hutchinson PJ. Chronic subdural haematoma: modern management and emerging therapies. Nat Rev Neurol. 2014;10(10):570–8.
30. Laberge S, Crizzle AM. A literature review of psychotropic medications and alcohol as risk factors for falls in community dwelling older adults. Clin Drug Investig. 2019;39(2):117–39.
31. Landi F, Onder G, Cesari M, Barillaro C, Russo A, Bernabei R. Psychotropic medications and risk for falls among community-dwelling frail older people: an observational study. J Gerontol A Biol Sci Med Sci. 2005;60(5):622–6.
32. Laporte S, Chapelle C, Caillet P, Beyens MN, Bellet F, Delavenne X, Mismetti P, Bertoletti L. Bleeding risk under selective serotonin reuptake inhibitor (SSRI) antidepressants: a meta-analysis of observational studies. Pharmacol Res. 2017;118:19–32.

33. Lazarus A. Neuroleptic malignant syndrome and preexisting brain damage. J Neuropsychiatry Clin Neurosci. 1992;4(2):185–7.
34. Levine SR, Brust JC, Futrell N, Ho KL, Blake D, Millikan CH, Brass LM, Fayad P, Schultz LR, Selwa JF, et al. Cerebrovascular complications of the use of the "crack" form of alkaloidal cocaine. N Engl J Med. 1990;323(11):699–704.
35. Machulda MM, Haut MW. Clinical features of chronic subdural hematoma: neuropsychiatric and neuropsychologic changes in patients with chronic subdural hematoma. Neurosurg Clin N Am. 2000;11(3):473–7.
36. McEvoy AW, Kitchen ND, Thomas DG. Intracerebral haemorrhage and drug abuse in young adults. Br J Neurosurg. 2000;14(5):449–54.
37. Nagele EP, Ross A, Then RK, Kavi T. Interhemispheric subdural and subarachnoid haemorrhage in a patient with amphetamine-induced vasculitis. BMJ Case Rep. 2017;2017:bcr2017222918.
38. Nutt D. Alcohol and the brain. Pharmacological insights for psychiatrists. Br J Psychiatry. 1999;175:114–9.
39. Pencalet P. [Clinical forms and prognostic factors of chronic subdural hematoma in the adult]. Neurochirurgie. 2001;47(5):469–72.
40. Pozzi M, Roccatagliata D, Sterzi R. Drug abuse and intracranial hemorrhage. Neurol Sci. 2008;29(Suppl 2):S269–70.
41. Renoux C, Vahey S, Dell'Aniello S, Boivin JF. Association of selective serotonin reuptake inhibitors with the risk for spontaneous intracranial hemorrhage. JAMA Neurol. 2017;74(2):173–80.
42. Saha D, Bisui B, Thakurta RG, Ghoshmaulik S, Singh OP. Chronic subdural hematoma following electro convulsive therapy. Indian J Psychol Med. 2012;34(2):181–3.
43. Schlaeppi M, Prica A, de Torrente A. Cerebral hemorrhage and "ecstasy" (in German). Praxis (Bern 1994). 1999;88(13):568–72.
44. Taylor S. Electroconvulsive therapy: a review of history, patient selection, technique, and medication management. South Med J. 2007;100(5):494–8.
45. Taylor D, Barnes TRE, Young AH. The Maudsley prescribing guidelines in psychiatry. 13th ed. New York: Wiley; 2018.
46. Thapa PB, Gideon P, Cost TW, Milam AB, Ray WA. Antidepressants and the risk of falls among nursing home residents. N Engl J Med. 1998;339(13):875–82.
47. Toi H, Kinoshita K, Hirai S, Takai H, Hara K, Matsushita N, Matsubara S, Otani M, Muramatsu K, Matsuda S, Fushimi K, Uno M. Present epidemiology of chronic subdural hematoma in Japan: analysis of 63,358 cases recorded in a national administrative database. J Neurosurg. 2018;128(1):222–8.
48. Uno M, Toi H, Hirai S. Chronic subdural hematoma in elderly patients: is this disease benign? Neurol Med Chir (Tokyo). 2017;57(8):402–9.
49. van de Wiel A. Diabetes mellitus and alcohol. Diabetes Metab Res Rev. 2004;20(4):263–7.
50. Vitry AI, Hoile AP, Gilbert AL, Esterman A, Luszcz MA. The risk of falls and fractures associated with persistent use of psychotropic medications in elderly people. Arch Gerontol Geriatr. 2010;50(3):e1–4.
51. Wijeratne C, Shome S. Electroconvulsive therapy and subdural hemorrhage. J ECT. 1999;15(4):275–9.
52. Wong S, Afshani M. Intracranial vascular complications of "molly" usage: case report and review of the literature. Conn Med. 2016;80(8):467–9.

Chapter 12
Chronic Subdural Hematoma in the Pediatric Population

Murat Ö. Yay, Daniel Wittschieber, and Mehmet Turgut

12.1 Introduction

Chronic subdural hematoma (CSDH) is accepted as one of the most frequent entities in neurosurgical practice [20]. The first reports of chronic subdural collections date back to 1916. Payr described a case with subdural hygroma (SDHy), which he called as "meningitis serosa traumatica" [65]. Cohen reported on the same clinical entity and referred to it as a "subdural fluid collection" in 1927 [15]. In 1932, Dandy started to use the term SDHy which today is considered a separate clinical entity [16, 65, 90].

CSDH is usually a disease of the elderly and in rare cases it may also be encountered in infants. This condition usually occurs as the consequence of trauma [28, 78]. Although the exact incidence of CSDH is unknown, it is more commonly seen in males [28, 54, 63]. Despite a significant mass effect seen on radiological studies, interestingly, clinical symptoms and signs can be silent in some cases in the pediatric population [1, 63]. They can be applied to different clinics in infants and in older

M. Ö. Yay (✉)
Department of Neurosurgery, Aydın Adnan Menderes University Faculty of Medicine, Efeler, Aydın, Turkey

D. Wittschieber
Institute of Legal Medicine, Jena University Hospital, Friedrich Schiller University Jena, Jena, Germany
e-mail: daniel.wittschieber@med.uni-jena.de

M. Turgut
Department of Neurosurgery, Aydın Adnan Menderes University Faculty of Medicine, Efeler, Aydın, Turkey

Department of Histology and Embryology, Aydın Adnan Menderes University Health Sciences Institute, Efeler, Aydın, Turkey

M. Turgut et al. (eds.), *Subdural Hematoma*,
https://doi.org/10.1007/978-3-030-79371-5_12

children. From the pediatricians' point of view, the term chronic subdural fluid collection is used for a group of conditions characterized by fluid excess within the extracerebral or extra-axial regions [20]. Fortunately, current neuroimaging techniques have greatly advanced our understanding of these conditions, but their exact pathogenesis and proper management are still controversial [36, 78]. In this chapter, our purpose is to present the anatomy, pathophysiology, etiology, diagnosis, and treatment of CSDH.

12.2 Anatomy and Pathophysiology

The subdural space or subdural cavity is a potential space that can be opened under pathological conditions by the separation of the arachnoid mater from the dura mater and a CSDH will develop in this space [68]. Out of the three extracerebral spaces, normally, the subdural and extradural regions do not exist as a physiological space, unlike the subarachnoid space, and accumulation of fluid within these spaces is pathological [30, 78]. Anatomically, subdural hematomas (SDHs) can appear in any intracranial location which cross suture margins. Internal dural attachments like the falx cerebri and tentorium cerebelli limit the extent of the SDH. Therefore, it typically appears as a crescent-shaped or concave extra-axial lesion on nonenhanced computed tomography (NECT) [68].

Basically, from a pathophysiological point of view, the following six different main entities of subdural fluid collections should be considered: (a) acute SDH; (b) SDHy; (c) subdural hematohygroma (SDHHy); (d) CSDH (as an independent entity); (e) subdural effusion; and (f) subdural empyema [90, 91]. Even today, however, the pathogenesis and mechanisms of development of different chronic subdural fluid collections provided above are not fully understood, although it is well known that it is a delayed process [71].

There is no doubt that many aspects of the relationship between subdural and subarachnoid spaces still remain a puzzle, although rebleeding from subdural neomembranes is a well-known disorder to neuropathologists [23, 75]. In CSDH, following the hemorrhage within the subdural space in approximately 2 weeks, the synthesis of collagen in the dura mater is stimulated and many fibroblasts move to the inner surface of the dura mater for the production of a thickened outer dural membrane [51, 72]. Subsequently, a thinner inner membrane develops, resulting in the encapsulation of the clot [51]. This ability to estimate the age of a CSDH is often used as forensic evidence when child abuse due to an inflicted head injury, mostly in form of a "shaken baby syndrome" (SBS) which is a common variant of the so-called "abusive head trauma" (AHT), is suspected [68]. Over time, the SDH may liquefy, resolve, or form a SDHy or SDHHy which is regarded as the precursor of the CSDH and the neomembranes may calcify in some cases [51, 90, 91]. It has been suggested that the vast majority of all SDHs liquefy [84]. In this event, the SDH generally tends to enlarge as opposed to remaining solid and stable in size [84].

Table 12.1 Pathophysiology of the development of CSDHs

	Causes	Suggested pathologic mechanisms
1	Following acute SDH	Repeated hemorrhage from the fragile neovessels of the granulating (neo) membrane of an acute SDH into the subdural space [38, 48, 90, 91]. However, a direct transformation of acute SDH into CSDH is observed very rarely and there may be an intermediate transient product called "SDHy" or "SDHHy" between acute SDH and CSDH [90, 91]
2	Leakage of CSF	Leakage of CSF through an opening in the subarachnoid membrane allows CSF to enter the subdural space. The CSF mixes with blood and results in a thin xanthochromic subdural fluid collection, known as "SDHy" or "SDHHy," respectively [85, 90, 91]
3	Cerebral atrophy	Babies with cerebral atrophy may be more susceptible to development of an CSDH as a result of tension on the dural border layer as the arachnoid collapses with the shrinking brain [30]
4	Infection or inflammatory process	After an infection or inflammatory process; subdural empyemas can result from sinusitis or otitis media [41]

Abbreviations: *CSDH* chronic subdural hematoma, *CSF* cerebrospinal fluid, *SDH* subdural hematoma, *SDHHy* subdural hematohygroma, *SDHy* subdural hygroma

Today, it has been suggested that a constant accumulation of fluid within the subdural space may develop depending on the following pathological mechanisms described below in detail (Table 12.1) [30, 38, 41, 48, 71, 85, 90, 91].

12.2.1 Following Acute SDH

Many authors consider rebleeding as the main reason causing persistence of the acute SDH [55]. It has been suggested that vascularized membranes with small fragile vessels are found around an acute SDH and the vessels in the membranes may bleed into the cavity of the hematoma with persistent trauma and changes in intravascular pressure [78]. In fact, however, this pathomechanism is considered rare and failed to be reproducible in studies [90, 91]. More likely, there is an intermediate transient developmental step called SDHy or SDHHy between SDH and CSDH [90, 91].

Many authors have suggested that repeated bleeding will trigger the formation of septations that may develop within the subdural space in order to organize the clot (or the clot changed by serum separation over time) [55, 91]. Generally, all of the liquefied blood may be resorbed; in some unfortunate cases, however, it may produce more severe symptoms than that of the original acute SDH. In such cases, the volume of the thick viscous fluid increases, in a similar way to that of crankcase fluid, as a result of high gradients in oncotic pressure and fluid volume caused by changes in oncotic pressure [78].

12.2.2 Leakage of CSF

This mechanism has been previously described thoroughly by one of the authors of this chapter [91]. Some authors suggested that the laceration of the arachnoid mater may behave as a valve against the backflow of CSF [9, 44]. This type of fluid collection within the subdural space, known as SDHy, may occur after the tearing of the arachnoid mater and may then allow CSF to enter the subdural space where it is the main precursor of the CSDH [90, 91]. SDHys may also occur in the expanded subdural space after shunting of the ventricular system [78] (Fig. 12.1). In general, septations are not seen within SDHys [78]. In these cases, it is possible to distinguish the subdural fluid from both subarachnoid and intraventricular fluids, considering its xanthochromic properties [34]. It has been speculated that the bridging draining veins are ruptured as a result of persistent mild trauma or spontaneously where small bleeding foci may be observed at the cortical surface [78].

12.2.3 Cerebral Atrophy

Some children with mitochondrial and lysosomal diseases display only cerebral atrophy on their magnetic resonance imaging (MRI) studies [45, 73]. Type 1 glutaric aciduria is characterized by microencephalic macrocephaly and an acute SDH

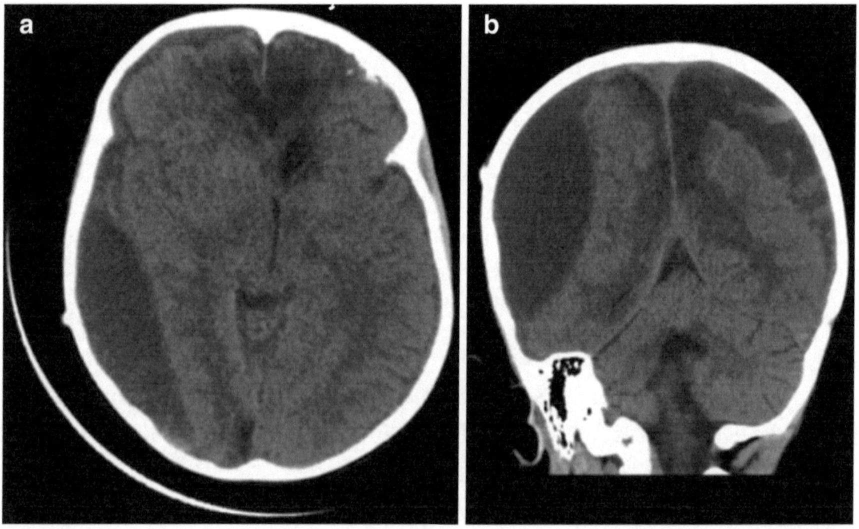

Fig. 12.1 Axial (**a**), coronal (**b**) non-enhanced computed tomography (NECT) sections demonstrating bilateral chronic subdural hematoma (CSDH) on post-shunt imaging of a 10-year-old male patient

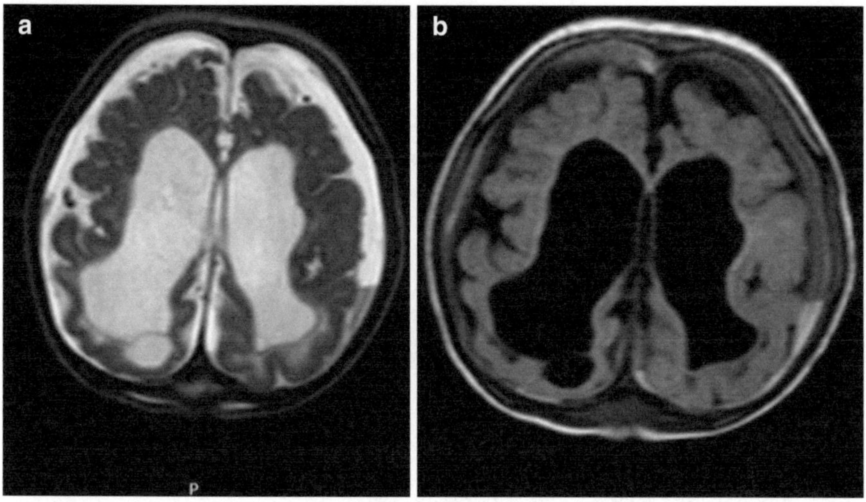

Fig. 12.2 A 2-year-old patient with a metabolic disease. The T2-weighted magnetic resonance imaging (MRI) scan (**a**) showed a CSDH overlying both cerebral hemispheres as hyperintense and isointense to cerebrospinal fluid (CSF); however, on the FLAIR image (**b**), the signal intensity is higher than CSF, indicating a different protein content

may develop in these children, possibly due to stretching of the bridging veins as a result of cerebral atrophy, as noted by one of the authors of this chapter in a previous review regarding the imaging of SBS [54, 89] (Fig. 12.2).

12.2.4 Infection or Inflammatory Process

The fourth type of purulent fluid accumulation within the subdural space is secondary to either an infectious or inflammatory process or both [71]. Subdural empyema, also known as subdural effusion, may develop from extension of infection from the middle ear or paranasal sinuses first into the extradural space and then into the subdural space by neighborhood way [78]. These infections are also seen following bacterial meningitis caused by *Streptococcus* spp. or *Pneumococcus* spp. [22, 33, 46, 60] (Fig. 12.3). In such cases, cultures of purulent subdural fluid may reveal a causative microorganism if antibiotic therapy is not given before taking a sample for culture [78].

12.3 Etiology

Terminologically, a CSDH is classified as a persistent intracranial hemorrhage between the dura mater and the arachnoid mater. CSDH is primarily a disease of the elderly and is a rare neurosurgical entity for children [1]. CSDH in the elderly is out

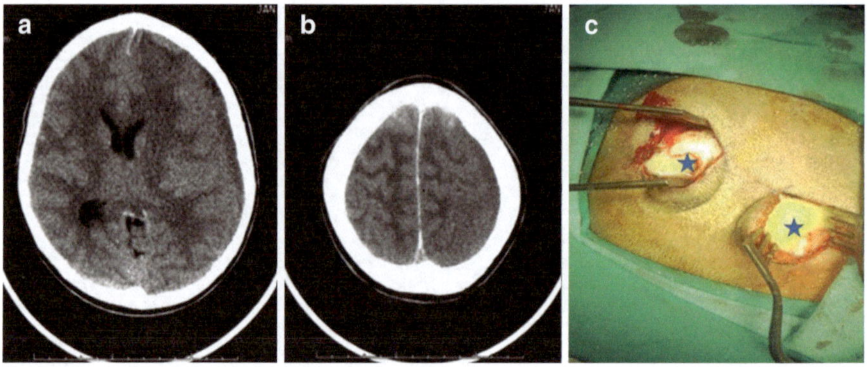

Fig. 12.3 NECT (**a**, **b**) demonstrated a left-sided subdural collection, and a purulent collection via burr-hole trephination (**c**)

of the scope of this chapter, but several etiologies for CSDH in infancy, including birth injury, vitamin K deficiency, child abuse, and coagulopathy, have been reported [2, 3, 42, 50, 93]. Etiologically, there are many causes for the development of CSDH, but the most frequent cause of CSDH in the pediatric population is head trauma which is more common in the male children [63, 66]. As a type of head trauma, AHT has an incidence of 14–30/100,000 live births in the infant age group [21, 31, 40]. In fact, the term AHT is used for head injuries caused by nonaccidental (inflicted) trauma in the pediatric population [14, 31, 40, 49]. According to some authors, the "SBS" is a frequent variant of AHT [14, 49].

The incidences of acute SDH in the pediatric population (infant age group and those under the age of 2 years) are 20–25/100,000 and 12/100,000, respectively [7, 10, 32, 39, 52]. Traumatic causes may be either accidental or nonaccidental, with the most frequent cause of SDH in children less than 2 years of age being nonaccidental [63, 81]. In general, the traumatic episode is overlooked; in fact, the CSDH is seen without remembering its acute form [78]. As mentioned above, the SDH does not appear to be the direct precursor of the CSDH [90, 91]. The further etiological discussion within this chapter currently addresses etiological aspects of the SDH, not the CSDH. As described below in detail, arachnoid cyst (AC) and benign enlargement of the subarachnoid spaces (BESS) are causes of the SDH, which may then develop to CSDHs via SDHy [90, 91].

Clinically, the other causes of SDH include hematological coagulopathies and various intracranial morphological anomalies such as an AC [78, 92]. Firstly, coagulation status of the patients should always be evaluated [78]. In the majority of such cases, however, an example of such an intracranial anomaly which may be a risk factor for the development of SDH is an AC of the middle cranial fossa [78]. It has been reported that epidemiology, demography, and clinical characteristics of cases with CSDH seen together with an AC are different from those counterparts without an AC [92]. The true incidence of bleeding in patients with an AC is not known, but rupture of the outer wall of the AC may allow CSF into the subdural space [64, 78]. Today, it is well known that ACs are intra-arachnoidal CSF collections, congenital or acquired, occurring rarely and any rupture of pre-existing ACs may develop as a result of minor but identifiable AHT or SBS or a sudden short-term increased intracranial pressure (IICP) [24, 69, 90,

91]. Importantly, it has been speculated that such a rupture may cause the development of SDHys rather than SDHs, although this has not been observed in infants to date [69, 90, 91]. In a review of the literature, Gelabert-González et al. reported that the ages of occurrence ranged from 5 to 25 years [24]. Based on this information, it is logical that ACs also rupture in infants as a result of AHT, SBS, or possibly spontaneously [90, 91].

Even today, there is still an ongoing discussion on whether the so-called BESS may predispose to SDH. Macroscopically, this condition is manifested with macrocephaly and bulging of the anterior fontanel in the pediatric population, and it is has been speculated that this mild form of communicating hydrocephalus is related to the delayed maturation of the arachnoid villi [78].

In clinical practice, birth trauma is considered a cause of CSDH [67]. It has been suggested that infants who have symptoms or macrocephaly starting from the newborn period may have birth-related CSDH [5]. Even more there have also been examples of CSDH occurring in utero [5, 13, 17]. Apart from in utero trauma, inherited coagulopathy, intracranial vascular malformations, and metabolic disorders should be considered among the causes of neonatal CSDH [27, 47, 57, 79, 83].

12.4 Clinical Presentation

Clinically, the presentation of a CSDH in the pediatric population differs due to the two conditions: the age of the patient and the cause of the hemorrhage [78]. The acute and chronic period symptoms of the patients are different. For example, an acute presentation is characterized by apnea or seizures, but a chronic presentation with a history of vomiting, irritability, poor feeding, or macrocephaly is common in infants (Table 12.2). As a rule, a careful examination for external signs of trauma as well as for retinal hemorrhages is necessary for all infants with unexplained SDH [78]. It is vital to remember that retinal hemorrhages can only be found with acute trauma in children with AHT or SBS [90, 91]. If the acute SDH has changed into a CSDH via SDHy or SDHHy, the retinal hemorrhages have usually already resolved [90, 91].

Table 12.2 Clinical symptoms of patients with CSDHs according to their age groups[a]

Age groups of children	
Infants	Older children
Apnea	Headache
Seizures	Cushing triad
Vomiting	Hemiparesis
Lethargy	Sensory deficit
Irritability	Reflex asymmetry
Macrocephaly	Sixth nerve palsy
Poor feeding	Papilledema
	Language disturbances

[a]Data in this table was taken from Emmahadi et al. [20] and Swift and McBride [78]

Older children generally present with chronic headaches and signs of IICP [78]. Headache is a more common presentation in younger patients than in the elderly [86]. The other symptoms that develop are lateralizing neurological signs such as hemiparesis or reflex asymmetry. Interestingly, CSDHs usually occur unilaterally in older children, but bilateral CSDH is frequent in infant age group [1].

Clinically, CSDHs may present as recurrent bleeding after minor trauma or even spontaneously without any trauma [82]. In a literature survey investigating CSDH, different predisposing factors were found in some case reports [8, 25, 76, 87]. Shrestha and You reported a 16-year-old female with headache and dizziness for 2 months; physical examination and blood profile were normal and there was no history of trauma [76]. In their case, the computed tomography (CT) scan revealed a left fronto-temporal CSDH with an AC of the middle cranial fossa [76]. Now, an AC is accepted as a risk factor for the development of CSDH following head injury in the pediatric age group [20].

In a previous study, Basmaci et al. described a 2-year-old patient, who was known to have acute myeloid leukemia, presenting with seizure, vomiting, and agitation [8]. In their case, the complete blood count revealed a platelet count of 48,000/mm^3 and there was no history of head trauma [8]. In their study, they reported that an incidence of tumor-related SDH is 0.5–4% [8]. Based on their observation, they concluded that head trauma, hematological coagulopathy, and chemotherapeutic agents increased the risk of intracranial hemorrhage in the pediatric population [8].

In 2013, Wang et al. described a 14-year-old female who was a music student with a history of headache for 2 weeks after visual blurring and bilateral papilledema was found [87]. Interestingly, they suggested that SDH can be triggered by an increased intravenous pressure during the Valsalva maneuver in the absence of any predisposing risk factors [87]. They also added another similar example, a 9-year-old male with a history of playing dodgeball at school, as a cause of CSDH in children [86].

Recently, Glen et al. described a healthy 45-day-old female with head trauma due to falling from a chair where the NECT revealed the presence of bilateral fronto-parietal hypodense fluid accumulation [25]. They operated on their case several times for subdural collections and the last MRI scan revealed multiple heterogeneous contrast enhancing areas in the right frontal, occipital, and parietal lobes [25]. Surprisingly, pathological examination of the surgical specimen demonstrated mitotically active high-grade sarcomatous proliferation and neoplastic proliferation; they concluded that MRI is useful for differentiating CSDH from sarcoma [25].

12.5 Diagnosis

The diagnosis of CSDH first begins with the clinical evaluation and a percutaneous aspiration is made from the anterior fontanel [63]. This method, called a "subdural tap," may cause bleeding to spread in the subarachnoid and/or subdural space. Hence, this can lead to misleading results.

CSDH is best diagnosed with neuroimaging techniques such as CT and MRI. In addition, neuroimaging is the best way to distinguish CSDH from other extracerebral fluid accumulations [61]. NECT is performed as the first imaging examination that distinguishes the differential diagnosis of subarachnoid hemorrhage from that of CSDH [61]. Radiologically, CT is also valuable in distinguishing between acute and chronic SDHs [5]. CSDH typically is isointense with CSF on MRI [61].

Today, MRI is the best imaging method for diagnosis of CSDH and it is often hyperintense on T1- and T2-weighted fluid attenuated inversion recovery (FLAIR) images [61]. In particular, a SDH is differentiated from subarachnoid hemorrhage using T1-weighted sequences [78]. On both T1- and T2-weighted sequences, CSDH is isointense with CSF. Recurrent hemorrhage is hyperintense on T1 and hypointense on T2 imaging with CSF [61]. On neuroimaging, CSDH is diffusely spread over the deflected cerebral hemisphere with multiple septations and contrast enhancement of the extra-axial collection of membranes [61]. Since MRI can better show hemorrhages of different ages, it is especially useful for the evaluation of nonaccidental trauma cases; in addition, membranes and clot are better shown on MRI [61].

Ultrasonography (USG) is the initial preferred imaging method to evaluate CSDH in infants because it is easy and cheap. Septations within a CSDH can be demonstrated with USG, but SDH and subarachnoid hemorrhage cannot be distinguished [78].

12.6 Treatment

The goals of treatment in pediatric cases with CSDH and macrocephaly are to relieve the IICP, to counteract the mass effect, and to allow normal head growth [78]. Various surgical procedures including repeated percutaneous subdural taps, subdural-peritoneal shunting (SPS), burr-hole evacuation, twist-drill craniostomy, temporary subdural external drainage, craniotomy, and wide resection of neomembranes have been suggested over the years [4, 6, 11, 12, 26, 42, 53, 56, 59, 61, 70, 78, 80]. Unfortunately, medical treatments for patients with CSDH are very limited.

As alternative procedures via craniotomy, various invasive procedures, such as wide excision of subdural membranes, as first suggested by Ingraham and Matson, lowering of the superior sagittal sinus, and extensive cranioplasty to reduce the craniocerebral disproportion have been suggested for infants [29, 37, 58]. Instead, however, less invasive treatment options for control of the IICP, such as subdural tapping, subdural drainage, and SPS, have been widely accepted [4, 62]. McLaurin et al. also proposed treatment with repeated subdural tapping to eliminate IICP with more satisfactory results [54]. In Aoki's series, subdural tapping was used primarily on the thickest area, but 43% of patients subsequently required SPS [1]. The most popular definitive treatment of CSDHs and SDHys is placement of a subdural shunt to the peritoneal cavity, called SPS. Technically, the shunts are usually placed unilaterally despite the presence of bilateral hematomas in infants [13].

Today, some neurosurgeons prefer to use burr-hole drainage for the treatment of CSDH, but recurrent hematoma after this technique occurs in 3–33% of the patients [19]. Huang et al. used various medical agents such as atorvastatin and low-dose dexamethasone for four relapsing cases with CSDH; they suggested that these agents are effective for patients with relapsing CSDH [35].

In 1998, Gruber et al. introduced endoscopic washout as another surgical technique for children with CSDHs [28]. They suggested that endoscopic washout is safe in these cases [28]. Today, minimally invasive techniques including endoscopic washout are popular in contrast to more extensive procedures such as craniotomy with membranectomy or repositioning of the sagittal sinus [29].

On the other hand, surgical treatment of cases of CSDH together with an AC is controversial [32]. Some authors have advocated only burr hole drainage [18, 77, 88], whereas others have suggested fenestration or removal of the AC membrane through craniotomy [43, 74, 94]. However, SDH may be treated conservatively with only clinical follow-up, in particular for patients with comorbidities (Fig. 12.4).

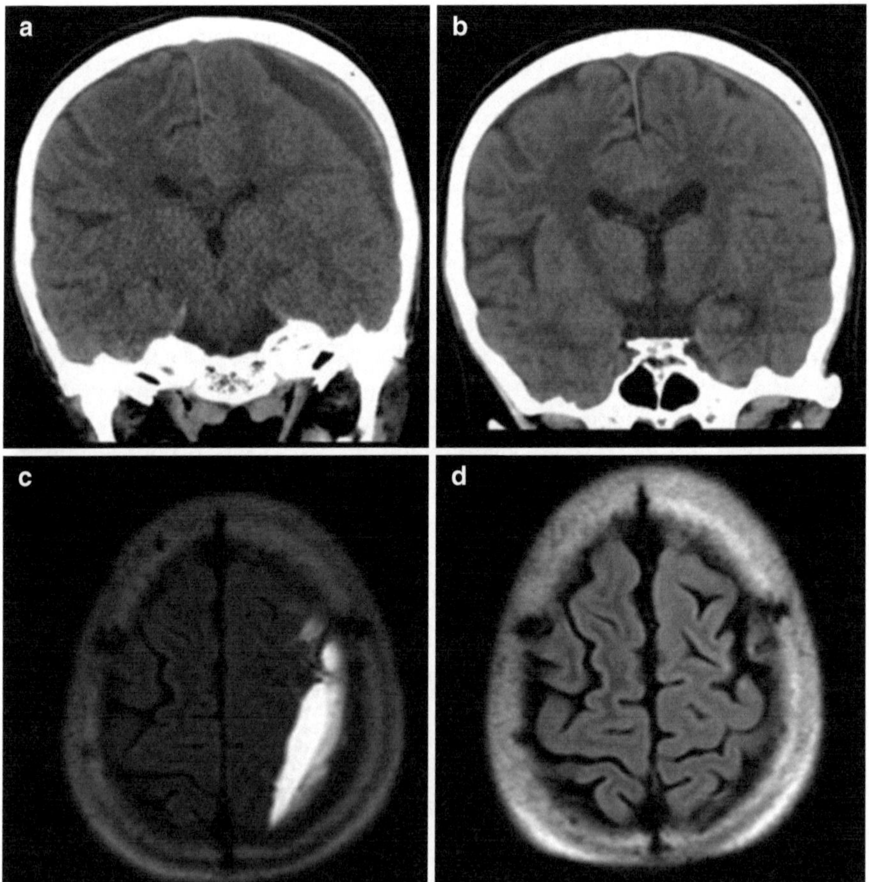

Fig. 12.4 Incidentally detected left-sided CSDH of a patient with aplastic anemia who has no clinical symptoms. Coronal NECT sections (**a**) and axial MRI sections (**c**) revealed the presence of CSDH. At a follow-up of 2 months, coronal sections on NECT (**b**) and axial MRI sections (**d**) showed regression of the hematoma

12.7 Conclusion

It is well known that CSDH in infants and older children is most commonly due to trauma. Clinically, CSDH rarely presents as an acute emergency; however, there may be a danger of herniation and permanent neurologic impairment after trauma if IICP is significant and various neurologic deficits with developmental delay, spasticity, and seizures may occur in about half of these children. Therefore, recognition without delay and appropriate management are necessary to minimize long-term sequelae in the pediatric population. Based on the current literature, it is concluded that the diagnosis of CSDH in this age group is very rare and imaging methods such as MRI and CT are the most widely used diagnostic tools. Today, the standard therapy is surgical evacuation by various surgical procedures such as twist-drill craniostomy, craniotomy, burr-hole drainage, SPS, and endoscopic removal of CSDH in the pediatric population.

References

1. Aoki N, Masuzawa H. Bilateral chronic subdural hematomas without communication between the hematoma cavities: treatment with unilateral subdural-peritoneal shunt. Neurosurgery. 1988;22:911–3.
2. Aoki N, Masuzawa H. Subdural hematomas in abused children: report of six cases from Japan. Neurosurgery. 1986;18:475–7.
3. Aoki N, Mizutani H, Masuzawa H. Unilateral subdural-peritoneal shunting for bilateral chronic subdural hematomas in infancy. J Neurosurg. 1985;63:134–7.
4. Aoki N. Chronic subdural hematoma in infancy. Clinical analysis of 30 cases in the CT era. J Neurosurg. 1990;73:201–5.
5. Atluru V, Kumar I. Intrauterine chronic subdural hematoma with postoperative tension pneumocephalus. Pediatr Neurol. 1987;3(5):306–9.
6. Balser D, Rodgers SD, Johnson B, Shi C, Tabak E, Samadani U. Evolving management of symptomatic chronic subdural hematoma: experience of a single institution and review of the literature. Neurol Res. 2013;35:233–42.
7. Barlow KM, Minns RA. Annual incidence of shaken impact syndrome in young children. Lancet. 2000;356:1571–2.
8. Basmaci M, Hasturk AE. Chronic subdural hematoma in a child with acute myeloid leukemia after leukocytosis. Indian J Crit Care Med. 2012;16:222–4.
9. Borzone M, Capuzzo T, Perria C, Rivano C, Tercero E. Traumatic subdural hygromas: a report of 70 surgically treated cases. J Neurosurg Sci. 1983;27:161–5.
10. Caffey J. Multiple fractures in the long bones of infants suffering from chronic subdural hematoma. Am J Roentgenol. 1946;56:163–7.
11. Caldarelli M, Di Rocco C, Romani R. Surgical treatment of chronic subdural hygromas in infants and children. Acta Neurochir. 2002;144:581–8.
12. Camel M, Grubb RL Jr. Treatment of chronic subdural hematoma by twist-drill craniostomy with continuous catheter drainage. J Neurosurg. 1986;65:183–7.
13. Capella L, Pierre-Karin A, Sainte Rose C, Renier D, Hoppe-Hirsch E, Hirsch JF. Treatment of chronic subdural collection in infants by subdural peritoneostomy. Neurochirurgie. 1989;35:404–6.
14. Christian CW, Block R, Committee on Child Abuse and Neglect, American Academy of Pediatrics. Abusive head trauma in infants and children. Pediatrics. 2009;123:1409–11.

15. Cohen I. Chronic subdural accumulation of cerebrospinal fluid after cranial trauma. Report of a case. Arch Neurol Psychiatry (Chicago). 1927;18:709–23.
16. Dandy WE. Chronic subdural hygroma and serous meningitis (pachymeningitis serosa; localized external hydrocephalus). In: Lewis D, editor. Practice of surgery. Hagerstown: W. F. Prior; 1952. p. 291–3.
17. Dias A, Taha S, Vinikoff L, Andriamamonjy C, Leriche B, Bintner M. Chronic subdural hematoma in utero. Case report with literature review. Neurochirurgie. 1998;44:124–6.
18. Domenicucci M, Russo N, Giugni E, Pierallini A. Relationship between supratentorial arachnoid cyst and chronic subdural hematoma: neuroradiological evidence and surgical treatment. J Neurosurg. 2009;110:1250–5.
19. Ducruet AF, Grobelny BT, Zacharia BE, Hickman ZL, DeRosa PL, Anersen KN, Sussman E, Carpenter A, Connolly ES Jr. The surgical management of chronic subdural hematoma. Neurosurg Rev. 2012;35:155–69.
20. Emmahadi M, Chadok SY, Alijani B, Behzadnia H, Rasoulian J, Andalib S. Chronic subdural hematoma in pediatrics: a case report and literature review of rare cases. Trauma Mon. 2016:38529.
21. Fanconi M, Lips U. Shaken baby syndrome in Switzerland: results of a prospective follow-up study, 2002-2007. Eur J Pediatr. 2010;169:1023–8.
22. Forman PM, Chipps BE, Meyer GA. Managing chronic subdural hematomas and effusions in infants: a continuing dilemma. Tex Med. 1974;70:62–6.
23. Friede RL. Hemorrhages in asphyxiated premature infants. In: Friede R, editor. Developmental neuropathology. Gottingen: Springer; 1989. p. 44–58.
24. Gelabert-Gonzalez M, Fernandez-Villa J, Cutrín-Prieto J, Allut AG, Martinez-Rumbo R. Arachnoid cyst rupture with subdural hygroma: report of three cases and literature review. Childs Nerv Syst. 2002;18:609–13.
25. Glenn CA, Fung KM, Tullos HJ, McNall-Knapp RY, Gunda D, Mapstone TB. Primary intracranial sarcoma presenting as chronic subdural fluid collections in a child. World Neurosurg. 2015;86(514):13–8.
26. Goodman JM, Mealey J Jr. Postmeningitic subdural effusions: the syndrome and its management. J Neurosurg. 1969;30:658–63.
27. Green PM. Idiopathic intracranial haemorrhage in the fetus. Fetal Diagn Ther. 1999;14:275–8.
28. Gruber DP, Crone KR. Endoscopic washout: a new tecnique for treatment chronic subdural hematomas in infants. Pediatr Neurosurg. 1997;27:292–5.
29. Gutierrez FA, McLone DG, Raimondi AJ. Physiopathology and a new treatment of chronic subdural hematoma in children. Childs Brain. 1976;5:216–32.
30. Haines DE, Harkey HL, al-Mefty O. The "subdural" space: a new look at an outdated concept. Neurosurgery. 1993;32:111–20.
31. Herrmann B. Epidemiologie, Klinik und Konzept des Schütteltrauma-Syndroms. Pädiatr Praxis. 2016;86:*297*–12.
32. Hobbs C, Childs AM, Wynne J, Livingston J, Seal A. Subdural haematoma and effusion in infancy: an epidemiological study. Arch Dis Child. 2005;90:952–5.
33. Hollenhorst RW, Stein HA, Keith HM, MacCarty LS. Subdural hematoma, subdural hygroma and subarachnoid hemorrage among infants and children. Neurosurgery. 1957;7:813–9.
34. Hoppe-Hirsch E, Sainte Rose C, Renier D, Hirsch JF. Pericerebral collections after shunting. Childs Nerv Syst. 1987;3:97–102.
35. Huang J, Li J, Zhang J, Gao C, Quan W, Tian Y, Sun J, Tian Q, Wang D, Dong J, Zhang J, Jiang R. Treatment of relapsed chronic subdural hematoma in four young children with atorvastatin and low-dose dexamethasone. Pharmacotherapy. 2019;39:783–9.
36. Hwang SK, Kim SL. Infantile head injury, with special reference to the development of chronic subdural hematoma. Childs Nerv Syst. 2000;16:590–4.
37. Ingraham FD, Matson DD. Subdural hematoma in infancy. J Pediatr. 1944;24:1–37.
38. Ito H, Yamamoto S, Komai T, Mizukoshi H. Role of local hyperfibrinolysis in the etiology of chronic subdural hematoma. J Neurosurg. 1976;45:26–31.

39. Jayawant S, Rawlinson A, Gibbon F, Price J, Schulte J, Sharples P, Sibert JR, Kemp AM. Subdural haemorrhages in infants: population based study. BMJ. 1998;317:1558–61.
40. Keenan HT, Runyan DK, Marshall SW, Nocera MA, Merten DF, Sinal SH. A population-based study of inflicted traumatic brain injury in young children. JAMA. 2003;290:621–6.
41. Kobayashi M, Toshinami N, Maeda T, Ito K, Hisada K. Post-meningitis subdural hygroma in a child showing abnormal RI accumulation in 169Yb-DTPA RI cisternography (in Japan). Kaku Igaku. 1976;13:553–7.
42. Kolias AG, Chari A, Santarius T, Hutchinson PJ. Chronic subdural haematoma: modern management and emerging therapies. Nat Rev Neurol. 2014;10:570–8.
43. Kwak YS, Hwang SK, Park SH, Park JY. Chronic subdural hematoma associated with the middle fossa arachnoid cyst: pathogenesis and review of its management. Childs Nerv Syst. 2013;29:77–82.
44. Lee KS. The pathogenesis and clinical significance of traumatic sub-dural hygroma. Brain Inj. 1998;12:595–603.
45. Levy PA. Inborn errors of metabolism: part 1: specific disorders. Pediatr Rev. 2009;30:131–7.
46. Litofsky NS, Raffel C, McComb JG. Management of symptomatic chronic extra-axial fluid collections in pediatric patients. Neurosurgery. 1992;31:445–50.
47. Lutschg J, Vassella F. Neurological complications in hemophilia. Acta Paediatr Scand. 1981;70:235–41.
48. Markwalder TM. Chronic subdural hematomas: a review. J Neurosurg. 1981;54:637–45.
49. Matschke J, Herrmann B, Sperhake J, Körber F, Bajanowski T, Glatzel M. Shaken baby syndrome: a common variant of non-accidental head injury in infants. Dtsch Arztebl Int. 2009;106:211–7.
50. Matson DD. Neurosurgery of infancy and childhood. 2nd ed. Springfield: Charles C Thomas; 1969. p. 328–51.
51. Mayer S, Rowland L. Head injury. In: Merritt's neurology, Rowland L (Ed). Philadelphia: Lippincott Williams & Wilkins, 2000, pp. 401.
52. McLaurin RL, Crone RK. Subdural hematomas and effusions in children. In: Wilkins RH, Rengachary SS, editors. Neurosurgery. New York: McGraw-Hill; 1996. p. 3741–4.
53. McLaurin RL, Isaacs E, Lewis HP. Results of nonoperative treatment in 15 cases of infantile subdural hematoma. J Neurosurg. 1971;34:753–9.
54. McLaurin RL. Subdural hematomas and effusions in children. In: Wilkins RH, Rengachary SS, editors. Neurosurgery. New York: McGraw-Hill; 1985. p. 2211–4.
55. McLone DC, Cutierrir FA, Itaimondi A. Ultrastructure of subdural membranes in children. Concepts in pediatric neurosurgery, vol. 1. Basel: Karger; 1981. p. 174–37.
56. Mizoi K, Takaku A, Suzuki J. Subdural efusion following radical surgery for chiasmal region tumors in children. Childs Brain. 1981;8:307–15.
57. Morris AA. Glutaric aciduria and suspected child abuse. Arch Dis Child. 1999;80:404–5.
58. Nakamura N. Head injuries: its mechanism and diagnosis at the acute stage. Tokyo: Bunkodo; 1986. p. 723–33.
59. Njiokiktjien CJ, Valk J, Ponssen H. Subdural hygroma: results of treatment by ventriculo-abdominal shunt. Childs Brain. 1980;7:285–302.
60. Oka H, Motomochi M, Suzuki Y, Ando K. Subdural hygroma after head injury. A review of 26 cases. Acta Neurochir (Wien). 1972;26:265–73.
61. Osborn AG. Chronic subdural hematoma. In: Osborn AG, Jhaveri MD, Salzman KL, editors. Diagnostic imaging: brain. Philadelphia: Elsevier; 2016. p. 164–7.
62. Otake G. Experience in external drainage of traumatic infantile subdural effusion. Shoni No No Shinkei. 1983;8:67–78.
63. Parent AT. Pediatric subdural hematoma: a retrospective comparative analysis. Pediatr Neurosurg. 1992;18:266–71.
64. Parsch CS, Krass I, Hoffmann E, Meixensberger J, Roosen K. Arachnoid cysts associated with subdural hematomas and hygromas: analysis of in cases, long-term follow-up, and review of literature. Neurosurgery. 1997;40:432–90.

65. Payr E. Meningitis serosa bei un nach Schaedelwerletzungen (traumatica). Med Klin. 1916;12:841–6.
66. Pereira C, Monterio J, Santos E, Dias L. Subdural hematoma in childhood: considerations about twenty cases and review of the literature. Internet J Pediatr Neonatol. 2004;5:1.
67. Powers CJ, Fuchs HE, George TM. Chronic subdural hematoma of the neonate: report of two cases and literature review. Pediatr Neurosurg. 2007;43:25–8.
68. Proctor MB. Neurosurgical aspects of nonaccidental trauma in children. In: Loftus B, editor. Neurological surgery principles and practice. Philadelphia: Lippincott Williams & Wilkins; 2003. p. 1065.
69. Punt J. Mechanisms and management of subdural hemorrhage. In: Minns RA, Brown JK, editors. Shaking and other non-accidental head injuries in children. London: Mac Keith Press; 2005. p. 290–313.
70. Rabe EF. Subdural effusions in infants. Pediatr Clin North Am. 1967;14:831–50.
71. Rutty GN, Squier MVW. Subdural hematoma in children. Essentials of autopsy practice: current methods and modern trends. 2006;4:131–53.
72. Sajanti J, Majamaa K. High concentrations of procollagen propeptides in chronic subdural haematoma and effusion. J Neurol Neurosurg Psychiatry. 2003;74:522–4.
73. Saudubray JM. Clinical approach to inborn errors of metabolism in pediatrics. In: Saudubray JM, Berghe GB, Walter JH, editors. Inborn metabolic disease. Berlin, Heidelberg: Springer; 2012. p. 3–52.
74. Servadei F, Vergoni G, Frattarelli M, Pasini A, Arista A, Fagioli L. Arachnoid cyst of middle cranial fossa and ipsilateral subdural haematoma: diagnostic and therapeutic implications in three cases. Br J Neurosurg. 1993;7:249–53.
75. Sherwood D. Chronic subdural hematoma in infants. Am J Dis Child. 1930;39:980–1021.
76. Shrestha R, You C. Spontaneous chronic subdural hematoma associated with arachnoid cyst in children and young adults. Asian J Neurosurg. 2014;9:168–72.
77. Sun J, Wang W, Wang D, An S, Xue L, Wang Y, Zhu SG, Jiang RC, Yang XJ, Yue SY. Clinical analysis of 10 patients of chronic subdural hematoma associated with arachnoid cyst. Zhonghua Yi Xue Za Zhi. 2017;97:1502–4.
78. Swift DM, McBride L. Chronic subdural hematoma in children. Neurosurg Clin N Am. 2000;11:439–46.
79. Sychlowy A, Pyda E. Toxic diarrhea in a heterozygote with galactosemia complicated by chronic subdural hematoma. Pol Tyg Lek. 1971;26:349–51.
80. Tsubokawa T, Nakamura S, Satoh K. Effect of temporary subdural-peritoneal shunt on subdural effusion with subarachnoid effusion. Childs Brain. 1984;11:47–59.
81. Tzioumi D, Oates RK. Subdural hematomas in children under 2 years. Accidental or inflicted? A ill year experience. Child Abuse Negl. 1998;22:1105–12.
82. Uscinski R. Shaken baby syndrome: fundamental questions. Br J Neurosurg. 2002;16:217–9.
83. Vapalahti PM. Intracranial arterial aneurysm in a three-month-old infant. Case report. J Neurosurg. 1969;30:169–71.
84. Victor M, Ropper A. Craniocerebral trauma. In: Victor M, Ropper A, editors. Adams and Victor's principles of neurology. 7th ed. New York: McGraw-Hill; 2001. p. 925.
85. Vinchon M, Defoort-Dhellemmes S, Noule N, Duhem R, Dhellemmes P. Accidental or nonaccidental brain injury in infants. Prospective study of 88 cases. Presse Med. 2004;33:1174–9.
86. Wang HK, Chen HJ, Lu K, Liliang PC, Liang CL, Tsai YD, Wang KW. A pediatric chronic subdural hematoma after dodgeball head injury. Pediatr Emerg Care. 2010;26:667–8.
87. Wang HS, Kim SW, Kim SH. Spontaneous chronic subdural hematoma in an adolescent girl. J Korean Neurosurg Soc. 2013;53:201–3.
88. Wang KD, Zhao JZ, Li JS, Zhang Y. Clinical study of patients of arachnoid cyst associated with chronic subdural hematoma. Zhonghua Yi Xue Za Zhi. 2011;9:460–3.
89. Wittschieber D, Kinner S, Pfeiffer H, Karger B, Hahnemann ML. Forensic aspects of imaging procedures in shaken baby syndrome—methodology, findings, differential diagnoses (in German). Rechtsmedizin. 2018;28:486–94.

90. Wittschieber D, Karger B, Niederstadt T, Pfeiffer H, Hahnemann ML. Subdural hygromas in abusive head trauma: pathogenesis, diagnosis, and forensic implications. AJNR Am J Neuroradiol. 2015;36:432–9.
91. Wittschieber D, Karger B, Pfeiffer H, Hahnemann ML. Understanding subdural collections in pediatric abusive head trauma. AJNR Am J Neuroradiol. 2019;40:388–95.
92. Wu X, Li G, Zhao J, Zhu X, Zhang Y, Hou K. Arachnoid cyst-associated chronic subdural hematoma: report of 14 cases and a systematic literature review. World Neurosurg. 2017;109:118–30.
93. Yasunaga A, Mori K, Matsusaka T. Intracranial hemorrhage due to vitamin K deficiency and chronic subdural hemorrhage in infants (in Japan). Proceedings of the 17th Annual Meeting of the Japanese Society of Pediatric Neurosurgery, In: Hayakawa I (ed.). Tokyo: Neuron, 1989, pp. 28–29.
94. Zhang H, Zhang JM, Chen G. Chronic subdural hematoma associated with arachnoid cyst: report of two cases. Chin Med J. 2007;120:2339–40.

Chapter 13
Imaging in Chronic Subdural Hematoma

Ersen Ertekin, Tuna Sahin, and Ahmet T. Turgut

13.1 Introduction

Chronic subdural hematoma (CSDH) is a disease characterized by the abnormal accumulation of blood products in the subdural space. Although its annual incidence varies according to different sources, it is between 1.72 and 20.6 per 100,000 and its incidence increases with aging [23, 50, 51].

The most important etiological factor in CSDH formation is trauma. A trauma history is evident in the vast majority of patients. The majority of these traumas are minor traumas. It has been reported that a CSDH develops in cases of intracranial hypotension developing after spontaneous or various surgical interventions that include spinal anesthesia application or after lumbar puncture. In addition, the conversion to CSDH as a result of capillary microhemorrhages in some subdural hygromas is significantly high [13, 31, 46]. Coagulopathies and the use of anticoagulants and antiplatelet drugs can contribute to the formation of CSDH by causing bleeding even in clinically insignificant traumas; specifically factor 8 deficiencies can cause spontaneous CSDH without trauma [4]. For this reason, especially in cases without any other underlying causative factors, patients should be evaluated for Factor 8 deficiency.

Some risk factors have been identified for the development and progression of CSHD, which is a dynamic process. Among these, advanced age is generally an accepted risk factor, and the more fragile vascular wall associated with age, the

E. Ertekin (✉) · T. Sahin
Department of Radiology, Aydın Adnan Menderes University Faculty of Medicine, Aydın, Turkey

A. T. Turgut
Department of Radiology, Yüksek İhtisas University Faculty of Medicine, Balgat, Ankara, Turkey

M. Turgut et al. (eds.), *Subdural Hematoma*,
https://doi.org/10.1007/978-3-030-79371-5_13

increase in the use of anticoagulant drugs due to concomitant systemic diseases, and the potential to fall more often than the general population are emphasized as the main factors [2, 21]. Because CSDH is rare in infants, the presence of bilateral CSDH should lead to the consideration of non-accidental trauma or type 1 glutaric aciduria [9, 36]. Male gender is considered among the risk factors due to the more frequent exposure to trauma and high alcohol use [2]. Another important risk factor for CSDH is anticoagulation or antiplatelet therapy [2, 21, 40]. CSDH generally displays a slow clinical course. Although the clinical presentation varies in its spectrum from asymptomatic patients to those in a coma, the most frequently observed symptoms are headache, seizure, and mental state changes.

Clinical presentations that may be observed include nausea/vomiting, weakness, dysarthria, gait disturbances, sensory disturbances, paralysis, and coma. The clinic findings usually develop secondary to increased intracranial pressure or brain compression as a result of the enlargement of the existing hematoma. Coma develops in 3–20% of the cases, and brain herniations are observed in 2%. CSDHs are aseptic collections, but they are also a potential focus for infections. Therefore, this possibility should be kept in mind if a patient has an underlying clinical infection [28, 41, 47].

The pathophysiology of CSDH remains unclear. Many hypotheses have been proposed with the most notable of the theories being an inflammatory response and the transformation from acute subdural hematoma (SDH) [13]. In his case report published in 1847, Virchow interpreted the findings of the inflammatory response on the inner surface of the dura as inflammatory in origin with the hemorrhage defined as pachymeningitis hemorrhage interna [48]. Trotter, on the other hand, supported the theory that CSDH transformed from an acute hemorrhage by arguing that a minor trauma was initially sustained, although in some cases the trauma history was not recalled on deeper investigation [45]. In addition, Holmes et al. supported the traumatic theory and stated that recurrent microtraumas can cause repeat rupture of the bridging vessels and that neovascularized vessels, which play a role in the growth of the existing hematoma, are less resistant to rupture [17]. On the contrary, Gardner and Zollinger suggested that the osmotic pressure difference between collections of blood products and blood vessels was responsible for the growth of the hematoma. However, the study by Weir et al. showed that there was no difference between hematoma osmolality and cerebrospinal fluid (CSF) or venous blood osmolality, which refuted this theory [15, 49, 53]. Recent studies believe that a chronic subdural hygroma is the main source for CSDH formation [14, 19, 24]. About half of the subdural effusions (SDE) eventually become CSDHs. The rupture of bridging vessels, hemorrhage from the hygroma wall due to neocapillaries, vascular hyperpermeability, increased fibrinolysis, and increased protein content in the hygroma are some of the explanations proposed for traumatic SDE pathogenesis transformed into CSDH [8, 11, 14]. We can categorize the clinical progression of CSDH in three distinct periods. The first period is the hemorrhage period in which there is one or more clinical/subclinical microtraumas that we can consider as seed removal. The latent period where the hematoma matures immediately follows. During this period, the hematoma continues to expand as a result of microhemorrhages from the fragile neovasculature while the capsule formation is manifested by the formation of neomembranes in the adjacent dura and arachnoid. Hematoma enlargement is aided by an increase in fibrinolytic activity. The latent period can asymptomatically last for years. The clinical period begins when intracranial compensation mechanisms are insufficient as a result of the continued enlargement. During this period, symptoms due to direct mass effect and/or global intracranial pressure increase begin to emerge [8, 11, 14, 19, 24].

The treatment of symptomatic CSDH is surgery. The size of the hematoma is the main factor in influencing surgical selection. While the approach through twist drill holes or burr hole openings is preferred in small-sized hematomas, craniotomy is the method used in large-sized hematomas and in cases where burr-hole treatment is inadequate. In asymptomatic patients, it is essential to correct an underlying coagulopathy due to underlying pathologies and medications in addition to providing symptomatic treatment [1, 3, 38].

Regarding prognosis, it has been reported in the literature that very few cases regress spontaneously. While the success rate of nonsurgical treatment is approximately 40%, 20% of the cases progress and require surgery [23, 50, 51]. Surgical treatment success rates approach 90%. Although CSDH recurrence rates are high (70%), only about 10–20% of these cases require repeat surgery [30, 35]. The location of the CSDH, its internal structure, its bilateral tendency, the patient's hospitalization status, advanced age, alcohol consumption, kidney and liver function disorders, and the presence of systemic diseases are considered risk factors for recurrence [22, 42]. The role of anticoagulant or antiplatelet drug use in the recurrence of CSDH is controversial. Recurrence rates also differ with respect to treatment methods. In general, the recurrence rates for burr hole techniques are higher than those for craniectomy [6, 22, 42]. There is a discrepancy between different studies in terms of recurrence rates of nonsurgical treatment, but it can be said that it is somewhat higher than for surgical treatment in general.

13.2 Radiological Imaging in CSDH: Basic Principles

Unenhanced computed tomography (CT) has become the accepted standard imaging method in the first investigation of patients with suspected SDH due to its widespread availability, rapid acquisition time, and noninvasive feature. While rapid scanning times can be obtained especially with multi-detector CT devices, a significant reduction in the radiation exposure dose is achieved thanks to dual-source and dual energy techniques and interactive methods. Although magnetic resonance imaging (MRI) has a restricted role in the investigation of acute SDH, it provides very useful information for revealing secondary causes such as dural tumors, evaluating pathologies in the cerebral parenchyma or cavities containing CSF, and detecting complications such as herniation [6].

13.2.1 General Imaging Characteristics of Subdural Hematoma

Generally, subdural hemorrhagic deposits are crescent-shaped extra-axial collections covering the cerebral hemispheres. Existing anatomical barriers are an important factor that determines the overall appearance of fluid or hematoma that accumulates in the subdural space. While the lesions do not cross the natural barriers formed by the dura at the interhemispheric fissure and tentorium level, unlike the epidural collections, they pass through the sutures since they have no association with the periosteum. Since SDHs tend to spread through the potential space between the dura mater and arachnoid mater, they do not extend into the sulci and cisterns in the absence of an accompanying subarachnoid hemorrhage. Another important factor affecting the appearance of SDHs is the age of the blood and the dissolution stage of the existing hematoma. Since CSDHs generally transform from acute SDH, it is necessary to mention the appearance of the age of the blood on imaging studies. Lesions on CT appear in shades of black and white, according to their density as specified by Hounsfield Units (HU). This is a standard method to describe a lesion by comparing it to another reference tissue, although one can have a general idea of the tissue type directly by measuring its density. If the lesions are of lower density compared to the reference tissue, they will appear in a more black tone and are referred to as "hypodense." If they are of equal density with the reference tissue, they are considered as "isodense," and if they are higher density than the reference tissue, they are regarded as "hyperdense" and have a more white tone. In general for cranial pathologies, cerebral gray matter is chosen as the reference tissue, and an acute phase SDH is mostly visible as homogeneously hyperdense. In the subsequent days, the lesion density decreases by an average of 1.5 HU per day and becomes isodense after 7–10 days. On the 10–14th days, the hematoma generally becomes hypodense and an uncomplicated CSDH usually decreases to CSF density after 2 weeks [25]. The evolution of the density of the SDH with respect to time is summarized in Table 13.1.

MRI appearance of SDHs is more complicated since many factors play a role in signal formation on MRI. The main markers determining the appearance of the hematoma are the structure of the hemoglobin within the lesion and its oxidation products. When the blood elements are out of the vein, the oxygenated hemoglobin in the red blood cell transforms first to deoxyhemoglobin and then later to

Table 13.1 CT appearance of subdural hematoma

Hematoma stage	Time	Computed tomography appearance
Hyperacute	<24 h	Hyperdense
Acute	1–3 days	Hyperdense
Early subacute	3–7 days	Hyperdense
Late subacute	7–14 days	Isodense
Chronic	>14 days	Hypodense

methemoglobin. This is followed by cell lysis with extracellular methemoglobin to lastly become ferritin and hemosiderin. These forms are associated with blood products in the hyperacute (<24 h), acute (24–72 h), early subacute (3–7 days), late subacute (7–14 days), and chronic stages (>14 days), respectively, and MRI determines the signal on the image. SDH, which is isointense in the acute and hyperacute period due to the lack of magnetic moment of oxyhemoglobin and deoxyhemoglobin, becomes hyperintense with the formation of methemoglobin, which is paramagnetic in the subacute phase. On T2-weighted images, the subdural collection is hyperintense due to a high water content. However, with the magnetic susceptibility effect of deoxyhemoglobin, intracellular methemoglobin, and hemosiderin, signal loss is observed and becomes hypointense on acute, late subacute, and chronic phases. Contrary to this complexity in the conventional sequences of MRI (T1- and T2-weighted images), the fluid attenuated inversion healing (FLAIR) images are frequently hyperintense in acute, subacute, and chronic stages. On gradient echo (GRE) T2 * and susceptibility-weighted images (SWI), acute hemorrhage or chronic hemosiderin rims often appear hypointense. These magnetic susceptibility sequences (GRE, T2 * and SWI) are extremely sensitive for the detection of chronic blood products (hemichromes and peripheric siderosis) [6, 43]. The views of SDHs according to time are summarized in Table 13.2.

In the natural course of a SDH, although radiological imaging features are well defined, it is not so easy to diagnose hematoma and determine its age in many cases. The most important reason for this is the intermittent recurrence or continuity of active bleeding. In many cases, due to the simultaneous presence of different stages of blood elements, a heterogeneous signal character is observed within the lesion. In addition, endogenous and exogenous factors that cause disruptions in the natural evolution of the hematoma can make the determination of the age difficult. The presence of coagulopathy or the use of anticoagulants, CSF leakage into the subdural space due to arachnoid membrane rupture, a low hematocrit due to profound anemia, or a superposed infection could affect by the density of the hematoma [10, 25, 43]. The role of radiology in CSDH is not limited to diagnosis. In addition to the diagnosis, evaluation of the possible secondary effects and the follow-up of CSDH with or without treatment are the most frequently used radiological imaging methods.

Table 13.2 MRI signals of the hematoma according to its stage

	MRI sequences		
Subdural hematoma stage	T1-weighted images	T2-weighted images	Fluid attenuation inversion recovery
Hyperacute	Isointense	Hyperintense	Hyperintense
Acute	Isointense	Hypointense	Hyperintense
Early subacute	Hyperintense	Hypointense	Hyperintense
Late subacute	Hyperintense	Hyperintense	Hyperintense
Chronic center rim	Isointense	Hyperintense Hypointense	Hyperintense

13.2.2 Classical Chronic Subdural Hematoma/Hygroma

As mentioned earlier, CSDHs refer to subdural hematomas that have existed for at least 2–3 weeks. In CSDHs that are formed as a result of acute bleeding, due to the destruction of blood products and progressive inflammation over time, the center will take the form of liquefied blood or a serosanguinous fluid with capsule formation at the periphery. At this stage, the radiological appearance of the CSDH is similar to that of CSF. Subdural hygromas resulting from traumatic arachnoid tearing or passive effusion in the case of spontaneous intracranial hypotension, dehydration, or brain atrophy are a collection of CSF without blood. At this stage, it is impossible to distinguish these two lesions from each other with CT, since both liquefied CSDH and subdural hygroma are seen as homogeneously hypodense on non-contrast CT (Fig. 13.1). In these cases, looking at the patient's previous imaging studies, if available, may help to determine the diagnosis. The diagnosis of CSDH can be made easily in cases with acute or subacute hemorrhage on the previous CT examination. Apart from this, the hematocrit effect due to gravity in some CSDHs contributes to the diagnosis in favor of a CSDH (Fig. 13.2). The hematocrit effect, which can be defined as the settling of the dense hemorrhagic components in the posterior aspect due to the effect of gravity with a liquid-sediment level with the CSF collection being superior, is an unexpected effect in hygroma without acute bleeding. The addition of acute bleeding to the event will not cause any difficulties in diagnosis since it will be hyperdense in the collection [5, 6, 43].

Unlike on CT, in MRI, CSDH is easy to distinguish from subdural hygroma, which appears in all MRI sequences with CSF characteristics. As a result of denaturation of extracellular methemoglobin in the chronic period, non-paramagnetic

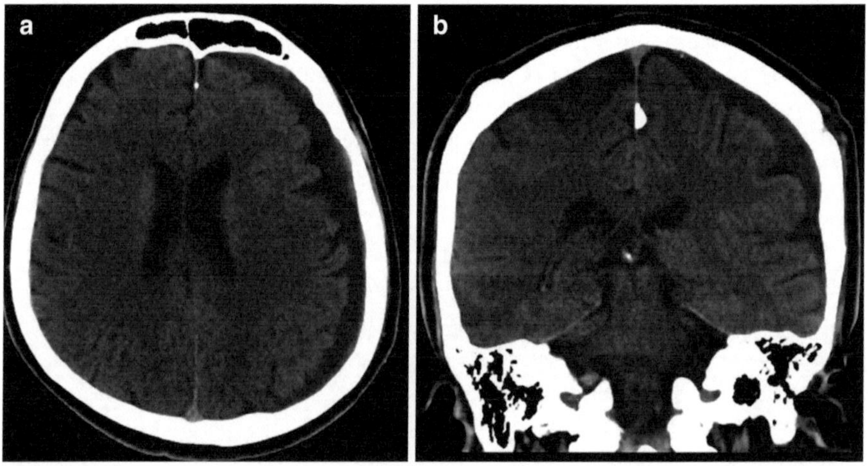

Fig. 13.1 A 60-year-old male patient; on reformatted CT images in axial (**a**) and coronal planes (**b**), a crescent-shaped, extra-axial hypodense collection (classical chronic subdural hematoma) is observed in the left frontoparietal region

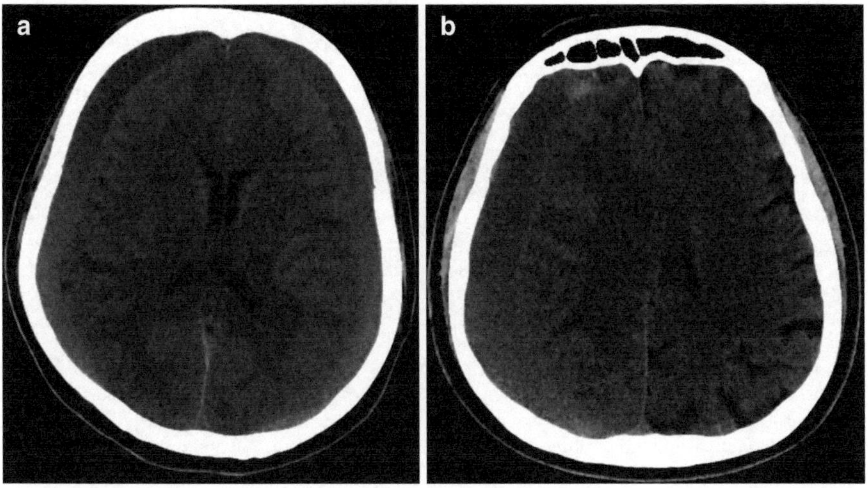

Fig. 13.2 Axial CT image of two different patients. (**a**) In the patient with bilateral subdural hemorrhage, fluid-fluid layering is observed in the bilateral frontoparietal region, as a result of the collapse of the dense hemorrhagic contents. (**b**) The patient with chronic subdural hematoma in the right frontoparietal region has hyperdensity of acute hemorrhage in the frontal region and hematocrit effect secondary to this in the posterior location

hemichromes, also known as "hemoglobin degradation products," are formed. The T1 signal of these hemichromes is less pronounced than that of methemoglobin, causing the hematoma intensity to decrease over time. However, because the protein content of SDH is higher than that of CSF, the T1 signal is always higher than that of CSF (hyperintense compared to CSF, isointense compared to gray matter). The T2 signal decreases slightly over time due to the magnetic sensitivity effect and high protein content, and it is seen as hyperintense compared to gray matter and isointense-hypointense compared to CSF. Unlike parenchymal hematomas, the hemosiderin ring is seen less frequently in SDHs, as the macrophages responsible for iron storage cannot remain in the axial spaces. Only in CSDHs, the peripheral siderosis ring can be identified as hypointense in GRE and SWI sequences that are sensitive to blood elements. Subdural hygromas do not show hemichromes and are therefore hypointense because they contain blood products and are observed with the same intensity as CSF. While normal CSF is suppressed in the FLAIR sequence, the SDH remains hyperintense and can thus be easily distinguished from a subdural hygroma (Fig. 13.3). A homogeneous and uncomplicated CSDH shows no diffusion restriction. The presence of diffusion restriction should suggest the presence of recurrent bleeding or a superposed infection [6, 43].

Thick internal septations may develop in some CSDHs. Both thick septa and the hematoma capsule are seen as hyperdense on CT. It is important to not confuse these hyperdense thick septa with active bleeding. On occasion in long-standing hematomas, diffuse thickened dural hyperdensity may appear as a result

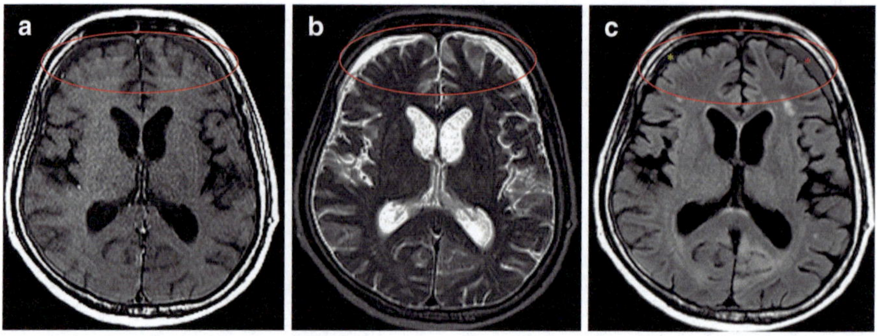

Fig. 13.3 Bifrontal extra-axial collections are observed in MR images of a 67-year-old male patient. The collections are hypointense on T1 (**a**) and hyperintense on T2 (**b**), but the collection density is higher on T1 than CSF on the left side. On FLAIR sequence (**c**), the collection signal on the right is suppressed (subdural hygroma), while the left collection is not suppressed due to its hemorrhagic content (chronic subdural hematoma)

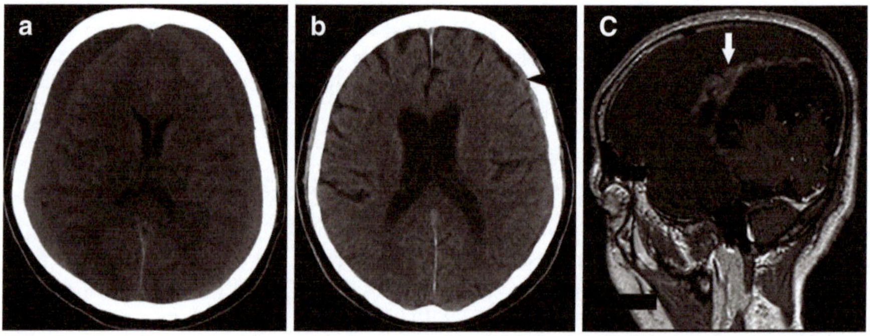

Fig. 13.4 Bilateral subdural hematoma is seen on the axial CT (**a**) image of a 56-year-old female patient. On follow-up CT imaging taken 3 months later (**b**), the collection was fully regressed on the right. On the left, while hemorrhagic content is fully resorbed, linear hyperdensity due to thickening of the dura is seen. On the sagittal contrast-enhanced T1 images (**c**) of another 70-year-old female patient, it is noteworthy that large chronic subdural hematoma is accompanied by irregular thickening of the dura (white arrow)

of complete resorption of liquefied hematoma. These thick septa and dura show significant contrast enhancement on contrast-enhanced CT or MRI (Fig. 13.4) [5, 6, 25, 43]. In long-standing hematomas, there are cases where the thickened dura is calcified. The best way to view calcifications is on CT where calcifications are hyperdense with a much higher density than acute blood elements [6, 25, 43]. On MRI, it is not possible to distinguish between calcification and hemichromes because they have signals similar to chronic blood destruction products. Therefore, it is recommended to image the case with CT when calcification is suspected.

The enlargements observed in the CSF spaces in patients with brain atrophy may pose a potential challenge in the diagnosis of CSDH and subdural hygroma [20].

Since no mass effect such as cortical buckling and sulcal effacement is observed in these patients, MRI should be preferred instead of CT in making the diagnosis and a careful examination will be useful for the diagnosis.

13.2.3 Acute on Chronic (Mixed Type) Subdural Hematomas

In CSDH, which is a dynamic process, things are not always uniform. Collection may become heterogeneous due to delays in hemoglobin degradation due to many endogenous and exogenous factors, or recurrent bleeding from rupture of bridging vessels and capsule membranes. In a chronic hematoma, acute blood elements or, less frequently, all three stages of blood elements can be observed in the same collection. A similar situation occurs in subdural hygroma with hemorrhages arising from the more fragile neovascular structures, which is not uncommon. CSF leakage into a hematoma collection is another entity that can make the image heterogeneous. All these situations may cause difficulties in diagnosis by causing a complex appearance of the CSDH on CT and MRI.

On unenhanced CT, the appearance of acute on chronic hematomas is seen as gravity-dependent hematocrit layering in a crescent-shaped subdural collection (Fig. 13.5). While hyperdense acute blood products are identified posteriorly with a dependent effect, liquefied chronic blood products are layered superiorly. Especially in chronic collections with septa, hyperdense acute blood elements may be visible in multiple diffuse locations. Hyperdense pockets containing acute blood products in multiloculated collections, multiple fluid-fluid level areas, and localized hyperdense collections can be seen [5].

Acute on CSDHs on MRI may show hematocrit leveling and compartmentalized acute blood product areas similar to those seen on CT. Mixed-type SDHs are highly variable depending on the amount of hemoglobin breakdown and the organization of different stage blood products. T1 and T2 signals are generally heterogeneous. FLAIR images are generally hyperdense while blooming artifact is seen on GRE and SWI (Fig. 13.5). Acute or subacute blood products usually show diffusion restriction on DWI. The fibrous capsule and internal septa show significant contrast enhancement on postcontrast T1-weighted images [5].

13.2.4 Secondary Effects of CSDH

Similarly important as the detection of SDH is the determination of the secondary effects that can be life-threatening and can guide treatment. The main mechanism responsible for secondary effects is the mass effect on the brain. Initially, the compression effect observed on the cerebral parenchyma, sulci, and ventricle cavities adjacent to the collection can also cause midline shift, herniation, obstructive

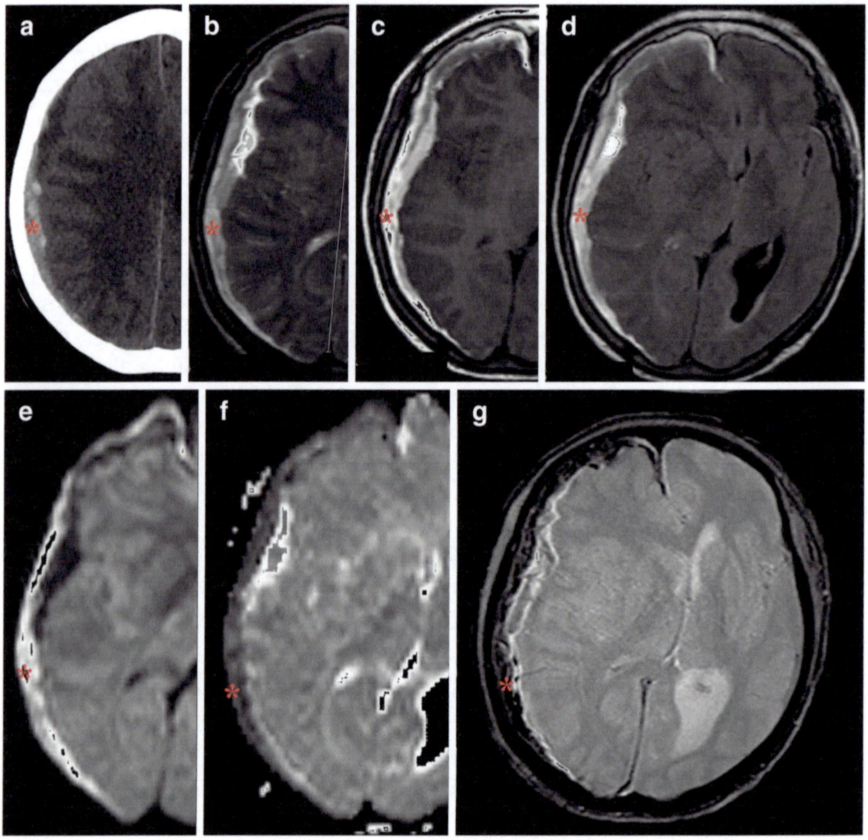

Fig. 13.5 In axial brain CT (**a**) of a 58-year-old male patient, a subdural collection due to acute on chronic hematoma in the right frontoparietal is observed. In the control MRI examination (**b–g**) taken 2 days later, an increase in the size of the hematoma was observed. Heterogeneous signal containing hypo-isointense areas on axial T2 (**b**), hyperintensities due to acute bleeding (red asterisk) in non-contrast T1 (**c**) are noticeable. In FLAIR images (**d**), the collection is viewed as hyperintense. Hyperintensity is observed in diffusion-weighted image (**e**) due to diffusion restriction in acute bleeding areas, and hypointensity on ADC map (**f**). Chronic blood products (hemichromes and hemosiderin) are selected as hypointense on gradient weighted T2 * images (**g**)

hydrocephalus, and ischemic events due to vascular compression by affecting more distant structures as the mass effect increases. Therefore, a detailed evaluation of all cases with CSDH with this consideration is important.

13.2.4.1 Mass Effect and Midline Shift

The collections observed in the subdural space first compress neighboring spaces. In the adjacent cerebral hemisphere, as a result of compression in the subarachnoid space, sulci are no longer visible, while the neighboring gyri are flattened. In radiological imaging methods, this situation manifests as the loss of visibility of the sulci

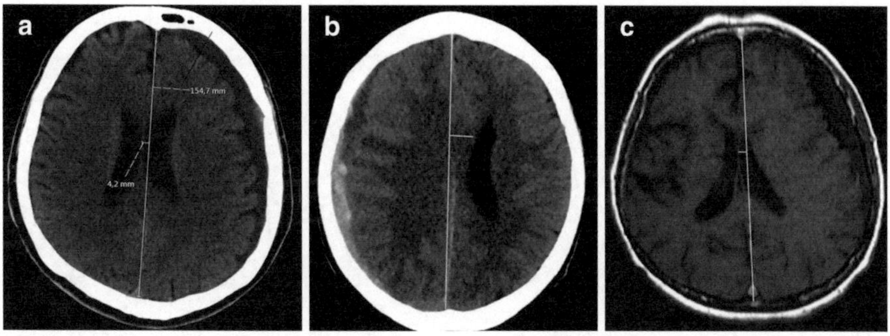

Fig. 13.6 Cases of midline shift secondary to the mass effect are observed on CT (**a**) and MRI (**c**) with chronic subdural hemorrhage and CT (**b**) images with chronic acute bleeding from different patients. On axial CT, a line is drawn between the most protruding areas of the frontal and occipital bone (midline line). The distance between this line and the septum pellicidum shows the degree of shift from the midline. Red asterisk (**b**) shows effacement in the cerebral sulcus due to the mass effect

and the cerebral parenchyma migrates toward the midline. In the next stage, cerebral edema begins to develop in the cerebral parenchyma due to vascular extravasation. Cortical thickening and loss of gray-white matter discrimination are observed due to cerebral edema. At this stage, the cerebral parenchyma appears hypodense on CT, hypointense on T1, and hyperintense on T2 and FLAIR sequences. Compression of the adjacent lateral ventricular horn and/or atrium accompanies the event. As the mass effect progresses, shift begins to occur toward the midline (Fig. 13.6). At this stage when herniation syndromes have not yet occurred, determining the presence and degree of the shift is of critical importance in the planning the appropriate patient treatment. In order to determine the shift on CT or MRI, the midline must first be drawn. For this, frontal and occipital peaks are identified and a straight line is drawn between the anterior and posterior points where the falx cerebrum joins the inner layer of the calvarium [6]. Then, the contralateral displacement of the midline structures is determined with a line perpendicular to this line. The septum pellicidum or interhemispheric fissure between the lateral ventricles can be used as midline markers.

13.2.4.2 Herniation Syndromes

As the mass effect increases in intensity, herniation syndromes, which are defined as the displacement of the brain parenchyma from the location in which it is present, to a different region may occur.

13.2.4.2.1 Subfalcine Herniation

The most common herniation syndrome, subfalcine herniation, is the displacement of the brain parenchyma and accompanying cerebral blood vessels underneath the free edge of the falx cerebri toward the opposite hemisphere. Subfalcine herniation occurs due to the mass effect of a lesion occupying space in the supratentorial com-

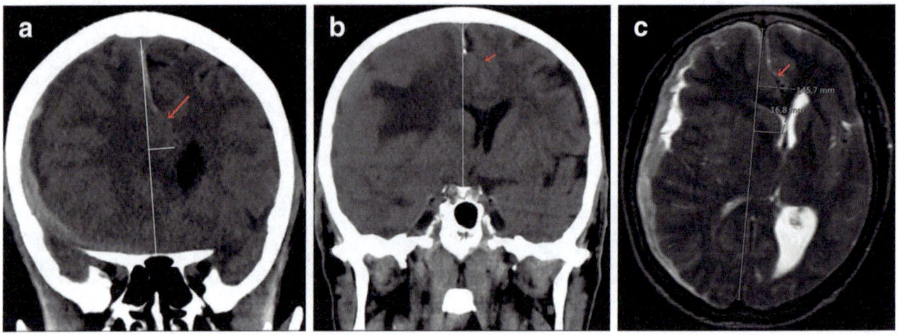

Fig. 13.7 Subfalcine herniation samples are observed on CT (**a**, **b**) in the coronal plane and T2 MRI (**c**) in the axial plane, in different patients. On coronal CT images (**a**, **b**), in addition to the midline shift, the right cingulate gyrus is displaced from under the free edge of the falx to the left (red arrow). In axial T2 MRI (**c**), in addition to the cingulate gyrus, the right anterior cerebral artery is also observed to be displaced to the left. In all cases, due to the compression of foramen Monro, enlargement of the contralateral lateral ventricle (hydrocephalus) is noted

partment where SDHs are among the most common causes. In the interhemispheric fissure, the advancing anterior cerebral arteries (ACAs) are often displaced by the herniated brain parenchyma (Fig. 13.7). One or both ACAs are compressed by the rigid free edge of the falx cerebri, leading to infarctions in the ACA perfusion territory. Therefore, careful evaluation of the brain parenchyma in ACA perfusion areas is very important in subfalcine herniation cases. In cases of severe subfalcine herniation, pressure and compression of the lateral ventricles may increase, and obstruction of the contralateral foramen of Monro may result in contralateral hydrocephalus. Ventricular dilatation is observed first in the frontal horn of the contralateral ventricle, followed by temporal horn and atrium enlargement [6, 29].

13.2.4.2.2 Descending Transtentorial Herniation

Transtentorial herniation is observed in the presence of a lesion that causes supratentorial mass effect similar to subfalcine herniation. In contrast, the direction of the mass effect is downward and medial. When there is sufficient downward pressure, the medial temporal lobe shifts downward from the free edge of the ipsilateral tentorial leaf toward the brainstem. First, obliteration of the ipsilateral ambient cistern is observed as a result of the medial displacement of the medial temporal lobe; as the mass effect increases, the loss of the quadrigeminal and suprasellar cisterns join the event (Fig. 13.8). In more severe cases, loss of consciousness, respiratory distress, cranial neuropathies, and eventually death may occur due to compression of the brainstem. Bilateral herniation can also be seen depending on the severity of the mass effect. In this case, where the brainstem is compressed from both sides, bilateral basal cistern obliteration occurs.

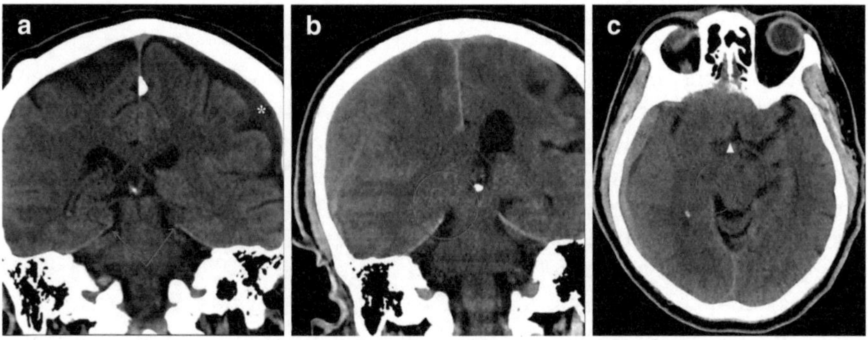

Fig. 13.8 (**a**) In a normal case, tentorium free edges, ambient systems, and temporal lobe relation (red arrows) are shown. (**b**) In the case with right subacute subdural hematoma (red asterisk), secondary to the mass effect, the right medial temporal lobe shifts to the midline and obliterates the right ambient cistern. (**c**) The axial CT image of the same patient shows obliteration of the right ambient (red circle) and suprasellar (white arrowhead) cisterns with the mass effect of the right subdural hematoma (red asterisk)

In descending transtentorial herniation, the P2 and P3 segments of the posterior cerebral arteries (PCA) may be compressed between the free edge of the tentorial leaflets and the temporal lobes during their passage through the basal cistern and may cause infarction in the PCA perfusion areas. Therefore, careful evaluation of the brain parenchyma in the ipsilateral PCA region in this type of herniation is important for early detection of infarction [6, 29].

Another clinically important point is that in severe herniation, the contralateral cerebral peduncle may become compressed with the contralateral medial temporal lobe. In this case, ipsilateral hemiparesis may develop. Pressure necrosis in the uncus and hippocampus secondary to severe herniation, infarction in the hypothalamus and basal ganglia as a result of compression of the perforating arteries originating from the proximal circle of Willis, and hemorrhagic infarctions called Duret hemorrhages in the ventral pons and midbrain as a result of compression and occlusion of the basilar perforating arteries can also be observed [6].

13.2.4.2.3 Ascending Transtentorial Herniation

Ascending transtentorial herniation is the least common type of herniation. Unlike the other two types of herniation, the source of the mass effect is in the posterior fossa. Parenchymal hemorrhages and SDHs may also lead to a similar picture, although they mostly result from mass lesions and edema that develop secondary to cerebellar infarction. There is upward displacement of the cerebellar vermis and medial cerebellar hemispheres through the tentorial opening due to the mass effect of the space-occupying lesion. As a result, the cerebellar structures that are displaced upwards push on the midbrain toward the ventral and basal cisterns that are obliterated due to the mass effect. Obstructive hydrocephalus may occur as a result of compression of the Aqueduct of Silvius and the fourth ventricle [6].

13.2.4.2.4 Acquired Tonsillar Herniation

Similar to ascending transtentorial herniation, acquired tonsillar herniation develops as a result of the mass effect of a space-occupying lesion in the posterior fossa. However, the herniation is caudally directed and the cerebellar tonsils are displaced down through the foramen magnum. Although the most common causes are edema due to posterior fossa tumors and ischemic cerebellar infarctions, parenchymal bleeding or SDHs may cause tonsillar herniation. In the imaging of tonsillar herniation, CT or MRI images in the sagittal plane are superior to axial slices. Complete filling of the foramen magnum by the cerebellar tonsils in axial cross-sectional images is a warning sign for tonsillar herniation [6, 29] (Fig. 13.9).

13.2.4.3 Obstructive Hydrocephalus

Obstructive hydrocephalus in CSDH generally occurs secondary to herniation syndromes. The most common form is contralateral ventricular hydrocephalus due to significant midline shift. While the entire contralateral ventricle may enlarge, frontal and temporal horn enlargement is more common. While hydrocephalus is expected in the third and bilateral lateral ventricles (triventricular) in transtentorial herniations, tonsillar herniations cause hydrocephalus in all ventricles (tetraventricular).

The enlargement of the temporal horns of the lateral ventricles may be the first sign of obstructive hydrocephalus [6]. Normally, temporal horns are either not visible at all or are seen as a thin line in young individuals due to their normal brain volume. In the elderly or in the presence of parenchymal atrophy for any other reason, the temporal horns become prominent, and as a result, the diagnosis of

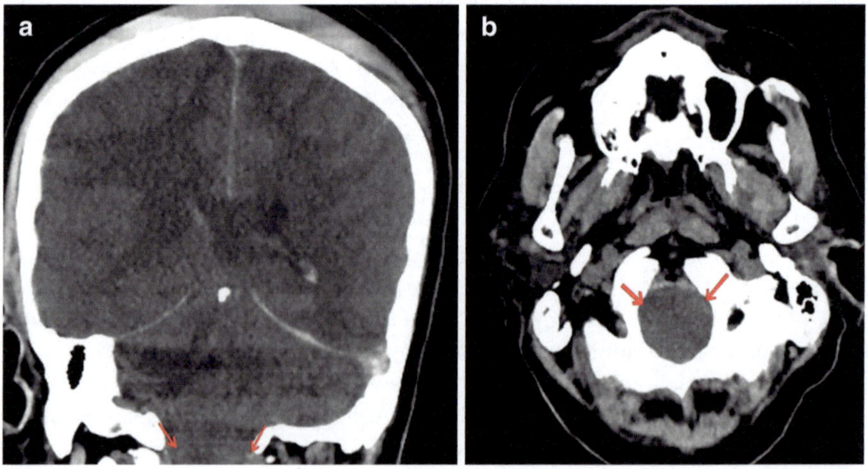

Fig. 13.9 In coronal (**a**) and axial (**b**) brain CT images, the plump appearance of the foramen magnum and compression of the medulla oblongata as a result of inferior displacement of the cerebellar tonsils draw attention

hydrocephalus becomes difficult to determine or overdiagnosis of hydrocephalus may occur. When diagnosing hydrocephalus in the presence of atrophy, it would be very useful to review and compare previous studies, if available.

13.2.5 Imaging Pitfalls and Differential Diagnosis

Normal anatomical structures and some pathologies can be confused with SDHs [7, 26]. In this section, we will briefly discuss these traps.

13.2.5.1 Prominent Venous Sinuses and Cortical Veins

Some sinuses and cortical veins can be confused with subacute and acute phase SDH, respectively, because of slow blood flow or when they are thrombosed, isodense, or hyperdense on non-contrast CT. The most common anatomical structure that causes this occurrence is the transverse sinus, followed by the sphenoparietal sinuses and cortical veins. Mastering the normal anatomical structures will be useful in avoiding this trap. Contrast-enhanced CT can be used in cases that cannot be determined. After contrast injection, normal venous sinuses and cortical veins can be safely distinguished from SDH by showing significant enhancement. Vascular structures that align parallel to the cross-section on MRI images, especially venous sinuses with slow flow rate, can be seen as hyperdense on T1 images. However, when the images obtained in other MRI sequences and in three orthogonal planes are reviewed, this distinction can be made easier than on CT (Fig. 13.10). In cases where venous structures are concerned, an accurate diagnosis can be made with magnetic resonance venography without or with contrast [7, 26].

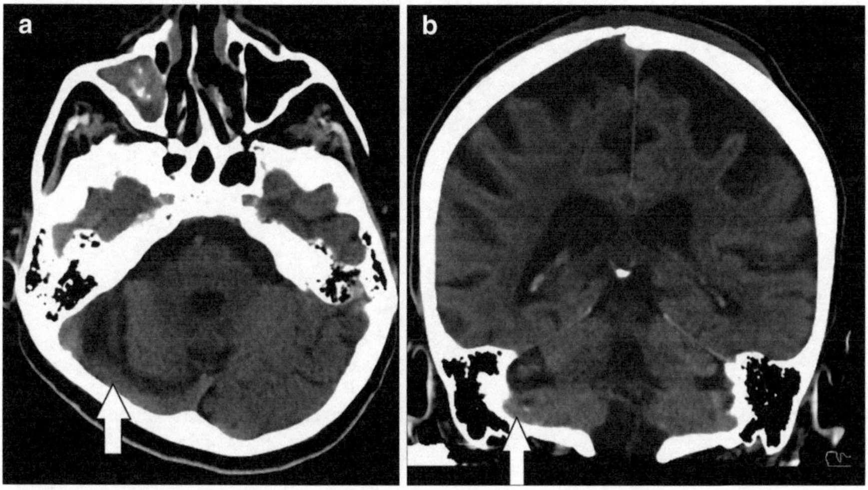

Fig. 13.10 In the case with increased CSF gaps secondary to cerebral atrophy, axial brain CT (**a**) right transverse sinus, coronal image (**b**) sigmoid sinus is observed as hyperdense due to slow flow

13.2.5.2 Cerebral Parenchyma Extensions

In axial images, the posterior part of the frontal lobe and cerebellar flocculi extending to the middle cranial fossa can give the impression of an extra-axial lesion (Fig. 13.11) [7, 32]. Selecting gray-white matter structures in tissue suspicious for lesions and demonstrating their continuity with the relevant cerebral/cerebellar tissue on reformatted CT or MRI scans in other orthogonal planes will be useful in preventing this mistake.

13.2.5.3 Artifacts

The most important artifact that can be confused with SDH is the Beam hardening artifact seen on CT. In this artifact, the X-ray may be scattered as it passes through the recessed bone surfaces, causing linear hyperdense views on the image. This artifact, which is frequently encountered in the anterior and posterior cranial fossa, can be minimized with various filtration and correction software. This artifact can be mistaken for acute period SDHs due to its hyperdense appearance. Patient movement can also be confused with aqua-subacute SDHs by causing linear miscoding, especially in MRI with long exposure times [7, 26].

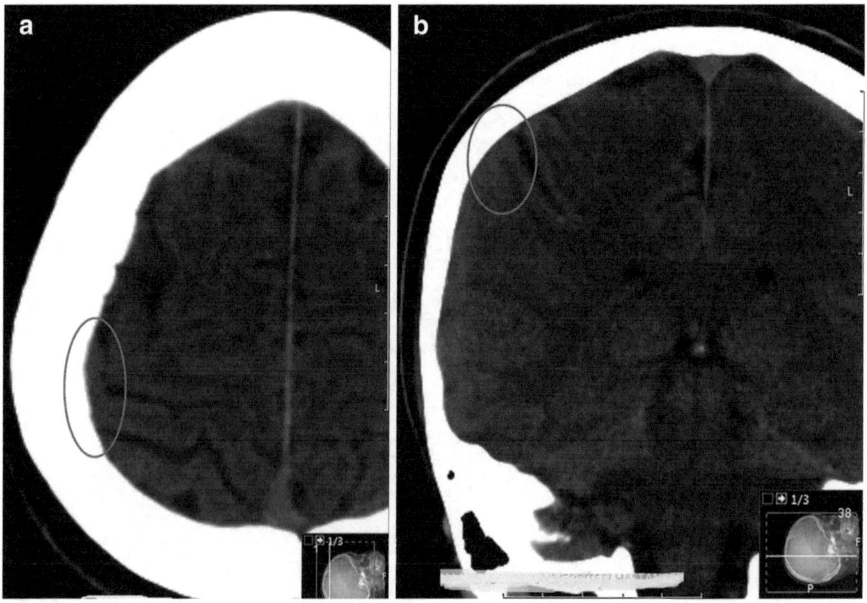

Fig. 13.11 In axial non-contrast brain CT (**a**) isodense appearance that can mimic a subdural hematoma adjacent to the right central sulcus, it is understood to be cerebral parenchyma since it shows continuity with the adjacent gray-white matter in the coronal reformatted image (**b**)

13.2.5.4 Tumors

The literature reviews show that many SDHs (from pure CSDH to acute or subacute SDH) are misdiagnosed as tumors. The main reason for this mistake seems to be that mixed density blood components increase the suspicion for an underlying lesion [44]. A known history of malignancy is the most important factor suggesting the presence of an underlying tumor. Failure of the natural evolution of the lesion or enlargement or a nodular appearance on follow-up imaging represent other suspicious findings [26]. Although the absence of a clear head injury seems suspicious, it is not a very assured way to diagnose a tumor. However, in a patient with a history of malignancy, even if there is a reasonable history of trauma, tumor suspicion should be kept in mind in the presence of subdural collections. Most of the lesions imitating SDH are metastatic tumors (breast, lung, and stomach), hematological malignancies, and meningiomas [34, 37].

Unenhanced CT, which is a first-line imaging modality, is generally insufficient to distinguish CSDH from a tumor, but it may contain some fine details that suggest the presence of a tumor. Neighboring skull involvement is an unexpected finding in CSDH. While the presence of hyperostosis may suggest meningioma, the presence of erosion in the bone should suggest the possibility of a metastasis. The contour properties of CSDH may also contain some useful hints. While CSDH normally has a smooth contour, a nodular or lobulated contour is more suggestive of the possibility of a tumor. Again, the possibility of tumor is higher in multifocal lesions. Although the different densities in the subdural collection suggest blood products from different periods, heterogeneity incompatible with blood stratification should also suggest the possibility of a tumor. While vasogenic edema with the effect of a mass in the cerebral parenchyma adjacent to the subdural collection supports the hematoma, focal cerebral edema may indicate the presence of a tumor [34, 37, 44] (Fig. 13.12).

Contrast imaging is a rational option in the presence of suspicion of a tumor. The imaging method recommended for contrast imaging is MRI. Contrast-enhanced CT may be an alternative in the case of an urgent need for surgery and MRI is not available immediately. While tumoral lesions usually show uniform distinct enhancement, CSDH does not show enhancement. Again, thickening and uniform enhancement of the pachymeninges should suggest dural metastases [26]. It should be kept in mind that dural thickening and enhancement may be observed especially in CSDH cases where blood products are almost completely resorbed.

13.2.5.5 Hypoxic-Ischemic Damage

The global hypoperfusion of the brain parenchyma is usually encountered as a result of myocardial infarction and traffic accidents. In this case, the hyperdense appearance in the subarachnoid and/or subdural space due to diffuse edema in the cerebral parenchyma is defined as pseudo-subarachnoid/subdural hemorrhage. Since pseudo-SAH is irrelevant, it will not be discussed here. In pseudo-SDH, it is thought

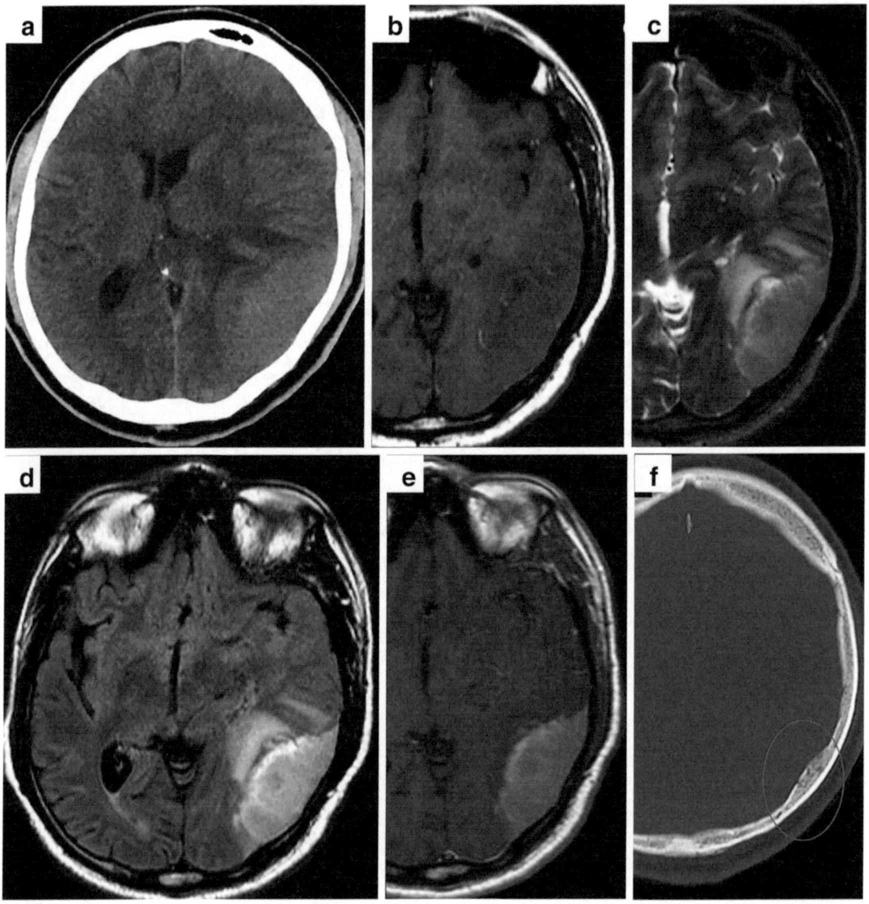

Fig. 13.12 Cranial CT (**a**, **f**) and MRI (**b**–**e**) images of a 55-year-old male patient. In the unenhanced axial CT image with a parenchyma window (**a**), an extra-axially located isodense (to the gray matter) lesion is observed in the left parieto-occipital region. The lesion is observed as isointense on T1 (**b**) with gray matter, iso-hyperintense on T2 (**c**), and hyperintense on FLAIR (**d**). A hyperintensity of edema due to mass effect is accompanied by T2 and FLAIR sequences in the adjacent cerebral parenchyma. On contrast-enhanced T1 (**e**), the lesion is observed to have a distinctly homogeneous enhancement. In the bone window axial CT image (**f**), the thickness of the adjacent bone is increased due to hyperostosis. Findings support the meningioma

that pathophysiologically, the decrease in the flow of the dural sinuses and the observation of hyperdensity at the falx and tentorium level are secondary to the decreased cerebral density. Hypoxic-ischemic damage, which is mostly confused with acute SDH, can also be confused with thickened dura mater in an almost completely resorbed CSDH. In hypoxic-ischemic damage, the loss of gray-white matter differentiation is accompanied by the loss of gray-white matter separation, the denser appearance of the basal gray matter structures (thalamus, caudate, and lentiform nuclei), and the reverse sign of the cerebellum, helping to distinguish it from CSDH. MRI will be useful in suspected cases [7, 26].

13.2.5.6 Hypertrophic Pachymeningitis

Hypertrophic pachymeningitis (HP) is a diffuse inflammatory disease characterized by thickening of the dura mater and adjacent leptomeninges. This entity progresses with thickening and enhancement as a result of dura mater inflammation idiopathically or with associated tumoral processes, systemic inflammatory diseases (sarcoidosis, Wegener, etc.), and infectious pathologies (tuberculosis, syphilis, Lyme disease, etc.) [16]. Detailed clinical investigation of systemic involvement findings is very important in this disease, which can be confused with CSDH with complete resorption of blood products. The nodular character of dural thickening and enhancement and accompanying leptomeninges enhancement may aid in establishing the differential diagnosis [26, 44].

13.2.5.7 Empyema

SDE, which is an emergency clinical condition, can occur by direct contiguous invasion or by a hematological route. SDE is frequently caused by sinusitis or middle ear infection, although trauma, an operation history, and meningitis are other common etiological factors [52]. SDE are usually seen as unilateral extra-axial isodense or hypodense collections on CT (Fig. 13.13). They contain a thick wall secondary to chronic inflammation. Gray-white matter differentiation may be lost in the adjacent cerebral parenchyma due to edema. On postcontrast CT, the wall is contrast enhancing. In this state, it is difficult to distinguish it from CSDH. The findings of sinusitis or otitis media, which are the source of infection, will contribute to the diagnosis. On MRI, most SDE seen on T1 imaging are isointense due to a high proteinaceous content, while on T2 the intensity is lower than that of CSF. SDE demonstrates dural enhancement on contrast-enhanced T1. The diffusion limitation in DWI is important in distinguishing it from CSDH. Observing the source of infection in neighboring structures on MRI also supports the diagnosis [52].

13.2.5.8 Subdural Hygroma

Subdural hygroma (SH) is the accumulation of CSF in the subdural space. Similar to CSDH, trauma can be observed as its etiology, or it can be observed for reasons such as spontaneous intracranial hypotension. Unlike CSDH, there are no blood products in pure SH. However, as mentioned in the pathophysiology of CSDH, bleeding into SHs may occur as a result of rupture of fragile neovascular formations due to growing expanding collections, and according to some authors, SHs play a role in the etiology of CSDH [12]. It is neither possible nor necessary to distinguish a naturally bleeding SH from CSDH. In this case, the resulting lesion is already a subdural hemorrhage. Pure SH is a mistaken pathology for CSDH. Both SH and CSDH are observed as hypodense on a CT without contrast and distinction is not

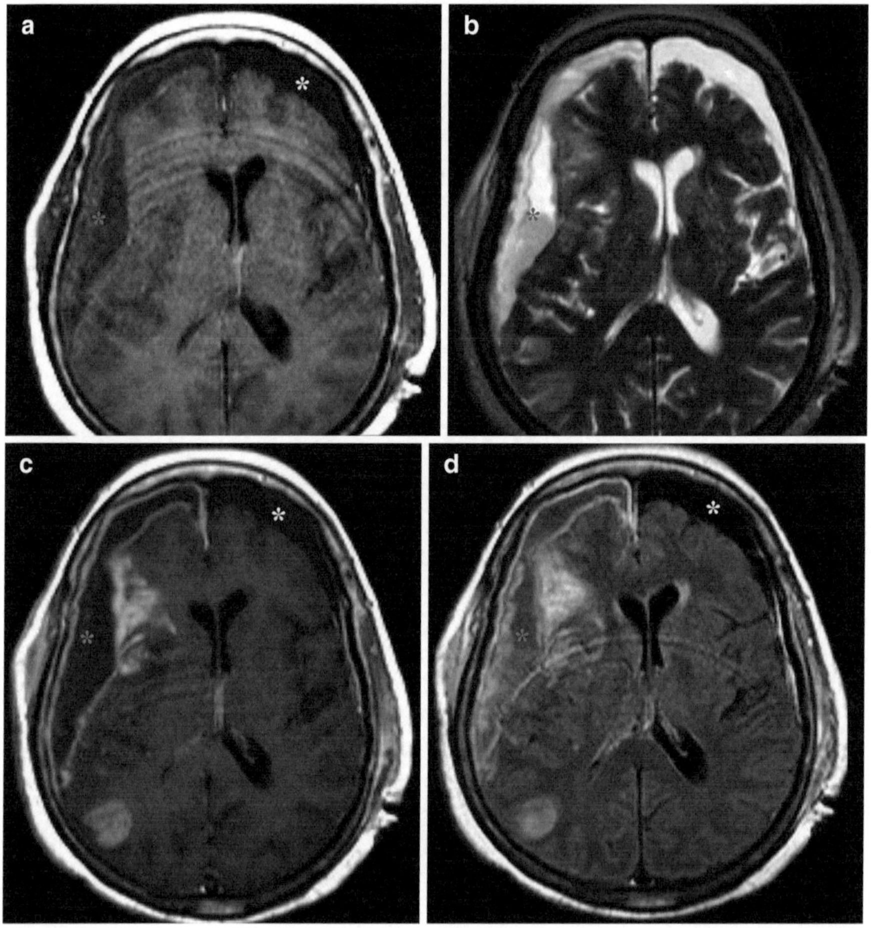

Fig. 13.13 Bilateral subdural collection is observed in the contrast-enhanced brain MRI examination of a 61-year-old male patient. Both collections are seen as (**a**) hypointense on T1 and hyperintense on T2 (**b**). It is noteworthy that the content of the collection on the right is more intense and gives fluid-fluid layering (red asterisk) due to hematocrit effect. On contrast-enhanced T1 (**c**), significant enhancement was observed in the dura accompanied by adjacent cerebral parenchymal and leptomeningeal enhancement. On postcontrast FLAIR image (**d**), thickening of the dura, a subdural collection with heterogeneous hyperintense to the CSF and signal increases due to parenchymal involvement were observed. The collection on the left side was homogeneously isointense with CSF in all sequences and did not show any enhancement. Findings show that the right-sided collection was an empyema secondary to meningo-encephalitis, and the left collection was subdural hygroma

possible. However, on MRI, as blood products are more intense than CSF, they are more hyperintense on T1 than CSF. Especially when CSF is suppressed on FLAIR sequence images, hyperintense appearance of the lesion in SCDH is very useful in the differential diagnosis [6, 26] (Fig. 13.3). SHs are mostly observed bilaterally, but bilaterality is not sufficient evidence for differentiation.

13.2.6 Radiological Recurrence Prediction

Surgical options are generally used in the treatment of CSDH in clinically symptomatic patients. There is a considerable amount of recurrence after surgery. The most important factors affecting the recurrence rates are the systemic reasons arising from the patient, as well as the surgical method utilized for treatment. For this reason, suspicious conditions in terms of recurrence should be determined in the preoperative period. Among the radiological risk factors for recurrence, the most important findings are bilaterality, midline shifts of more than 10 mm, and CSDH volume more than 150 mL. Apart from these, a positive correlation was found between CT density and recurrence rates [42]. The recurrence rates of hematomas with a homogeneous isodense or hypodense radiological appearance were lower than those with hyperdense or heterogeneous mixed density. It has been stated that recurrence rates are higher in laminar or separated CSDHs compared to those without. Presence of pressurized pneumocephaly in the postoperative period also increases the risk of recurrence [18, 27, 33, 39, 42].

13.2.7 Postoperative Imaging of Subdural Hematomas

The most commonly used imaging method to evaluate possible complications in the early postoperative period is cranial CT without contrast [5, 6, 26]. The most important factors in this are that it is a fast and a relatively inexpensive method, its prevalence, the presence of instrumentation in postoperative patients, and its ability for determining most of the postoperative complications. CT can accurately detect new bleeding, mass effect and herniation, tension pneumocephaly and calvarial fractures that may be observed in the early postoperative period. MRI is a frequently used imaging method because it is highly sensitive in detecting acute ischemia and infections. However, intracranial air, which is frequently observed in the postoperative period, may cause artifacts on MRI. Therefore, the choice to use MRI in the postoperative setting should be made according to the clinical scenario.

13.3 Conclusion

CSDH, a collection of blood products in the subdural space, is a dynamic process. It may present with an asymptomatic clinical picture or as a life-threatening coma. Radiologically, it can be a simple homogeneous fluid collection or have a complex heterogeneous appearance. There are some radiological pitfalls in making the diagnosis, and a good knowledge of the radioanatomy and imaging features according to the stage of the hematoma will help in making the differential diagnosis.

References

1. Almenawer SA, Farrokhyar F, Hong C, Alhazzani W, Manoranjan B, Yarascavitch B, Arjmand P, Baronia B, Reddy K, Murty N, Singh S. Chronic subdural hematoma management: a systematic review and meta-analysis of 34,829 patients. Ann Surg. 2014;259(3):449–57.
2. Baechli H, Nordmann A, Bucher HC, Gratzl O. Demographics and prevalent risk factors of chronic subdural haematoma: results of a large single-center cohort study. Neurosurg Rev. 2004;27(4):263–6.
3. Blaauw J, Jacobs B, den Hertog HM, van der Gaag NA, Jellema K, Dammers R, Lingsma HF, van der Naalt J, Kho KH, Groen RJM. Neurosurgical and perioperative management of chronic subdural hematoma. Front Neurol. 2020;11:550.
4. Bosche B, Molcanyi M, Noll T, Kochanek M, Kraus B, Rieger B, El Majdoub F, Dohmen C, Löhr M, Goldbrunner R, Brinker G. Occurrence and recurrence of spontaneous chronic subdural haematoma is associated with a factor XIII deficiency. Clin Neurol Neurosurg. 2013;115(1):13–8.
5. Broder JS. Head computed tomography interpretation in trauma: a primer. Psychiatr Clin North Am. 2010;33(4):821–54.
6. Carroll JJ, Lavine SD, Meyers PM. Imaging of subdural hematomas. Neurosurg Clin N Am. 2017;28(2):179–203.
7. Catana D, Koziarz A, Cenic A, Nath S, Singh S, Almenawer SA, Kachur E. Subdural hematoma mimickers: a systematic review. World Neurosurg. 2016;93:73–80.
8. Cecchini G. Chronic subdural hematoma pathophysiology: a unifying theory for a dynamic process. J Neurosurg Sci. 2017;61(5):536–43.
9. Chiesa A, Duhaime AC. Abusive head trauma. Pediatr Clin North Am. 2009;56(2):317–31.
10. Duy L, Badeeb A, Duy W, Alqahtani E, Champion W, Kim DH, Martin D, Vartanians V, Coffin P, Small JE. CT attenuation of acute subdural hematomas in patients with anemia. J Neuroimaging. 2019;29(4):536–9.
11. Edlmann E, Giorgi-Coll S, Whitfield PC, Carpenter KLH, Hutchinson PJ. Pathophysiology of chronic subdural haematoma: inflammation, angiogenesis and implications for pharmacotherapy. J Neuroinflammation. 2017;14(1):108.
12. Fan G, Ding J, Wang H, Wang Y, Liu Y, Wang C, Li Z. Risk factors for the development of chronic subdural hematoma in patients with subdural hygroma. Br J Neurosurg. 2021;35(1):1–6.
13. Feghali J, Yang W, Huang J. Updates in chronic subdural hematoma: epidemiology, etiology, pathogenesis, treatment, and outcome. World Neurosurg. 2020;141:339–45.
14. Feng JF, Jiang JY, Bao YH, Liang YM, Pan YH. Traumatic subdural effusion evolves into chronic subdural hematoma: two stages of the same inflammatory reaction? Med Hypotheses. 2008;70:1147–9.
15. Gardner WJ. Traumatic subdural hematoma. Arch Neurpsych. 1932;27(4):847–58.
16. Hahn LD, Fulbright R, Baehring JM. Hypertrophic pachymeningitis. J Neurol Sci. 2016;367:278–83.
17. Holmes WH. Chronic subdural hematoma. Arch Neurpsych. 1928;20(1):162–70.
18. Huang YH, Lin WC, Lu CH, Chen WF. Volume of chronic subdural haematoma: is it one of the radiographic factors related to recurrence? Injury. 2014;45(9):1327–31.
19. Jafari N, Gesner L, Koziol JM, Rotoli G, Hubschmann OR. The pathogenesis of chronic subdural hematomas: a study on the formation of chronic subdural hematomas and analysis of computed tomography findings. World Neurosurg. 2017;107:376–81.
20. Ju MW, Kim SH, Kwon HJ, Choi SW, Koh HS, Youm JY, Song SH. Comparison between brain atrophy and subdural volume to predict chronic subdural hematoma: volumetric CT imaging analysis. Korean J Neurotrauma. 2015;11(2):87–92.
21. Kostić A, Kehayov I, Stojanović N, Nikolov V, Kitov B, Milošević P, Kostić E, Zhelyazkov H. Spontaneous chronic subdural hematoma in elderly people—arterial hypertension and other risk factors. J Chin Med Assoc. 2018;81(9):781–6.

22. Kung WM, Lin MS. CT-based quantitative analysis for pathological features associated with postoperative recurrence and potential application upon artificial intelligence: a narrative review with a focus on chronic subdural hematomas. Mol Imaging. 2020;19:1536012120914773.
23. Lee KS. History of chronic subdural hematoma. Korean J Neurotrauma. 2015;11(2):27–34.
24. Lee KS. Natural history of chronic subdural haematoma. Brain Inj. 2004;18(4):351–8.
25. Lee KS, Bae WK, Bae HG, et al. The computed tomographic attenuation and the age of subdural hematomas. J Korean Med Sci. 1997;12(4):353–9.
26. Lim M, Kheok SW, Lim KC, Venkatanarasimha N, Small JE, Chen RC. Subdural haematoma mimics. Clin Radiol. 2019;74(9):663–75.
27. Liu LX, Cao XD, Ren YM, Zhou LX, Yang CH. Risk factors for recurrence of chronic subdural hematoma: a single center experience. World Neurosurg. 2019;132:e506–13.
28. Májovský M, Netuka D. Chronic subdural hematoma—review article. Rozhl Chir. 2018;97(6):253–7.
29. Matsumoto H, Hanayama H, Okada T, Sakurai Y, Minami H, Masuda A, Tominaga S, Miyaji K, Yamaura I, Yoshida Y. Clinical investigation of chronic subdural hematoma with impending brain herniation on arrival. Neurosurg Rev. 2018;41(2):447–55.
30. Matsuoka K, Nakai E, Kawanishi Y, Kadota T, Fukuda H, Ueba T. Acute deterioration in a patient with bilateral chronic subdural hematomas associated with intracranial hypotension treated with an epidural blood patch. World Neurosurg. 2020;141:331–4.
31. Mcdonald RL. Pathophysiology of chronic subdural hematomas. In: Winn HR, editor. Youmans and Winn neurological surgery. 7th ed. Amsterdam: Elsevier; 2017. p. 304–9.
32. McKinney AM. Cerebellar flocculus pseudomass. In: Atlas of normal imaging variations of the brain, skull, and craniocervical vasculature. Cham: Springer; 2017. p. 13–8.
33. Miah IP, Tank Y, Rosendaal FR, Peul WC, Dammers R, Lingsma HF, den Hertog HM, Jellema K, van der Gaag NA, Dutch Chronic Subdural Hematoma Research Group. Radiological prognostic factors of chronic subdural hematoma recurrence: a systematic review and meta-analysis. Neuroradiology. 2021;63(1):27–40.
34. Miki K, Kai Y, Hiraki Y, Kamano H, Oka K, Natori Y. Malignant meningioma mimicking chronic subdural hematoma. World Neurosurg. 2019;124:71–8.
35. Nakaguchi H, Tanishima T, Yoshimasu N. Factors in the natural history of chronic subdural hematomas that influence their postoperative recurrence. J Neurosurg. 2001;95(2):256–62.
36. Orman G, Kralik SF, Meoded A, Desai N, Risen S, Huisman TAGM. MRI findings in pediatric abusive head trauma: a review. J Neuroimaging. 2020;30(1):15–27.
37. Patil S, Veron A, Hosseini P, Bates R, Brown B, Guthikonda B, DeSouza R. Metastatic prostate cancer mimicking chronic subdural hematoma: a case report and review of the literature. J La State Med Soc. 2010;162(4):203–5.
38. Ragland JT, Lee K. Chronic subdural hematoma ICU management. Neurosurg Clin N Am. 2017;28(2):239–46.
39. Ridwan S, Bohrer AM, Grote A, Simon M. Surgical treatment of chronic subdural hematoma: predicting recurrence and cure. World Neurosurg. 2019;128:e1010–23.
40. Rust T, Kiemer N, Erasmus A. Chronic subdural haematomas and anticoagulation or antithrombotic therapy. J Clin Neurosci. 2006;13(8):823–7.
41. Sahyouni R, Goshtasbi K, Mahmoodi A, Tran DK, Chen JW. Chronic subdural hematoma: a historical and clinical perspective. World Neurosurg. 2017;108:948–53.
42. Shimizu Y, Park C, Tokuda K. Gradation density hematoma is a predictor of chronic subdural hematoma recurrence associated with inflammation of the outer membrane. Clin Neurol Neurosurg. 2020;194:105839.
43. Sieswerda-Hoogendoorn T, Postema FAM, Verbaan D, Majoie CB, van Rijn RR. Age determination of subdural hematomas with CT and MRI: a systematic review. Eur J Radiol. 2014;83(7):1257–68.
44. Tan LQ, Loh DD, Qiu L, Ng YP, Hwang PYK. When hoofbeats mean zebras not horses: tumour mimics of subdural haematoma—case series and literature review. J Clin Neurosci. 2019;67:244–8.

45. Trotter W. Chronic subdural haemorrhage of traumatic origin, and its relation to pachymeningitis hemorrhagica interna. Br J Surg. 1914;2:271–91.
46. Uno M, Toi H, Hirai S. Chronic subdural hematoma in elderly patients: is this disease benign? Neurol Med Chir (Tokyo). 2017;57(8):402–9.
47. Vega RA, Valadka AB. Natural history of acute subdural hematoma. Neurosurg Clin N Am. 2017;28(2):247–55.
48. Virchow R. Das ha'matom der dura mater. Verh Phys Med Ges. 1857;7:134–42.
49. Weir B. The osmolality of subdural hematoma fluid. J Neurosurg. 1971;34(4):528–33.
50. Yadav YR, Parihar V, Namdev H, Bajaj J. Chronic subdural hematoma. Asian J Neurosurg. 2016;11(4):330–42.
51. Yang W, Huang J. Chronic subdural hematoma: epidemiology and natural history. Neurosurg Clin N Am. 2017;28(2):205–10.
52. Yuan X, Shi X, Xiao H, Sun G, Bai Y, Zhao H, Gao M. Intracranial subdural empyema mimicking chronic subdural hematoma. J Craniofac Surg. 2016;27(2):529–30.
53. Zollinger R, Gross RE. Traumatic subdural hematoma. JAMA. 1934;103(4):245–9.

Chapter 14
Organized Chronic Subdural Hematoma

Mustafa Balevi, Ayşe M. Dumlu, and Mehmet Turgut

14.1 Introduction

Chronic subdural hematoma (CSDH) is a frequently encountered neurosurgical disease characterized by the progressive collection of blood and its breakdown products in the subdural space of the intracranial cavity [74]. Interestingly, CSDH may present a different architecture with multiple loculations and septations with thickened membranes and solid encapsulated areas, called an "organized" CSDH, in some patients [62, 80].

Von Rokitansky reported the first calcified CSDH in an autopsy in 1841 [89]. The first surgery for organized CSDH was performed in 1930 [26]. Feghali et al. reported that CSDH is a problematic disease with an incidence of 1.7–20.6 per 100,000 persons per year, with a greater incidence in the elderly [21]. The incidence of organization or calcification of CSDH is only 0.3–2.7% and its incidence has progressively increased over the years, in particular in the aged population using an anticoagulation/antiplatelet medication [9, 44, 59, 61]. CSDHs tend to develop in

M. Balevi (✉)
Department of Neurosurgery, Konya Numune State Hospital, Konya, Turkey

A. M. Dumlu
Department of Neurosurgery, Aydın Adnan Menderes University Faculty of Medicine, Aydın, Turkey

M. Turgut
Department of Neurosurgery, Aydın Adnan Menderes University Faculty of Medicine, Efeler, Aydın, Turkey

Department of Histology and Embryology, Aydın Adnan Menderes University Health Sciences Institute, Efeler, Aydın, Turkey

M. Turgut et al. (eds.), *Subdural Hematoma*,
https://doi.org/10.1007/978-3-030-79371-5_14

adults and elderly with brain atrophy [83]. Younger adults with compliant brains are far less prone to experience this complication. CSDH is usually seen in older patients or children under 2 years of age [83].

14.2 Dynamic Pathophysiology of Organized CSDH

Pathophysiologically, both formation and expansion of the CSDH are complicated with the formation of new membranes as a result of certain inflammatory events, including angiogenesis [21]. Later, it leads to fibrin deposition, formation of subdural membranes, and the development of fragile capillaries in the membranes [14, 19, 43]. Importantly, it has been suggested that the existence of plasminogen activator in the CSDH increases fibrolytic activity and failure of hemostasis, resulting in "rebleeding from the outer membranes" and "plasma effusion" within the subdural space [35, 39, 90]. More importantly, the degree of reabsorption of the blood collection in the subdural space is a vital factor for the resolution or progression of the CSDH [14, 22, 39, 76]. Furthermore, various coagulation disorders play a role in the development of the new membranes and fragile vessels at the junction of the inner and outer membranes over 6–12 months, resulting in recurrent hemorrhages and finally a solid fibrous structure with fusion of the inner and outer membranes [24, 36, 62, 66, 70, 84, 93].

In some patients, a CSDH may possess a liquefied hematoma within multiple cavities of different ages, as a result of the multiple recurrent bleedings into the cavity over a long period [19]. Afterwards, calcification, metaplastic or dystrophic, and ossification may develop within the CSDH, although its exact mechanism for development is not clear [3, 5, 53, 54]. Calcification may occur 6 months to several years after hemorrhage [17, 33, 60, 94]. After a few years of calcification, ossification of the CSDH may occur [47, 61].

Recently, the senior author and his colleagues on this chapter reported that patients with calcified or ossified CSDH, a rarely encountered disease, may remain asymptomatic for many years [87]. Unfortunately, it has been suggested that the capsule of calcified or ossified CSDH may be adherent to the leptomeninges and the underlying brain surface [44]. Interestingly, the clinical features of calcified or ossified CSDH are very similar to those of noncalcified or nonossified hematomas [18, 58].

An organized CSDH is rare in children [85]. Children with organized CSDH often have a history of ventriculoperitoneal shunt or subduroperitoneal shunt operations in infancy [17, 59]. Shunt procedures for hydrocephalus, meningitis, encephalitis, and epileptic seizures are the other predisposing factors for organized CSDH occurrence [17]. In the non-elderly, surgery should be considered in asymptomatic patients with organized CSDH for the prevention of possible future brain damage due to cerebral compression [30, 44, 46, 55, 58, 63, 64, 87].

14.3 Clinical Presentation of Organized CSDH

Clinically, headache, nausea and vomiting, lethargy, confusion, apathy, dizziness, weakness, behavioral changes, voiding dysfunction with decreased bladder capacity and the presence of high-amplitude overactive detrusor contractions but intact sphincteric response, and epileptic seizures are classical symptoms of patients with an organized CSDH [5, 28, 44, 58]. In some patients, an organized CSDH frequently presents with symptoms of dementia. Calcified or ossified CSDH may remain asymptomatic for many years. Organized CSDH generally occurs in the elderly although it may present in young patients but is rarely seen in infants.

14.4 Radiology of Organized CSDH

The appearance of an organized CSDH on computed tomography (CT) has a mixed density, is multiseptated, with signs of new hemorrhage, midline shift, and thickening, or calcification of the inner membrane (Fig. 14.1) [4, 6, 9–11, 13, 37, 44, 63, 82, 92]. On magnetic resonance imaging (MRI), an organized CSDH is hyperintense on both T1- and T2-weighted images, but it may be hypointense on T1 and hyperintense on T2 scans in some patients; however, it may have a hypointense web-like structure within the cavity of the CSDH (Figs. 14.2 and 14.3) [9–11, 23, 29, 42, 79]. MRI with contrast enhancement may reveal the existence of connective tissue as a sign of maturation of a calcified or ossified CSDH [5]. A thickened inner membrane may be seen on both MRI and CT (Figs. 14.1 and 14.4) [63, 94]. If the initial CT confirms that the CSDH is multiloculated and multilayered, MRI study with contrast enhancement is indicated [15]. The calcified or ossified CSDHs, though rare, could mimic a calvarial mass. Images with contrast administration are essential to determine whether there is any associated primary or metastatic dural disease [16].

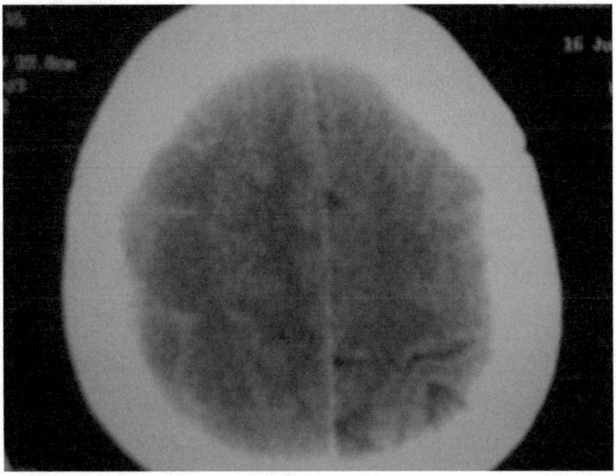

Fig. 14.1 Axial non-contrast computed tomography (CT) showing right, mixed density, multiseptated organized chronic subdural hematoma (CSDH), with signs of new hemorrhage, thickened inner membrane, and the presence of midline shift

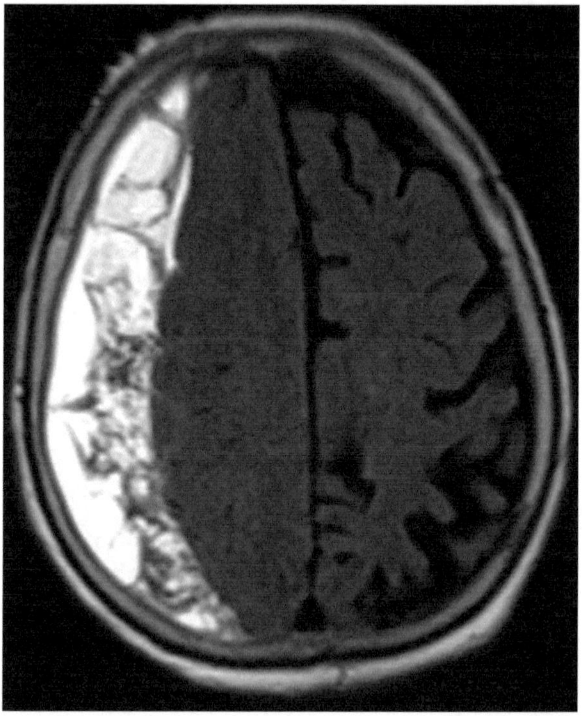

Fig. 14.2 Preoperative T1-weighted magnetic resonance imaging (MRI) demonstrating multiple loculations within the CSDH, which appear as hypointense web-like structures within the organized CSDH over the right cerebral hemisphere

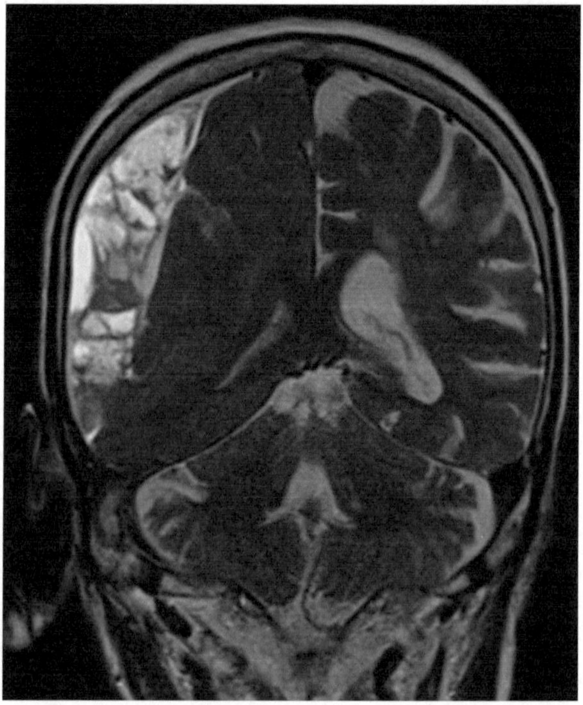

Fig. 14.3 Preoperative T2-weighted MRI showing multiple intrahematomal loculations with a hypointense web-like structure within the organized CSDH over the right cerebral hemisphere

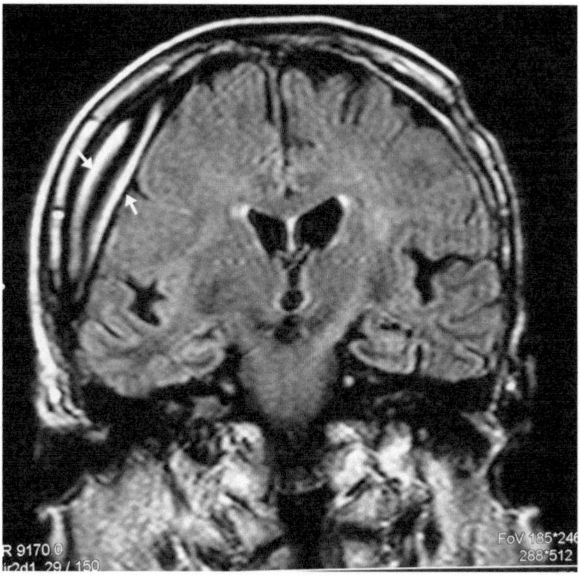

Fig. 14.4 Preoperative T1-weighted contrast-enhanced MRI showing a thickened inner and outer membrane within the right hemispheric organized CSDH (white arrows)

14.5 Risk Factors for Organized CSDH

Various risk factors including elderly age, alcohol consumption, systemic comorbidities such as hepatic and/or renal dysfunction, coagulopathies or anticoagulant drugs, and long-term use of aspirin or anti-inflammatory drugs have been suggested as reasons for recurrence of an organized CSDH [25].

14.6 Prophylaxis for Seizure

Although there is conflicting evidence about seizure prophylaxis in CSDH, antiepileptic drug prophylaxis may be given in patients with a high risk for seizures [12]. The mortality is high in postoperative seizure patients; therefore prophylaxis for seizures should be administered in high-risk patients [12].

14.7 Treatment and Complications

Many surgical treatment options have been suggested for the management of patients with CSDH, but the best choice of surgical technique for CSDH is still controversial [45, 49]. From the surgical point of view, burr hole irrigation or craniotomy with or without membranectomy are popular treatment options [88]. In clinical practice, burr hole craniostomy with closed system drainage is generally used in the majority of patients with CSDH, although it may be ineffective in some patients [2, 20, 25, 86].

Even today, the primary risk factor responsible for recurrence of a subdural collection in the postoperative period is not clear and the best option for the surgical treatment of patients with CSDH is still controversial. Some authors suggested that the development of subdural membranes may be an obstacle for re-expansion of the cerebral cortex and neurological recovery of the patient after surgery, resulting with postoperative complications such as recurrence in patients aged 70 years or more [7, 9, 45, 50].

In 2003, Weigel et al. reported that craniotomy for CSDH should be a last resort for reducing the recurrence rate, because of the fact that it has a higher morbidity (12.3%) in those treated with craniotomy in contrast to those treated with twist drill craniostomy (3%), and burr hole craniostomy (3.8%) [91]. In a similar study, Callovini et al. also reported that craniotomy should be used only in patients with recurrent CSDH or failure of expansion of the cerebral cortex after attempted drainage [15]. In 2011, Kim et al. reported that a large craniotomy with extended membranectomy as the initial treatment was successful in reducing the reoperation rate in patients with CSDH compared with a small craniotomy with partial membranectomy [37]. This surgical technique may be useful in elderly patients since the development of an acute subdural hematoma (SDH) or recurrence of a CSDH may be possible owing to the blood oozing from the membrane incision lines [51, 80, 87, 88].

On the other hand, Link et al. suggested that middle meningeal artery embolization is a minimally invasive technique for evacuation of CSDH after failure of conservative management or prophylactic treatment of recurrence of a CSDH following surgery, although its exact role remains unclear [41, 95].

Recently, some authors reported that the endoscopic removal of an organized CSDH has obtained good results [48, 67, 78]. Ishikawa et al. suggested that the drainage technique using a rigid endoscope and aspiration tube through a small craniotomy may be used in patients with multiloculated CSDH [33]. As a rule, a large craniotomy has been advocated for surgical treatment of an organized CSDH by many authors, although a craniotomy procedure may cause various postoperative hemorrhagic complications and recurrence of an organized CSDH [5, 32, 34, 37, 50, 65, 73]. Removal of thick or calcified membranes of the organized CSDH with a large craniotomy may provide re-expansion of the cerebral cortex following surgical evacuation of the hematoma [5, 38, 40, 50, 76, 79]. Old age, persistence of subdural air, and prior cerebral infarction are causative factors for poor brain re-expansion after surgery [52]. Importantly, some authors have suggested that brain compliance is a critical factor in the re-expansion of the cerebral cortex following the evacuation of a CSDH [45, 50]. There is no doubt that poor re-expansion of the brain tissue is associated with recurrence of a CSDH. From this perspective, influx of the air into the subdural space must be avoided during surgical intervention [52]. On the other hand, an extended membranectomy procedure for organized CSDH has a high risk of surgical damage to the underlying arachnoid surface and the potential for rebleeding from new capillary structures [13, 54, 55, 69]. However,

Acakpo-Satchivi and Luerssen suggested that partial inner membranectomy may cause brain herniation through the inner membrane in patients with a calcified or ossified CSDH [1].

Theoretically, re-accumulation of a CSDH within 3 months following the surgical intervention is considered an "early recurrence," while persistence or enlargement of a CSDH at 3 months or more after surgery represents a "late recurrence" [56]. The incidence of early recurrence is between 0 and 30% after surgery for an organized CSDH treated by craniotomy with membranectomy [32, 34, 40, 66, 79]. It has been stated that the main cause of recurrence in these patients treated by a large craniotomy was the fragile capillaries at the junction of the inner and outer membranes, resulting in repeated multifocal hemorrhages [11]. It has been speculated that recurrence is a result of stretching and rupturing bridging veins entering the venous sinuses such as the superior sagittal sinus [37, 76].

Basically, the meaning of the term "pneumocephalus" is the existence of air in the intracranial cavity (Fig. 14.5). It is known as "tension pneumocephalus" (TP), an important life-threatening complication after surgery, when intracranial air causes neurological deterioration due to increased intracranial pressure, in particular after evacuation of a CSDH [27, 31]. One of the authors of this chapter reported that the incidence rate of TP after a large craniotomy with membranectomy for OSDH was 28.5% [11, 71, 72, 77]. Clinical symptoms include headaches, nausea and vomiting, dizziness, depressed neurological status, and epileptic seizures [72]. The subdural air with high tension easily separates and compresses both frontal lobes, resulting in compression of the frontal lobes with a widened interhemispheric

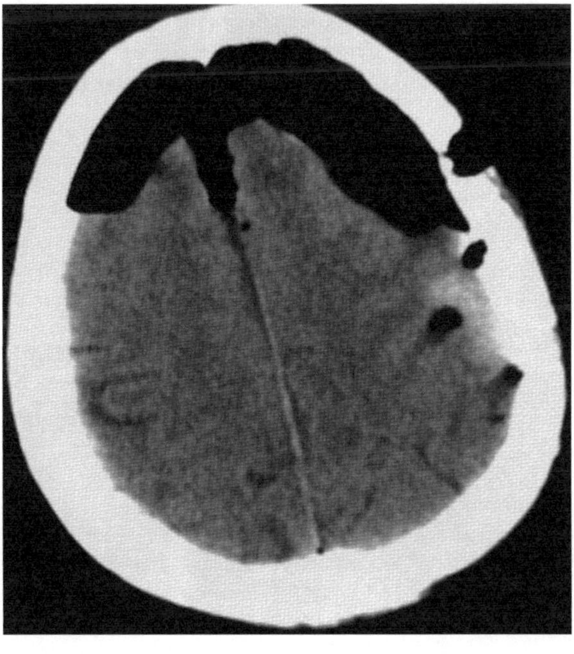

Fig. 14.5 Axial CT scan showing tension pneumocephalus

space between the frontal poles, thus mimicking the silhouette of Mt. Fuji on CT, called a "Mt. Fuji" sign [68]. The main mechanism for recurrence of CSDH is rupturing of stretched veins entering the venous sinuses such as the superior sagittal sinus [77]. Another sign of pneumocephalus is the existence of multiple small air bubbles in the subarachnoid space, particularly in the basal cisterns.

A controlled decompression through a closed water-seal drainage system was applied to the patients for 2 days [8, 81]. The most appropriate treatment of TP is lying in a straight position, fluid replacement therapy, and breathing 100% O_2 [57]. Postoperative epileptic seizures that are medically treated were reported in 25–50% patients undergoing large craniotomy with extended membranectomy [52].

14.8 Prognosis

The mortality rate in patients with organized CSDH varied from 0 to 15.6% [75]. Callovini et al. reported only one fatal case (3%) that was complicated by intraventricular and subarachnoid hemorrhage [15].

14.9 Conclusion

A large craniotomy with extended membranectomy for patients with organized CSDH should be undertaken as a main procedure, despite its high risk of complication. In patients with organized CSDH, the worst prognostic factors were the neurological condition before surgical intervention and the patient's age >70 [25]. TP and residual SDH are frequently seen complications in elderly patients.

References

1. Acakpo-Satchivi L, Luerssen TG. Brain herniation through an internal subdural membrane. A rare complication seen with chronic subdural hematomas in children. Case report. J Neurosurg. 2007;107:485–8.
2. Adam D, Iftimie D, Moisescu C. Recurrence of chronic subdural hematomas requiring reoperation: could small trephination be a valid alternative to conventional approaches? Rom Neurosurg. 2018;32:187–204.
3. Afra D. Ossification of subdural hematoma. Report of two cases. J Neurosurg. 1961;18:393–7.
4. Al Whoaibi M, Russell N, Al Ferayan A. A baby with an armoured brain. CMAJ. 2003;169:46–7.
5. Altinel F, Altin C, Gezmis E, Altinors N. Cortical membranectomy in chronic subdural hematoma: report of two cases. Asian J Neurosurg. 2015;10:236–9.
6. Aoki N, Sakai T. Computed tomography features immediately after replacement of haematoma with oxygen through percutaneous subdural tapping for the treatment of chronic subdural haematoma in adults. Acta Neurochir (Wien). 1993;120:44–6.

7. Araújo Silva DO, Matis GK, Costa LF, Kitamura MA, de Carvalho Junior EV, de Moura Silva M, et al. Chronic subdural hematomas and the elderly: surgical results from a series of 125 cases: old "horses" are not to be shot! Surg Neurol Int. 2012;3:150.
8. Arbit E, Shah J, Bedford R, Carlon G. Tension pneumocephalus: treatment with controlled decompression via a closed water-seal drainage system. Case report. J Neurosurg. 1991;74:139–42.
9. Asghar M, Adhiyaman V, Greenway MW, Bhowmick BK, Bates A. Chronic subdural haematoma in the elderly—a North Wales experience. J R Soc Med. 2002;95:290–2.
10. Baek HG, Park SH. Craniotomy and membranectomy for treatment of organized chronic subdural hematoma. Korean J Neurotrauma. 2018;14:134–7.
11. Balevi M. Organized chronic subdural hematomas treated by large craniotomy with extended membranectomy as the initial treatment. Asian J Neurosurg. 2017;12:598–604.
12. Battaglia F, Lubrano V, Ribeiro-Filho T, Pradel V, Roche PH. Incidence and clinical impact of seizures after surgery for chronic subdural haematoma. Neurochirurgie. 2012;58:230–4.
13. Bremer AM, Nguyen TQ. Tension pneumocephalus after surgical treatment of chronic subdural hematoma: report of three cases. Neurosurgery. 1982;11:284–7.
14. Byrne P, Bartlett J. Chronic subdural haematoma: editorial. Br J Neurosurg. 1991;5:459–60.
15. Callovini GM, Bolognini A, Callovini G, Gammone V. Primary enlarged craniotomy in organized chronic subdural hematomas. Neurol Med Chir (Tokyo). 2015;54:349–56.
16. Cheng YK, Wang TC, Yang JT, Lee MH, Su CH. Dural metastasis from prostatic adenocarcinoma mimicking chronic subdural hematoma. J Clin Neurosci. 2009;16:1084–6.
17. Cho HR, Kim Y, Sim HB, Lyo IU. An organized chronic subdural hematoma with partial calcification in a child. J Korean Neurosurg Soc. 2005;37:386–8.
18. Dammers R, ter Laak-Poort MP, Maas AI. Neurological picture. Armoured brain: case report of a symptomatic calcified cchronic subdural haematoma. J Neurol Neurosurg Psychiatry. 2007;78:542–3.
19. Drapkin AJ. Chronic subdural haematoma: pathophysiological basis for treatment. Br J Neurosurg. 1991;5:467–73.
20. El-Kadi H, Miele VI, Kaufman HH. Prognosis of chronic subdural hematomas. Neurosurg Clin N Am. 2000;11:553–67.
21. Feghali J, Yang W, Huang J. Updates in chronic subdural hematoma: epidemiology, etiology, pathogenesis, treatment and outcome. World Neurosurg. 2020;141:339–45.
22. Firsching R, Muller W, Thun F, Boop F. Clinical correlates of erythropoiesis in chronic subdural hematoma. Surg Neurol. 1990;33:173–7.
23. Fobben ES, Grossman RI, Atlas SW, Hackney DB, Goldberg HI, Zimmerman RA, Bilaniuk LT. MR characteristics of subdural hematomas and hygromas at 1.5 T. AJR Am J Roentgenol. 1989;153:589–95.
24. Fujioka M, Okuchi K, Miyamoto S, Sakaki T, Tsunoda S, Iwasaki S. Bilateral organized chronic subdural haematomas: high field magnetic resonance images and histological considerations. Acta Neurochir (Wien). 1994;131:265–9.
25. Gelabert-Gonzalez M, Iglesias-Pais M, García-Allut A, Martínez-Rumbo R. Chronic subdural haematoma: surgical treatment and outcome in 1000 cases. Clin Neurol Neurosurg. 2005;107:223–9.
26. Goldhahn R. Uber ein gosses, perative entferntes, verkalktes, intrakranielles hamatoma. Dtsch Z Chir. 1930;224:323.
27. Goyal S, Batra AM, Rohatgi A, Acharya R, Sharma AG. Tension pneumocephalus: a neurosurgical emergency. J Assoc Physicians India. 2008;56:985.
28. Hirakawa T, Tanaka A, Yoshinaga S, Ohkawa M, Tomonaga M. Calcified chronic subdural hematoma with intracerebral rupture forming a subcortical hematoma. A case report. Surg Neurol. 1989;32:51–5.
29. Hosoda K, Tamaki N, Masumura M, Matsumoto S, Maeda F. Magnetic resonance images of chronic subdural hematomas. J Neurosurg. 1987;67:677–83.
30. Ide M, Jimbo M, Yamamoto M, Umebara Y, Hagiwara S. Asymptomatic calcified chronic subdural hematoma—report of three cases. Neurol Med Chir (Tokyo). 1993;33:559–63.

31. Ihab Z. Pneumocephalus after surgical evacuation of chronic subdural hematoma: is it a serious complication? Asian J Neurosurg. 2012;7:66–74.
32. Imaizumi S, Onuma T, Kameyama M, Naganuma H. Organized chronic subdural hematoma requiring craniotomy-five case reports. Neurol Med Chir (Tokyo). 2001;41:19–24.
33. Ishikawa T, Endo K, Endo Y, Sato N, Ohta M. Neuro-endoscopic surgery for multi-lobular chronic subdural hematoma (in Japan). No Shinkei Geka. 2017;45:667–75.
34. Isobe N, Sato H, Murakami T, Kurokawa Y, Seyama G, Oki S. Six cases of organized chronic subdural hematoma. No Shinkei Geka. 2008;36:1115–20.
35. Ito H, Komai T, Yamamoto S. Fibrinolytic enzyme in the lining walls of chronic subdural haematoma. J Neurosurg. 1978;48:197–200.
36. Kawano N, Endo M, Saito M, Nakayama K, Beppu T. Origin and pathological significance of smooth muscle cells and myofibroblasts in the subdural neomembrane (in Japan). Neurol Med Chir (Tokyo). 1986;26:361–8.
37. Kim JH, Kang DS, Kim JH, Kong MH, Song KY. Chronic subdural hematoma treated by small or large craniotomy with membranectomy as the initial treatment. J Korean Neurosurg Soc. 2011;50:103–8.
38. Kondo S, Okada Y, Iseki H, Hori T, Takakura K, Kobayashi A, Nagata H. Thermological study of drilling bone tissue with a high-speed drill. Neurosurgery. 2000;46:1162–8.
39. Kwon TH, Park YK, Lim DJ, Cho TH, Chung YG, Chung HS, Suh JK. Chronic subdural hematoma: evaluation of the clinical significance of postoperative drainage volume. J Neurosurg. 2000;93:796–9.
40. Lee JY, Ebel H, Ernestus RI, Klug N. Various surgical treatments of chronic subdural hematoma and outcome in 172 patients: is membranectomy necessary? Surg Neurol. 2004;61:523–7.
41. Link TW, Boddu S, Paine SM, Kamel H, Knopman J. Middle meningeal artery embolization for chronic subdural hematoma: a series of 60 cases. Neurosurgery. 2019;85:801–7.
42. Liu W, Bakker NA, Groen RJ. Chronic subdural hematoma: a systematic review and meta-analysis of surgical procedures. J Neurosurg. 2014;121:665–73.
43. Maggio WW. Chronic subdural hematoma in adults. In: Apuzzo MCI, editor. Brain surgery, complication avoidance and management, vol. 2. New York: Churchill Livingstone; 1993. p. 1299–314.
44. Mahmoud B, Assiri A, Shaheen A. Excision of huge calcified chronic subdural hematoma: a case report and review of literature. Al-Azhar Assiut Med J. 2015;13:379.
45. Markwalder TM, Reulen HJ. Influence of neomembranous organisation, cortical expansion and subdural pressure on the post-operative course of chronic subdural haematoma-an analysis of 201 cases. Acta Neurochir (Wien). 1986;79:100–6.
46. Matsumura M, Nojiri K. Asymptomatic calcified chronic subdural hematoma in the elderly. Neurol Med Chir (Tokyo). 1984;24:504–6.
47. McLaurin RL, McLaurin KS. Calcified subdural hematomas in childhood. J Neurosurg. 1966;24:648–55.
48. Miki K, Oshiro S, Koga T, Inoue T. A case of organizing chronic subdural hematoma treated with endoscopic burr-hole surgery using a curettage and suction technique (in Japan). No Shinkei Geka. 2016;44:747–51.
49. Misra M, Salazar JL, Bloom DM. Subdural-peritoneal shunt: treatment for bilateral chronic subdural hematoma. Surg Neurol. 1996;46:378–83.
50. Mohamed EEH. Chronic subdural haematoma treated by craniotomy, durectomy, outer membranectomy and subgaleale suction drainage. Personal experience in 39 patients. Br J Neurosurg. 2003;17:244–7.
51. Moon KS, Lee JK, Kim TS, Jung S, Kim JH, Kim SH, et al. Contralateral acute subdural hematoma occurring after removal of calcified chronic subdural hematoma. J Clin Neurosci. 2007;14:283–6.
52. Mori K, Maeda M. Surgical treatment of chronic subdural hematoma in 500 consecutive cases: clinical characteristics, surgical outcome, complications, and recurrence rate. Neurol Med Chir. 2001;41:371–81.

53. Mori N, Nagao T, Nakahara A, Izawa M, Amano K, Kitamura K. A case of huge calcified subdural hematoma. No Shinkei Geka. 1982;10:1203–9.
54. Niwa J, Nakamura T, Fujishige M, Hashi K. Removal of a large asymptomatic calcified chronic subdural hematoma. Surg Neurol. 1988;30:135–9.
55. Oda S, Shimoda M, Hoshikawa K, Shiramizu H, Matsumae M. Organized chronic subdural haematoma with a thick calcified inner membrane successfully treated by surgery: a case report. Tokai J Exp Clin Med. 2010;35:85–8.
56. Oh HJ, Lee KS, Shim JJ, Yoon SM, Yun IG, Bae HG. Postoperative course and recurrence of chronic subdural hematoma. J Korean Neurosurg Soc. 2010;48:518–23.
57. Paiva WS, de Andrade AF, Figueiredo EG, Amorim RL, Prudente M, Teixeira MJ. Effects of hyperbaric oxygenation therapy on symptomatic pneumocephalus. Ther Clin Risk Manag. 2014;6:769–73.
58. Pappamikail L, Rato R, Novais G, Bernardo E. Chronic calcified subdural hematoma: case report and review of the literature. Surg Neurol Int. 2013;4:21.
59. Park J, Kwon TH, Park YK, Chung HS, Lee HK, Suh JK. Calcified chronic subdural hematoma: late sequelae of shunt operation in a child with hydrocephalus. J Korean Neurosurg Soc. 2000;29:968–72.
60. Park JS, Son EI, Kim DW, Kim SP. Calcified chronic subdural haematoma associated with intracerebral haematoma. J Korean Neurosurg. 2003;34:177–8.
61. Per H, Gümüş H, Tucer B, Akgün H, Kurtsoy A, Kumandaş S. Calcified chronic subdural hematoma mimicking calvarial mass: a case report. Brain Dev. 2006;28:607–9.
62. Prieto R, Pascual JM, Subhi-Issa I, Yus M. Acute epidural-like appearance of an encapsulated solid non-organized chronic subdural hematoma. Neurol Med Chir (Tokyo). 2010;50:990–9.
63. Rahman A, Haque M, Bhandari PB. Calcified chronic subdural haematoma. BMJ Case Rep. 2012;2012:5499.
64. Rao ZX, Li J, Yin H, You C. Huge calcified chronic subdural haematoma. Br J Neurosurg. 2010;24:722–3.
65. Richter HP, Klein HJ, Schäfer M. Chronic subdural haematomas treated by enlarged burr hole craniotomy and closed system drainage. Retrospective study of 120 patients. Acta Neurochir (Wien). 1984;71:179–88.
66. Rocchi G, Caroli E, Salvati M, Delfini R. Membranectomy in organized chronic subdural hematomas: indications and technical notes. Surg Neurol. 2007;67:374–80.
67. Rodziewicz GS, Chuang WC. Endoscopic removal of organized chronic subdural hematoma. Surg Neurol. 1995;43:569–72.
68. Sadeghian H. Mount Fuji sign in tension pneumocephalus. Arch Neurol. 2000;57:1366.
69. Sakamoto T, Hoshikawa Y, Hayashi T, Taguchi Y, Sekino H. Inner membrane preservation surgery for organized or calcified chronic subdural hematoma. Jpn J Neurosurg (Tokyo). 2000;9:541–6.
70. Sato S, Suzuki J. Ultrastructural observations of the capsule of chronic subdural hematoma in various clinical stages. J Neurosurg. 1975;43:569–78.
71. Schirmer CM, Heilman CB, Bhardwaj A. Pneumocephalus: case illustrations and review. Neurocrit Care. 2010;13:152–8.
72. Sharma BS, Tewari MK, Khosla VK, Pathak A, Kak VK. Tension pneumocephalus following evacuation of chronic subdural haematoma. Br J Neurosurg. 1989;3:381–7.
73. Shigeki I, Takehide O, Motonobu K, Hiroshi N. Organized chronic subdural hematoma requiring craniotomy-five case report. Neurol Med Chir. 2001;41:19–24.
74. Shim YS, Park CO, Hyun DK, Park HC, Yoon SH. What are the causative factors for a slow, progressive enlargement of a chronic subdural hematoma? Yonsei Med J. 2007;48:210–7.
75. Slater JP. Extramedullary hematopoiesis in chronic subdural hematoma. Case report. J Neurosurg. 1966;25:211–4.
76. Stroobandt G, Fransen P, Thauvoy C, Menard E. Pathogenetic factors in chronic subdural haematoma and causes of recurrence after drainage. Acta Neurochir (Wien). 1995;137:6–14.

77. Suda K, Sato M, Matsuda M, Handa J. Subdural tension pneumocephalus after trephination for chronic subdural hematoma. No To Shinkei. 1984;36:127–30.
78. Takahashi S, Yazaki T, Nitori N, Kano T, Yoshida K, Kawase T. Neuroendoscope-assisted removal of an organized chronic subdural hematoma in a patient on bevacizumab therapy—case report. Neurol Med Chir (Tokyo). 2011;51:515–8.
79. Tanikawa M, Mase M, Yamada K, Yamashita N, Matsumoto T, Banno T, Miyati T. Surgical treatment of chronic subdural hematoma based on intrahematomal membrane structure on MRI. Acta Neurochir (Wien). 2001;143:613–8.
80. Tatli M, Guzel A, Altinors N. Spontaneous acute subdural hematoma following contralatera calcified chronic subdural hematoma surgery: an unusual case. Pediatr Neurosurg. 2006;42:122–4.
81. Tommiska P, Lönnro K, Raj R, Luostarinen T, Kivisaari R. Transition of a clinical practice to use of subdural drains after burr hole evacuation of chronic subdural hematoma: the Helsinki experience. World Neurosurg. 2019;129:614–26.
82. Topsakal C, Yıldırım H, Erol FS, Akdemir I, Tiftikçi M. Mixed-density subdural hematoma on CT: case report and review of subdural hematoma classification. Turk Neurosurg. 2002;12:39–45.
83. Tsutsumi K. Chronic subdural hematoma (letter). J Neurosurg. 1998;88:937–8.
84. Tsutsumi K, Maeda K, Iijima A, Usui M, Okada Y, Kirino T. The relationship of preoperative magnetic resonance imaging findings and closed system drainage in the recurrence of chronic subdural hematoma. J Neurosurg. 1997;87:870–5.
85. Turgut M, Palaoglu S, Saglam S. Huge ossified crust-like subdural hematoma covering the hemisphere and causing acute signs of increased intracranial pressure. Childs Nerv Syst. 1997;13:415–7.
86. Turgut M, Akalan N, Saglam S. A fatal acute subdural hematoma occurring after evacuation of "contralateral" chronic subdural hematoma. J Neurosurg Sci. 1998;42:61–3.
87. Turgut M, Akhaddar A, Turgut AT. Calcified or ossified chronic subdural hematoma: a systematic review of 114 cases reported during last century with a demonstrative case report. World Neurosurg. 2020;134:240–63.
88. Tyson G, Strachan WE, Newman P, Winn HR, Butler A, Jane J. The role of craniectomy in the treatment of chronic subdural hematomas. J Neurosurg. 1980;52:776–81.
89. Von Rokitansky C. Anatomie, vol. 2. Wien: Braunmuller und Seidel; 1884. p. 717.
90. Wang R, Gao L, Fu H, Shi W. Treatment of organized chronic subdural hematoma using urokinase. Int J Clin Exp Med. 2017;10:14834–40.
91. Weigel R, Schmiedek P, Krauss JK. Outcome of contemporary surgery for chronic subdural haematoma: evidence based review. Neurol Neurosurg Psychiatry. 2003;74:937–43.
92. Yamada K, Ohta T, Takatsuka H, Yamaguchi K. High-field magnetic resonance image of a huge calcified chronic subdural hematoma, so-called "armoured brain". Acta Neurochir (Wien). 1992;114:151–3.
93. Yamashima T. The inner membrane of chronic subdural hematomas: pathology and pathophysiology. Neurosurg Clin N Am. 2000;11:413–24.
94. Yang HZ, Tseng SH, Chen Y, Lin SM, Chen CJ. Calcified chronic subdural haematoma—case report. Tzu Chi Med J. 2004;16:261–5.
95. Yokoya S, Nishii S, Takezawa H, Katsumor HT. Organized chronic subdural hematoma treated with middle meningeal artery embolization and small craniotomy: two case reports. Asian J Neurosurg. 2020;15:421–5.

Chapter 15
Calcified or Ossified Chronic Subdural Hematoma

Mehmet Turgut

15.1 Introduction

A collection of blood between the meningeal layers (dura mater and arachnoid mater) covering the cerebral hemisphere due to the rupture of the bridging veins is one of the most common neurosurgical conditions in clinical practice [46]. However, calcification or ossification of a chronic subdural hematoma (CSDH) is very rare and the majority of these cases are described in single case reports [30, 33, 49, 63, 83]. CSDH commonly occur in children and adolescents rather than adults [83]. As a result of the introduction of new radiology modalities including computed tomography (CT) and magnetic resonance imaging (MRI), the outcome for patients with CSDH has been improved in spite of relatively little progress in its treatment [12]. Unfortunately, there is still no surgical or nonsurgical treatment that has become standardized in randomized controlled trials. Even today the debate regarding the management of calcified or ossified CSDH is ongoing, and the final decision has not yet been made.

In this chapter, the clinical characteristics, surgical and histopathological findings, complications, and outcome for patients with calcified or ossified CSDHs are discussed in detail.

M. Turgut (✉)
Department of Neurosurgery, Aydın Adnan Menderes University Faculty of Medicine, Efeler, Aydın, Turkey

Department of Histology and Embryology, Aydın Adnan Menderes University Health Sciences Institute, Efeler, Aydın, Turkey

M. Turgut et al. (eds.), *Subdural Hematoma*,
https://doi.org/10.1007/978-3-030-79371-5_15

15.2 History

Bull reported that Sir Prescott Hewitt described the first bilateral case of CSDH in 1845 [9]. The surgical resection of CSDH was first performed by Goldhahn in 1930 [23], although von Rokitansky reported the first patient with calcified/ossified CSDH after an autopsy in 1884 [38, 39, 64]. Recently, in a systematic review of the literature, we found a total of 114 such CSDH cases that have been reported in the English language [70].

15.3 Pathogenesis

Pathogenetically, CSDH is a progressively enlarging intracranial lesion having both inner and outer membranes with many capillaries as a result of rebleeding into the subdural space, caused by angiogenesis, inflammation, and fibrinolysis, in addition to its delayed resorption [4, 5, 33, 66, 67, 79, 82]. In addition to hypoxia-inducible factor-1a and cyclooxygenase-2 pathway, angiogenic growth factors, like vascular endothelial growth factor and basic fibroblast growth factor, matrix metalloproteinase, and various inflammatory cytokines have been suggested to cause expansion and recurrence of CSDH, as a result of fragile microvessels with increased permeability in the outer membrane of the hematoma mass [25, 27, 48, 79].

In some cases, the outer capsule of the intrameningeal blood collection may gradually first undergo "hyalinization," then "calcification," and finally "ossification" processes, although it usually resolves over time. Interestingly, the condition may infrequently progress to the formation of an encased brain, called an armo(u)red brain and Matrioska head in the presence of the extensive bilateral calcifications or ossifications involving the entire hemisphere, known as "crust-like," "double skull," or "bone under bone," although the underlying exact mechanism for the production of calcification or ossification in cases of CSDH remains poorly understood [2, 3, 15, 19, 22, 24, 32, 33, 40, 54, 57, 60, 61, 63, 67–69, 71, 75, 80]. Macroscopically, the ipsilateral cerebral hemisphere becomes atrophic as a result of chronic compression from the calcified or ossified CSDH [46]. In these cases, the time interval between the initial acute hemorrhage and the development of the calcified or ossified CSDH ranges from 3 months to 46 years [1, 3, 7, 14, 34, 46].

15.4 Risk Factors

Risk factors of the development of CSDH include use of alcohol, aspirin, anti-inflammatory drugs, anticoagulant medications for a long duration, sports where head injury is common, arachnoid cyst, hematological diseases with a reduced ability for blood clotting, and old age [45, 77, 79].

15.5 Etiology

Although the majority of calcified or ossified CSDHs are due to traumatic head injury, intracranial hypotension (spontaneous, traumatic, or iatrogenic) and coagulation disorders (coagulopathy, anticoagulants, and antiplatelet drugs) could also be responsible causes. Interestingly, the majority of cases with calcified or ossified CSDHs have mild head injury, although repeated traumatic head injuries sustained while playing have been suggested for children and adolescents [79]. Development of iatrogenic intracranial hypotension following shunting for hydrocephalus, lumbar puncture, spinal anesthesia, spine surgery, or sudden decompression of an intracranial lesion should also be considered as a potential cause of CSDH [79].

Numerous studies have shown that the most frequent etiologic factors for calcified or ossified CSDH are traumatic injury and shunting for hydrocephalus, either ventriculoperitoneal (VP) or ventriculoatrial (VA) [1–3, 6, 7, 10, 14, 15, 17, 19, 21, 22, 24, 26, 29–33, 35, 38–40, 42, 51, 53–55, 57, 60, 63, 64, 66, 68, 69, 71, 75, 86].

15.6 Anatomic Location

Anatomical locations of calcified or ossified CSDHs are more common in the frontoparietal and temporoparietal areas, although they can occupy any location over the surface of the cerebral hemisphere in the intracranial compartment. In contrast to the subarachnoid space, the fragile nature of bridging veins in the subdural space and a lack of arachnoid trabeculations have been suggested for the development of CSDHs in these regions [79].

15.7 Clinical Presentation

The clinical symptoms and signs of calcified or ossified CSDH are generally related to increased intracranial pressure (IICP), including headache, papilledema, and loss of consciousness, localized neurologic deficits such as hemiparesis or hemihypoesthesia, vision and/or memory loss, developmental delay, and/or epilepsy, although cases with calcified or ossified CSDH may also be asymptomatic [46, 52, 82]. Unfortunately, the diagnosis for these patients may be difficult in some cases because their clinical presentation is slowly progressive and nonspecific [10, 14, 53, 55, 78].

15.8 Radiological Findings

Many patients with calcified or ossified CSDH are incidentally diagnosed using various radiological modalities such as X-ray examination, CT, and MRI. Radiologically, a giant calcified or ossified CSDH involving the entire

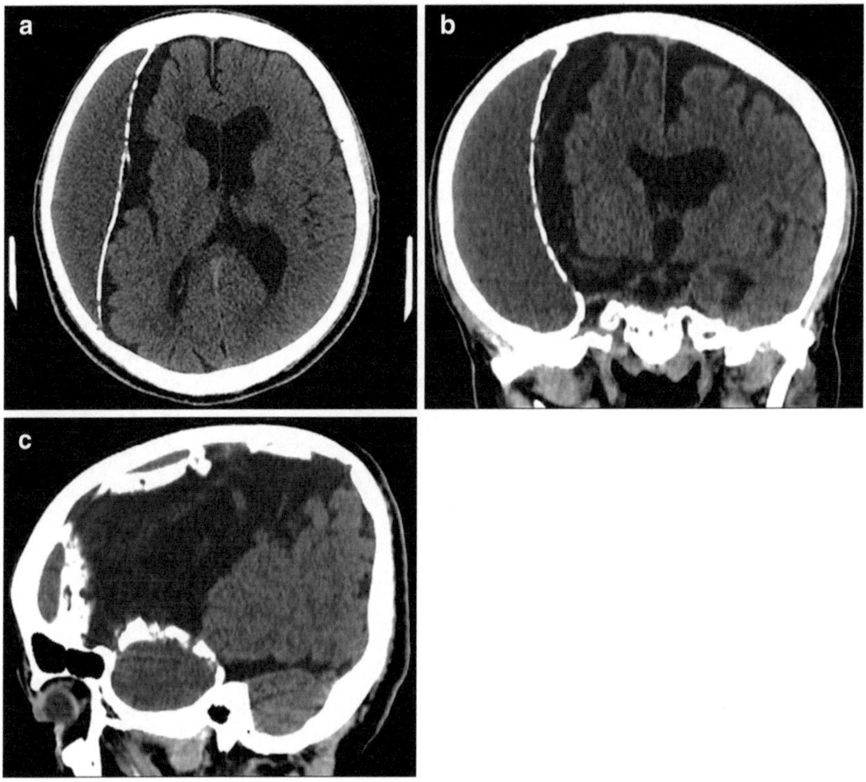

Fig. 15.1 Axial (**a**), coronal (**b**), and sagittal (**c**) CT scans of a 59-year-old man, who had a history of epileptic seizures after head trauma about 4 years ago and an unremarkable neurological examination with the exception of left hemihypoesthesia, showing a giant ossified and calcified chronic subdural hematoma (CSDH) covering the cerebral hemisphere involving the right frontotemporoparietal region with compression of the lateral ventricle, confirmed by histopathological examination of the mass after complete microsurgical resection [70, 73]

cerebral convexity, called "Matrioska head" or "double skull" with hyperdense outer and inner layers separated by a hypodense area on CT scan, has very rarely been reported in the literature (Fig. 15.1) [40, 61, 69, 70, 73]. In some cases, the calcified or ossified CSDH can present itself as space occupying lesion with midline shift toward the contralateral side (Fig. 15.1) [70, 73]. The most convenient method for the estimation of volume in all types of hematomas, including CSDH, is the formula 2/3*Sh* (the largest axial hematoma slice area (S) × depth (h) are multiplied by 2/3), instead of the formula 1/2*abc* [87]. Following contrast administration, CT and/or MRI are essential for differentiating primary or metastatic dural disease from a calcified or ossified CSDH [11]. Among the various imaging techniques, MRI is more sensitive for demonstrating the internal content of CSDHs that include membranes, septations, and web-like structures that are hyperintense on both T1- and T2-weighted images [8]. Recently, it has been suggested that diffusion-weighted imaging and enhanced MRI are useful for the detection of neomembranes and the diagnosis of infected subdural hematoma [79].

15.9 Differential Diagnosis

CT and/or MRI is necessary for the differential diagnosis of other extra-axial lesions such as calcification of an extradural hematoma, calcification of an arachnoid cyst, calcification of the cranial convexity dura mater, calcified empyema, benign or malignant neoplasms, and various metastatic tumors [14, 34, 53, 55, 69, 81].

15.10 Surgery

A conservative treatment with/without corticosteroids is generally sufficient in the absence of progressive neurological findings in cases with calcified or ossified CSDH [18, 33, 41, 52, 85]. Today, surgical intervention is indicated in infants, children, and adolescents with progressive neurological findings related to calcified or ossified CSDH [28, 33, 52, 82]. From a technical point of view, surgery under general anesthesia has a low recurrence rate and few complications [20, 29, 31, 33, 50, 71, 72, 76]. A "large craniotomy with an extended membranectomy technique" may be necessary to reduce the recurrence rate in calcified or ossified CSDH, as compared to a "small craniotomy with a partial membranectomy technique" [36]. More recently, a new technique called multiple tenting procedure has also been reported for the obliteration of the dead space in cases with calcified or ossified CSDH [31]. With the help of microsurgical dissection technique, a calcified or ossified membrane can be excised from the cerebral surface without any difficulty and pulsation of the brain through the inner membrane may be observed after excision of the calcified or ossified plaques [33, 49, 50]. However, it should be kept in mind that there is a high risk for acute hemorrhage due to traumatic injury to the underlying cerebral tissue during the surgical intervention [29, 44]. Therefore, many neurosurgeons are content with only incomplete excision of inner calcified membranes because of potential risk of permanent neurological deficit owing to cerebral contusion [1, 30, 44, 49, 53, 56, 63, 71, 80]. Despite the progress in surgical techniques, there is still a high risk of postoperative epileptic seizure activity and/or recurrence in these cases because of inadequate expansion of atrophic brain tissue after removal of the extensive calcified or ossified CSDH [46, 58, 59]. In hydrocephalic pediatric patients with shunt overdrainage, many authors also suggest that revision surgery should also be considered in addition to direct surgical excision of the calcified or ossified CSDH [2, 3, 6, 15, 17, 19, 21, 22, 24, 26, 31, 32, 40, 51, 54, 57, 60, 63, 64, 66, 68, 75].

15.11 Complications

Postoperatively, there are potential risks for recurrence, infection, development of a new intracranial hematoma, seizure, cerebral edema, and inadequate expansion of the brain as a result of cranio-cerebral disproportion [16, 79]. Following evacuation of a CSDH, there is also a potential risk of pneumocephalus or tension pneumocephalus in about 11% of cases with calcified or ossified CSDH [13, 62, 65, 79]. In particular, the presence of subdural air causing peaking of the compressed frontal lobes, called the "Mount Fuji" sign, is pathognomonic in such patients with findings of IICP and/or epileptic seizures [37, 74]. So far, numerous factors such as prolonged surgical intervention, use of nitrous oxide and/or osmotherapy, hyperventilation, overdrainage of cerebrospinal fluid, and rupture of leptomeningeal layers have been suggested as causes for the development of tension penumocephalus in these cases [43]. Therefore, saline replacement, slow and simultaneous decompression, use of suction drainage, position of the burr hole at the highest point during closure, Valsalva maneuver, and gravity in a 30° Trendelenburg position are recommended to prevent tension pneumocephalus [79].

15.12 Pathology

There is no doubt that the definitive distinction of ossification from calcification is possible with histopathological examination of the excised material in these cases. Histologically, sequential stages of hyalinization, calcification, and ossification of the other membranes are observed following proliferation of fibroblasts and collagen fibrils, and new capillaries [47, 52]. Furthermore, distorted nerve fibers, reduced cerebral blood flow, and vasogenic cerebral edema have been documented in patients with calcified or ossified CSDHs [33, 84].

15.13 Prognosis

Although the vast majority of cases with CSDH are often thought of as relatively benign entities, a large craniotomy and extended excision with a potential of high rate of mortality and morbidity may be necessary for some cases of calcified or ossified CSDHs [65]. Today, some authors therefore recommend surgical intervention only in the presence of progressive neurological symptoms or signs, confirming the principle of "*no injury no surgery*" [50, 81]. Postoperatively, an incidence of recurrence ranging from 5 to 33% following surgical intervention of calcified or ossified CSDH has been reported [65].

15.14 Conclusion

Calcified or ossified CSDH is one of rarely reported entities in neurosurgical practice. From the etiological point of view, cranial trauma is more common in adult patients, while a shunting procedure is more common in children and adolescents.

Surgical intervention is only indicated in the presence of calcified or ossified CSDH with progressively symptomatic patients, but the debate regarding this topic is ongoing and a final decision should be determined on an individualized basis. In the postoperative period, a high index of suspicion for the diagnosis of life-threatening tension pneumocephalus is vital for the correct diagnosis and proper management.

References

1. Afra D. Ossification of subdural hematoma. Report of two cases. J Neurosurg. 1961;18: 393–7.
2. Al Wohaibi M, Russell N, Al Ferayan A. A baby with armoured brain. CMAJ. 2003;169:46–7.
3. Amr R, Maraqa L, Choudry Q. 'Armoured brain'. A case report of a calcified chronic subdural haematoma. Pediatr Neurosurg. 2008;44:88–9.
4. Aoki N, Sakai T. Computed tomography features immediately after replacement of haematoma with oxygen through percutaneous subdural tapping for the treatment of chronic subdural haematoma in adults. Acta Neurochir (Wien). 1993;120:44–6.
5. Arbit E, Shah J, Bedford R, Carlon G. Tension pneumocephalus: treatment with controlled decompression via a closed water-seal drainage system. Case report. J Neurosurg. 1991;74:139–42.
6. Barmeir EP, Stern D, Harel S, Holtzman M, Krijie TJ. Calcified subdural hematomas associated with arrested hydrocephalus-late sequale of shunt operation in infancy. Eur J Radiol. 1985;3:186–9.
7. Boyd DA, Merrell P. Calcified subdural hematoma. J Nerv Ment Dis. 1943;98:609–17.
8. Bremer AM, Nguyen TQ. Tension pneumocephalus after surgical treatment of chronic subdural hematoma: report of three cases. Neurosurgery. 1982;11:284–7.
9. Bull JWD. The radiological diagnosis of chronic subdural haematoma. Proc R Soc Med. 1940;33:203–24.
10. Celik H, Karatay M, Erdem Y, Bayar MA. Ossified chronic subdural hematoma which is present with epilepsy. J Neurol Sci [Turk]. 2014;31:361–5.
11. Cheng YK, Wang TC, Yang JT, Lee MH, Su CH. Dural metastasis from prostatic adenocarcinoma mimicking chronic subdural hematoma. J Clin Neurosci. 2009;16:1084–6.
12. Cote DJ, Karhade AV, Larsen AM, Burke WT, Castlen JP, Smith TR. United States neurosurgery annual case type and complication trends between 2006 and 2013: an American College of Surgeons National Surgical Quality Improvement Program analysis. J Clin Neurosci. 2016;31:106–11.
13. Cummins A. Tension pneumocephalus is a complication of chronic subdural hematoma evacuation. J Hosp Med. 2009;4:E3–4.
14. Debois V, Lombaert A. Calcified chronic subdural hematoma. Surg Neurol. 1980;14:455–8.
15. Dimogerontas G, Rovlias A. Bilateral huge calcified chronic subdural hematomas (armoured brain) in an adult patient with a coexistent VA shunt infection. Br J Neurosurg. 2006;6:435–6.
16. Dinc C, Iplikcioglu AC, Bikmaz K, Navruz Y. Intracerebral haemorrhage occurring at remote site following evacuation of chronic subdural haematoma. Acta Neurochir (Wien). 2008;150:497–9.
17. Djoubairou BO, Gazzaz M, Dao I, Mostarchid BE. Chronic calcified extradural and subdural hematoma following a ventriculoperitoneal shunt placement. Neurol India. 2015;63:282–3.
18. Ducruet AF, Grobelny BT, Zacharia BE, Hickman ZL, Derosa PL, Anderson K, et al. The surgical management of chronic subdural hematoma. Neurosurg Rev. 2012;35:155–69.
19. Evans SJ. Armored brain. Neurology. 2007;68:1954.
20. Fang J, Liu Y, Jiang X. Ossified chronic subdural hematoma in children: case report and review of literature. World Neurosurg. 2019;126:613–5.

21. Gandolfi A, Matelli M, Cusmano F. Calcified chronic subdural hematoma following ventriculo-atrial shunting operation for infantile hydrocephalus. Acta Neurol (Napoli). 1983;2:130–7.
22. Garg K, Singh PK, Singla R, Chandra PS, Singh M, Satyarthhe GD, et al. Armored brain-massive bilateral calcified chronic subdural hematoma in a patient with ventriculoperotoneal shunt. Neurol India. 2013;61:548–50.
23. Goldhahn R. Uber ein grobes, operativ entferntes, verkalktes, intrakranielles Hamatom. Dtsch Z Chir. 1930;224:323–31.
24. Gupta SK, Pandia MP. Anesthetic management of a case of armored brain. Saudi J Anaesth. 2015;9:89–90.
25. Hara M, Tamaki M, Aoyagi M, Ohno K. Possible role of cyclooxygenase-2 in developing chronic subdural hematoma. J Med Dent Sci. 2009;56:101–6.
26. He XS, Zhang X. Giant calcified chronic subdural hematoma: a long term complication of shunted hydrocephalus. J Neurol Neurosurg Psychiatry. 2005;76:367.
27. Hong HJ, Kim YJ, Yi HJ, Ko Y, Oh SJ, Kim JM. Role of angiogenic growth factors and inflammatory cytokine on recurrence of chronic subdural hematoma. Surg Neurol. 2009;71:161–5.
28. Ide M, Jimbo M, Yamamoto M, Umebara Y, Hagiwara S. Asymptomatic calcified chronic subdural hematoma-report of three cases. Neurol Med Chir (Tokyo). 1993;33:559–63.
29. Imaizumi S, Onuma T, Kameyama M, Naganuma H. Organized chronic subdural hematoma requiring craniotomy-five case reports. Neurol Med Chir (Tokyo). 2001;41:19–24.
30. Iplikcioglu AC, Akkas O, Sungur R. Ossified chronic subdural hematoma: case report. J Trauma. 1991;31:272–5.
31. Juan WS, Tai SH, Hung YC, Lee EJ. Multiple tenting techniques improve dead space obliteration in the surgical treatment for patients with giant calcified chronic subdural hematoma. Acta Neurochir (Wien). 2012;154:707–10.
32. Kanu OO, Igwilo AI, Daini O. Armoured brain: a case of bilateral calcified chronic subdural haematoma complicating infantile hydrocephalus. Rom Neurosurg. 2012;XIX:1.
33. Kaplan M, Akgün B, Seçer HI. Ossified chronic subdural hematoma with armored brain. Turk Neurosurg. 2008;18:420–4.
34. Kaspera W, Bierzynska-Macyszyn G, Majchrzak H. Chronic calcified subdural empyema occurring 46 years after surgery. Neuropathology. 2005;25:99–102.
35. Kavcic A, Meglic B, Meglic NP, Vodusek DB, Mesec A. Asymptomatic huge calcified subdural hematoma in a patient on oral anticoagulant therapy. Neurology. 2006;66:758.
36. Kim JH, Kang DS, Kim JH, Kong MH, Song KY. Chronic subdural hematoma treated by small or large craniotomy with membranectomy as the initial treatment. J Korean Neurosurg Soc. 2011;50:103–8.
37. Lega BC, Danish SF, Malhotra NR, Sonnad SS, Stein SC. Choosing the best operation for chronic subdural hematoma: a decision analysis. J Neurosurg. 2010;113:615–21.
38. Li H, Mao X, Tao XG, Li JS, Liu BY, Wu Z. A tortuous process of surgical treatment for a large calcified chronic subdural hematoma. World Neurosurg. 2017;108:996.e1–6.
39. Li X, Wan Y, Qian C, Yang S, Zhu X, Wang Y. Double-loculated calcification chronic subdural hematoma: case report and literature review. Neurosurg Q. 2015;25:167–73.
40. Ludwig B, Nix W, Lanksch W. Computed tomography of the armored brain. Neuroradiology. 1983;25:39–43.
41. Marcikić M, Hreckovski B, Samardzić J, Martinović M, Rotim K. Spontaneous resolution of post-traumatic chronic subdural hematoma: case report. Acta Clin Croat. 2010;49:331–4.
42. Matsumura M, Nojiri K. Asymptomatic calcified chronic subdural hematoma in the elderly. Neurol Med Chir (Tokyo). 1984;24:504–6.
43. Miranda LB, Braxton E, Hobbs J, Quigley MR. Chronic subdural hematoma in the elderly: not a benign disease. J Neurosurg. 2011;114:72–6.
44. Moon KS, Lee JK, Kim TS, Jung S, Kim JH, Kim SH, et al. Contralateral acute subdural hematoma occurring after removal of calcified chronic subdural hematoma. J Clin Neurosci. 2007;14:283–6.

45. Mori K, Yamamoto T, Horinaka N, Maeda M. Arachnoid cyst is a risk factor for chronic subdural hematoma in juveniles: twelve cases of chronic subdural hematoma associated with arachnoid cyst. J Neurotrauma. 2002;19:1017–27.
46. Mosberg WH Jr, Smith GW. Calcified solid subdural hematoma; review of literature and report of an unusual case. J Nerv Ment Dis. 1952;115:163–73.
47. Moskala M, Goscinski I, Kaluza J, Polak J, Krupa M, Adamek D, et al. Morphological aspects of the traumatic chronic subdural hematoma capsule: SEM studies. Microsc Microanal. 2007;13:211–9.
48. Nanko N, Tanikawa M, Mase M, Fujita M, Tateyama H, Miyati T, et al. Involvement of hypoxia-inducible factor-1a and vascular endothelial growth factor in the mechanism of development of chronic subdural hematoma. Neurol Med Chir (Tokyo). 2009;49:379–85.
49. Niwa J, Nakamura T, Fujishige M, Hashi K. Removal of a large asymptomatic calcified chronic subdural hematoma. Surg Neurol. 1988;30:135–9.
50. Oda S, Shimoda M, Hoshikawa K, Shiramizu H, Matsumae M. Organized chronic subdural haematoma with a thick calcified inner membrane successfully treated by surgery: a case report. Tokai J Exp Clin Med. 2010;35:85–8.
51. Papanikolaou PG, Paleologos TS, Triantafyllou TM, Chatzidakis EM. Shunt revision after 33 years in a patient with bilateral calcified chronic subdural hematomas. Case illustration. J Neurosurg. 2008;108:401.
52. Park JS, Son EI, Kim DW, Kim SP. Calcified chronic subdural hematoma associated with intracerebral hematoma: case report. J Korean Neurosurg Soc. 2003;34:177–8.
53. Per H, Gumus H, Tucer B, Akgun H, Kurtsoy A, Kumandas S. Calcified chronic subdural hematoma mimicking calvarial mass: a case report. Brain Dev. 2006;28:607–9.
54. Petraglia AL, Moravan MJ, Jahromi BS. Armored brain: a case report and review of the literature. Surg Neurol Int. 2011;2:120.
55. Rahman A, Haque M, Bhandari PB. Calcified chronic subdural haematoma. BMJ Case Rep. 2012;2012. pii: bcr0120125499.
56. Sakamoto T, Hoshikawa Y, Hayashi T, Taguchi Y, Sekino H. Inner membrane preservation surgery for organized or calcified chronic subdural hematoma. Jpn J Neurosurg (Tokyo). 2000;9:541–6.
57. Salunke P, Aggarwal A, Madhivanan K, Futane S. Armoured brain due to chronic subdural collections masking underlying hydrocephalus. Br J Neurosurg. 2013;27:524–5.
58. Sandhu K, Dash HH. Anesthesia related neurological complication. Indian J Anaesth. 2004;48:439–45.
59. Santarius T, Kirkpatrick PJ, Kolias AG, Hutchinson PJ. Working toward rational and evidence-based treatment of chronic subdural hematoma. Clin Neurosurg. 2010;57:112–22.
60. Satyarthee GD, Lalwani S. Armored brain associated with secondary craniostenosis development at 7-year following ventriculoperitoneal shunt surgery during infancy: extremely unusual association and review. Asian J Neurosurg. 2018;13:1175–8.
61. Sgaramella E, Sotgiu S, Miragliotta G, Fotios Kalfas Crotti FM. "Matrioska head". Case report of calcified chronic subdural hematoma. J Neurosurg Sci. 2002;46:28–31.
62. Shaikh N, Masood I, Hanssens Y, Louon A, Hafiz A. Tension pneumocephalus as complication of burr-hole drainage of chronic subdural hematoma: a case report. Surg Neurol Int. 2010;1:27.
63. Sharma RR, Mahapatra A, Pawar SJ, Sousa J, Athale SD. Symptomatic calcified subdural hematomas. Pediatr Neurosurg. 1999;31:150–4.
64. Siddiqui SA, Singh PK, Sawarkar D, Singh M, Sharma BS. Bilateral ossified chronic subdural hematoma presenting as diabetes insipidus-case report and literature review. World Neurosurg. 2017;98:520–4.
65. Sikahall-Meneses E, Salazar-Pérez N, Sandoval-Bonilla B. Chronic subdural hematoma. Surgical management in 100 patients. Cir Cir. 2008;76:199–203.
66. Spadaro A, Ambrosio D, Moraci A, Albanese V. Nontumoral aqueductal stenosis in children affected by von Recklinghausen's disease. Surg Neurol. 1986;26:487–95.

67. Spadaro R, Rotondo M, Di Celmo D, Simpatico S, Parlato C, Zotta DC, Albanese V. Bilateral calcified chronic subdural hematoma. Further pathogenetic and clinical consideration on the so-called armored brain. J Neurosurg Sci. 1987;2:49–52.
68. Taha MM. Armored brain in patients with hydrocephalus after shunt surgery: review of the literatures. Turk Neurosurg. 2012;22:407–10.
69. Tandon V, Garg K, Mahapatra AK. 'Double skull' appearance due to calcifications of chronic subdural hematoma and cephalhematoma: a report of two cases. Turk Neurosurg. 2013;23:815–7.
70. Turgut M, Akhaddar A, Turgut AT. Calcified or ossified chronic subdural hematoma: a systematic review of 114 cases reported during last century with a demonstrative case report. World Neurosurg. 2020;134:240–63.
71. Turgut M, Palaoglu S, Sağlam S. Huge ossified crust-like subdural hematoma covering the hemisphere and causing acute signs of increased intracranial pressure. Childs Nerv Syst. 1997;13:415–7.
72. Turgut M, Samancoğlu H, Ozsunar Y, Erkuş M. Ossified chronic subdural hematoma. Cent Eur Neurosurg. 2010;71:146–8.
73. Turgut M, Yay MO. A rare case of ossified chronic subdural hematoma complicated with tension pneumocephalus. J Neurol Surg Rep. 2019;80:e44–5.
74. Tyson G, Strachan WE, Newman P, Winn HR, Butler A, Jane J. The role of craniectomy in the treatment of chronic subdural hematomas. J Neurosurg. 1980;52:776–81.
75. Viozzi I, van Baarsen K, Grotenhuis A. Armored brain in a young girl with a syndromal hydrocephalus. Acta Neurochir (Wien). 2017;159:81–3.
76. Weigel R, Schmiedek P, Krauss JK. Outcome of contemporary surgery for chronic subdural haematoma: evidence based review. J Neurol Neurosurg Psychiatry. 2003;74:937–43.
77. Wester K, Helland CA. How often do chronic extra-cerebral haematomas occur in patients with intracranial arachnoid cysts? J Neurol Neurosurg Psychiatry. 2008;79:72–5.
78. Xiao ZY, Chen XJ, Li KZ, Zhang ZP. Calcified chronic subdural hematoma: a case report and literature review. Transl Neurosci Clin. 2017;3:220–3.
79. Yadav YR, Parihar V, Namdev H, Bajaj J. Chronic subdural hematoma. Asian J Neurosurg. 2016;11:330–42.
80. Yamada K, Ohta T, Takatsuka H, Yamaguchi K. High-field magnetic resonance image of a huge calcified chronic subdural haematoma, so-called "armoured brain". Acta Neurochir (Wien). 1992;114:151–3.
81. Yan HJ, Lin KE, Lee ST, Tzaan WC. Calcified chronic subdural hematoma: case report. Changgeng Yi Xue Za Zhi. 1998;21:521–5.
82. Yang X, Qian Z, Qiu Y, Li X. Diagnosis and management of ossified chronic subdural hematoma. J Craniofac Surg. 2015;26:e550–1.
83. Yang HZ, Tseng SH, Chen Y, Lin SM, Chen CJ. Calcified chronic subdural haematoma—case report. Tzu Chi Med J. 2004;16:261–5.
84. Yokoyama K, Matsuki M, Shimano H, Sumioka S, Ikenaga T, Hanabusa K, et al. Diffusion tensor imaging in chronic subdural hematoma: correlation between clinical signs and fractional anisotropy in the pyramidal tract. AJNR Am J Neuroradiol. 2008;29:1159–63.
85. Zarkou S, Aguilar MI, Patel NP, Wellik KE, Wingerchuk DM, Demaerschalk BM. The role of corticosteroids in the management of chronic subdural hematomas: a critically appraised topic. Neurologist. 2009;15:299–302.
86. Zhang S, Wang X, Liu Y, Mao Q. Resection of a huge calcified chronic subdural haematoma: case report. Br J Neurosurg. 2018;14:1–3.
87. Zhao KJ, Zhang RY, Sun QF, Wang XQ, Gu XY, Qiang Q, et al. Comparisons of 2/3Sh estimation technique to computer-assisted planimetric analysis in epidural, subdural and intracerebral hematomas. Neurol Res. 2010;32:910–7.

Chapter 16
Cranial Chronic Subdural Hematoma Following Traumatic Subdural Hygroma

Ali Akhaddar

16.1 Introduction

The origins of cranial chronic subdural hematoma (CSDH) are multiple. Among them, traumatic subdural hygroma (SDHG) may be the precursor of CSDH (Fig. 16.1). Although the relationship between these two entities is well recognized, the pathogenesis of conversion is not completely understood.

Traumatic subdural hydroma is defined as the accumulation of cerebrospinal fluid (CSF) in the subdural space because of a tear in the arachnoid membrane of the brain following a head injury. First designated by Dandy in 1932 as a "subdural hydroma," the currently preferred expression is "subdural hygroma" [1–3]. Hygroma comes from the Greek "hygros" which literally means wet. Other names have been used in the literature for the same conditions such as "subdural fluid accumulation," "subdural fluid collection," or "subdural effusion" [4–9]. Most SDHGs are habitually associated with a modified CSF composition [5, 6, 10, 11]. Progressively, hygroma may increase in size secondary to a flap-valve mechanism, causing a mass effect on the brain parenchyma and subsequent neurological manifestations. Both CSDH and SDHG occur in the subdural space usually after trauma; however, CSDH differs from subdural hygroma in many aspects such as the content of subdural fluid collection, neuroimaging appearance, and clinical manifestations [5, 12–16]. In some cases, distinction between these two entities is not easy because the subdural contents within SDHG are habitually a mixture of blood and CSF [3, 7, 8, 17, 18].

Yamada et al. were the first to report their experience with three cases in which a traumatic SDHG progressed to a CSDH [11]. Since this first publication in 1979, many studies were published especially from Asia [3, 4, 6, 9, 10, 12, 15–17, 19–26].

A. Akhaddar (✉)
Avicenne Military Hospital of Marrakech, Department of Neurosurgery,
Mohammed V University in Rabat, Rabat, Morocco

M. Turgut et al. (eds.), *Subdural Hematoma*,
https://doi.org/10.1007/978-3-030-79371-5_16

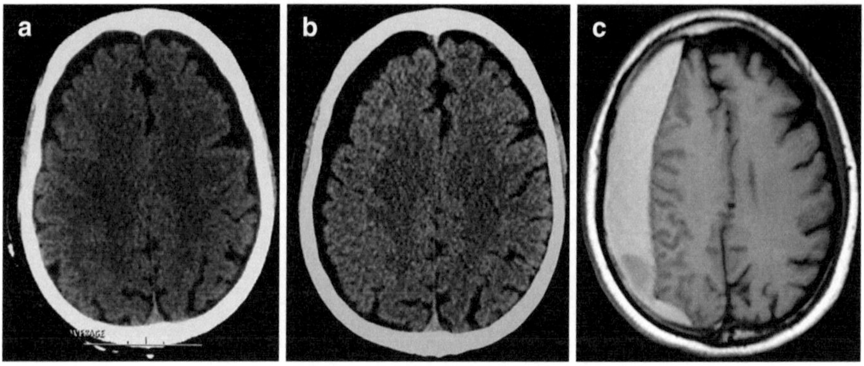

Fig. 16.1 Case 1. Initial CT-scan in a 64-year-old man who sustained a mild head injury on the right side (**a**). Six weeks later, a small right subdural hygroma can be seen (**b**). Three months from trauma, chronic subdural hematoma was evident on T1-weighted MRI (**c**)

Indeed, the role of posttraumatic SDHG in the development of CSDH seems to be overlooked, especially in Western countries.

This chapter provides a comprehensive overview of the role of posttraumatic subdural hygroma in the development of chronic subdural hematomas.

16.2 Incidence of Traumatic Subdural Hygromas Transforming into CSDH

Overall incidence rates of traumatic SDHG developing into a CSDH vary from 4 to 48.8% (Table 16.1). Furthermore, 4.7 to 24.2% of cases of CSDH originated from traumatic SDHG (Table 16.2). The reason for all these varying incidences is not clear. Also, there is some unpredictability among different series of cases concerning criteria of data collection. For example, some patients had developed SDHG following the head injury while others had a "collection of subdural fluid" at the time of initial brain imaging.

The relatively high incidence in the Japanese and South Korean publications can be explained by the advanced age of the patients as well as the practice of vigilance and regular follow-up of head-injured patients by successive computed tomography scan (CT-scan) in these two Asian countries [9, 29, 30, 34]. As suggested by Ohno et al., such patients may be ignored in other countries if there is no exhaustive neuroimaging control [9, 11, 29]. On the opposite, very few series were reported from Western countries compared to those from Asia [28, 32]. For Park and coworkers, perhaps most of the cases with acute SDHG reported by Western neurosurgeons received surgical treatment rather than conservative measures [25, 30]. SDHG developing into CSDH: rare or unreported entity? More epidemiologic studies will be necessary in Europe and North America in order to clarify this association/conversion. Regarding developing countries, with the wide use of CT-scan in patients

Table 16.1 Literature review on patients with cranial chronic subdural hematoma among those of posttraumatic subdural hygroma

Authors [reference]	Year	Countries	Incidence rate (%)	Results
Yamada et al. [27]	1980	Japan	25	6 CSDHs among 24 cases of traumatic SDHG
St John and Dila [28]	1981	USA	4	1 CSDH among 25 cases of traumatic SDHG
Ohno et al. [29]	1987	Japan	46.5	20 CSDHs among 43 cases of traumatic SDHG
Koizumi et al. [4]	1987	Japan	1.8[a]	3 CSDHs among 169 cases of SDHG after craniotomy
Murata [8]	1993	Japan	26.9	29 CSDHs among 108 cases of traumatic SDHG
Lee et al. [17]	1994	South Korea	8.2	5 CSDHs among 61 cases of traumatic SDHG
Parker et al. [30]	1994	South Korea	8.9	13 CSDHs among 145 cases of traumatic SDHG
Lee et al. [24]	2000	South Korea	32.8	19 CSDHs among 58 cases of traumatic SDHG
Kumar et al. [22]	2008	India	5[b]	1 CSDH among 20 children with traumatic SDHG
Liu et al. [16]	2009	China	22.7	32 CSDHs among 192 cases of traumatic SDHG
Wang et al. [26]	2015	China	16.7	10 CSDHs among 44 cases of traumatic SDHG
Ahn et al. [19]	2016	South Korea	44.4	20 CSDHs among 45 cases of traumatic SDHG
Fan et al. [20]	2020	China	48.8	22 CSDHs among 45 cases of traumatic SDHG

CSDH Chronic subdural hematoma, *SDHG* Subdural hygroma
[a]Following craniotomy
[b]Pediatric population

with head injury, more cases with CSDH secondary to SDHG will be surely identified as shown in our personal experience (Figs. 16.1, 16.2, 16.3, 16.4, and 16.5).

16.3 Mechanisms of Evolution and Risk Factors for Conversion

Subdural hygromas are considered to occur as a result of separation of the dura/arachnoid interface after trauma; this looks like a small subdural fluid collection. A leptomeningeal (arachnoid membrane) tear and flap valve action are generally accepted as the pathogenic mechanism [4, 35–41]. Also, a sufficient potential subdural space (especially cerebral atrophy in the elderly) represents a crucial

Table 16.2 Literature review of patients in which chronic subdural hematoma was preceded by posttraumatic subdural hygroma on initial brain imaging

Authors [reference]	Year	Countries	Incidence rate (%)	Results
Park et al. [25]	2008	South Korea	15	24 cases of SDHG with CT-scan at initial injury among 160 CSDHs
Akhaddar et al. [31]	2009	Morocco (Rabat)	7.2	8 cases of SDHG with CT-scan at initial injury among 110 CSDHs[a]
Olivero et al. [32]	2017	USA	18.9	7 cases of SDHG with CT-scan or MRI at initial injury among 37 CSDHs
Komiyama et al. [21]	2019	Japan	13.3	23 cases of SDHG with CT-scan at initial injury among 172 CSDHs
Akhaddar et al.[b]	2020	Morocco (Marrakech)	4.7	4 cases of SDHG with CT-scan or MRI at initial injury among 84 CSDHs
Chen et al. [33]	2020	China	24.2	17 cases of SDHG with CT-scan at initial injury among 70 CSDHs

CSDH Chronic subdural hematoma, *SDHG* Subdural hygroma, *CT* Computed tomography, *MRI* Magnetic resonance imaging

[a]One patient was initially operated on for a contralateral spontaneous brain hematoma

[b]Unpublished personnel study (84 patients managed in our department between Oct 2013 and Oct 2020)

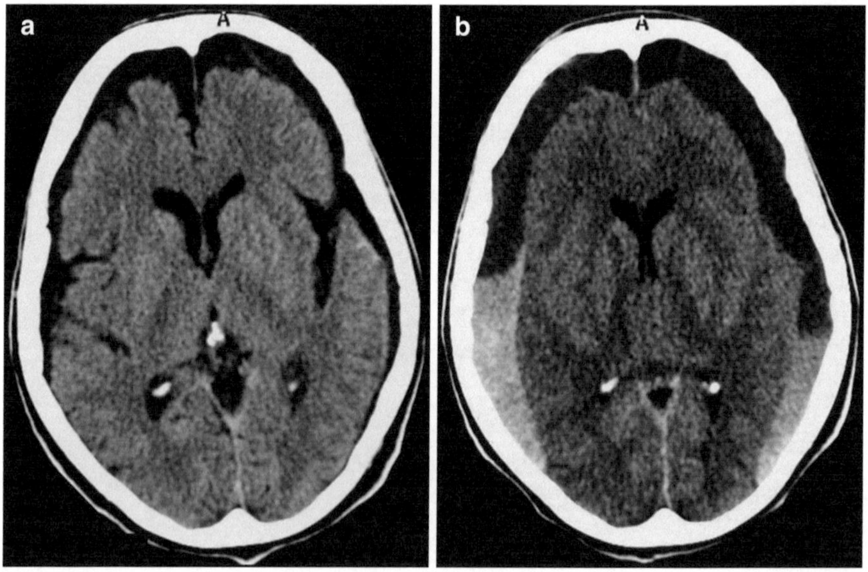

Fig. 16.2 Case 2. This 60-year-old woman with psychiatric illness had a fall. Initial CT-scan on the third day after trauma shows small bifrontal subdural hygromas (**a**). Here neurological status worsened 2 months later. Bilateral chronic subdural hematomas mixed with acute bleeding were evident on the control CT-scan (**b**)

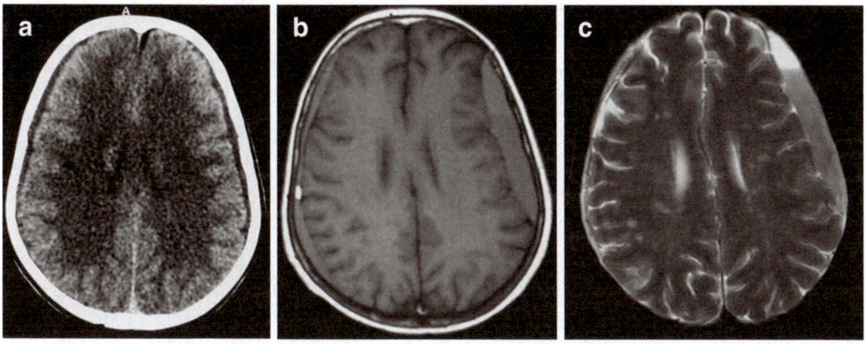

Fig. 16.3 Case 3. Initial CT-scan in a 48-year-old woman after 2 days from trauma (**a**). There is a small bilateral subdural hygroma (**a**). Follow-up T1 (**b**) and T2-weighted MRI (**c**) images demonstrated newly developed chronic subdural hematoma on the left side

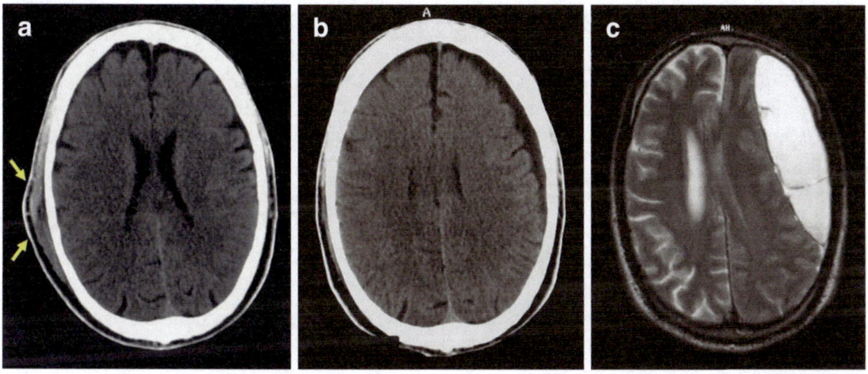

Fig. 16.4 Case 4. Initial CT-scan in a 44-year-old man who sustained a head injury (**a**). There is no intracranial lesion but a scalp contusion was present on the right side (arrows) (**a**). Ten days later, a small left (contralateral) subdural hygroma can be seen (**b**). Two months from trauma, a voluminous chronic subdural hematoma was evident on T2-weighted MRI [on the opposite side of the initial trauma] (**c**)

condition for the expansion of SDHG [3, 6, 17, 23, 36]. Classically, brain atrophy occurs mainly in the frontal areas lobes and this loss of brain parenchyma is compensated by around an 11% increase in the CSF volume principally close to the frontal lobes [28]. Consequently, most hygromas occur around the frontal lobe convexities and the Sylvian fissure.

Presently, various mechanisms for the development of CSDH from a SDHG have been suggested. Some authors have advanced that premorbid circumstance, like cerebral atrophy in elderly (due to a decrease in brain weight and increase in subdural space with age) may contribute to the transformation of SDHG into CSDH [3, 9, 17, 20, 25, 29, 42]. Park and colleagues did not agree with this hypothesis. In their work published in 1994, they had found that advanced age and brain atrophy on

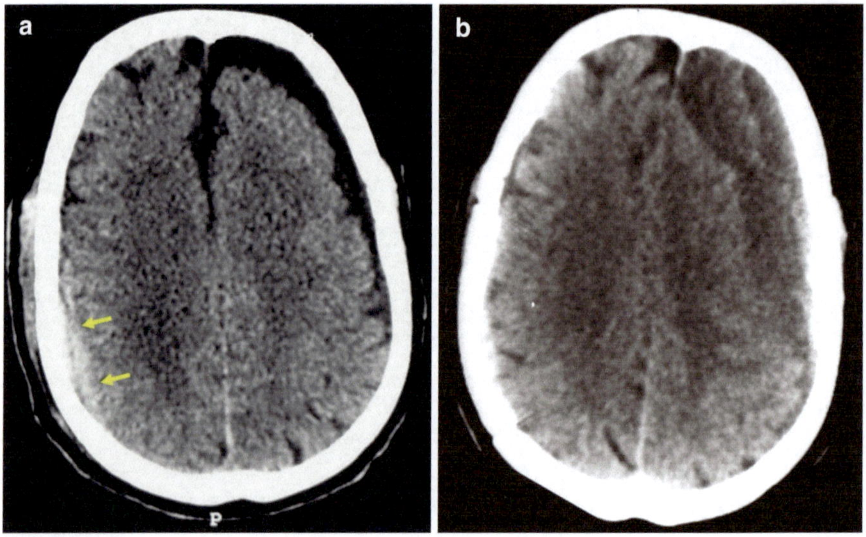

Fig. 16.5 Case 5. Chronic subdural hematoma proceeded by traumatic subdural hygroma in a 69-year-old man following a traffic accident. The initial CT-scan on admission showed a mild acute subdural hematoma on the right side (arrows) and a small subdural hygroma on the opposite side (**a**). Ten weeks later, a heterogeneous chronic subdural hematoma was present on control CT-scan on the left side [on the opposite side of the initial trauma] (**b**)

CT-scans do not appear to be contributing factors in the transformation of SDHG into CSDH in their 13 patients [30].

Other mechanisms are hypothesized to explain the conversion of SDHG into CSDH: persistent subdural fluid collection can be the source of neomembrane formation, and the rupture of bridging veins or micro-hemorrhage of cyst wall can be the cause of growing hygromas [3, 9, 22]. Also, excessive fibrinolysis process into the hygroma may cause a coagulation disorder. It is well known that fibrinogen is a marker of rebleeding, thrombin is an indicator of coagulation, and both tissue plasminogen activator (tPA) and fibrin degradation product (FDP) are indicators of fibrinolysis action [10, 13, 25, 43]. This phenomenon is accompanied by an inflammatory response that may induce CSDH [10, 12, 44, 45]. Another mechanism is about the protein or blood components that mix in the hygroma and will allow the SDHG to evolve into CSDH [9, 20, 44].

For many authors, the prediction of transformation of SDHG into CSDH in CT-scan could be an increase of subdural collection at an early period followed by an increase in density accumulation at a later phase [25, 34].

Ohno and others showed that posttraumatic SDHGs tend to occur bilaterally at first. If they persist for a long time, a CSDH may develop on either side [9, 17, 25, 29]. Two of our patients also support this hypothesis (Figs. 16.4 and 16.5). For Ahn et al., the potential to progress into CSDH should be considered in patients with traumatic SDHG, mostly in patients with bilateral SDHG [19]. Recently, a new study performed by Fan and coworkers found that bilateral SDHG and hygroma thickness were independent risk factors for SDHG evolution into CSDH. A SDHG thickness superior to 11.37 mm had a high risk of SDHG transformation [20].

Two previous study reported meningeal enhancement on post-gadolinium magnetic resonance imaging (MRI) in some patients with traumatic SDHG [19, 37]. In Ahn's experience, seven among nine patients with pachymeningeal enhancement developed CSDH [19]. For Hasegawa, microscopic examination of the enhanced pachymeninge in five patients showed a vascularized neomembrane in which the vessel endothelium demonstrated numerous pinocytic vesicles and fenestrations, signifying that SDHG with meningeal enhancement is likely to transform into CSDH [37].

The role of male predominance in the conversion of SDHG into CSDH has been suggested by several authors [19, 25, 30, 34]. However, it is obvious that men usually have greater exposure to trauma. In studies of intracranial hemorrhage or subdural hemorrhage, hypertension was reported to be a risk factor for SDHG conversion to CSDH. Indeed, high blood pressure may increase the risk of bleeding [17, 23, 25, 30]. On the contrary, others find that hypertension, diabetes mellitus, and coronary heart disease are not risk factors of SDHG conversion [20].

16.4 Clinical Features and Management

As mentioned above, most patients with SDHG transformed into CSDH have an advanced age. However, young people should not be ignored [18, 22, 26]. In Wang's experience, 10 cases among 32 with SDHG which developed into CSDH were between 2 months and 10 years old and 50% of patients were under 40 years old [26].

In most of the patients, the time for conversion of posttraumatic SDHG into CSDH was more than 1 month. More accurately, the mean time was between 50 and 68 days [9, 12, 20, 25, 30, 31]. Generally, all patients had signs and symptoms related to CSDH [46–48]. Also, surgical management and outcome do not differ in any way from those of the usual forms of classic CSDH. It is important to point out that, as reported in many studies and in our personal experience, spontaneous resolution of CSDH may occur without any surgical evacuation or medical treatment [17, 23, 25, 30, 49]. However, the conservatively treated cases of CSDH took several months to be completely resolved.

16.5 Future Prospects

Further prospective studies performed by neuroradiologists and/or neurosurgeons, from multiple institutions worldwide, are needed to ascertain the role of abovementioned risk factors. Also, additional epidemiologic studies with larger number of patients from outside Asia will be appreciated. Moreover, supplementary investigations focusing on histological changes of posttraumatic SDHG should be conducted for a better understanding of the processing mechanism in the transformation of SDHG into CSDH.

16.6 Conclusion

Chronic subdural hematoma may develop as a consequence of posttraumatic SDHG. This potential of development must be considered when the brain fails to expand, especially in aging population. Up to 50% of SDHG in head-injured patients may later develop to a CSDH and this is more common in men, older persons with bilateral SDHG, and those with hygroma thickness superior to 11.37 mm, as well as in patients with meningeal enhancement on post-gadolinium MRI.

All the patients with a posttraumatic SDHG should be carefully followed up by a neurosurgeon to decide on the appropriate treatment when a CSDH develops.

In the future, supplementary investigations, especially epidemiologic, neuroradiologic, and histopathologic, should be conducted for a better understanding of the processing mechanism in the transformation of SDHG into CSDH.

References

1. Dandy WE. Chronic subdural hydroma and serous meningitis (pachymeningitis serosa; localized external hydrocephalus). In: Lewis D, editor. Practice of surgery. Hagerstown: WF Prior Co.; 1932. p. 306–9.
2. Dandy WE. Chronic subdural hydroma and serous meningitis (pachymeningitis serosa; localized external hydrocephalus). In: Lewis D, editor. Practice of surgery. Hagerstown: WF Prior Co.; 1955. p. 291–3.
3. Lee KS. Chronic subdural hematoma in the aged, trauma or degeneration? J Korean Neurosurg Soc. 2016;59:1–5. https://doi.org/10.3340/jkns.2016.59.1.1.
4. Koizumi H, Fukamachi A, Nukui H. Postoperative subdural fluid collections in neurosurgery. Surg Neurol. 1987;27:147–53. https://doi.org/10.1016/0090-3019(87)90286-2.
5. Kristof RA, Grimm JM, Stoffel-Wagner B. Cerebrospinal fluid leakage into the subdural space: possible influence on the pathogenesis and recurrence frequency of chronic subdural hematoma and subdural hygroma. J Neurosurg. 2008;108:275–80. https://doi.org/10.3171/JNS/2008/108/2/0275.
6. Lee KS. The pathogenesis and clinical significance of traumatic subdural hygroma. Brain Inj. 1998;12:595–603. https://doi.org/10.1080/026990598122359.
7. McConnell AA. Traumatic subdural effusions. J Neurol Psychiatry. 1941;4:237–56. https://doi.org/10.1136/jnnp.4.3-4.237.
8. Murata K. Chronic subdural hematoma may be preceded by persistent traumatic subdural effusion. Neurol Med Chir (Tokyo). 1993;33:691–6. https://doi.org/10.2176/nmc.33.691.
9. Ohno K, Suzuki R, Masaoka H, Matsushima Y, Inaba Y, Monma S. Role of traumatic subdural fluid collection in developing process of chronic subdural hematoma. Bull Tokyo Med Dent Univ. 1986;33:99–106.
10. Tao Z, Lin Y, Hu M, Ding S, Li J, Qiu Y. Mechanism of subdural effusion evolves into chronic subdural hematoma: IL-8 inducing neutrophil oxidative burst. Med Hypotheses. 2016;86:43–6. https://doi.org/10.1016/j.mehy.2015.11.027.

11. Yamada H, Nihei H, Watanabe T, Shibui S, Murata S. Chronic subdural hematoma occurring consequently to the posttraumatic subdural hygroma—on the pathogenesis of the chronic subdural hematoma (author's transl). No To Shinkei. 1979;31:115–21.
12. Feng JF, Jiang JY, Bao YH, Liang YM, Pan YH. Traumatic subdural effusion evolves into chronic subdural hematoma: two stages of the same inflammatory reaction? Med Hypotheses. 2008;70:1147–9. https://doi.org/10.1016/j.mehy.2007.11.014.
13. Fujisawa H, Ito H, Saito K, Ikeda K, Nitta H, Yamashita J. Immunohistochemical localization of tissue-type plasminogen activator in the lining wall of chronic subdural hematoma. Surg Neurol. 1991;35(6):441–5. https://doi.org/10.1016/0090-3019(91)90177-b.
14. Fujisawa H, Nomura S, Kajiwara K, Kato S, Fujii M, Suzuki M. Various magnetic resonance imaging patterns of chronic subdural hematomas: indicators of the pathogenesis? Neurol Med Chir (Tokyo). 2006;46:333–8. https://doi.org/10.2176/nmc.46.333.
15. Liu Y, Zhu S, Jiang Y, Li G, Li X, Su W, et al. Clinical characteristics of chronic subdural hematoma evolving from traumatic subdural effusion. Zhonghua Wai Ke Za Zhi. 2002;40: 360–2.
16. Liu Y, Gong J, Li F, Wang H, Zhu S, Wu C. Traumatic subdural hydroma: clinical characteristics and classification. Injury. 2009;40:968–72. https://doi.org/10.1016/j.injury.2009.01.006.
17. Lee KS, Bae WK, Park YT, Yun IG. The pathogenesis and fate of traumatic subdural hygroma. Br J Neurosurg. 1994;8:551–8. https://doi.org/10.3109/02688699409002947.
18. Nguyen VN, Wallace D, Ajmera S, Akinduro O, Smith LJ, Giles K, et al. Management of subdural hematohygromas in abusive head trauma. Neurosurgery. 2020;86:281–7. https://doi.org/10.1093/neuros/nyz076.
19. Ahn JH, Jun HS, Kim JH, Oh JK, Song JH, Chang IB. Analysis of risk factor for the development of chronic subdural hematoma in patients with traumatic subdural hygroma. J Korean Neurosurg Soc. 2016;59:622–7. https://doi.org/10.3340/jkns.2016.59.6.622.
20. Fan G, Ding J, Wang H, Wang Y, Liu Y, Wang C, et al. Risk factors for the development of chronic subdural hematoma in patients with subdural hygroma. Br J Neurosurg. 2020;29:1–6. https://doi.org/10.1080/02688697.2020.1717444.
21. Komiyama K, Tosaka M, Shimauchi-Ohtaki H, Aihara M, Shimizu T, Yoshimoto Y. Computed tomography findings after head injury preceding chronic subdural hematoma. Neurosurg Focus. 2019;47:E12. https://doi.org/10.3171/2019.8.
22. Kumar R, Singhal N, Mahapatra AK. Traumatic subdural effusions in children following minor head injury. Childs Nerv Syst. 2008;24:1391–6. https://doi.org/10.1007/s00381-008-0645-1.
23. Lee KS, Bae WK, Doh JW, Bae HG, Yun IG. Origin of chronic subdural haematoma and relation to traumatic subdural lesions. Brain Inj. 1998;12:901–10. https://doi.org/10.1080/026990598121972.
24. Lee KS, Bae WK, Bae HG, Yun IG. The fate of traumatic subdural hygroma in serial computed tomographic scans. J Korean Med Sci. 2000;15:560–8. https://doi.org/10.3346/jkms.2000.15.5.560.
25. Park SH, Lee SH, Park J, Hwang JH, Hwang SK, Hamm IS. Chronic subdural hematoma preceded by traumatic subdural hygroma. J Clin Neurosci. 2008;15:868–72. https://doi.org/10.1016/j.jocn.2007.08.003.
26. Wang Y, Wang C, Liu Y. Chronic subdural haematoma evolving from traumatic subdural hydroma. Brain Inj. 2015;29:462–5. https://doi.org/10.3109/02699052.2014.990513.
27. Yamada H, Watanabe T, Murata S, Shibui S, Nihei H, Kohno T, et al. Developmental process of chronic subdural collections of fluid based on CT scan findings. Surg Neurol. 1980;13: 441–8.
28. St John JN, Dila C. Traumatic subdural hygroma in adults. Neurosurgery. 1981;9:621–6. https://doi.org/10.1227/00006123-198112000-00002.
29. Ohno K, Suzuki R, Masaoka H, Matsushima Y, Inaba Y, Monma S. Chronic subdural haematoma preceded by persistent traumatic subdural fluid collection. J Neurol Neurosurg Psychiatry. 1987;50:1694–7. https://doi.org/10.1136/jnnp.50.12.1694.
30. Park CK, Choi KH, Kim MC, Kang JK, Choi CR. Spontaneous evolution of posttraumatic subdural hygroma into chronic subdural haematoma. Acta Neurochir. 1994;127:41–7. https://doi.org/10.1007/BF01808545.

31. Akhaddar A, Bensghir M, Abouqal R, Boucetta M. Influence of cranial morphology on the location of chronic subdural haematoma. Acta Neurochir. 2009;151:1235–40. https://doi.org/10.1007/s00701-009-0357-7.
32. Olivero WC, Wang H, Farahvar A, Kim TA, Wang F. Predictive (subtle or overlooked) initial head CT findings in patients who develop delayed chronic subdural hematoma. J Clin Neurosci. 2017;42:129–33. https://doi.org/10.1016/j.jocn.2017.03.005.
33. Chen S, Peng H, Shao X, Yao L, Liu J, Tian J, et al. Prediction of risk factors for the evolution of traumatic subdural effusion into chronic subdural hematoma. Neuropsychiatr Dis Treat. 2020;16:943–8. https://doi.org/10.2147/NDT.S245857.
34. Takahashi Y, Sato H, Inoue Y, Takeda S, Ohkawara S. CT findings and the evaluation of chronic subdural hematoma (Part I)–forecast of chronic subdural hematoma (author's transl). Neurol Med Chir (Tokyo). 1981;21:485–90.
35. Asano Y, Hasuo M, Takahashi I, Shimosawa S. Surgical outcome of 32 cases in traumatic subdural hygroma. No To Shinkei. 1992;44:1127–31.
36. Haines DE, Harkey HL, al-Mefty O. The "subdural" space: a new look at an outdated concept. Neurosurgery. 1993;32:111–20. https://doi.org/10.1227/00006123-199301000-00017.
37. Hasegawa M, Yamashima T, Yamashita J, Suzuki M, Shimada S. Traumatic subdural hygroma: pathology and meningeal enhancement on magnetic resonance imaging. Neurosurgery. 1992;31:580–5. https://doi.org/10.1227/00006123-199209000-00024.
38. Ishibashi A, Yokokura Y, Miyagi J. Clinical analysis of nineteen patients with traumatic subdural hygromas. Kurume Med J. 1994;41:81–5. https://doi.org/10.2739/kurumemedj.41.81.
39. Kamezaki T, Yanaka K, Fujita K, Nakamura K, Nagatomo Y, Nose T. Traumatic acute subdural hygroma mimicking acute subdural hematoma. J Clin Neurosci. 2004;11:311–3. https://doi.org/10.1016/j.jocn.2003.10.013.
40. So SK, Ogawa T, Gerberg E, Sakimura I, Wright W. Tracer accumulation in a subdural hygroma: case report. J Nucl Med. 1976;17:119–21.
41. Zanini MA, de Lima Resende LA, de Souza Faleiros AT, Gabarra RC. Traumatic subdural hygromas: proposed pathogenesis based classification. J Trauma. 2008;64:705–13. https://doi.org/10.1097/TA.0b013e3180485cfc.
42. Cotton F, Euvrard T, Durand-Dubief F, Pachai C, Cucherat M, Ramirez Rozzi F, et al. Correlation between cranial vault size and brain size over time: preliminary MRI evaluation. J Neuroradiol. 2005;32:131–7. https://doi.org/10.1016/s0150-9861(05)83128-1.
43. Yamashita K, Sekino H, Hayashi T. Systemic and local activation of coagulofibrinolysis in the etiology of chronic subdural hematoma. Jpn J Neurosurg. 1994;3:390–7.
44. Suzuki M, Endo S, Inada K, Kudo A, Kitakami A, Kuroda K, et al. Inflammatory cytokines locally elevated in chronic subdural haematoma. Acta Neurochir (Wien). 1998;140:51–5. https://doi.org/10.1007/s007010050057.
45. Suzuki M, Kudo A, Kitakami A, Doi M, Kubo N, Kuroda K, et al. Local hypercoagulative activity precedes hyperfibrinolytic activity in the subdural space during development of chronic subdural haematoma from subdural effusion. Acta Neurochir. 1998;140:261–5. https://doi.org/10.1007/s007010050093.
46. Stanisic M, Lund-Johansen M, Mahesparan R. Treatment of chronic subdural hematoma by burr-hole craniostomy in adults: influence of some factors on postoperative recurrence. Acta Neurochir. 2005;147:1249–56. https://doi.org/10.1007/s00701-005-0616-1.
47. Su TM, Shih TY, Yen HL, Tsai YD. Contralateral acute subdural hematoma occurring after evacuation of subdural hygroma: case report. J Trauma. 2001;50:557–9. https://doi.org/10.1097/00005373-200103000-00025.
48. Sucu HK, Gökmen M, Bezircioglu H, Tektaş S. Contralateral development of chronic subdural hematoma after evacuation of chronic subdural hematoma. A case report. J Neurosurg Sci. 2006;50:71–4.
49. Zanini MA, Resende LA, Freitas CC, Yamashita S. Traumatic subdural hygroma: five cases with changed density and spontaneous resolution. Arq Neuropsiquiatr. 2007;65:68–72. https://doi.org/10.1590/s0004-282x2007000100015.

Chapter 17
Subdural Hemorrhage Secondary to Cerebrospinal Fluid Shunting and Endoscopic Neurosurgery

Alexander E. Braley and Walter A. Hall

17.1 Introduction

Cerebrospinal fluid (CSF) diversion is the primary treatment for most forms of hydrocephalus and consists of creating a shunt between the ventricular system and another bodily cavity or space. Ventriculoperitoneal shunting (VPS) is the most common and well-studied variation of CSF diversion but there are innumerable ways of diverting CSF which include (in no particular order) shunting from the ventricle to the abdomen, pleural space, ureter, urinary bladder, gallbladder, systemic venous system (or directly into atrium), and even into the subdural or subgaleal spaces. Diverting CSF from the lumbar subarachnoid cistern such as in lumbar-peritoneal shunting is an additional method of CSF diversion. There are several risks of CSF shunts which include direct parenchymal injury, stroke, over/under drainage, bleeding, and infection, among other risks. The risk of infection is compounded by the presence of implanted hardware, which may become colonized by microbes during the infection which create a biofilm that is very difficult to eradicate and most often necessitates its removal and subsequent replacement, with an intervening period of external ventricular drainage.

Although not typically referred to as a shunt, endoscopic third ventriculostomy does create a pathway that diverts CSF from the intraventricular space to the

A. E. Braley (✉)
Department of Neurosurgery, State University of New York, Upstate Medical University, Syracuse, NY, USA
e-mail: Braleya@upstate.edu

W. A. Hall
Department of Neurosurgery, SUNY Upstate Medical University, Syracuse, New York, USA
e-mail: Hallw@upstate.edu

M. Turgut et al. (eds.), *Subdural Hematoma*,
https://doi.org/10.1007/978-3-030-79371-5_17

subarachnoid space just inferior to the floor of the third ventricle, with the added benefit of typically requiring no implanted hardware. This procedure negates the aforementioned risks of infection and results in fewer return trips to the operating room for removal or replacement following infection [5]. This advantage is because, in the unfortunate event of an infection such as meningitis, there is no implanted hardware to remove or replace. The overall complication rates between ETV and shunting are comparable with some studies reporting that ETV has more perioperative complications but less delayed complications [5].

Subdural collections, including subdural hematoma and subdural hygroma, are known complications of CSF shunting. Although less likely, subdural collections are possible complications of ETV as well [5]. These collections may be asymptomatic or may cause neurologic symptoms such as headache, weakness, numbness, and seizures. The symptomatology largely is determined by the size and the acuity of the development of these collections and may result from trauma such as falls and become particularly dangerous if combined with anticoagulation or antiplatelet therapy that is especially common in the idiopathic normal pressure hydrocephalus (iNPH) patient population [1, 15].

17.2 Etiology of Subdural Collections After CSF Diversion

Subdural collections after CSF diversion are thought to develop from two interrelated and often co-existent sources, CSF accumulation in the form of a hygroma secondary to decreased size of the ventricles, and hemorrhage that can develop when bridging veins are disrupted. Subdural CSF accumulation can occur in any patient that has large ventricles who subsequently has a dramatic decrease in the size of their dilated ventricles. This development occurs because the brain and blood volumes stay relatively constant, and as the ventricles decrease in size through direct drainage, they require less space and cause another space to enlarge as compensation. This increase in the subdural space can lead to hemorrhage in a manner similar to how ex-vacuo atrophy results in hemorrhage; bridging veins are stretched as the subdural space increases in size and small traumatic events or rotation of the brain can lead to hemorrhage. This hemorrhage can vary from small, repeat hemorrhages that accumulate over prolonged periods of time prior to causing symptoms or can manifest as an acute subdural hemorrhage that leads to the abrupt and potentially catastrophic onset of symptoms.

The core mechanism leading to subdural collection formation is the overdrainage of CSF. This overdrainage may be secondary to a shunt opening pressure that is too low, but also may be the consequence of continued drainage in the setting of resolution of the initial pathology that necessitated placement of the shunt. Additional reasons for subdural collections with a similar mechanism for development to that of CSF overdrainage is intracranial hypotension secondary to a spinal CSF leak [2, 12]. These entities often manifest in a similar fashion, with bilateral subdural collections/hemorrhage accumulating until the CSF leak is repaired or spontaneously occludes [2, 6, 9].

17.3 Management of Subdural Collections

Prevention of these subdural collections is thought to be critical for avoiding hemorrhage that requires surgical intervention. Appropriate selection of the shunt valve opening pressure and the consideration of the placement of a programmable shunt are key contributing factors for the avoidance of this unfortunate complication [11]. Shunt valve opening pressures can be estimated by ventricular or lumbar cisternal pressure measurements pre- or intraoperatively to guide the choice of the initial or subsequent valve pressure setting [11].

With this point addressed, it is worth noting that subdural hemorrhage/collection accumulation secondary to overdrainage can occur even if the pressure setting was appropriately chosen at the time of shunt placement or can persist even when the shunt setting is increased. This occurrence can result secondary to the siphoning effect [4, 13]. CSF Shunts rely on relatively simple pressure gradients to open and close the valve; this finding is true for programmable and fixed pressure valves. The pressure gradient functions based on the assumption that the intrabdominal pressure is low or negligible and that the intracranial pressure is at a higher level. During postural change to an erect position, the intra-abdominal pressure becomes much lower than that of the intracranial pressure due to the differences in height. This variability in location leads to shunt drainage based on supine or erect positioning. Indeed, some patients who are bedridden may experience shunt failure due to the loss of the additional flow that results during erect positioning [3, 4]. The opposite effect is also true, patients who are upright may develop neurological symptoms secondary to overdrainage and may develop subdural collections and/or hemorrhage in a similar fashion to those that have too low of a shunt valve opening pressure [4]. This can be particularly hard to treat because simply increasing the opening pressure will be insufficient. Anti-siphon valves were introduced to address this issue specifically and some literature reports decreased overdrainage complications for patients that have had anti-siphon valves placed [13]. These anti-siphon devices can be incorporated into the valve mechanism or may be an in-line additional component placed between the valve and the distal catheter.

The traditional treatment for subdural collections has primarily been surgical in nature, requiring various interventions such as burr hole drainage, craniotomy for evacuation, and even subdural shunting [15]. The persistent drainage of CSF from the ventricles can further promote subdural hemorrhage and subdural fluid enlargement and as such the drainage should be reduced or discontinued, at least temporarily [15].

The method of reducing CSF drainage after subdural hemorrhage is limited by the initial hardware chosen for the initial shunt placement. Use of fixed pressure valves has only realistically two options for reducing CSF flow, ligation or replacement of the valve for a higher-pressure system [8]. Lumbar-peritoneal shunts are in a similar situation necessitating ligation or introduction of a different pressure valve. The introduction and increasing popularity of programmable shunts have provided a nonsurgical option for temporarily and percutaneously changing the CSF opening pressure which can allow for reduced flow or complete cessation of CSF drainage [8]. This capability has been shown to allow for the nonoperative treatment of subdural hematomas/hygromas that were previously treated mainly with surgery [8, 15]. With programmable valves, the opening pressure can be increased such that less CSF drains or none at all [1, 7, 8, 11]. This shunt valve can then be maintained at an increased pressure until clinical stabilization occurs or resolution of the hemorrhage is attained and then the valve pressure setting can be noninvasively decreased back down to a level that addresses the underlying need for CSF diversion. To reduce the risk of future subdural collections of a nontraumatic etiology, it is suggested to consider utilizing a baseline opening pressure slightly higher than previously chosen. The follow-up for these patients should be frequent to allow for early identification of subdural fluid re-accumulation prior to clinical symptoms developing which enhances the chances of nonoperative intervention being successful.

Although most subdural collections secondary to shunt drainage are subclinical or demonstrate clinical symptoms that do not necessitate surgical intervention, there are situations where the symptoms do create an indication for surgery. These symptoms may include refractory headache, weakness, numbness, seizures, lethargy, coma, etc. When present, surgical drainage of the collection should be accomplished in the least invasive manner. Subdural evacuating port system (SEPS) placement at the bedside is a minimally invasive way of evacuating subdural collections and typically involves only local anesthesia or moderate sedation, further diminishing patient risks [10, 14]. This technique is best utilized for chronic subdural hematomas or hygromas, but there are good data that support SEPS drainage in subacute and even mixed-acute hemorrhages [10]. Loculations decrease the likelihood of SEPS success but this method of drainage is still worth attempting as the risks are minimal and avoiding a trip to the OR is a desirable goal [10]. Operative interventions may include simple burr hole craniotomy, double burr hole placement with irrigation, or open craniotomy for evacuation of hematoma. As expected, the rate of effectiveness increases with the degree of invasiveness of the procedure; however complication rates are similarly more likely with more extensive procedures [10, 14]. Additional risks of open surgery compared to SEPS include a slightly higher risk of infection given a larger incision and the need for implanted hardware in the form of craniotomy plating systems [10].

17.4 Conclusion

Subdural collections may include hemorrhage or hygroma and are an unfortunate and difficult-to-treat complication of CSF diversion. These entities can manifest themselves with a wide variety of clinical presentations from asymptomatic collection/hemorrhage to life-threatening massive subdural bleeding causing brain compression. The primary goal of treatment is reduced CSF diversion, via surgical or nonsurgical methods in addition to the possible surgical evacuation of the hemorrhage. Prevention techniques include careful consideration of initial opening pressure of the CSF diverting shunt valve, opting for a programmable valve, and the utilization of an anti-siphon valve all of which are intended to prevent overdrainage of CSF. More investigation and research are necessary to highlight the optimal strategy for the prevention and management of this avoidable complication (Figs. 17.1, 17.2, and 17.3).

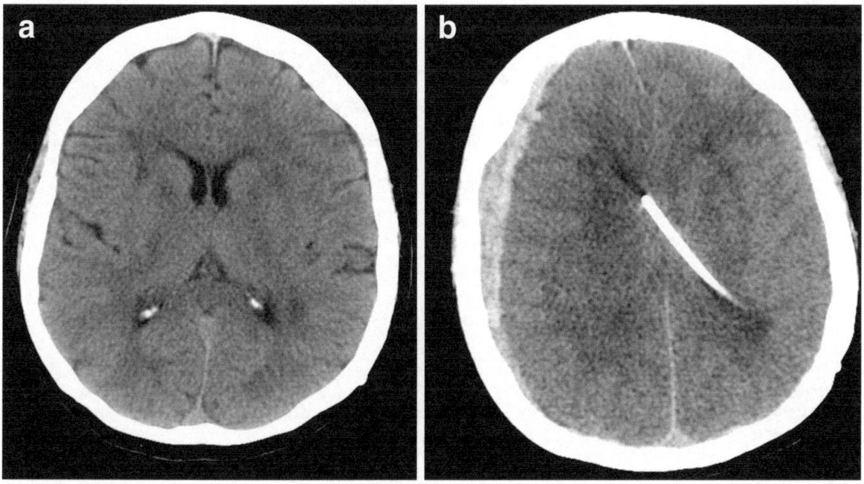

Fig. 17.1 Axial non-contrast CT of a 63-year-old male with moderate ventricles prior to left parietal shunt insertion (**a**). Interval development of a right acute subdural hematoma after cerebrospinal fluid overdrainage resulting in slit ventricles (**b**)

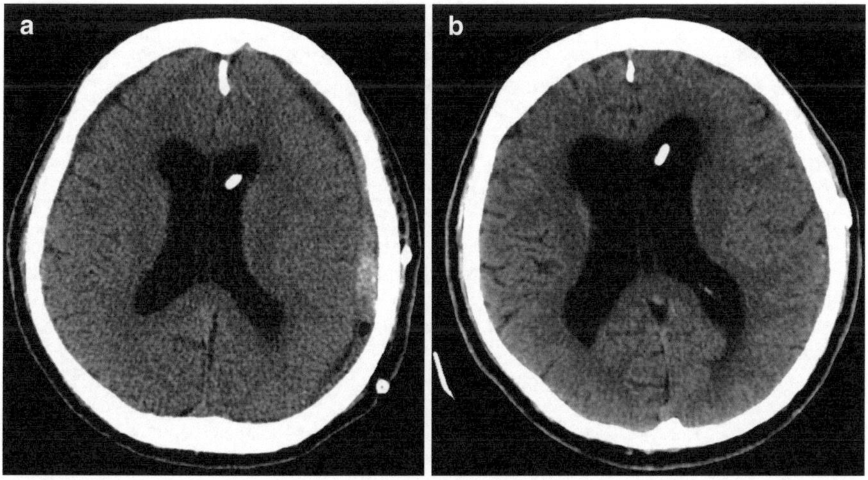

Fig. 17.2 58-year-old female with normal pressure hydrocephalus treated with a ventriculoperitoneal (VP) shunt with a programmable valve. (**a**) A left-sided acute on chronic subdural hemorrhage is visible after placement of a VP shunt. (**b**) The hemorrhage has resolved at 6 month follow-up after SEPS drainage and adjusting the valve to a higher pressure. Note the increased ventricular size

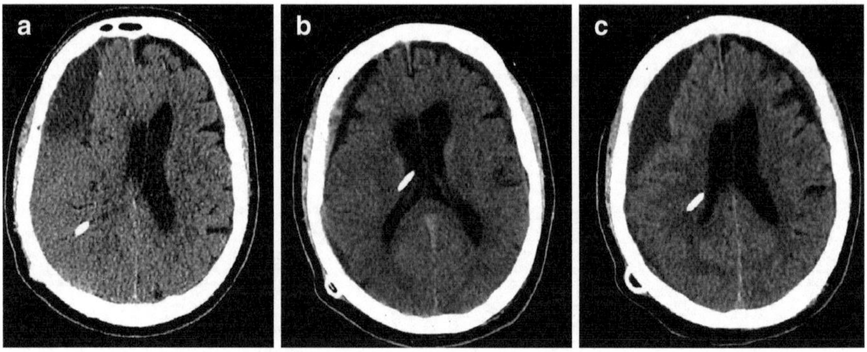

Fig. 17.3 84-year-old male with normal pressure hydrocephalus that developed a mixed density right subdural hematoma after insertion of a medium pressure shunt (**a**). Reduced size of the hemorrhage after subdural evacuating port system placement without changing the shunt valve (**b**). Three months later the patient had asymptomatic partial re-accumulation of the subdural fluid since the valve pressure was not changed (**c**)

References

1. Berger A, Constantini S, Ram Z, Roth J. Acute subdural hematomas in shunted normal-pressure hydrocephalus patients—management options and literature review: a case-based series. Surg Neurol Int. 2018;9:238.
2. Chan SM, Chodakiewitz YG, Maya MM, Schievink WI, Moser FG. Intracranial hypotension and cerebrospinal fluid leak. Neuroimaging Clin N Am. 2019;29:213–26.
3. Craven CL, Toma AK, Watkins LD. Persistent hydrocephalus due to postural activation of a ventricular shunt anti-gravity device. J Clin Neurosci. 2017;37:91–5.
4. Czosnyka Z, Czosnyka M, Richards HK, Pickard JD. Posture-related overdrainage: comparison of the performance of 10 hydrocephalus shunts in vitro. Neurosurgery. 1998;42(2):327–34.
5. Dewan MC, Lim J, Shannon CN, Wellons JC. The durability of endoscopic third ventriculostomy and ventriculoperitoneal shunts in children with hydrocephalus following posterior fossa tumor resection: a systematic review and time-to-failure analysis. J Neurosurg Pediatr. 2017;19:578–84.
6. Dillon WP. Challenges in the diagnosis and treatment of spontaneous intracranial hypotension. Radiology. 2018;289:773–4.
7. Feletti A, d'Avella D, Wikkelsø C, Klinge P, Hellström P, Tans J, et al. Ventriculoperitoneal shunt complications in the European idiopathic normal pressure hydrocephalus multicenter study. Oper Neurosurg. 2019;17:97–102.
8. Hayes J, Roguski M, Riesenburger RI. Rapid resolution of an acute subdural hematoma by increasing the shunt valve pressure in a 63-year-old man with normal-pressure hydrocephalus with a ventriculoperitoneal shunt: a case report and literature review. J Med Case Rep. 2012;6:393.
9. He F-F, Li L, Liu M-J, Zhong T-D, Zhang Q-W, Fang X-M. Targeted epidural blood patch treatment for refractory spontaneous intracranial hypotension in China. J Neurol Surg B Skull Base. 2018;79:217–23.
10. Hoffman H, Ziechmann R, Beutler T, Verhave B, Chin LS. First-line management of chronic subdural hematoma with the subdural evacuating port system: institutional experience and predictors of outcomes. J Clin Neurosci. 2018;50:221–5.

11. Kim KH, Yeo IS, Yi JS, Lee HJ, Yang JH, Lee IW. A pressure adjustment protocol for programmable valves. J Korean Neurosurg Soc. 2009;46:370–7.
12. Mokri B. Spontaneous CSF leaks. Neurol Clin. 2014;32:397–422.
13. Pereira RM, Suguimoto MT, de Oliveira MF, Tornai JB, Amaral RA, Teixeira MJ, et al. Efeito da válvula de pressão fixa com antisifão SPHERA® no tratamento da hidrocefalia de pressão normal e prevenção de hiperdrenagem. Arq Neuropsiquiatr. 2016;74:55–61.
14. Singla A, Jacobsen WP, Yusupov IR, Carter DA. Subdural evacuating port system (SEPS)—minimally invasive approach to the management of chronic/subacute subdural hematomas. Clin Neurol Neurosurg. 2013;115:425–31.
15. Sundstrom N, Lagebrant M, Eklund A, Koskinen L-O, Malm J. Subdural hematomas in 1846 patients with shunted idiopathic normal pressure hydrocephalus: treatment and long-term survival. J Neurosurg. 2018;129:797–804.

Chapter 18
Chronic Subdural Hematoma Following Lumbar Puncture and Spinal Anesthesia

Hatim Belfquih, Hassan Baallal, and Ali Akhaddar

Abbreviations

CN	Cranial nerve
CSDH	Chronic subdural hematoma
CSF	Cerebrospinal fluid
CT	Computed tomography
EBP	Epidural blood patch
ICHD-II	International Classification of Headache Disorders-II
LP	Lumbar puncture
MRI	Magnetic resonance imaging
PDPH	Postdural puncture headache

18.1 Introduction

Spinal anesthesia is widely used for many obstetric, gynecological, orthopedic, and urological operations. Epidural anesthesia involves the injection of an anesthetic solution into the epidural space of the spine [7], which offers the advantages of avoiding general anesthesia and allowing patients to remain awake during surgical procedures. Unintentional dural puncture during epidural anesthesia is not uncommon, occurring with an estimated frequency of up to 3.6% [18]. Intentional dural puncture occurs with spinal anesthesia, where the anesthetic is injected into the subarachnoid space. Spinal anesthesia offers the same advantages as epidural anesthesia with a shorter time of onset [32].

H. Belfquih (✉) · H. Baallal
Department of Neurosurgery, Avicenne Military Hospital of Marrakech, Cady Ayyad University in Marrakech and Mohammed V University in Rabat, Rabat, Morocco

A. Akhaddar
Avicenne Military Hospital of Marrakech, Department of Neurosurgery, Mohammed V University in Rabat, Rabat, Morocco

M. Turgut et al. (eds.), *Subdural Hematoma*,
https://doi.org/10.1007/978-3-030-79371-5_18

The safety of spinal and epidural anesthesia is well documented; however, complications are occasionally related to these procedures and include back pain, postdural puncture headache (PDPH), infection, hematoma, nerve injury, and intracranial hemorrhage which occur in approximately 0.05% of cases [5]. The most common benign complication is a PDPH [49]. Chronic subdural hematoma (CSDH) is among the rare, most severe, and potentially fatal complications that may be misdiagnosed as PDPH [23]. Raising clinicians' awareness regarding the signs and symptoms of CSDH will result in the prevention of unwanted outcomes through urgent intervention.

18.2 Incidence

The incidence of inadvertent dural puncture as a result of epidural anesthesia ranges from 0.4 to 6% [1–5]. PDPH develops in approximately one-third of those who have had dural puncture for any reason, whether it is intentional or inadvertent [11, 22]. It is estimated that 74% of obstetric patients develop PDPH that typically spontaneously resolves [4].

There is little data about CSDH that is caused by spinal anesthesia. As the symptomatology frequently mimics PDPH, a number of them are probably not identified. According to the literature, CSDH incidence ranges between 1/500,000 and 1/1,000,000 [31]. A Swedish retrospective study published in 2004 and spanning a decade (1990–1999) identified 127 cases of neurological complications following spinal anesthesia, the risk of which was determined to be 1/20,000 to 1/30,000, among which 2 cases of CSDH were reported [29]. The incidence of CSDH specifically caused by epidural anesthesia used in obstetric practice has been estimated to be 1:500,000. The recent study from Canada published in 2019 collected 22,130,815 childbirths after neuraxial anesthesia, where there were 68,374 deliveries identified with PDPH, for an overall rate of 309 per 100,000 women; the number of cases of postpartum CSDH was 342, for an incidence of 1.5 per 100,000 deliveries [30].

Finally, the true incidence of CSDH after dural puncture or spinal anesthesia may be greater than published because patients are often treated without further investigation.

18.3 Pathophysiology

Both PDPH and postdural puncture CSDH are caused by CSF leakage through the dural breach.

18.3.1 Consequences of Dural Puncture

Puncture of the dura has the potential to allow for the development of excessive leakage of CSF. The rate of CSF loss through the dural perforation (0.084–4.5 mL s^{-1}) is generally greater than the rate of CSF production (0.35 mL min^{-1}), particularly with needle sizes larger than 25G. Excess loss of CSF leads to intracranial hypotension and a demonstrable reduction in CSF volume where the adult subarachnoid pressure of 15 ± 5 cm H_2O is reduced to 4.0 cm H_2O or less [36].

18.3.2 PDPH

Although the loss of CSF and lowering of CSF pressure is not disputed, the actual mechanism that causes the PDPH is unclear. There are two possible explanations. First, the lowering of CSF pressure causes traction on the intracranial structures in the upright position; these structures are pain sensitive, leading to the characteristic headache. Secondly, the loss of CSF produces a compensatory venodilatation. The sum of the volumes in the intracranial compartment for CSF and intracranial blood is constant; therefore the consequence of a decrease in CSF volume leads to a compensatory increase in blood volume through venous dilatation and the venodilatation is then responsible for the headache [37].

18.3.3 CSDH

The primary mechanism for CSDH after spinal anesthesia is the same as PDPH with some minor differences. A leak of CSF at the level of the arachnoid tear probably induces a lowering of intraspinal and intracranial pressure. The resulting dynamic alteration of CSF flow leads to a relative ventricular collapse and a rostrocaudal movement of the central nervous system. As a consequence, sensitive meningeal structures or meningeal pain sensors, cranial nerves and bridging-veins are stretched. The sudden decrease in the CSF volume may also activate adenosine receptors, thus producing arterial and venous vasodilatation and the subsequent clinical symptoms of PDPH. If the traction exerted on the bridging veins is substantial, it may cause a rupture at their weakest point in the subdural space, leading to CSDH formation (Fig. 18.1) [28].

Electron microscopic data on human bridging veins show thin walls of variable thickness, circumferential arrangement of collagen fibers, and the lack of outer reinforcement by arachnoid trabecules. All this contributes to render the subdural portion of the vein more fragile than its subarachnoid portion. These features explain the laceration of veins and the subdural location of resultant hematomas, which can evolve in various ways, acute or chronic [47].

18.4 Predisposing Factors

The risk factors of postdural puncture headache and CSDH include the size and design of the spinal needle used, the experience of the personnel performing the dural puncture, and the patient factors or clinical conditions.

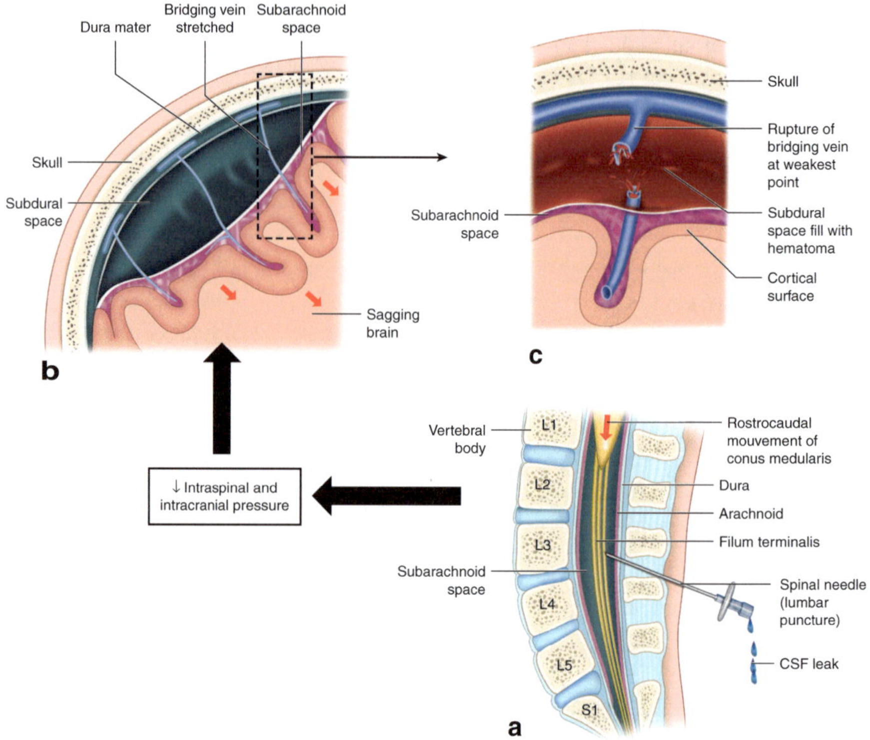

Fig. 18.1 The mechanism for CSDH after dural puncture. Leakage of cerebrospinal fluid from a dural perforation at the spinal level (**a**) results in decreased intraspinal and intracranial pressure with sagging of the brain (**b**). This places tension on the bridging veins between the dura and the arachnoid (**b**). If the traction exerted on the bridging veins is substantial, it may cause a rupture at their weakest point in the subdural space, leading to formation (**c**)

18.4.1 Size and Design of the Spinal Needle

Zeidan et al. [50] state that CSDH, like PDPH, enlarges due to the leakage of CSF from the hole created by the spinal needle, so the size of the needle and degree of the dural tear have a direct correlation with PDPH and CSDH. In the case of using a large needle diameter and making more attempts at inserting the needle, loss of CSF may be over 200 mL per day.

Anesthetists have been active in attempting to reduce the incidence of PDPH by reducing the size of the spinal needle; the incidence is 40% with a 22G needle, 25% with a 25G needle [12], 2% ± 12% with a 26G Quincke needle [13], and <2% with a 29G needle [16]. Needle modifications, such as the Whitacre, the Sprotte, and Atraucan needles, promise further reductions in PDPH (Fig. 18.2).

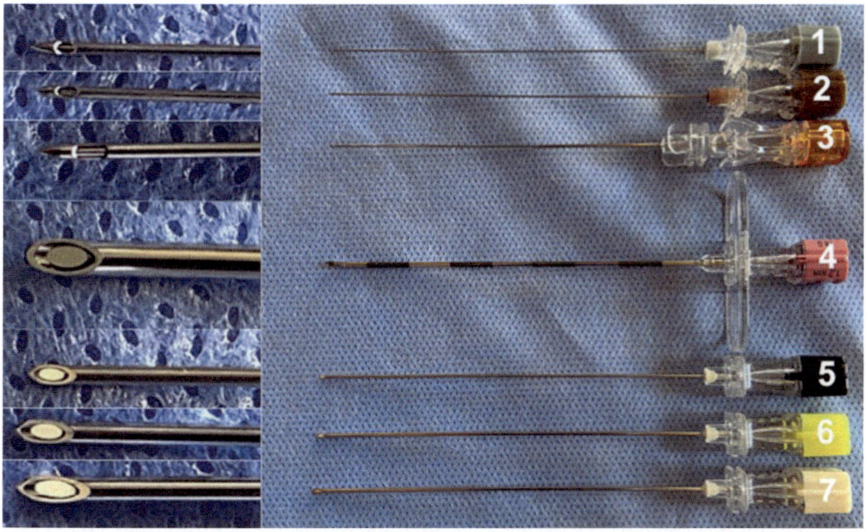

Fig. 18.2 Photograph of epidural needle (needle 4) and other different spinal needle tip design for lumbar puncture and spinal anesthesia. 1: 27G Sprotte Style Pencil Point; 2: 26G Sprotte Style Pencil Point; 3: 25G Sprotte Style Pencil Point; 4: 18G Tuohy epidural needle; 5: 22G Quincke type spinal needle for lumbar puncture; 6: 20G Quincke type spinal needle for lumbar puncture, 7: 19G Quincke type spinal needle for lumbar puncture

18.4.2 Factors Related to the Puncture Technique

It has been proposed that coming in contact with bone during insertion or repeated puncture attempts may lead to spinal needle tip deformation whereby damaged needle tips could lead to an increase in the size of the subsequent dural perforation. Recent in vivo studies have demonstrated that the cutting type of the spinal needle is more likely to become deformed after bony contact than comparable sized pencil-point needles. When used, the cutting-edge needle (Quincke type) should be inserted parallel to the orientation of the longitudinal arachnoid fibers to decrease the risk of PDPH by 50% compared with a perpendicular insertion [20].

Some studies have demonstrated that the puncture orifice can remain opened for up to 18 weeks and extravasation of CSF can reach up to 240 mL.day^{-1} in orifices of 0.6 mm of diameter, which causes loss of the autoregulation mechanisms of intracranial pressure and provides an explanation for the prolonged evolution of the PDPH episode [36].

18.4.3 Factors Related to the Patient Conditions

Susceptibility of pregnant patients to postdural puncture CSDH might be attributed to the frequent use of epidural analgesia during labor [3]. A review of the literature demonstrated that 20 out of 22 cases [43, 48] of CSDH after inadvertent dural puncture during epidural block were in obstetric patients. Some authors believe that due to hemostatic imbalance, differences in elasticity of the dura and possibly gender-based differences in cranial morphology, CSDH may occur more frequently in pregnant patients in comparison to other patients [2, 46]. Cesarean delivery was also negatively associated with CSDH. This may be because of the absence of pushing efforts during labor or the usage of smaller-gauge spinal needles for spinal anesthesia. Moreover, the presence of presumed PDPH after neuraxial anesthesia in childbirth, compared with no headache, was associated with a small but statistically significant absolute increase in the risk of being diagnosed with CSDH [2]. Further research is needed to establish if this association is causal for this rare outcome.

Other possible risk factors that are apparently unrelated to spinal anesthesia but may coexist in patients undergoing CSDH included head trauma, coagulopathy, cerebral aneurysm, arteriovenous malformation, tumors, cerebral atrophy, chronic alcoholism, cardiovascular disease, meningovascular syphilis, and diabetes mellitus.

Gender is believed to be an independent risk factor for the development of postdural puncture headache. A systematic review examined a total of 18 trials (2163 males, 1917 females), the odds of developing a postdural puncture headache were significantly lower for males than nonpregnant female subjects (odds ratio = 0.55). In addition, the incidence of PDPH seems to increase in females relative to male subjects after the onset of puberty [9, 21, 34]. Estrogen has been shown to mediate cerebral artery tone and may dilate cerebral pial vessels [14, 27].

18.5 Clinical Symptoms

The clinical manifestations of CSDH depend on age, size, location, speed of formation of the blood collection, compression of intracranial structures, and the clinical condition of the patient. According to the onset of the symptoms, it may be hard to differentiate a CSDH from PDPH, the most frequent benign complication of spinal anesthesia that improves within a few days if treated with analgesics and bed rest.

PDPH presents as a diffuse headache commonly described as throbbing and positional: worsening upon standing and improving upon recumbency. Maneuvers that increase intracranial pressure, such as coughing or straining, may worsen the symptoms.

International Classification of Headache Disorders-II (ICHD-II) criteria [41] for PDPH specifies that all of the following be met:

1. The headache worsens within 15 min of sitting or standing, improves within 15 min of lying.
2. The headache is accompanied by at least one of the following: neck stiffness, tinnitus, hypacusia, photophobia, and/or nausea.

3. The headache develops within 5 days after a dural puncture.
4. The headache resolves either spontaneously within 1 week or within 48 h after effective treatment of the spinal fluid leak, usually by an epidural blood patch (EBP).

The changing characteristics of PDPH includes symptoms of nonpostural headaches along with focal neurological abnormalities such as consciousness disorder, nausea, vomiting, dizziness, hemiplegia, cranial nerve palsies, visual disturbance, diplopia, photophobia, rarely seizures [42], and unresponsiveness of the headache to ordinary treatments are warning signs and should arouse the suspicion to evaluate for a CSDH [33, 35]. Reported symptoms and signs for a CSDH caused by dural puncture present at the time of diagnosis are listed in Table 18.1 [2, 6, 26].

The previous reports of cranial nerve (CN) palsy in CSDH suggested that the downward traction of the brain and compression of the CN leads to the neurologic deficit [25]; abducens palsy is the most common CN affected in post-LP CSDH, in comparison to other cranial nerves due to its long intracranial course. Abducens palsy usually occurs 4–14 days after LP and spinal anesthesia. The deficit can be unilateral or bilateral and is usually associated with PLPH. Bradycardia has also been described and is thought to occur due to rostral migration of the brain with subsequent compression of the hypothalamus. Mass effect on the hypothalamus can cause alterations in autonomic outflow [10].

Based on the interval between anesthesia and the onset of symptoms, subdural hematomas may be acute and subacute/chronic. Most reported acute cases develop within the first 2 days with a severe and persistent nonpostural headache, unresponsive to analgesics, with symptoms of acute neurological deterioration, suggesting a sudden increase in intracranial pressure, such as anisocoria, hemiparesis, and altered level of consciousness. Subacute/chronic subdural bleeding may develop over a period of days or weeks, posing diagnostic problems. A CSDH may be confused with PDPH, causing an initial orthostatic headache, responsive to analgesics, bed rest, and fluid replacement. With time these symptoms may go through alternate phases of improvements and exacerbations, losing their relation to position and accompanied by neurological signs. According to a published study, the duration of time from dural puncture to the diagnosis of SDH ranges widely from 4 h to 29 weeks [11]. In case series, 37% of cases were diagnosed within 1 week of dural puncture, and 85% were diagnosed within 1 month [23].

Table 18.1 Symptoms and signs with CSDH caused by dural puncture [2, 6, 25]

Symptom/sign	Occurrence rate
Headache	74–91%
Nausea/vomiting	31–41%
Altered mental status	31–40%
Focal motor deficit	23–28%
Diplopia/visual changes	14–20%
Aphasia/dysarthria	11–13%

Nakanuno et al. [31] studied 69 cases of intracranial CSDH after dural puncture for the purpose of anesthesia, diagnosis, or treatment. They classified the duration of headache associated with CSDH into three patterns with patients reporting the onset of a headache within 4 days after dural puncture. The pain persisted until subdural hemorrhage occurred. Other patients complained about a headache that occurred early after dural puncture. The pain disappeared or was alleviated temporarily but reappeared and worsened, followed by the onset of subdural hemorrhage. The third category of patients suffered from a headache that did not occur early after dural puncture but appeared later with the onset of subdural hemorrhage. In their study, the first pattern was found in 47% (33 cases), the second in 44% (30 cases), and the third pattern in 6% (4 cases); 3% (2 cases) were unknown. Most of the cases had a headache early after the dural puncture. The third pattern, with an acute onset and no early-stage headache, was rare.

In the study of Cuypers et al. [6], the headache that is not consistent with PDPH occurs in 83% of 56 patients with CSDH following neuraxis anesthesia. PDPH symptoms alone, without other serious neurologic symptoms, may be accompanied by clinically insidious CSDH.

18.6 Imaging

Using a magnetic resonance imaging (MRI) technique, Grant et al. measured the volume of intracranial CSF in 20 patients before and 24 h after LP. The total brain quantity of CSF, the ventricular CSF volume, cortical sulcal CSF volume, and the posterior fossa CSF volume measurements were performed. They showed the occurrence of headache in patients with very variable alterations in intracranial CSF volume. This study also demonstrated that the total intracranial CSF volume is almost always reduced following LP and the majority of the deficit is due to a loss of cortical sulcal CSF. This finding may explain why CSDH can occur as a complication of LP [17]. MRI can also detect further classical signs of intracranial hypotension due to the excess loss of CSF, namely, slit-like lateral ventricles, an enlarged pituitary gland, and aseptic pachymeningitis [45].

Computed tomography (CT) scan is a safe, easy, and low-cost method of detecting CSDH. Patients with severe, prolonged, or atypical headaches must first be examined with CT scan to avoid catastrophic results [30].

Most previously reported cases of CSDH were unilateral; however, few cases involved bilateral subdural hematomas. This finding may be attributable to the greater loss of CSF, which is caused by the use of larger needles in epidural anesthesia. Zeidan and Baraka [48] made a similar comment on this issue as some of the patients in that review also developed bilateral hematomas.

Spinal MRI or spinal CT may detect the CSF leaking area. Spinal MRI, performed with T1 and T2 sequences and fat saturation on sagittal and coronal planes, may detect the fistula causing CSF leaking; more often, it only detects the area of extradural CSF collection. In the acute phase, spinal CT has a higher sensitivity and specificity in comparison to spinal MRI [8].

18.7 Treatment

Treatment of CSDH after LP or spinal anesthesia is conservative therapy or surgical evacuation. The size of the hematoma and the patient's neurological status are important in influencing treatment selection.

A conservative approach has been recommended for patients with CSDH without mental status changes, no seizure activity, absent intracranial mass effect, and when the hematoma is <1 cm in maximum thickness, and causing a midline shift <5 mm. This approach requires bed rest, analgesia including opioids, intravenous hydration, and close neurological and neuroradiological follow-up to recognize potential clinical and radiographic worsening as early as possible [38]. Furthermore, some have advocated for the use of EBP in the treatment of CSDH caused by dural tears resulting in chronic CSF leaks. EBP was performed at the level of the dural puncture with a midline approach, and 15 cc of a solution composed of the patient's autologous blood and fibrin glue was introduced through a Tuohy needle under fluoroscopic control, with the aim to develop a blood clot to close the dural fistula. After the procedure, the patient is required to lie down for 2 h. The success rate of EBP in patients with PDPH is 60–90% [39]. However, recent studies have shown that the probability of success depends on the timing of the patch placement. Better results are achieved if the EBP is performed within 72 h after dural puncture [44]. The EBP should be considered in cases of failure of standard conservative treatment for small hematomas. In the study of Nakanuno et al., 83% of patients recovered completely, while the remaining 17% died or had permanent neurological deficits. For several bad outcomes, delayed diagnosis was implicated [31]. Even though sealing of the dural defect and restoration of the CSF pressure are expected by EBP, there is a possibility that the CSDH may enlarge or reoccur and may require hematoma evacuation [19].

Surgical intervention for CSDH is indicated if the hematoma thickness exceeds 10 mm, there is a midline shift of greater than 5 mm, or there is neurologic deterioration. Acute SDH often causes a rapid neurological deterioration that indicates surgical evacuation of the hematoma by craniotomy or burr holes to reduce the intracranial pressure and preserve brain function is necessary [15]. EBP might be performed at the same time of surgical evacuation especially for the patient with recurrent hematomas after surgical evacuation. Rates of surgical intervention for CSDH after dural puncture vary from 9 to 80% [39, 51] with death reported in 7–10% of cases [24].

18.8 Prevention

Prevention of CSDH involves meticulous guidelines for the performance of lumbar punctures, including the use of non-cutting (pencil-edge) needles. Bed rest, hydration, and blood patch placement do not always prevent the occurrence of a CSDH.

Based on the literature data, there are some ways to potentially mitigate the occurrence and to make an early diagnosis of CSDH particularly after labor epidural anesthesia:

- Utilize the smallest possible pencil point gauge spinal needle for subarachnoid access [40].
- Maintain close contact with patients who develop PDPH.
- Offer EBP early in cases of PDPH that is refractory to conservative management and the possibility of repeating EBP in cases where the dural hole may be large [24].
- Reserve the performance of head imaging by CT or MRI for cases of postpartum headache that do not fit ICHD-II criteria for PDPH [41].

18.9 Conclusion

We must take heed of the seriousness of CSDH as a corollary of LP or spinal anesthesia. Prolonged and nonpostural PDPH, worsening clinical condition after an epidural blood patch, and the development of neurological symptoms should be regarded as warning signs of CSDH which necessitate an immediate diagnosis and treatment.

References

1. Acharya R, Chhabra SS, Ratra M, Sehgal AD. Cranial subdural haematoma after spinal anaesthesia. Br J Anaesth. 2001;86:893–5. https://doi.org/10.1093/bja/86.6.893.
2. Amorim JA, Valença MM. Postdural puncture headache is a risk factor for new postdural puncture headache. Cephalalgia. 2008;28(1):5–8. https://doi.org/10.1111/j.1468-2982.2007.01454.x. Epub 2007 Oct 23.
3. Amorim JA, Remígio DS, Damázio Filho O, de Barros MA, Carvalho VN, Valença MM. Intracranial subdural hematoma post-spinal anesthesia: report of two cases and review of 33 cases in the literature. Rev Bras Anestesiol. 2010;60(6):620–9, 344–9. English, Portuguese, Spanish. https://doi.org/10.1016/S0034-7094(10)70077-5.
4. Angle P, Thompson D, Halpern S, Wilson DB. Second stage pushing correlates with headache after unintentional dural puncture in parturients. Can J Anaesth. 1999;46(9):861–6. https://doi.org/10.1007/BF03012976.
5. Cruvinel MG, Barbosa PR, Teixeira VC, Castro CH. Tampão peridural com dextran 40 na profilaxia da cefaléia pós-punção acidental da duramáter em paciente HIV positivo: relato de caso [Epidural patch with dextran 40 to prevent postdural puncture headache in an HIV patient: case report]. Rev Bras Anestesiol. 2002;52(6):712–8. Portuguese.
6. Cuypers V, Van de Velde M, Devroe S. Intracranial subdural haematoma following neuraxial anaesthesia in the obstetric population: a literature review with analysis of 56 reported cases. Int J Obstet Anesth. 2016;25:58–65. https://doi.org/10.1016/j.ijoa.2015.09.003.
7. de Lange JJ, Cuesta MA, Cuesta de Pedro A. Fidel Pagés Miravé (1886-1923). The pioneer of lumbar epidural anaesthesia. Anaesthesia. 1994;49(5):429–31. https://doi.org/10.1111/j.1365-2044.1994.tb03480.x.
8. De Lipsis L, Belmonte R, Cusano M, Giannetti MA, Muccio CF, Mancinelli M. Subdural hematoma as a consequence of labor epidural analgesia. Asian J Neurosurg. 2018;13(3):931–4.

9. Ebinger F, Kosel C, Pietz J, Rating D. Headache and backache after lumbar puncture in children and adolescents: a prospective study. Pediatrics. 2004;113(6):1588–92. https://doi.org/10.1542/peds.113.6.1588.
10. Evans RW. Complications of lumbar puncture. Neurol Clin. 1998;16(1):83–105. https://doi.org/10.1016/s0733-8619(05)70368-6.
11. Evans RW, Armon C, Frohman EM, Goodin DS. Assessment: prevention of post-lumbar puncture headaches: report of the therapeutics and technology assessment subcommittee of the american academy of neurology. Neurology. 2000;55(7):909–14. https://doi.org/10.1212/wnl.55.7.909.
12. Flaatten H, Rodt S, Rosland J, Vamnes J. Postoperative headache in young patients after spinal anaesthesia. Anaesthesia. 1987;42(2):202–5. https://doi.org/10.1111/j.1365-2044.1987.tb03001.x.
13. Flaatten H, Rodt SA, Vamnes J, Rosland J, Wisborg T, Koller ME. Postdural puncture headache. A comparison between 26- and 29-gauge needles in young patients. Anaesthesia. 1989;44(2):147–9. https://doi.org/10.1111/j.1365-2044.1989.tb11167.x.
14. Geary GG, Krause DN, Duckles SP. Estrogen reduces mouse cerebral artery tone through endothelial NOS- and cyclooxygenase-dependent mechanisms. Am J Physiol Heart Circ Physiol. 2000;279(2):H511–9. https://doi.org/10.1152/ajpheart.2000.279.2.H511.
15. Gerard C, Busl KM. Treatment of acute subdural hematoma. Curr Treat Options Neurol. 2014;16(1):275. https://doi.org/10.1007/s11940-013-0275-0.
16. Geurts JW, Haanschoten MC, van Wijk RM, Kraak H, Besse TC. Post-dural puncture headache in young patients. A comparative study between the use of 0.52 mm (25-gauge) and 0.33 mm (29-gauge) spinal needles. Acta Anaesthesiol Scand. 1990;34(5):350–3. https://doi.org/10.1111/j.1399-6576.1990.tb03101.x.
17. Grant R, Condon B, Hart I, Teasdale GM. Changes in intracranial CSF volume after lumbar puncture and their relationship to post-LP headache. J Neurol Neurosurg Psychiatry. 1991;54(5):440–2. https://doi.org/10.1136/jnnp.54.5.440.
18. Gurudatt CL. Unintentional dural puncture and postdural puncture headache-can this headache of the patient as well as the anaesthesiologist be prevented? Indian J Anaesth. 2014;58(4):385–7. https://doi.org/10.4103/0019-5049.138962.
19. Hashizume K, Watanabe K, Kawaguchi M, Fujiwara A, Furuya H. Evaluation on a clinical course of subdural hematoma in patients undergoing epidural blood patch for spontaneous cerebrospinal fluid leak. Clin Neurol Neurosurg. 2013;115(8):1403–6. https://doi.org/10.1016/j.clineuro.2013.01.022.
20. Jokinen MJ, Pitkänen MT, Lehtonen E, Rosenberg PH. Deformed spinal needle tips and associated dural perforations examined by scanning electron microscopy. Acta Anaesthesiol Scand. 1996;40(6):687–90. https://doi.org/10.1111/j.1399-6576.1996.tb04511.x.
21. Karnik R, Valentin A, Winkler WB, Khaffaf N, Donath P, Slany J. Sex-related differences in acetazolamide-induced cerebral vasomotor reactivity. Stroke. 1996;27(1):56–8. https://doi.org/10.1161/01.str.27.1.56.
22. Kim EJ, Chang IY. Intracerebral hemorrhage after vesicolitholapaxy under spinal anesthesia. Korean J Anesthesiol. 2006;51:379–82.
23. Kuntz KM, Kokmen E, Stevens JC, Miller P, Offord KP, Ho MM. Post-lumbar puncture headaches: experience in 501 consecutive procedures. Neurology. 1992;42(10):1884–7. https://doi.org/10.1212/wnl.42.10.1884.
24. Landau R, Ciliberto CF, Goodman SR, Kim-Lo SH, Smiley RM. Complications with 25-gauge and 27-gauge Whitacre needles during combined spinal-epidural analgesia in labor. Int J Obstet Anesth. 2001;10(3):168–71. https://doi.org/10.1054/ijoa.2000.0834.
25. Liegl O. Neuroophthalmologische Komplikationen durch Liquor=leckage nach diagnostischen bzw. therapeutischen Eingriffen am Spinalkanal [Neuroophthalmological complications through liquor leakage after surgical operation on the spinal canal for diagnostic i.e. therapeutic purposes (author's transl)]. Klin Monbl Augenheilkd. 1977;171(4):526–30. German.

26. Lim G, Zorn JM, Dong YJ, DeRenzo JS, Waters JH. Subdural hematoma associated with labor epidural analgesia: a case series. Reg Anesth Pain Med. 2016;41(5):628–31. https://doi.org/10.1097/AAP.0000000000000455.
27. Littleton-Kearney MT, Agnew DM, Traystman RJ, Hurn PD. Effects of estrogen on cerebral blood flow and pial microvasculature in rabbits. Am J Physiol Heart Circ Physiol. 2000;279(3):H1208–14. https://doi.org/10.1152/ajpheart.2000.279.3.H1208.
28. Macon ME, Armstrong L, Brown EM. Subdural hematoma following spinal anesthesia. Anesthesiology. 1990;72(2):380–1.
29. Moen V, Dahlgren N, Irestedt L. Severe neurological complications after central neuraxial blockades in Sweden 1990-1999. Anesthesiology. 2004;101(4):950–9.
30. Moore AR, Wieczorek PM, Carvalho JCA. Association between post-dural puncture headache after neuraxial anesthesia in childbirth and intracranial subdural hematoma. JAMA Neurol. 2020;77(1):65–72. https://doi.org/10.1001/jamaneurol.2019.2995.
31. Nakanuno R, Kawamoto M, Yuge O. [Intracranial subdural hematoma following dural puncture]. Masui. 2007;56(4):395–403. Japanese.
32. Ng K, Parsons J, Cyna AM, Middleton P. Spinal versus epidural anaesthesia for caesarean section. Cochrane Database Syst Rev. 2004;(2):CD003765.
33. Nolte CH, Lehmann TN. Postpartum headache resulting from bilateral chronic subdural hematoma after dural puncture. Am J Emerg Med. 2004;22(3):241–2.
34. Oláh L, Valikovics A, Bereczki D, Fülesdi B, Munkácsy C, Csiba L. Gender-related differences in acetazolamide-induced cerebral vasodilatory response: a transcranial Doppler study. J Neuroimaging. 2000;10(3):151–6.
35. Ozdemir N, Ari MK, Gelal MF, Bezircioğlu H. Intracranial chronic subdural haematoma as a complication of epidural anesthesia. Turk Neurosurg. 2009;19(3):285–7.
36. Parker RK, White PF. A microscopic analysis of cut-bevel versus pencil-point spinal needles. Anesth Analg. 1997;85(5):1101–4.
37. Ready LB, Cuplin S, Haschke RH, Nessly M. Spinal needle determinants of rate of transdural fluid leak. Anesth Analg. 1989;69(4):457–60.
38. Rocchi R, Lombardi C, Marradi I, Di Paolo M, Cerase A. Intracranial and intraspinal hemorrhage following spinal anesthesia. Neurol Sci. 2009;30(5):393–6.
39. Safa-Tisseront V, Thormann F, Malassiné P, Henry M, Riou B, Coriat P, et al. Effectiveness of epidural blood patch in the management of post-dural puncture headache. Anesthesiology. 2001;95(2):334–9.
40. Santanen U, Rautoma P, Luurila H, Erkola O, Pere P. Comparison of 27-gauge (0.41-mm) Whitacre and Quincke spinal needles with respect to post-dural puncture headache and non-dural puncture headache. Acta Anaesthesiol Scand. 2004;48(4):474–9.
41. Silberstein SD, Olesen J, Bousser MG, Diener HC, Dodick D, First M, et al. The International Classification of Headache Disorders, 2nd Edition (ICHD-II)—revision of criteria for 8.2 Medication-overuse headache. Cephalalgia. 2005;25(6):460–5.
42. Suess O, Stendel R, Baur S, Schilling A, Brock M. Intracranial haemorrhage following lumbar myelography: case report and review of the literature. Neuroradiology. 2000;42(3):211–4.
43. Vaughan DJ, Stirrup CA, Robinson PN. Cranial subdural haematoma associated with dural puncture in labour. Br J Anaesth. 2000;84(4):518–20.
44. Verdu MT, Martínez-Lage JF, Alonso B, Sánchez-Ortega JL, Garcia-Candel A. Non-surgical management of intracranial subdural hematoma complicating spinal anesthesia. Neurocirugia (Astur). 2007;18(1):40–3.
45. Vien C, Marovic P, Ingram B. Epidural anesthesia complicated by subdural hygromas and a subdural hematoma. Case Rep Anesthesiol. 2016;2016:5789504.
46. Wu CL, Rowlingson AJ, Cohen SR, Michaels RK, Courpas GE, Joe EM, et al. Gender and post-dural puncture headache. Anesthesiology. 2006;105(3):613–8.
47. Yamashima T, Friede RL. Why do bridging veins rupture into the virtual subdural space? J Neurol Neurosurg Psychiatry. 1984;47(2):121–7.

48. Zeidan A, Baraka A. Is bilateral cerebral subdural hematoma more frequent after epidural anesthesia than spinal anesthesia? Anesthesiology. 2006;105(6):1277–8; author reply 1278.
49. Zeidan A, Chaaban M, Farhat O, Baraka A. Cerebral rebleeding by spinal anesthesia in a patient with undiagnosed chronic subdural hematoma. Anesthesiology. 2006;104(3):613–4.
50. Zeidan A, Farhat O, Maaliki H, Baraka A. Does postdural puncture headache left untreated lead to subdural hematoma? Case report and review of the literature. Int J Obstet Anesth. 2006;15(1):50–8.
51. Zhang J, Jin D, Pan KH. Epidural blood patch for spontaneous intracranial hypotension with chronic subdural haematoma: a case report and literature review. J Int Med Res. 2016;44(4):976–81.

Chapter 19
Intracranial Hypotension

Justin Oh, Timothy Beutler, and Satish Krishnamurthy

19.1 Introduction

Intracranial hypotension (IH) is a rare cause of chronic subdural hematomas (CSDHs). The most common clinical presentation is headaches that often have a positional component and worsen when upright. According to the International Classification of Headache Disorders (ICHD-3), the diagnosis of IH requires a temporal relation of headaches to low cerebrospinal fluid (CSF) pressures [16]. Patients should be evaluated for low CSF pressures as well as for evidence of spinal fluid leaks on imaging.

There are several etiologies associated with IH, including post-traumatic, iatrogenic, and spontaneous. Post-traumatic, degenerative, and iatrogenic causes often have an identifiable cause of the spinal fluid leak, while cases of spontaneous IH may require more diagnostic workup. Spontaneous IH is rare and described most often in small retrospective reviews and literature reviews. Best estimates place the incidence of spontaneous IH at 5 per 100,000 per year [40].

Regardless of the etiology, diagnosis is difficult because the most common presenting symptom of IH is headaches. Both clinically and radiographically there are several other pathologies that present similarly and can confound the diagnosis. The focus of this chapter is IH presenting as CSDHs or hygromas. IH is an important etiology on the differential for CSDHs because they are managed differently from other subdural collections. While traditionally, CSDHs are managed with surgical evacuation, if IH is present surgery can result in worsened symptoms.

In this chapter we will review the presenting symptoms, clinical findings, radiology findings, and management of subdural hematomas (SDHs)/collections in the setting of IH.

J. Oh (✉) · T. Beutler · S. Krishnamurthy
Department of Neurosurgery, SUNY Upstate Medical University, Syracuse, NY, USA
e-mail: ohj@upstate.edu; beutlert@upstate.edu; krishnsa@upstate.edu

M. Turgut et al. (eds.), *Subdural Hematoma*,
https://doi.org/10.1007/978-3-030-79371-5_19

19.2 Pathogenesis

While IH can be spontaneous in nature, many cases described in the literature are secondary to invasive procedures. Some of the common iatrogenic causes include lumbar punctures, durotomies during spine surgery, and intradural spinal and cranial surgery [11, 22, 23, 53]. Any surgery or procedure where the dura is opened or breached can potentially result in IH if a spinal fluid leak persists. Likewise, traumatic etiologies of IH are secondary to dural injury. Some cases of traumatic IH have been linked to innocuous trauma [39]. There have also been case reports of degenerative spinal pathology that has resulted in dural defects leading to IH [6, 46, 49].

On the other hand, spontaneous cases of IH are thought to be secondary to an underlying weakness in the dura that results in a spinal fluid leak. Spontaneous cases of IH have been associated with connective tissue disorders but they are not linked directly to a specific disease process. Spontaneous etiologies have also been associated with spinal meningeal diverticula. These are outpouchings of the dura at the nerve root sheath which are thought to be susceptible to rupture and injury. However, interestingly, a recent retrospective series showed there was no difference in the presence and number of diverticula seen in patients with IH compared to those without it [20].

Regardless of the etiology, the mechanism through which low intracranial pressure develops is through a spinal fluid leak. One consequence of IH is the development of subdural fluid collections or hematomas. The data regarding the prevalence of subdural collections in the setting of IH is limited to retrospective reviews and ranges from 19.8 to 50% [5, 10, 22, 39, 45, 50].

The mechanism through which subdural collections or hematomas develop in the setting of IH is not well studied. One hypothesis is that there is a relative loss of pressure and buoyancy in the intracranial space that causes stretching of bridging veins making them susceptible to shear forces [22]. Another theory is that IH causes the development of thin-walled and fragile vessels within the dura that are prone to rupture. A small sample of six meningeal biopsies of diffusely enhancing dura showed small thin vessels on the subdural side of the dura in a loose amorphous fibroblastic matrix [22, 32]. CSDHs have also been shown to be encapsulated and divided by membranes in which there is neovasculature that has been associated with re-bleeding and expansion [17, 18, 51].

19.3 Clinical Presentation

The most common presentation of IH is headaches. Sometimes the headaches can have a positional component and worsen when patients are upright. However, when patients develop subdural collections from IH, there are a variety of additional

Table 19.1 Symptoms of intracranial hypotension

Headaches (postural or non-postural)
Neck stiffness
Dizziness or vertigo
Focal weakness or paresthesia
Visual deficits (such as diplopia)
Hearing disturbances (such as tinnitus)
Depressed level of consciousness

symptoms that can develop (Table 19.1). These symptoms range from mild focal neurologic deficits to severe alterations in mental status. Additional symptoms that patients may present with include but are not limited neck stiffness, dizziness, vertigo, focal neurological deficits such as weakness or paresthesia, visual field deficits, diplopia, hearing disturbance, tinnitus, and depressed level of consciousness [25, 41, 45]. In very rare cases, IH may mimic neurodegenerative disease such as dementia, Parkinsonism, and memory deficits [3].

The presenting symptoms are often nonspecific for IH. Therefore, a thorough clinical history can be very helpful in raising clinical suspicion for the diagnosis. Some clinical histories that have been associated with spontaneous IH include weight lifting, straining, violent sneezing or coughing, increased intra-abdominal pressure, and chiropractic manipulation [37, 38].There are reports in the literature that attribute up to 50% of patients presenting with SDHs due to IH to prior lumbar puncture [22]. There are also a number of reports of IH developing after spine or posterior fossa surgery [23, 49, 53].

A recent retrospective study showed that patients that presented with SDHs due to IH tended to have fewer underlying medical comorbidities, additional radiological signs of spontaneous IH such as meningeal enhancement, and had smaller volume of subdural hemorrhage compared to SDHs secondary to other pathologies [19]. Age is a demographic factor that has been studied as a risk factor for SDHs but studies conflict whether or not younger or older patients are at more risk for SDHs due to IH [19, 50].

One rare presentation of IH described in the literature is spontaneous cerebral venous thrombosis. Although venous sinus thrombosis itself is rare, there are several case reports in the literature that attribute the etiology to IH [35, 52, 54]. Treating venous sinus thrombosis secondary to IH can become challenging when CSDHs are present. The pathophysiology is not well understood, but one theory is that decreased intracranial pressure increases cerebral blood volume and leads to stasis in the venous system [52]. Standard venous sinus thrombosis treatment requires systemic anticoagulation; however, in the setting of IH and subdural hemorrhage, it may place patients at increased risk for complications. The successful treatment of cerebral venous thrombosis in the setting of IH requires identifying and treating the underlying cause of the IH [54].

19.4 Radiographic Imaging

Imaging plays an important role first in diagnosing IH and also identifying the cause. Because the clinical history can have an insidious onset, cranial imaging often plays an important role in establishing the diagnosis. If the clinical history does not reveal an obvious etiology for IH, then additional imaging of the spine may be needed in order to establish a diagnosis.

19.4.1 Cranial Imaging

Computed tomography (CT) of the head is often the first imaging completed in patients presenting with neurological symptoms or deficits. In IH, CT scans are often negative for any pathology, however can reveal subdural collections. Most commonly, subdural collections secondary to IH will appear hypodense (Fig. 19.1). They will often appear as bilateral collections and their appearance will be similar to chronic subdural hematomas or hygromas. They can be difficult to detect on CT imaging if the collections are small or appear isodense to the brain. Sometimes, the collections will appear subacute and have a mixed density, loculated appearance.

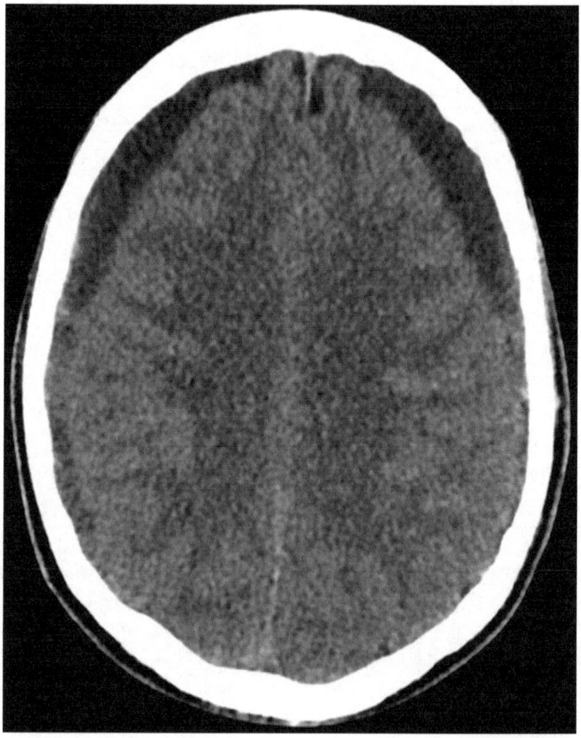

Fig. 19.1 Axial CT head of bilateral chronic subdural hematomas secondary to intracranial hypotension

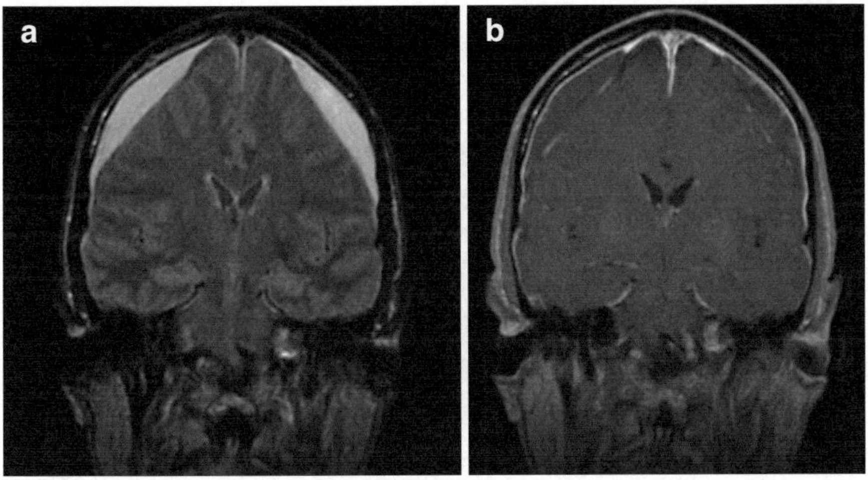

Fig. 19.2 Coronal MRI brain findings for intracranial hypotension. (**a**) FLAIR imaging revealing bilateral chronic subdural hematomas with compression of the frontal lobes. (**b**) T1 contrast weighted imaging with diffuse dural enhancement

CT imaging can also sometimes detect brain descent. This can be visualized by the appearance of cerebellar tonsillar crowding around the foramen magnum, obscured cisternal spaces, or ventral brainstem crowding. These findings can be misdiagnosed as a Chiari malformation.

Magnetic resonance imaging (MRI) of the brain in the setting of IH often reveals classic and reproducible findings. T1 contrasted sequences may reveal diffuse dural or pachymeningeal enhancement (Fig. 19.2). This finding can be considered pathognomonic. In some retrospective studies this finding was observed in 95% of the patients that were diagnosed with IH [1, 25, 31, 50]. The reason for which dural contrast enhancement occurs is not well understood but it is a finding that can also be seen in patients after shunting procedures [7].

A proportion of patients with IH may also have small subdural collections or hematomas that can be visualized on MRI of the brain that may not be apparent on CT imaging. These collections are often bilateral in nature but can present as unilateral subdural collections or hematomas [15, 34]. These collections can be subdural hygromas or CSF collections or can be hemorrhage that is chronic in nature. In a cohort of 40 patients, Schievenk et al. describes that 50% of patients had abnormal subdural collections and of those patients 60% had subdural hygromas while 40% had SDHs [41]. The underlying mechanism and explanation of why some patients will develop hematomas while others hygromas is not well understood.

MRI is more sensitive than CT imaging for detecting features of IH and a variety of additional imaging findings have been described (Fig. 19.3). Classically there is pontine flattening that can be quantified as a pontomesencephalic angle less than 50° or as a mammillopontine distance less than 5.5 mm. Crowding the basal cisterns and be present as well as an interpeduncular angle at the level of the mammillary

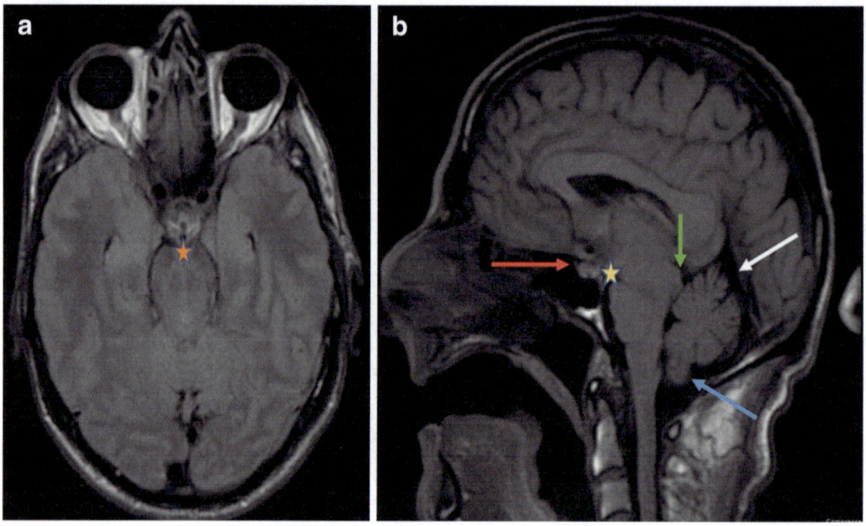

Fig. 19.3 Additional MRI findings associated with intracranial hypotension. (**a**) T1 axial imaging at the level of the mammillary bodies can show an interpeduncular angle <40° (orange star). (**b**) Venous engorgement and congestion of the straight sinus (white arrow), tectum displaced below the level of the tentorium (green arrow), cerebellar tonsillar descent (blue arrow), enlargement of the pituitary gland (red arrow), continue flattening with a pontomesencephalic angle <50° and mammillopontine distance less than 5.5 mm (yellow star)

bodies less than 40°. Both cerebellar tonsilar descent and descent of the tectum below the level of the tentorium are also suggestive of IH.

IH is a state of low pressures within the calvarium due to CSF hypovolemia and it is thought that a hyperemic compensatory mechanism occurs that results in venous engorgement [10]. Kim et al. describes that congestion and engorgement of both the straight dural sinus and the transverse dural sinus can be useful in the detection of IH [19]. Also venous sinus thrombosis has been associated as a complication of IH and may be visualized in these cases [35, 36, 54]. Finally, the pituitary gland may be conspicuously hyperemic or contrast enhancing on a post contrast sequence on MRI adding to the theory that these findings are related to a hyperemic state within the brain in the setting of low pressures [11, 25, 31].

19.4.2 Spinal Imaging

Once the diagnosis of IH has been established, additional spinal imaging may be needed if there is not a clear etiology from the patient's history. CSF leaks can have an insidious presentation. They may present as intermittent, low flow, or high flow leaks and the choice of imaging modality can affect the visualization and localization of these leaks [21]. CT myelogram, radionuclide cisternogram, digital subtraction myelography, and magnetic resonance imaging with or without myelography are all modalities that have been used in order to detect the source of CSF leak. All of these imaging modalities involve the injection of intrathecal contrast with the exception of the T2-weighted fat saturation MRI. CSF leaks can have a variety of appearances such as epidural collections, small collections around nerve roots, or paraspinal collections.

CT myelography has been regarded as the traditional study for identifying CSF leaks because of its widespread availability and familiarity [21]. This involves the injection of iodinated contrast into the thecal sac through a lumbar puncture and subsequent or concurrent CT imaging of the spine. CSF leak rates can be variable. High flow leaks can show widespread extravasation of contrast from the thecal sac and localizing the egress point can be difficult. In these cases, dynamic CT myelography can be used. Using this technique serial CT scans of the spine are obtained both during and after injection of contrast allowing the visualization of early extravasation of contrast [27].

Spinal MRI has been more recently described in the literature as a comparable method to CT myelography for identifying spinal CSF leaks. Because CSF as well as fat is hyperintense on T2-weighted imaging, fat suppressed T2-weighted imaging can be used to identify CSF leaks. Spinal MRI has been useful in identifying high flow leaks which appear as an abnormal fluid (T2 hyperintense) epidural collection or collection adjacent to a nerve root [44]. There is some evidence to support that MRI is comparable to CT myelography. Starling et al. reported that 91.7% of patients with confirmed CSF leak on CT myelogram were also identified to have a CSF leak on spinal MRI [44]. Wang et al. also showed a high concordance rate between the two modalities [47]. MR myelography using intrathecal gadolinium has also been described; however, intrathecal injection of gadolinium is considered off-label use by the FDA [4].

Finally, both radionuclide cisternogram and digital subtraction myelography are less commonly used modalities for identifying CSF leaks. Digital subtraction myelography may be useful in the real-time detection, and localization of CSF leaks however is time and resource intensive. Radionuclide cisternogram seems to have fallen out of favor as an imaging modality for detecting spinal CSF leaks due to CT and MR imaging modalities having higher imaging resolution [21].

While spinal imaging can often identify a discrete leak that can be targeted for treatment. Sometimes there is no overt leak that can be identified. One pathology that has been found in association with spontaneous IH is perineural cysts (Fig. 19.4). These are spinal meningeal diverticula that occur at the nerve root sheath. They are thought to be a weakened portion of the dura that can be susceptible to elevated intracranial pressure or shear injury.

19.5 Treatment

The primary treatment for IH is to repair an identifiable CSF leak. Because IH is a rare entity and subdural collections only occur in a subset of patients, the literature regarding treatment algorithms is sparse. However, there have been a number of retrospective studies addressing treatment strategies and their effectiveness.

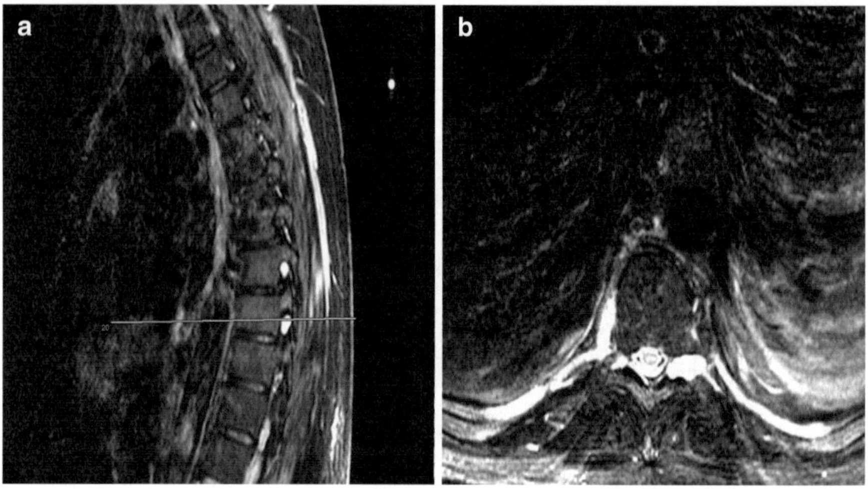

Fig. 19.4 T2-weighted imaging of the spine. Sagittal (**a**) and axial (**b**) imaging showing a perineural cyst

19.5.1 Conservative Management

Conservative management for IH involves bed rest and adequate hydration. The head of the bed is often kept flat. Effort is made to avoid straining, and analgesics may be employed for symptom control. Takahashi et al. describe that in a retrospective analysis of 55 patients with subdural hematomas in the setting of IH, 23.6% of patients were successfully treated via conservative measures [45].

19.5.2 Epidural Blood Patch

Epidural blood patches are an effective treatment modality for IH. Epidural blood patches can be performed under fluoroscopic guidance to inject autologous blood into the epidural space. These procedures can be targeted to a specific level if a discrete leak or abnormality is discovered on imaging. Numerous retrospective studies have shown that epidural blood patches are not only effective in relieving symptoms of IH but also can result in radiographic improvement on follow-up imaging. The literature describes the success rate of epidural blood patches to be anywhere between 46.8 and 100% and including patients that required multiple or repeat blood patch procedures [13, 14, 26, 30].

However, not all patients diagnosed with IH may be diagnosed with a targetable CSF leak [41, 42, 45]. Epidural blood patches can be performed as a "targeted" or "blind" procedure. Targeted epidural blood patches are performed precisely at the identified level of a CSF leak while blind epidural blood patches are performed at the level of the lumbar spine [2, 28]. The efficacy of targeted versus blind epidural blood patches has not been well studied but reported efficacy in both groups appears promising. He et al. demonstrated that 87.9% of patients had symptomatic relief after the first targeted epidural blood patch one or two vertebral levels below the identified leak [14]. Levi et al. showed also that 89.1% of patients had symptomatic relief after blind lumbar epidural blood patches and included patients who underwent repeat procedures [24].

19.5.3 Fibrin Glue

Fibrin glue epidural injections have also been described in the literature as an alternative or adjunct to epidural blood patches. There have been reports described of fibrin glue mixed with autologous blood, fibrin glue alone, or fibrin glue use after epidural blood patch failure for the treatment of IH [8, 29, 43]. However, the literature on its use is sparse and further investigation is needed to evaluate its efficacy and safety.

19.5.4 Open Surgical Repair

Conservative measures and epidural patches can be effective treatment options; however, refractory cases IH may require an open surgical approach if there is an identifiable source of CSF leak. There are very few cases reported in the literature for open surgical repairs of CSF leaks for IH [12, 15, 46, 49]. The specific method of repair varies depending on the location of the leak, but even in the case reports, open surgical methods are reserved as a therapeutic modality in patients that fail multiple epidural blood patches or for those who present with acute neurological decline. Also, the majority of these cases involve ventral degenerative pathologies of the spine such as disc osteophyte complexes. Both anterior and posterior approaches to the spine have been described. Some interventions even required a partial corpectomy in order to reach the dural defect for primary or secondary repair.

19.5.5 Subdural Evacuation

CSDHs and collections have been shown to radiographically improve after the underlying cause of IH has been treated. These collections have been shown to resolve without surgical evacuation [9]. However, some CSDHs caused by IH can enlarge to a significant enough size to cause midline shift, altered level of consciousness, and herniation. In these cases, where patients present in neurologic extremis, subdural evacuation may be indicated. However, subdural evacuation without addressing the underlying etiology may provide little benefit and can result in worsened outcomes.

Schievenk et al. and Ferrante et al. describe patients that underwent subdural evacuations alone, some due to delayed diagnoses, and reported that these patients had no improvement in symptoms or had significant neurological decline [9, 15, 41]. Fortunately, the majority of patients in these studies did have neurological recovery after the underlying IH was addressed.

There is no consensus or guidelines on how to manage large symptomatic CSDHs in the setting of IH. Takahashi et al. and Yoon et al. describe their clinical experience and recommend utilizing a combination of blind or targeted epidural blood patches with evacuation of the SDH in sequence [45, 52]. Whether or not the SDH should be evacuated before or after the underlying IH is addressed has not been studied. Extreme cases of IH may present with downward herniation syndrome. When downward herniation is suspected in the setting of IH, basic steps should be taken to reverse the pathology. The patient should be positioned with the head down in trendelenberg position. Intravascular volume should be expanded. Two case reports also describe that infusion of saline into the thecal sac can be a useful salvage maneuver in patients that show signs of downward herniation [33, 48].Then the underlying etiology should be addressed.

19.6 Conclusion

CSDHs are commonly encountered in the field of neurosurgery. While CSDHs caused by IH is a rare entity, recognizing the diagnosis is important in order to provide patients with the appropriate treatment. Because IH is rare, there are often delays in diagnosis. The clinical history is important in raising suspicion for IH. The diagnosis often requires multimodal cranial and spinal imaging. The vast majority of subdural collections will resolve by addressing the underlying cause of IH. Except for patients presenting in neurologic extremis with rapidly declining exams, caution should be given towards surgical evacuation until the source of the CSF leak has been identified and treated. Surgical intervention on SDHs secondary to IH can result in worsened neurologic symptoms.

References

1. Barahona ML, Mora-Encinas JP, Gonzalez-Montano VM, Pozo-Zamorano T, Fernandez-Gil MA. [Intracranial hypotension syndrome: a review of the magnetic resonance findings]. Rev Neurol. 2011;52:676–80.
2. Berroir S, Loisel B, Ducros A, Boukobza M, Tzourio C, Valade D, et al. Early epidural blood patch in spontaneous intracranial hypotension. Neurology. 2004;63:1950–1.
3. Capizzano AA, Lai L, Kim J, Rizzo M, Gray L, Smoot MK, et al. Atypical presentations of intracranial hypotension: comparison with classic spontaneous intracranial hypotension. Am J Neuroradiol. 2016;37:1256–61.

4. Chazen JL, Talbott JF, Lantos JE, Dillon WP. MR myelography for identification of spinal CSF leak in spontaneous intracranial hypotension. Am J Neuroradiol. 2014;35:2007–12.
5. Chen YC, Wang YF, Li JY, Chen SP, Lirng JF, Hseu SS, et al. Treatment and prognosis of subdural hematoma in patients with spontaneous intracranial hypotension. Cephalalgia. 2016;36:225–31.
6. Cornips E, Grouls M, Bekelaar K. Transdural thoracic disk herniation with longitudinal slitlike dural defect causing intracranial hypotension: report of 2 cases. World Neurosurg. 2020;140:e311–9.
7. Gupta M, Patidar Y, Khwaja GA, Chowdhury D, Batra A, Dasgupta A. Intracranial hypotension due to shunt overdrainage presenting as reversible dorsal midbrain syndrome. Neurology Asia. 2014;19(1):107–110.
8. Elwood J, Dewan M, Smith J, Mokri B, Mauck W, Eldrige J. Efficacy of epidural blood patch with fibrin glue additive in refractory headache due to intracranial hypotension: preliminary report. Springerplus. 2016;5:317.
9. Ferrante E, Rubino F, Beretta F, Regna-Gladin C, Ferrante MM. Treatment and outcome of subdural hematoma in patients with spontaneous intracranial hypotension: a report of 35 cases. Acta Neurol Belg. 2018;118:61–70.
10. Ferrante E, Savino A, Sances G, Nappi G. Spontaneous intracranial hypotension syndrome: report of twelve cases. Headache. 2004;44:615–22.
11. Gilmour GS, Scott J, Couillard P. Leaking the diagnosis: a case of convulsive status epilepticus due to intracranial hypotension. Neurocrit Care. 2019;31:562–6.
12. Hasiloglu ZI, Abuzayed B, Imal AE, Cagil E, Albayram S. Spontaneous intracranial hypotension due to intradural thoracic osteophyte with superimposed disc herniation: report of two cases. Eur Spine J. 2012;21(Suppl 4):383.
13. Hazama A, Loree J, Braley A, Awawdeh F, Swarnkar A, Chin L, et al. Spontaneous Intracranial Hypotension and the durability of Epidural Blood Patch. World Neurosurg. 2019;66(1):90. https://doi.org/10.1093/neuros/nyz310_353.
14. He FF, Li L, Liu MJ, Zhong TD, Zhang QW, Fang XM. Targeted epidural blood patch treatment for refractory spontaneous intracranial hypotension in China. J Neurol Surg B Skull Base. 2018;79:217–23. Thieme Medical Publishers, Inc.
15. Inamasu J, Moriya S, Shibata J, Kumai T, Hirose Y. Spontaneous intracranial hypotension manifesting as a unilateral subdural hematoma with a marked midline shift. Case Rep Neurol. 2015;7:71–7.
16. International Classification of Headache Disorders. 3rd ed. Headache attributed to non-vascular intracranial disorder. 2019. https://ichd-3.org/7-headache-attributed-to-non-vascular-intracranial-disorder/7-2-headache-attributed-to-low-cerebrospinal-fluid-pressure/7-2-3-headache-attributed-to-spontaneous-intracranial-hypotension/. Accessed 14 Jan 2021.
17. Ito H, Komai T, Yamamoto S. Fibrinolytic enzyme in the lining walls of chronic subdural hematoma. J Neurosurg. 1978;48:197–200.
18. Killeffer JA, Killeffer FA, Schochet SS. The outer neomembrane of chronic subdural hematoma. Neurosurg Clin N Am. 2000;11:407–12.
19. Kim JH, Roh H, Yoon WK, Kwon TH, Chong K, Hwang SY, et al. Clinical features of patients with spontaneous intracranial hypotension complicated with bilateral subdural fluid collections. Headache. 2019;59:775–86.
20. Kranz PG, Stinnett SS, Huang KT, Gray L. Spinal meningeal diverticula in spontaneous intracranial hypotension: analysis of prevalence and myelographic appearance. Am J Neuroradiol. 2013;34:1284–9.
21. Kranz PG, Luetmer PH, Diehn FE, Amrhein TJ, Tanpitukpongse TP, Gray L. Myelographic techniques for the detection of spinal CSF leaks in spontaneous intracranial hypotension. Am J Roentgenol. 2016;206:8–19.
22. Lai TH, Fuh JL, Lirng JF, Tsai PH, Wang SJ. Subdural haematoma in patients with spontaneous intracranial hypotension. Cephalalgia. 2007;27:133–8.

23. Lau D, Lin J, Park P. Cranial nerve III palsy resulting from intracranial hypotension caused by cerebrospinal fluid leak after paraspinal tumor resection: etiology and treatment options. Spine J. 2011;11:e10–3.
24. Levi V, Di Laurenzio NE, Franzini A, Tramacere I, Erbetta A, Chiapparini L, et al. Lumbar epidural blood patch: effectiveness on orthostatic headache and MRI predictive factors in 101 consecutive patients affected by spontaneous intracranial hypotension. J Neurosurg. 2020;132:809–17.
25. Li C, Raza HK, Chansysouphanthong T, Zu J, Cui G. A clinical analysis on 40 cases of spontaneous intracranial hypotension syndrome. Somatosens Mot Res. 2019;36:24–30.
26. Loya JJ, Mindea SA, Yu H, Venkatasubramanian C, Chang SD, Burns TC. Intracranial hypotension producing reversible coma: a systematic review, including three new cases. A review. J Neurosurg. 2012;117:615–28.
27. Luetmer PH, Schwartz KM, Eckel LJ, Hunt CH, Carter RE, Diehn FE. When should i do dynamic CT myelography? Predicting fast spinal CSF leaks in patients with spontaneous intracranial hypotension. Am J Neuroradiol. 2012;33:690–4.
28. Madsen SA, Fomsgaard JS, Jensen R. Epidural blood patch for refractory low CSF pressure headache: a pilot study. J Headache Pain. 2011;12:453–7.
29. Mammis A, Agarwal N, Mogilner AY. Alternative treatment of intracranial hypotension presenting as postdural puncture headaches using epidural fibrin glue patches: two case reports. Int J Neurosci. 2014;124:863–6.
30. Martin R, Louy C, Babu V, Jiang Y, Far A, Schievink W. A two-level large-volume epidural blood patch protocol for spontaneous intracranial hypotension: retrospective analysis of risk and benefit. Reg Anesth Pain Med. 2020;45:32–7.
31. Michali-Stolarska M, Bladowska J, Stolarski M, Sąsiadek MJ. Diagnostic imaging and clinical features of intracranial hypotension—review of literature. Pol J Radiol. 2017;82:842–9.
32. Mokri B, Parisi JE, Scheithauer BW, Piepgras DG, Miller GM. Meningeal biopsy in intracranial hypotension: meningeal enhancement on MRI. Neurology. 1995;45:1801–7.
33. Muram S, Yavin D, DuPlessis S. Intrathecal saline infusion as an effective temporizing measure in the management of spontaneous intracranial hypotension. World Neurosurg. 2019;125:37–41.
34. Osada Y, Shibahara I, Nakagawa A, Sakata H, Niizuma K, Saito R, et al. Unilateral chronic subdural hematoma due to spontaneous intracranial hypotension: a report of four cases. Br J Neurosurg. 2020;34:632–7.
35. Paris D, Rousset D, Bonneville F, Fabre N, Faguer S, Huguet-Rigal F, et al. Cerebral venous thrombosis and subdural collection in a comatose patient: do not forget intracranial hypotension. A case report. Headache. 2020;60:2583–8.
36. Perry A, Graffeo CS, Brinjikji W, Copeland WR, Rabinstein AA, Link MJ. Spontaneous occult intracranial hypotension precipitating life-threatening cerebral venous thrombosis: case report. J Neurosurg Spine. 2018;28:669–78.
37. Pettyjohn EW, Donlan RM, Breck J, Clugston JR. Intracranial hypotension in the setting of post-concussion headache: a case series. Cureus. 2020;12:e10526.
38. Sarrafzadeh AS, Hopf SA, Gautschi OP, Narata AP, Schaller K. Intracranial hypotension after trauma. Springerplus. 2014;3:1–7.
39. Schievink WI. Spontaneous spinal cerebrospinal fluid leaks and intracranial hypotension. J Am Med Assoc. 2006;295:2286–96.
40. Schievink WI, Maya MM, Moser F, Tourje J, Torbati S. Frequency of spontaneous intracranial hypotension in the emergency department. J Headache Pain. 2007;8:325–8.
41. Schievink WI, Meyer FB, Atkinson JLD, Mokri B. Spontaneous spinal cerebrospinal fluid leaks and intracranial hypotension. J Neurosurg. 1996;84:598–605.
42. Schievink WI, Morreale VM, Atkinson JLD, Meyer FB, Piepgras DG, Ebersold MJ. Surgical treatment of spontaneous spinal cerebrospinal fluid leaks. J Neurosurg. 1998;88:243–6.
43. Schievink WI, Maya MM, Moser FM. Treatment of spontaneous intracranial hypotension with percutaneous placement of a fibrin sealant. Report of four cases. J Neurosurg. 2004;100:1098–100.

44. Starling A, Hernandez F, Hoxworth JM, Trentman T, Halker R, Vargas BB, et al. Sensitivity of MRI of the spine compared with CT myelography in orthostatic headache with CSF leak. Neurology. 2013;81:1789–92.
45. Takahashi K, Mima T, Akiba Y. Chronic subdural hematoma associated with spontaneous intracranial hypotension: therapeutic strategies and outcomes of 55 cases. Neurol Med Chir (Tokyo). 2016;56:69–76.
46. Veeravagu A, Gupta G, Jiang B, Berta SC, Mindea SA, Chang SD. Spontaneous intracranial hypotension secondary to anterior thoracic osteophyte: resolution after primary dural repair via posterior approach. Int J Surg Case Rep. 2013;4:26–9.
47. Wang YF, Lirng JF, Fuh JL, Hseu SS, Wang SJ. Heavily T2-weighted MR myelography vs CT myelography in spontaneous intracranial hypotension. Neurology. 2009;73:1892–8.
48. Watanabe A, Takai H, Ogino S, Ohki T, Ohki I. Intracranial subdural hematoma after resection of a thoracic spinal cord tumor. J Spinal Disord Tech. 2002;15:533–6.
49. Witiw CD, Fallah A, Muller PJ, Ginsberg HJ. Surgical treatment of spontaneous intracranial hypotension secondary to degenerative cervical spine pathology: a case report and literature review. Eur Spine J. 2012;21(Suppl 4):S422–7.
50. Xia P, Hu X-Y, Wang J, Hu B-B, Xu Q-L, Zhou Z-J, et al. Risk factors for subdural haematoma in patients with spontaneous intracranial hypotension. PLoS One. 2015;10:e0123616.
51. Yamashima T, Yamamoto S. How do vessels proliferate in the capsule of a chronic subdural hematoma? Neurosurgery. 1984;15:672–8.
52. Yoon KW, Cho MK, Kim YJ, Lee SK. Sinus thrombosis in a patient with intracranial hypotension: a suggested hypothesis of venous stasis. A case report. Interv Neuroradiol. 2011;17:248–51.
53. Zakaria AF, Tsuji M. Intracranial subdural hematoma after lumbar spine surgery: a case report. Malays Orthop J. 2019;13:85–7.
54. Zhang D, Wang J, Zhang Q, He F, Hu X. Cerebral venous thrombosis in spontaneous intracranial hypotension: a report on 4 cases and a review of the literature. Headache. 2018;58:1244–55.

Chapter 20
Chronic Subdural Hematoma Following Electroconvulsive Therapy: A Rare but Serious Complication

Anil Kalyoncu, Ali Saffet Gonul, and Mehmet Turgut

20.1 Introduction

Electroconvulsive therapy (ECT) is a widely used treatment that is based on electrical conduction through the skull to induce a therapeutic seizure. ECT is a common choice for treating various psychiatric conditions, including depression, mania, catatonia, and schizophrenia. ECT is generally considered for patients who have not responded to standard medical therapy or patients with severe symptoms such as suicidality and life-treating functional impairments. The Food and Drug Administration (FDA) regulates the application of ECT with approximately one million patients worldwide and 100,000 patients in the US receiving ECT every year [2, 20]. The administration technique changes with the method of electrode placement. Electrode placement could be unilateral or bilateral. Unilateral ECT is most often administered to the right side of the brain, which is usually the non-dominant hemisphere. Bilateral electrode placements are bifrontal or bitemporal, where they are administered to the anterior left and right temporal lobes [22].

A. Kalyoncu (✉)
Department of Psychiatry, Ege University Faculty of Medicine, Izmir, Turkey

A. S. Gonul
Department of Psychiatry, Ege University Faculty of Medicine, Izmir, Turkey

Department of Psychiatry and Behavioral Sciences, Mercer University School of Medicine, Macon, GA, USA
e-mail: ali.saffet.gonul@ege.edu.tr

M. Turgut
Department of Neurosurgery, Aydın Adnan Menderes University Faculty of Medicine, Efeler, Aydın, Turkey

Department of Histology and Embryology, Aydın Adnan Menderes University Health Sciences Institute, Efeler, Aydın, Turkey

M. Turgut et al. (eds.), *Subdural Hematoma*,
https://doi.org/10.1007/978-3-030-79371-5_20

Although the exact mechanism of action is not yet well defined, the neurophysiological effects of ECT include an increase in the cerebral blood flow and the blood-brain barrier permeability during seizure activity. In addition to cerebral blood flow changes, ECT increases hippocampal volume and enhances brain-derived neurotrophic factor levels that play a role in the treatment [17, 18, 23].

20.2 Side Effects of ECT

Today it is well known that ECT is considered a safe treatment option for patients, and there is no absolute contraindication for its use [1]. The mortality rate is 2.4 per 100,000 treatments on the first day of ECT but increases to 18 per 100,000 within 14 days [11]. From a global perspective, the risk of mortality is almost the same as the risk of using short-acting barbiturate anesthetics [13]. There are various side effects of ECT recorded in the literature. ECT complications and side effects can be divided into two groups based on their sources: side effects due to seizures and side effects due to general anesthesia [3]. Common side effects of ECT include headache, dry mouth, nausea, confusion, and myalgia. These side effects are usually of low severity and transient in nature. Other side effects develop due to the use of general anesthesia, such as prolonged apnea, malignant hyperthermia, and hyperkalemia. Cardiac side effects may be associated with ECT. High blood pressure, myocardial infarction, and cardiomyopathy can be seen due to ECT [9]. Neurological complications of ECT vary from common side effects such as memory loss and cognitive impairment to rare side effects as cerebrovascular events [3].

20.3 ECT and Chronic Subdural Hematoma

Chronic subdural hematoma (CSDH) is accepted as a major neurological side effect of ECT. This complication is very rare and, to the best of our knowledge, there are only five cases of CSDH following ECT in the literature (Table 20.1) [6, 10, 13, 21, 27]. The ages of patients reported in the literature are between 38 and 76 years. Out of these cases, two patients had a diagnosis of bipolar disorder, and three patients had treatment-resistant depression. Two patients abstained from anticoagulant or antiplatelet treatment, while there was no information provided for the other patients. In contrast, acquired information suggests that warfarin treatment is safe in ECT with respect to intracerebral hemorrhage [8, 16]. Thus, there is no clear evidence that anticoagulant treatment can cause CSDH in ECT patients. The number of ECT sessions varied from 1 to 12 before subdural hematoma (SDH) was diagnosed. In two cases, pre-ECT neuroimaging was not available; therefore, the bleeding could have resulted from a new lesion that developed during the ECT, or the ECT could have caused bleeding from preexisting lesions. One patient was diagnosed with a left-sided CSDH before the ECT. This patient received unilateral

Table 20.1 Summary of five cases with chronic subdural hematoma following electroconvulsive therapy reported in the English literature to date

Author(s), year/ref.#	Sex	Age	Psychiatric diagnosis	Antico-agulant/ antiplatelet drug	ECT technique	Initial dose of ECT	Number of ECT sessions	Neuro-imaging before	Neurologic symptoms/ GCS	Neuroimaging after ECT	Neuro-imaging: brain shift	Treatment of SDH	Outcome
Wijeratne et al., 1999 [27]	Male	76	Persistent depression	NS	R unilateral	378mC	6	CSDH, L	Reduced consciousness	CSDH (parietal), L	No	Medical	Died within 28 days
Awasthy et al., 2005 [6]	Male	63	Bipolar disorder	NS	NS	NS	10	NS	E3V3M6	CSDH (frontoparietal), L	Yes	Surgery: Burr-hole	Recovered completely
Saha et al., 2012 [21]	Female	38	Bipolar disorder	NS	NS	NS	12	NS	R hemiparesis	CSDH (temporo-parietal), L	Yes	Surgery	NS
Kulkarni et al., 2012 [13]	Male	42	Persistent depression	No	Bitemporal	120mC	1	No cortical atrophy	E2V4M2	Acute SDH (frontoparietal, R; and parietal, L), bilateral	Yes	Surgery: Burr-hole	NS
Dauleac et al., 2019 [10]	Female	64	Persistent depression	No	Bitemporal	176mC	4	Cortical atrophy	E1V2M4	CSDH (frontoparietal), R	Yes	Surgery: Burr-hole	Recovered completely

Abbreviations: *R* right, *L* left, *CSDH* chronic subdural hematoma, *SDH* subdural hematoma, *GCS* Glasgow Coma Scale, *NS* not stated right-sided ECT because of the presence of the CSDH. Two patients received bitemporal ECT before they were diagnosed with SDH. All patients were symptomatic after they were diagnosed with SDH. In the elderly population, SDH tends to be asymptomatic, and as such the numbers of SDH after ECT could be much more common than are recorded in published reports [10, 26]. All but one patient were treated with surgical intervention. One patient had a 6 mm left-sided SDH without brain shift that was treated with medications only. That patient died within 28 days after ECT without any expansion of the SDH on the post-treatment CT. The other two patients recovered without neurological sequelae.

20.4 Management of SDH Following ECT

Patients with a history of cerebral atrophy and patients who undergo anticoagulation/antiplatelet treatment are included in the risk group for ECT. For this reason, SDH should be evaluated with pre-ECT brain imaging to determine whether there is a risk for these patients [10]. ECT may cause side effects that can be confused with the signs of a cerebrovascular incident, including nausea, postictal confusion, and Todd paresis [14, 24]. Patients showing signs of cerebrovascular incidents such as a persistent change in the level of consciousness, focal neurological signs, recurrent epileptic convulsions, intractable vomiting, and incontinence should undergo a neuroimaging evaluation [13]. The relationship between cerebrovascular events and ECT might be explained by a transient increase in blood pressure and blood-brain barrier permeability during the seizure that can contribute to an increased intracranial pressure (IICP) [4]. Hence, IICP can induce SDH or increase the size of an existing SDH [27]. Even though the mechanism of ECT includes intracranial pressure alteration, there are patients with CSDH treated successfully without increasing the SDH size [5, 15, 27]. Prior to ECT, hyperventilation can reduce cerebrospinal fluid (CSF) pressure and lower the intracranial pressure. Thus, hyperventilation may help to prevent the development of SDH [7, 13]. The other major factors that contribute to the side effects are the electrode placement and the dosage of ECT. The width between electrodes determines the seizure of activated area. Wider distance between electrode placement increases the size of the affected brain region. According to long-standing studies that compare unilateral and bilateral electrode placement, unilateral electrode placement is less effective with fewer side effects than bilateral electrode placement [19, 25]. Stimulus dosage is another major factor that has an impact on the side effects and efficacy. More neuronal depolarization, seizure foci, and stronger seizure generalization are induced by greater electrical dosage [22]. Wijeratne and Shome recommended dose titration with unilateral ECT administration to the contralateral side of a preexisting SDH [27]. In this way, it has been claimed that the underlying cortex of the side on ECT administration would not be affected by current flow [12]. Considering that the effectiveness of unilateral ECT is lower and requires a higher dose than bitemporal ECT, bilateral ECT could be administered in severe cases of psychiatric conditions without negative consequences [27]. The previous history of a CSDH is not an absolute contraindication for ECT; however, neurosurgical follow-up is recommended during treatment [10]. CSDH is a known and rare complication of ECT where the development is not easy to predict. However, early detection and treatment of CSDH is crucial to prevent further neurological damage.

20.5 Conclusion

ECT is a fundamental treatment option for specific psychiatric patients and has been used safely for more than 80 years. Even when considered safe, complications can occur due to ECT. SDH is one of these complications which has been reported in the literature. Although the SDH is a very rare complication of ECT, it should be kept in mind in high-risk populations especially in those patients who show clinical symptoms several days after ECT. Therefore, the pre-ECT assessment of patients is essential in order to determine whether any post-ECT complications have occurred as a result of treatment.

References

1. American Psychiatric Association. The practice of electroconvulsive therapy: recommendations for treatment, training, and privileging. Washington, DC: APA Press; 1990.
2. American Psychiatric Association. The practice of electroconvulsive therapy. Recommendations for treatment, training, and privileging: a task force report of APA. Washington, DC: American Psychiatric Association; 2002.
3. Andrade C, Arumugham SS, Thirthalli J. Adverse effects of electroconvulsive therapy. Psychiatr Clin North Am. 2016;39:513–30.
4. Andrade C, Bolwig TG. Electroconvulsive therapy, hypertensive surge, blood-brain barrier breach, and amnesia: exploring the evidence for a connection. J ECT. 2014;30:160–4.
5. Anwar N, Brakoulias V. Safety of electroconvulsivetherapy after subdural hemorrhage. Aust N Z J Psychiatry. 2010;44:294.
6. Awasthy N, Chand K. Subdural hematoma: as complication of electroconvulsive therapy. Pak J Med Sci. 2005;21:491–3.
7. Bryson EO, Kellner CH. Chronic subdural hematoma following electroconvulsive therapy. Indian J Psychol Med. 2013;35:220.
8. Bleich S, Degner D, Scheschonka A, Ruther E, Kropp S. Electroconvulsive therapy and anticoagulation [letter]. Can J Psychiatry. 2000;45:87–8.
9. Cristancho MA, Alici Y, Augoustides JG, O'Reardon JP. Uncommon but serious complications associated with electroconvulsive therapy: recognition and management for the clinician. Curr Psychiatry Rep. 2008;10:474–80.
10. Dauleac C, Vinckier F, Bourdillon P. Subdural hematoma and electroconvulsive therapy: a case report and review of the literature. Neurochirurgie. 2019;65:40–2.
11. Dennis NM, Dennis PA, Shafer A, Weiner RD, Husain MM. Electroconvulsive therapy and all-cause mortality in Texas, 1998-2013. J ECT. 2017;33:22–5.
12. Hsiao JK, Evans DL. ECT in a depressed patient after craniotomy. Am J Psychiatry. 1984;141:442–4.

13. Kulkarni RR, Melkundi S. Subdural hematoma: an adverse event of electroconvulsive therapy case report and literature review. Case Rep Psychiatry. 2012;2012:585303.
14. Liff JM, Bryson EO, Maloutas E, Garruto K, Pasculli RM, Briggs MC, Kellner CH. Transient hemiparesis (Todd's paralysis) after electroconvulsive therapy (ECT) in a patient with major depressive disorder. J ECT. 2013;29:247–8.
15. Malek-Ahmadi P, Beceiro JR, McNeil BW, Weddige RL. Electroconvulsive therapy and chronic subdural hematoma. Convuls Ther. 1990;6:38–41.
16. Mehta V, Mueller PS, Gonzalez-Arriaza HL, Pankratz VS, Rummans TA. Safety of electroconvulsive therapy in patients receiving long-term warfarin therapy. Mayo Clin Proc. 2004;79:1396–401.
17. Nordanskog P, Dahlstrand U, Larsson MR, Larsson EM, Knutsson L, Johanson A. Increase in hippocampal volume after electroconvulsive therapy in patients with depression: a volumetric magnetic resonance imaging study. J ECT. 2010;26:62–7.
18. Rocha RB, Dondossola ER, Grande AJ, Colonetti T, Ceretta LB, Passos IC, Quevedo J, da Rosa MI. Increased BDNF levels after electroconvulsive therapy in patients with major depressive disorder: a meta-analysis study. J Psychiatr Res. 2016;83:47–53.
19. Sackeim HA, Prudic J, Devanand DP, Kiersky JE, Fitzsimons L, Moody BJ, McElhiney MC, Coleman EA, Settembrino JM. Effects of stimulus intensity and electrode placement on the efficacy and cognitive effects of electroconvulsive therapy. N Engl J Med. 1993;328:839–46.
20. Sadock, Sadock VA. Kaplan & Sadock's comprehensive textbook of psychiatry. Philadelphia: Lippincott Williams & Wilkins; 2009.
21. Saha D, Bisui B, Thakurta RG, Ghoshmaulik S, Singh OP. Chronic subdural hematoma following electroconvulsive therapy. Indian J Psychol Med. 2012;34:181–3.
22. Swartz CM, Nelson AI. Rational electroconvulsive therapy electrode placement. Psychiatry (Edgmont). 2005;2:37–43.
23. Taylor S. Electroconvulsive therapy: a review of history, patient selection, technique, and medication management. South Med J. 2007;100:494–8.
24. Tzabazis A, Schmitt HJ, Ihmsen H, Schmidtlein M, Zimmermann R, Wielopolski J, Münster T. Postictal agitation after electroconvulsive therapy: incidence, severity, and propofol as a treatment option. J ECT. 2013;29:189–95.
25. UK ECT Review Group. Efficacy and safety of electroconvulsive therapy in depressive disorders: a systematic review and meta-analysis. Lancet. 2003;361:799–808.
26. Uno M, Toi H, Hirai S. Chronic subdural hematoma in elderly patients: is this disease benign? Neurol Med Chir (Tokyo). 2017;57:402–9.
27. Wijeratne C, Shome S. Electroconvulsive therapy and subdural hemorrhage. J ECT. 1999;15:275–9.

Chapter 21
Chronic Subdural Hematoma Caused by Hematological Diseases

Alican Tahta, Yaşar B. Turgut, and Gökhan Pektaş

21.1 Introduction

The overall incidence of chronic subdural hematoma (CSDH) is 5 per 100,000 in the US population [51]. This risk increases to 58 per 100,000 for people over 70 years old [50]. The incidence of CSDH will increase in the future considering that the elderly population increases day by day [15]. In previous studies, it was determined that the most common cause of CSDH is head trauma. However, the increase in the average age of the population, the increase in cancer and the use of antithrombotic agents reduce the proportion of those patients with head trauma due to CSDH [17, 33, 50, 62]. Brain atrophy is common in the elderly and increases the probability of bleeding from bridging veins placed under stretch [8]. Repeated absorption and recurrent hemorrhage within the hematoma cavity are the most accepted theories for the pathophysiology of CSDH [37]. Two burr holes and burr-hole craniostomy with or without a drainage system are well-known surgical procedures for treatment of CSDH. The reoperation rate in patients with CSDH is between 2.3 and 38.7% [63]. There is a significant relationship between recurrence and outcome; prognosis worsens with increasing recurrence of the CSDH [38]. Older patients are at higher risk for recurrence [5]. Also, the higher rates of antithrombotic agent use in elderly patients pose another risk for recurrence of the CSDH.

A. Tahta
Department of Neurosurgery, Istanbul Medipol University Faculty of Medicine, Istanbul, Turkey

Y. B. Turgut (✉)
Department of Internal Medicine, Muğla Sıtkı Koçman University Faculty of Medicine, Muğla, Turkey

G. Pektaş
Department of Hematology, Muğla Sıtkı Koçman University Faculty of Medicine, Muğla, Turkey

M. Turgut et al. (eds.), *Subdural Hematoma*, https://doi.org/10.1007/978-3-030-79371-5_21

21.2 Antithrombotic Drugs

Since the use of antithrombotic agents for chronic diseases is more common in elderly patients, the effects of these agents on CSDH and the precautions that should be taken and the follow-up for patients during the postoperative period are very important. Various studies have been conducted on the relationship between antithrombotic agents and the recurrence of CSDH, but the results are inconsistent [1, 13, 16]. According to the systematic review published by Nathan et al. in 2017, the effects of combined anticoagulant and antiplatelet use on the recurrence of CSDH were examined in four articles [41]. Three studies showed that combined use was not significant risk factor for the recurrence of CSDH [5, 6, 20]. However, they found that the combined use was a significant factor for recurrence in one study [24]. According to a meta-analysis conducted by Wang et al. in 2019, patients who use antiplatelet and anticoagulant drugs together have a higher recurrence risk for CSDH (OR: 1.30, 95% CI, 1.11–1.52, $p = 0.001$), but the combined use did not increase the rate of mortality in patients with CSDH [63]. Also, Motoie et al. stated that severe complications such as acute epidural hematoma and acute subdural hematoma (SDH) are related to the use of oral antithrombotic agents at the time of admission, but they do not increase recurrence rates in these patients [39].

21.3 Anticoagulation

Warfarin inhibits the vitamin K epoxide reductase complex 1 (VKORC1), which is an enzyme that stimulates the vitamin K available in the body; thus it may consume the reserves of vitamin K through this mechanism and the synthesis of active clotting factors is reduced [45]. Neurosurgeon should consider the diagnosis of CSDH in elderly patients receiving warfarin (Fig. 21.1).

Results of the activated prothrombin time (aPTT) and international normalized ratio (INR) must be normalized before surgery in order to prevent complications, particularly recurrence [37]. If emergent surgical intervention is required, the INR can be reduced to normal values by giving a total of four factor prothrombin complex concentrates (PCC) that include factors 2, 7, 9, and 10. Fresh frozen plasma (FFP) contains all of the coagulation factors, but it can only partially reverse warfarin according to the factor concentration and it takes a long time for warfarin reversal due to the intravenous volume burden [22, 30]. PCCs are generally preferred for administration because of the higher quantity of factors, with the aim of inhibition by an influx of factors involved in the coagulation. Also, vitamin K can be administered intravenously to stimulate synthesis of cofactors. Vitamin K is usually an adjuvant treatment with PCCs and/or FFP [21]. Warfarin should be discontinued at least 5 days before elective surgery. The INR value should be reviewed on the day of surgery.

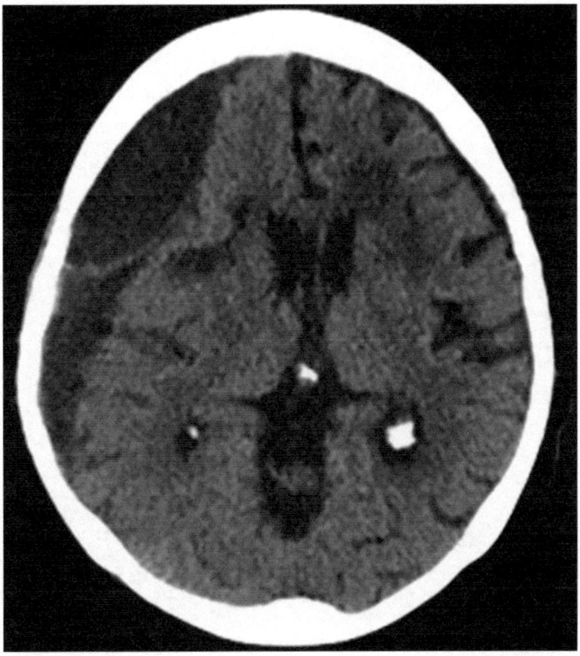

Fig. 21.1 Axial non-contrast computed tomography showing a right frontoparietal chronic subdural hematoma (CSDH) in an 86-year-old female patient using warfarin

Both unfractionated heparin and low molecular weight heparin (LMWH) enhance the activity of antithrombin-3, which inhibits thrombin formation [19]. Both types of heparin are monitored by the aPTT levels and can be reversed with protamine. However, LMWH cannot be reversed completely. Therefore, the neurosurgeon should consider persistent coagulopathy in patients receiving LMWH.

The target of novel oral anticoagulation agents (NOACs) is directed at factor Xa or thrombin [55]. Surgery can be a challenge due to the absence of reversing agents for NOACs. PraxBind is a reversal agent for dabigatran. This drug has been shown to normalize laboratory values in 11 h [66]. Although PCC and/or FFP can be used before surgery, these agents have not been found to improve outcome [40]. Rivaroxaban is cleared at 32 h, apixaban is cleared at 28 h, and dabigatran at 56 h [61]. Since there is an absence of an effective reversing agent, NOACs should be discontinued for an appropriate period of time under elective conditions. However, Motoie et al. found that the CSDH recurrence rate did not increase in 21 patients using NOACs [39]. These drugs have been shown to increase recurrence rates in a study conducted by Arai et al. [4].

Ohba et al. and Chon et al. found increased odds of recurrence in patients with CSDH [13, 42]. However, only Chon et al. found recurrence that had statistical significance [13]. In addition, the use of anticoagulants increases the risk of recurrence rates according to the meta-analysis of Wang et al. [63]. However, it has not been shown to increase the risk of mortality [63].

21.4 Antiplatelet

Acetylsalicylic acid (ASA, aspirin) is the most commonly used antiplatelet drug. ASA irreversibly inhibits COX_2, causing platelet dysfunction when it is used at low doses [58]. In clinical practice, every neurosurgeon should consider the diagnosis of CSDH in patients on antiplatelet treatment (Fig. 21.2). The average platelet life span

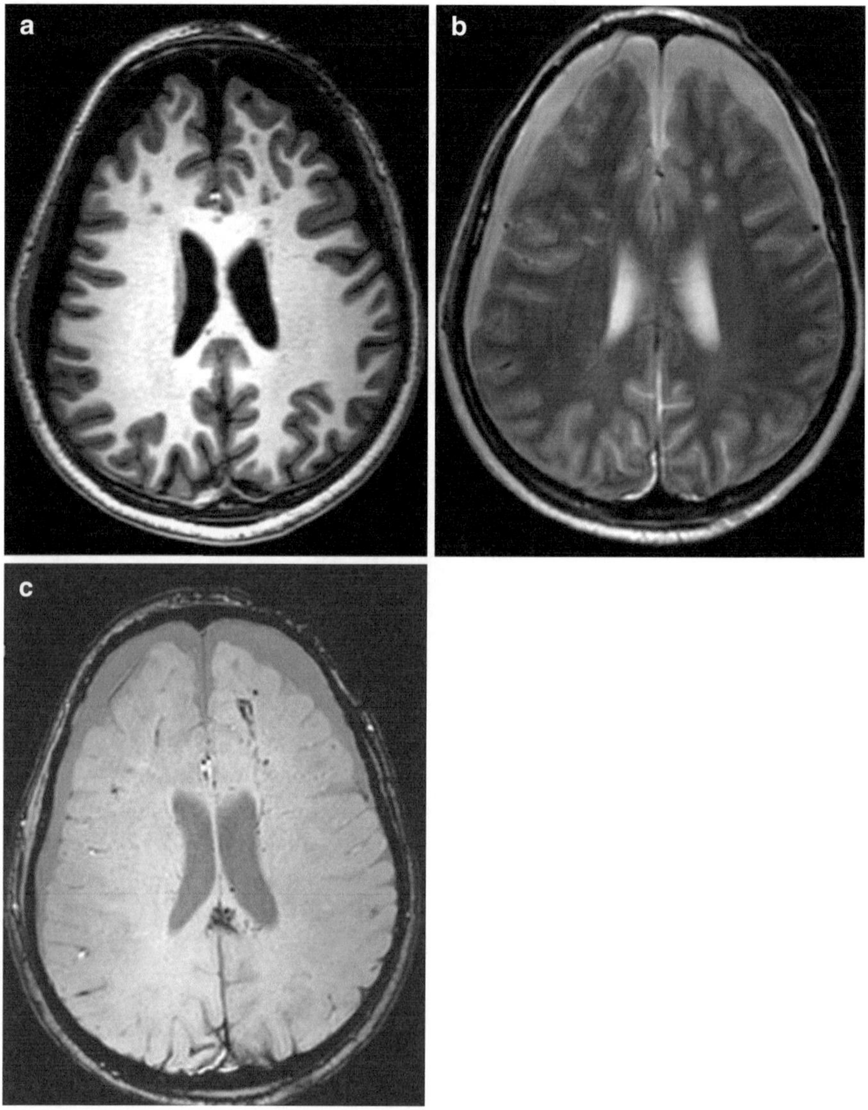

Fig. 21.2 Axial T1WI (**a**), axial T2WI (**b**), and axial SWI (**c**) demonstrating bilateral CSDH in a 74-year-old male patient on antiplatelet treatment

is 5–7 days. Therefore, ASA should be discontinued 5–7 days before surgery in elective cases. Platelet transfusion is an appropriate option in emergent conditions [57]. Taylor et al. showed that platelet transfusion was an effective treatment for ASA utilization [57]. Clopidogrel, prasugrel, ticagrelor, ticlopidine, and cangrelor are inhibitors of P2Y12 [37]. They bind or block the platelet ADP receptor, causing platelet dysfunction. There are no reversal agents for these drugs. All of them, except Ticagrelor, are irreversible. Ticagrelor is removed from the circulation within 28 h. It is recommended to wait for 5–10 days after discontinuation of the drug in elective surgeries and to perform platelet transfusion in emergent surgeries involving other agents [37].

Ohba et al. found that the CSDH recurrence rate was 15.2% in patients using antiplatelet agents [42]. The recurrence rate was 10.4% in patients who did not use antiplatelet agents, but there was no statistically significant difference between the two groups [42]. Chon et al. did not find a significant difference in terms of re-bleeding rates among patients using and those not using antiplatelet agents [13]. In a meta-analysis conducted by Wang et al., antiplatelet use has been shown to increase recurrence rates for CSDH [63]. However, most of the studies showed that the use of antiplatelet agents did not increase CSDH recurrence [7, 16, 36, 59].

21.5 Time to Restart

The rate of ischemic complications within 7 days after discontinuation of warfarin is 2.6–4.8% [65]. Guha et al. compared the incidence of thromboembolism following surgery for CSDH in patients receiving antithrombotic therapy and those not undergoing antithrombotic therapy [20]. All of the antithrombotic agents were discontinued and about half of the patients who had a history of taking antithrombotic agents resumed taking them at a median of 52 days following neurosurgical intervention [20]. They reported a trend toward an increased incidence of thromboembolic complications in patients receiving antithrombotic therapy (2.6% vs. 0.8%) [20]. Amano et al. found a significantly increased prevalence of thromboembolic complications in patients with CSDH undergoing antithrombotic therapy compared to those not undergoing antithrombotic therapy (9.1% vs. 0.9%) [3]. The rate of thromboembolic complications was lower in patients that resumed antithrombotic therapy than in patients that had not resumed antithrombotic therapy in a meta-analysis published by Phan et al. (2.9% vs. 15.3%) [46]. According to these results, thromboembolism is an important complication in patients with CSDH undergoing antithrombotic therapy.

Even today, the timing of the restarting of antithrombotic agents after surgery in patients with CSDH is not clear. Most of the studies have shown that CSDH recurrences occur in the first month after surgery [11]. Phan et al. advised restarting antithrombotic agents after this period [46]. Amano et al. stated that antithrombotic agents must be resumed as soon as possible after confirmation of an absence of hemorrhagic complications following surgery [3]. So, they advise resuming antithrombotic agents on the day after surgical treatment [3]. However, there are no randomized controlled trials regarding the optimal time to restart these agents. Future studies are required to fully understand the effect of different periods of time over which treatment is restarted. The decision to restart antithrombotic agents is complex, so the resumption of antithrombotic drugs should be based on an individualized approach.

21.6 Hematological Malignancies

Patients with hematological malignancies are more likely to develop intraparenchymal intracerebral hemorrhage (ICH) and subarachnoid hemorrhage compared to SDH. However, as the life expectancy of patients with leukemia and lymphoma increases with new treatment alternatives, these patients are more likely to develop CSDH [9, 10, 29]. Hematopoietic stem-cell transplantation (HSCT), diagnostic and therapeutic lumbar puncture, chemotherapy administration, coagulopathy, and platelet dysfunction are all risk factors for CSDH development and recurrence after treatment in this patient group [25, 43, 60]. Patients with acute myeloid leukemia (AML) have an increased risk of ICH compared to other hematological malignancies [12]. Primary central nervous system (CNS) lymphoma, intravascular lymphoma, and myeloma are other malignancies that have an increased risk of ICH [12]. SDHs are detected more often in older patients compared to ICHs [12]. Also, symptoms have slower clinical onset in patients with SDHs than in those with ICHs.

Recurrence, surgical morbidity, and mortality are increased in SDHs due to hematological malignancies compared to SDHs secondary to trauma or antithrombotic agent use [29]. Patients with hematological malignancies are at a high risk for surgery. Shortening the bleeding time and correcting the coagulopathy with appropriate transfusions are necessary prior to surgery. But this preoperative intervention is usually temporary. Patients with hematological malignancy are usually older, immunosuppressed, and they also have additional clinical disorders and a prolonged bleeding time. So surgical treatment options are difficult to select and require a multidisciplinary approach. In a study published by Reichman et al., surgery was performed in 32% of patients with hematological malignancies and SDH [48]. In the series of Owattanapanich et al., 10% of the patients underwent surgery and it was revealed that the survival for the patients that had surgery was better than that of those who did not [44]. Wright et al. revealed that the prognosis for patients with SDH was better in patients with hematological malignancy compared to those with ICHs [64]. However, the median survival of patients was <5 months despite all treatment options [64]. The recurrence rate in patients undergoing surgery was 9–30% [34, 52]. Low hemoglobin and platelet levels, prolonged prothrombin time, and advanced age were associated with increased mortality [12, 64].

Clinical awareness of the neurological symptoms and signs is important in elderly patients. In the case of a symptom or sign that may cause a suspicion for a SDH, neuroimaging should be done quickly and a diagnosis should be determined. The expected life span is usually less than 5 months. So, a discussion should be held between the hematologist, oncologist, neurosurgeon, and the patient's family regarding surgery in the last 6 months of a patient's life [64].

21.7 Intractable Thrombocytopenia

CSDH evacuation is not a major neurosurgical intervention. No major blood loss is anticipated during surgery and operations can be performed even under local anesthesia [2]. It is recommended that the platelet count should be >100,000 per microliter before major neurosurgical operations [35]. If the platelet count is below this value, the risk of acute bleeding increases in the postoperative period. In emergent operations, it is recommended that the platelet count should be at least 80,000 [2]. In a study by Abdelfatah et al., 41 patients with CSDH and intractable thrombocytopenia were evaluated [2]. The platelet count of all patients on admission was <60,000 per microliter. Despite random donor pooled platelet infusion, patients' platelet values could not be increased above 80,000. SDHs of the patients that were evacuated with two burr holes and a subgaleal drain was placed at surgery. Clinical improvement was observed in all patients and an acute SDH was not detected in the early postoperative period. Only two patients had recurrence of a CSDH within 1 month and re-evacuation was performed [2]. Although there are not many studies demonstrating the effect of intractable thrombocytopenia in patients with CSDH, it appears that it is sufficient to increase the platelet count above 50,000 using random donor platelet transfusion.

21.8 Hematopoietic Stem Cell Transplantation

CSDH after HSCT is a rare but serious and life-threatening complication [14, 47]. The diagnosis can be difficult to make because symptoms and signs are not always pathognomonic. In 5–9% of patients with non-Hodgkin lymphoma, leptomeningeal infiltration or a parenchymal mass can be detected [32]. Especially when thrombocytopenia is present in the aplastic phase of HSCT, where the risk of developing a CSDH is quite high. Although there are a few case reports mentioning CSDH after HSCT, CSDH should be considered in the differential diagnosis when patients develop headache, hemiparesis, dysphasia, or altered consciousness after HSCT. The diagnosis and treatment should be performed using a multidisciplinary approach including hematologists and neurosurgeons [23, 26].

21.9 Idiopathic Thrombocytopenic Purpura

Idiopathic thrombocytopenic purpura (ITP) is an autoimmune disorder. Antibody-coated platelets are destroyed by the immune system [27]. Intracranial hemorrhages are a rare source of bleeding that occurs in 1% of patients with ITP [18]. Bleeding is usually seen as intraparenchymal or subarachnoid hemorrhage, but CSDH is rare. A small number of patients are reported in case reports in the current literature [28, 53, 54, 56].

Patients with CSDH usually have trauma in their medical history. However, trauma is less common in the history of patients with ITP and CSDH [54]. Clinical features such as headache, hemiparesis, and altered consciousness are usually accompanied by mucocutaneous bleeding [49]. Neurological signs and symptoms are more common in patients under 20 years of age. Surgical evacuation of the SDH should be performed after correcting the hematological profile of the patients. Conservative treatment can be considered in patients with no neurological deficits or with no increase in the hematoma size. The hematological status of the patients can be optimized with corticosteroids, IVIG, and splenectomy [54]. In a study conducted by Lee and Kim, splenectomy was shown to be beneficial in 2 of the 3 ITP patients with a CSDH [31]. Also, it has been shown that corticosteroids and IVIG are beneficial in increasing platelet levels in most patients [49]. Corticosteroids have an effect on preventing the progression of CSDH. Surgical treatment should be reserved for emergent conditions, patients with progressive neurological deficits or an increasing hematoma size.

21.10 Conclusion

Various studies have been conducted on the relationship between antithrombotic agents and CSDH recurrence. However, the results are inconsistent. Patients who use antiplatelet and anticoagulant drugs together have a higher risk of CSDH recurrence. However, combined use did not increase the risk of mortality in patients with CSDH. The use of anticoagulants increases the risk of recurrence of CSDHs. As the life expectancy for patients with leukemia and lymphoma increases with new treatment alternatives, these patients are more likely to develop a CSDH rather than an ICH. Also, ITP, thrombocytopenia, and HSCT are all risk factors for developing a CSDH.

References

1. Abboud T, Dhrsen L, Gibbert C, Westphal M, Martens T. Influence of antithrombotic agents on recurrence rate and clinical outcome in patients operated for chronic subdural hematoma. Neurocirugía (English Edition). 2018;29:86–92.

2. Abdelfatah M. Management of chronic subdural hematoma in patients with intractable thrombocytopenia. Turk Neurosurg. 2018;28:400–4.
3. Amano T, Takahara K, Maehara N, Shimogawa T, Mukae N, Sayama T, Arihiro S, Arakawa S, Morioka T, Haga S. Optimal perioperative management of antithrombotic agents in patients with chronic subdural hematoma. Clin Neurol Neurosurg. 2016;151:43–50.
4. Arai N, Mine Y, Kagami H, Maruyama M, Daikoh A, Inaba M. Safe burr hole surgery for chronic subdural hematoma using dabigatran with idarucizumab. World Neurosurg. 2018;109:432–5.
5. Aspegren OP, Åstrand R, Lundgren MI, Romner B. Anticoagulation therapy a risk factor for the development of chronic subdural hematoma. Clin Neurol Neurosurg. 2013;115:981–4.
6. Baraniskin A, Steffens C, Harders A, Schmiegel W, Schroers R, Spangenberg P. Impact of prehospital antithrombotic medication on the outcome of chronic and acute subdural hematoma. J Neurol Surg A Cent Eur Neurosurg. 2014;75:031–6.
7. Bartek J, Sjåvik K, Kristiansson H, Ståhl F, Fornebo I, Förander P, Jakola AS. Predictors of recurrence and complications after chronic subdural hematoma surgery: a population-based study. World Neurosurg. 2017;106:609–14.
8. Beck J, Gralla J, Fung C, Ulrich CT, Schucht P, Fichtner J, Andereggen L, Gosau M, Hattingen E, Gutbrod K. Spinal cerebrospinal fluid leak as the cause of chronic subdural hematomas in nongeriatric patients. J Neurosurg. 2014;121:1380–7.
9. Bower H, Björkholm M, Dickman PW, Höglund M, Lambert PC, Andersson TM-L. Life expectancy of patients with chronic myeloid leukemia approaches the life expectancy of the general population. J Clin Oncol. 2016;34:2851–7.
10. Bureau UC. An aging nation: projected number of children and older adults. In: The United States Census Bureau. https://www.census.gov/library/visualizations/2018/comm/historic-first.html. Accessed 3 July 2020.
11. Chari A, Clemente Morgado T, Rigamonti D. Recommencement of anticoagulation in chronic subdural haematoma: a systematic review and meta-analysis. Br J Neurosurg. 2014;28:2–7.
12. Chen CY, Tai CH, Cheng A, Wu HC, Tsay W, Liu JH, Chen PY, Huang SY, Yao M, Tang JL, Tien HF. Intracranial hemorrhage in adult patients with hematological malignancies. BMC Med. 2012;10:97.
13. Chon K-H, Lee J-M, Koh E-J, Choi H-Y. Independent predictors for recurrence of chronic subdural hematoma. Acta Neurochir. 2012;154:1541–8.
14. Colosimo M, McCarthy N, Jayasinghe R, Morton J, Taylor K, Durrant S. Diagnosis and management of subdural haematoma complicating bone marrow transplantation. Bone Marrow Transplant. 2000;25:549–52.
15. Ducruet AF, Grobelny BT, Zacharia BE, Hickman ZL, DeRosa PL, Anderson K, Sussman E, Carpenter A, Connolly ES. The surgical management of chronic subdural hematoma. Neurosurg Rev. 2012;35:155–69.
16. Fornebo I, Sjåvik K, Alibeck M, Kristiansson H, Ståhl F, Förander P, Jakola AS, Bartek J. Role of antithrombotic therapy in the risk of hematoma recurrence and thromboembolism after chronic subdural hematoma evacuation: a population-based consecutive cohort study. Acta Neurochir (Wien). 2017;159:2045–52.
17. Forster M, Mathé A, Senft C, Scharrer I, Seifert V, Gerlach R. The influence of preoperative anticoagulation on outcome and quality of life after surgical treatment of chronic subdural hematoma. J Clin Neurosci. 2010;17:975–9.
18. George JN, Woolf SH, Raskob GE, Wasser JS, Aledort LM, Ballem PJ, Blanchette VS, Bussel JB, Cines DB, Kelton JG, Lichtin AE, McMillan R, Okerbloom JA, Regan DH, Warrier I. Idiopathic thrombocytopenic purpura: a practice guideline developed by explicit methods for the American Society of Hematology. Blood. 1996;88:3–40.
19. Gray E, Hogwood J, Mulloy B. The anticoagulant and antithrombotic mechanisms of heparin. Handb Exp Pharmacol. 2012;207:43–61.
20. Guha D, Coyne S, Macdonald RL. Timing of the resumption of antithrombotic agents following surgical evacuation of chronic subdural hematomas: a retrospective cohort study. J Neurosurg. 2016;124:750–9.
21. Hanley JP. Warfarin reversal. J Clin Pathol. 2004;57:1132–9.

22. Harrison NE, Gottlieb M. Comparison of fresh frozen plasma with prothrombin complex concentrate for warfarin reversal. Ann Emerg Med. 2017;69:777–9.
23. Hilgendorf I, Wilhelm S, Prall F, Junghanss C, Steiner B, Wolff D, Freund M, Casper J. Headache after hematopoietic stem cell transplantation: being aware of chronic bilateral subdural hematoma. Leuk Lymphoma. 2006;47:2247–9.
24. Honda Y, Sorimachi T, Momose H, Takizawa K, Inokuchi S, Matsumae M. Chronic subdural haematoma associated with disturbance of consciousness: significance of acute-on-chronic subdural haematoma. Neurol Res. 2015;37:985–92.
25. Jourdan E, Dombret H, Glaisner S, Micléa JM, Castaigne S, Degos L. Unexpected high incidence of intracranial subdural haematoma during intensive chemotherapy for acute myeloid leukaemia with a monoblastic component. Br J Haematol. 1995;89:527–30.
26. Kannan K, Koh LP, Linn YC. Subdural hematoma in two hematopoietic stem cell transplant patients with post-dural puncture headache and initially normal CT brain scan. Ann Hematol. 2002;81:540–2.
27. Karpatkin S. Autoimmune thrombocytopenic purpura. Semin Hematol. 1985;22:260–88.
28. Kolluri VR, Reddy DR, Reddy PK, Naidu MR, Kumari CS. Subdural hematoma secondary to immune thrombocytopenic purpura: case report. Neurosurgery. 1986;19:635–6.
29. Krok-Schoen JL, Fisher JL, Stephens JA, Mims A, Ayyappan S, Woyach JA, Rosko AE. Incidence and survival of hematological cancers among adults ages ≥75 years. Cancer Med. 2018;7(7):3425–33. https://doi.org/10.1002/cam4.1461.
30. Le Roux P, Pollack CV, Milan M, Schaefer A. Race against the clock: overcoming challenges in the management of anticoagulant-associated intracerebral hemorrhage. J Neurosurg. 2014;121(Suppl):1–20.
31. Lee MS, Kim WC. Intracranial hemorrhage associated with idiopathic thrombocytopenic purpura: report of seven patients and a meta-analysis. Neurology. 1998;50:1160–3.
32. Levitt LJ, Dawson DM, Rosenthal DS, Moloney WC. CNS involvement in the non-Hodgkin's lymphomas. Cancer. 1980;45:545–52.
33. Lindvall P, Koskinen L-OD. Anticoagulants and antiplatelet agents and the risk of development and recurrence of chronic subdural haematomas. J Clin Neurosci. 2009;16:1287–90.
34. Liu W, Bakker NA, Groen RJM. Chronic subdural hematoma: a systematic review and meta-analysis of surgical procedures. J Neurosurg. 2014;121:665–73.
35. Liumbruno G, Bennardello F, Lattanzio A, Piccoli P, Rossetti G, Italian Society of Transfusion Medicine and Immunohaematology (SIMTI) Work Group. Recommendations for the transfusion of plasma and platelets. Blood Transfus. 2009;7:132–50.
36. Matsumoto H, Hanayama H, Okada T, Sakurai Y, Minami H, Masuda A, Tominaga S, Miyaji K, Yamaura I, Yoshida Y, Yoshida K. Clinical investigation of refractory chronic subdural hematoma: a comparison of clinical factors between single and repeated recurrences. World Neurosurg. 2017;107:706–15.
37. Mehta V, Harward SC, Sankey EW, Nayar G, Codd PJ. Evidence based diagnosis and management of chronic subdural hematoma: a review of the literature. J Clin Neurosci. 2018;50:7–15.
38. Motiei-Langroudi R, Stippler M, Shi S, Adeeb N, Gupta R, Griessenauer CJ, Papavassiliou E, Kasper EM, Arle J, Alterman RL. Factors predicting reoperation of chronic subdural hematoma following primary surgical evacuation. J Neurosurg. 2017;129:1143–50.
39. Motoie R, Karashima S, Otsuji R, Ren N, Nagaoka S, Maeda K, Ikai Y, Uno J, Gi H. Recurrence in 787 patients with chronic subdural hematoma: retrospective cohort investigation of associated factors including direct oral anticoagulant use. World Neurosurg. 2018;118:e87–91.
40. Nagalla S, Thomson L, Oppong Y, Bachman B, Chervoneva I, Kraft WK. Reversibility of apixaban anticoagulation with a four-factor prothrombin complex concentrate in healthy volunteers. Clin Transl Sci. 2016;9:176–80.
41. Nathan S, Goodarzi Z, Jette N, Gallagher C, Holroyd-Leduc J. Anticoagulant and antiplatelet use in seniors with chronic subdural hematoma: systematic review. Neurology. 2017;88:1889–93.
42. Ohba S, Kinoshita Y, Nakagawa T, Murakami H. The risk factors for recurrence of chronic subdural hematoma. Neurosurg Rev. 2013;36:145–9.

43. Openshaw H, Ressler JA, Snyder DS. Lumbar puncture and subdural hygroma and hematomas in hematopoietic cell transplant patients. Bone Marrow Transplant. 2008;41:791–5.
44. Owattanapanich W, Auewarakul CU. Intracranial hemorrhage in patients with hematologic disorders: prevalence and predictive factors. J Med Assoc Thai. 2016;99:15–24.
45. Patel S, Singh R, Preuss CV, Patel N. Warfarin. StatPearls; 2020.
46. Phan K, Abi-Hanna D, Kerferd J, Lu VM, Dmytriw AA, Ho Y-T, Fairhall J, Reddy R, Wilson P. Resumption of antithrombotic agents in chronic subdural hematoma: a systematic review and meta-analysis. World Neurosurg. 2018;109:e792–9.
47. Pomeranz S, Naparstek E, Ashkenazi E, Nagler A, Lossos A, Slavin S, Or R. Intracranial haematomas following bone marrow transplantation. J Neurol. 1994;241:252–6.
48. Reichman J, Singer S, Navi B, Reiner A, Panageas K, Gutin PH, Deangelis LM. Subdural hematoma in patients with cancer. Neurosurgery. 2012;71:74–9.
49. Rodeghiero F. Idiopathic thrombocytopenic purpura: an old disease revisited in the era of evidence-based medicine. Haematologica. 2003;88:1081–7.
50. Rust T, Kiemer N, Erasmus A. Chronic subdural haematomas and anticoagulation or antithrombotic therapy. J Clin Neurosci. 2006;13:823–7.
51. Santarius T, Hutchinson P. Chronic subdural haematoma: time to rationalize treatment? Br J Neurosurg. 2004;18:328–32.
52. Schwarz F, Loos F, Dünisch P, Sakr Y, Safatli DA, Kalff R, Ewald C. Risk factors for reoperation after initial burr hole trephination in chronic subdural hematomas. Clin Neurol Neurosurg. 2015;138:66–71.
53. Sebe A, Ohshima T, Ebisudani D, Oka H, Matsumoto K, Yoshizima S. A case of chronic subdural hematoma associated with idiopathic thrombocytopenic purpura (ITP) (in Japan). No Shinkei Geka. 1990;18:761–5.
54. Seçkin H, Kazanci A, Yigitkanli K, Simsek S, Kars HZ. Chronic subdural hematoma in patients with idiopathic thrombocytopenic purpura: a case report and review of the literature. Surg Neurol. 2006;66:411–4.
55. da Silva RMFL. Novel oral anticoagulants in non-valvular atrial fibrillation. Cardiovasc Hematol Agents Med Chem. 2014;12:3–8.
56. Sreedharan PS, Rakesh S, Sajeev S, Pavithran K, Thomas M. Subdural haematoma with spontaneous resolution—rare manifestation of idiopathic thrombocytopenic purpura. J Assoc Physicians India. 2000;48:432–4.
57. Taylor G, Osinski D, Thevenin A, Devys J-M. Is platelet transfusion efficient to restore platelet reactivity in patients who are responders to aspirin and/or clopidogrel before emergency surgery? J Trauma Acute Care Surg. 2013;74:1367–9.
58. Tohgi H, Konno S, Tamura K, Kimura B, Kawano K. Effects of low-to-high doses of aspirin on platelet aggregability and metabolites of thromboxane A2 and prostacyclin. Stroke. 1992;23:1400–3.
59. Toi H, Kinoshita K, Hirai S, Takai H, Hara K, Matsushita N, Matsubara S, Otani M, Muramatsu K, Matsuda S, Fushimi K, Uno M. Present epidemiology of chronic subdural hematoma in Japan: analysis of 63,358 cases recorded in a national administrative database. J Neurosurg. 2018;128:222–8.
60. Ureshino H, Nishioka A, Kojima K, Kizuka H, Sano H, Shindo T, Kubota Y, Ando T, Kimura S. Subdural hematoma associated with dasatinib and intrathecal methotrexate treatment in Philadelphia Chromosome-positive Acute Lymphoblastic Leukemia. Intern Med. 2016;55:2703–6.
61. Vílchez JA, Gallego P, Lip GYH. Safety of new oral anticoagulant drugs: a perspective. Ther Adv Drug Saf. 2014;5:8–20.
62. Wada M, Yamakami I, Higuchi Y, Tanaka M, Suda S, Ono J, Saeki N. Influence of antiplatelet therapy on postoperative recurrence of chronic subdural hematoma: a multicenter retrospective study in 719 patients. Clin Neurol Neurosurg. 2014;120:49–54.
63. Wang H, Zhang M, Zheng H, Xia X, Luo K, Guo F, Qian C. The effects of antithrombotic drugs on the recurrence and mortality in patients with chronic subdural hematoma: a meta-analysis. Medicine (Baltimore). 2019;98:e13972.

64. Wright CH, Wright J, Alonso A, Raghavan A, Momotaz H, Burant C, Zhou X, Selman W, Sajatovic M, Hoffer A. Subdural hematoma in patients with hematologic malignancies: an outcome analysis and examination of risk factors of operative and nonoperative management. World Neurosurg. 2019;130:e1061–9.
65. Yeon JY, Kong D-S, Hong S-C. Safety of early warfarin resumption following burr hole drainage for warfarin-associated subacute or chronic subdural hemorrhage. J Neurotrauma. 2012;29:1334–41.
66. Yogaratnam D, Ditch K, Medeiros K, Doyno C, Fong JJ. Idarucizumab for reversal of dabigatran-associated anticoagulation. Ann Pharmacother. 2016;50:847–54.

Chapter 22
Acute and Chronic Subdural Hematoma Related to Intracranial Vascular Malformations

Haydn Hoffman and Grahame C. Gould

22.1 Introduction

The most common cause of subdural hematoma (SDH) is trauma, but a subset of spontaneous SDHs may be attributed to vascular malformations. Intracranial vascular malformations include arteriovenous malformations (AVM) and cavernous malformations (CM). AVMs are abnormal connections of arteries to veins without the presence of intervening capillaries that grossly appear as dilated tangles of blood vessels. Their rupture typically results in intraparenchymal hemorrhage (IPH) with or without subarachnoid hemorrhage (SAH) or intraventricular hemorrhage (IVH), but SDH may also occur. CMs are abnormal collections of dilated blood vessels within brain parenchyma that comprise 10–20% of intracranial vascular malformations. Their rupture usually results in an intralesional IPH; however extralesional SDH may also occur with peripherally located CMs. Although not true malformations, dural arteriovenous fistulas (dAVF) are frequently considered with other intracranial vascular malformations and will be included in this chapter. dAVFs are fistulous connections between dural arteries and veins that account for 10–15% of intracranial vascular malformations and are believed to be acquired. They have heterogenous presentations including headache, ocular symptoms, tinnitus, and non-hemorrhagic neurologic deficits (NHND). Their rupture may cause IPH, SAH, or, less commonly, SDH. In Lasjaunias's review of 191 dAVFs, 41 bled and of these 5 (12.2%) led to SDH [9]. In a more recent series, SDH occurred in 18% of those with dAVF-related hemorrhage [5].

H. Hoffman · G. C. Gould (✉)
Department of Neurosurgery, State University of New York Upstate Medical University, Syracuse, NY, USA
e-mail: hoffmanh@upstate.edu; gouldg@upstate.edu

M. Turgut et al. (eds.), *Subdural Hematoma*,
https://doi.org/10.1007/978-3-030-79371-5_22

22.2 Epidemiology

AVMs are rare and population-based prevalence data are lacking, but detection rates have been estimated between 0.55–1.21 per 100,000 person-years [18]. They are slightly more common in men and have an average age of presentation of 33 years. There is an association with Osler-Weber-Rendu syndrome (hereditary hemorrhagic telangiectasia). CMs are present in 0.02–0.16% of the population and may be sporadic or hereditary, with multiple lesions frequently seen in the latter. They do not have a sex preponderance. dAVFs are most often diagnosed in the fifth or sixth decade and they do not have a sex predilection [15].

22.3 Natural History

The natural history of AVMs is controversial. The often-cited 4% annual hemorrhage rate was derived from a large prospective study of symptomatic angiographically confirmed AVMs [13]. Given the population's symptomatic nature, 4% is probably an overestimate and not applicable to all AVMs. More recent studies have identified annual hemorrhage rates closer to 2–3% [6, 8]. Risk factors for AVM rupture include prior hemorrhage, deep venous drainage, an associated aneurysm (present in approximately 7% of patients with AVMs), and venous outflow stenosis.

Incidentally discovered CMs are associated with low annual hemorrhage rates of 0.3% for non-brainstem locations and 2.8% for those in the brainstem [20]. As with AVMs, prior hemorrhage greatly increases the risk of future hemorrhage. In addition, CMs may demonstrate a temporal clustering phenomenon in which they are prone to repeated hemorrhages shortly after an initial bleed [2].

The natural history of dAVFs is dictated by the presence or absence of cortical venous drainage (CVD). dAVFs without CVD are regarded as benign lesions without risk of hemorrhage and a low likelihood of transformation. Presence of CVD portends a higher risk of hemorrhage, ranging from 1.5 to 8% [15]. Among those with CVD, prior hemorrhage or NHND increase the chance of rupture.

22.4 Anatomy

The dural convexities are primarily supplied by the anterior meningeal artery (AMA), middle meningeal artery (MMA), and posterior meningeal artery (PMA). The largest contributor to meningeal blood supply is the MMA, which is a proximal branch of the internal maxillary artery. The MMA may be hypertrophied in patients with chronic SDH, as demonstrated in Fig. 22.1. Most dAVFs include arterial input from the MMA, and this is a common route for embolization given its relatively straight, easily navigable course. Embolization of the MMA is an increasingly popular treatment for chronic SDH. Due to their fragile, hypervascular membranes, chronic SDH has a characteristic angiographic appearance. Figure 22.2 shows contrast stasis

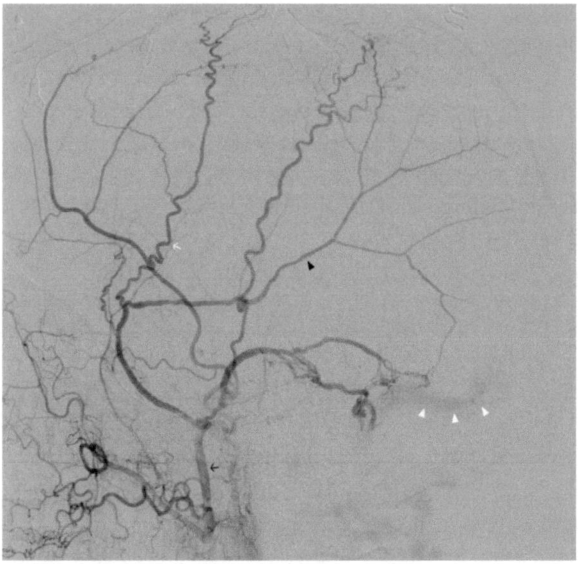

Fig. 22.1 Lateral mid-arterial phase right external carotid artery injection in a patient with recurrent bilateral chronic subdural hematomas who presented for middle meningeal artery (MMA) embolization. Early retrograde opacification of the transverse-sigmoid sinus junction from enlarged petrous branches of the MMA is present, consistent with a Cognard 2a dural arteriovenous fistula (black arrow: proximal MMA trunk; white arrow: frontal branch of MMA; black arrowhead: parietal branch of MMA; white arrowhead: early transverse sinus opacification)

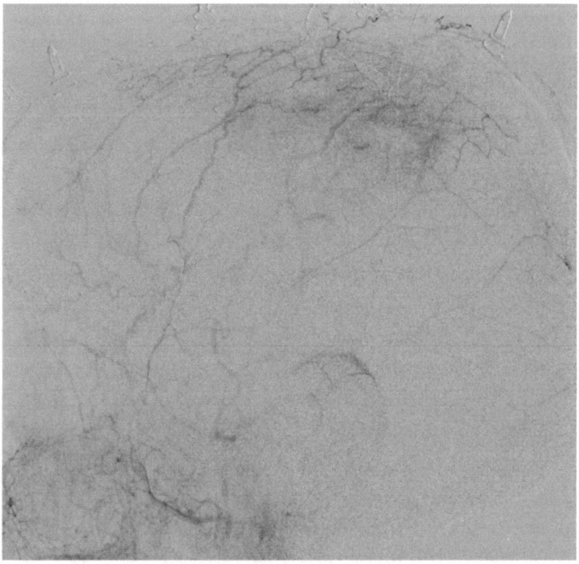

Fig. 22.2 Lateral capillary phase left external carotid artery injection in the same patient as Fig. 22.1 demonstrating dense contrast blush within the chronic subdural hematoma

within the membranes of a chronic SDH with supply from the MMA. The PMA, which is usually a branch of the V3 segment of the vertebral artery, supplies the dura of the posterior fossa. The posterior fossa dura also has variable supply from the occipital, ascending pharyngeal, and posterior auricular arteries. The petrosquamosal region is in hemodynamic equilibrium with the MMA. Posterior fossa dAVFs may include arterial input from any number of these vessels. The AMA arises from the ethmoid arteries (branches of the ophthalmic artery) and travels within the wall of the superior sagittal sinus to supply the frontal convexity dura. The meningohypophyseal trunk, which is a branch of the cavernous segment of the internal carotid artery, supplies the tentorium cerebri and the clival dura via the artery of the tentorium (Bernasconi and Cassinari) and the dorsal meningeal artery, respectively.

22.5 Classifications

AVMs are usually classified by Spetzler-Martin grade. This scale assigns points based on size (1: <3 cm; 2: 3–6 cm; 3: >6 cm), presence of deep venous drainage (0: absent; 1: present), and eloquent location (0: absent; 1: present). The grade ranges from 1 to 5 and is directly proportional to operative morbidity and mortality. Spetzler and Ponce derived a three-tier classification from the Spetzler-Martin grade with recommendations for treatment. Grade 1 and 2 were combined (Class A) with a recommendation for surgical resection, Grade 3 (Class B) was deemed most suitable for multimodal treatment, and Grade 4 and 5 were combined (Class C) with a recommendation for observation [17]. Finally, Lawton and Young supplemented the existing Spetzler-Martin grading scheme to include points for age (1: <20 years; 2: 20–40 years; 3: >40 years), unruptured presentation (0: ruptured; 1: unruptured), and nidal morphology (0: compact; 1: diffuse) [10]. When these components were added to the Spetzler-Martin grade and a threshold of 6 was applied (1–6: low–moderate risk; >6: high risk), they were able to predict surgical outcome with greater accuracy than the Spetzler-Martin grade alone [10].

A classification for CMs with wide clinical application does not exist, but a radiographic classification based on MRI appearance that is associated with hemorrhage risk has been proposed. Zabramski et al. described: Type 1 lesions are hyperintense on T1 and hyper- or hypointense on T2 sequences, type 2 have a classic "popcorn" appearance with a reticulated core, type 3 are isointense on T1 and T2 indicative of chronic hemorrhage, and type 4 are characterized by a punctate hypointensity only seen on GRE sequences [21]. Type 4 lesions are usually seen in familial subtypes. Type 1 and 2 CMs have higher hemorrhage rates than types 3 and 4 [12].

The most commonly used classification schemes for dAVFs are the Borden and Cognard scales. Both are influenced by the pattern of venous drainage, which is the most important determinant of a dAVF's propensity for hemorrhage. The Borden classification includes type 1: anterograde drainage into a dural sinus or meningeal vein, type 2: anterograde drainage into a dural sinus with retrograde cortical venous drainage, and type 3: isolated retrograde cortical venous drainage directly into a cortical vein or through a trapped segment of sinus [3]. The Cognard classification includes type 1: anterograde drainage into a dural sinus, type 2a: retrograde drainage into a dural sinus, type 2b: anterograde drainage into a dural sinus with cortical venous reflux, type 2a + b: retrograde drainage into a dural sinus with cortical venous reflux, type 3: direct cortical venous drainage, type 4: direct cortical venous drainage with venous ectasia, type 5: drainage into spinal perimedullary veins [4].

22.6 Diagnosis

Vascular imaging is warranted when a patient presents with an acute SDH in the absence of trauma. Delayed expansion of a SDH without another cause may also prompt evaluation for a vascular malformation [14]. Older patients may present with a chronic SDH due to remote minor trauma that they are unable to recall. In these situations, we typically do not obtain vascular imaging unless there are other findings that raise suspicion for an underlying structural vascular etiology.

When an investigation of the cranial vasculature is indicated, noninvasive imaging such as CT angiography (CTA) or MR angiography (MRA) is typically performed first. AVMs appear as an abnormal tangle of blood vessels with tortuous dilated feeding arteries and draining veins entering and exiting the region of hypervascularity, respectively. CMs are angiographically occult and not well visualized on CT, CTA, or MRA, but a developmental venous anomaly may be detected. The imaging modality of choice for CMs is MRI. Their typical appearance on MRI is that of different-aged blood products surrounded by a hemosiderin ring often described as a "popcorn" appearance, although this only applies to Zabramski type 2 lesions. Susceptibility weighted imaging sequences are highly sensitive to blood products and well suited for detecting CMs. Most dAVFs are suboptimally evaluated with CTA and MRA but may appear as dilated arterial feeders or ectatic draining veins exiting the fistula with or without venous congestion. Time of flight MRA is useful for detecting early venous drainage. When noninvasive imaging yields a newly diagnosed AVM or dAVF, digital subtraction angiography (DSA) is performed to confirm the diagnosis, obtain more details about its angioarchitecture, and plan treatment. DSA is the gold standard for evaluating these lesions, while CMs do not appear on DSA.

22.7 Treatment

Acute SDHs causing mass effect and impaired mental status require emergent evacuation before an associated vascular etiology is addressed. Chronic SDHs may also necessitate urgent evacuation if severe midline shift and neurologic deficits are noted, although their presentations are usually more insidious. Once the patient is stabilized, work-up for an etiology of the hemorrhage can proceed if indicated.

AVMs may be treated with surgical resection, endovascular embolization, stereotactic radiosurgery, or any combination of these. When the perceived risk of postoperative morbidity is acceptably low, surgical resection is preferred because it is the treatment most likely to achieve a cure. As described by Spetzler and Ponce, this corresponds to Spetzler-Martin grade I and II AVMs [17]. Spetzler-Martin grade III AVMs carry greater surgical risk and are frequently embolized preoperatively or treated with radiosurgery with or without embolization. The latter is associated with a 2–3-year latency period before AVM obliteration, which limits its use in ruptured lesions. Spetzler-Martin grade IV and V AVMs are high risk for any treatment modality and generally should not be treated unless symptomatic. As with grade III AVMs, treatment is typically multimodal.

Surgical resection of CMs is indicated if the lesion has bled and is in a surgically accessible location. In the case of a SDH, the CM would likely be superficial and amenable to resection at the time of hematoma evacuation. In one report, the CM was attached to the dura and resected en bloc at the time of SDH evacuation [19]. Radiosurgery has been described as a treatment option for CMs but does not convincingly alter their natural history.

dAVFs are most commonly treated with endovascular techniques, but certain locations are favorable for microsurgical interruption of the fistulous connection. These include anterior skull base, tentorium, and foramen magnum. In a literature review of dAVFs causing isolated SDHs, lesions were roughly evenly distributed among the anterior fossa, middle fossa, and frontal, temporal, parietal, or occipital regions [11].

22.8 Outcome

Outcome after AVM rupture depends on the size and location of the hemorrhage, presence of IVH, presence of an associated aneurysm, and age [1, 7]. Patients with AVMs in the posterior fossa and eloquent locations have poorer outcomes [1]. Overall, hemorrhage results in approximately 20% mortality and only 35% complete recovery [7]. Surgical outcomes are closely linked to Spetzler-Martin grade, and the incidence of a poor outcome increases from 4% with grade 1 lesions to 37% with grade 5 lesions [16]. Outcomes after CM hemorrhage are related to the lesion's location, with eloquent and brainstem regions yielding poorer outcomes and fixed neurologic deficits. Surgical treatment of brainstem CMs often results in transient worsening of neurologic deficits with eventual improvement. Outcomes for ruptured dAVFs are predominantly favorable, with more than two-thirds recovering with minimal or no symptoms [5].

22.9 Conclusion

Vascular malformations are rare causes of SDH, but their investigation may be warranted in the absence of trauma. In the setting of a large SDH causing herniation, the hematoma should be evacuated before evaluating for a vascular malformation. CMs causing SDH are typically superficial or exophytic and likely can be resected at the time of hematoma evacuation. AVMs and dAVFs require DSA to characterize their morphology and devise a treatment strategy. Successful treatment of these lesions requires a thorough understanding of their natural history, angioarchitecture, and the available treatment modalities.

References

1. Abla AA, Nelson J, Rutledge WC, Young WL, Kim H, Lawton MT. The natural history of AVM hemorrhage in the posterior fossa: comparison of hematoma volumes and neurological outcomes in patients with ruptured infra- and supratentorial AVMs. Neurosurg Focus. 2014;37:E6.
2. Barker FG 2nd, Amin-Hanjani S, Butler WE, Lyson S, Ojemann RG, Chapman PH, et al. Temporal clustering of hemorrhages from untreated cavernous malformations of the central nervous system. Neurosurgery. 2001;49:15–24.
3. Borden JA, Wu JK, Schucart WA. A proposed classification for spinal and cranial dural arteriovenous fistulous malformations and implications for treatment. J Neurosurg. 1995;82:166–79.
4. Cognard C, Gobin YP, Pierot L, Bailly AL, Houdart E, Casasco A, et al. Cerebral dural arteriovenous fistulas: clinical and angiographic correlation with a revised classification of venous drainage. Radiology. 1995;194:671–80.
5. Daniels DJ, Vellimana AK, Zipfel GJ, Lanzino G. Intracranial hemorrhage from dural arteriovenous fistulas: clinical features and outcome. Neurosurg Focus. 2013;34:E15.
6. Gross BA, Du R. Natural history of cerebral arteriovenous malformations: a meta-analysis. J Neurosurg. 2013;118:437–43.
7. Karlsson B, Jokura H, Yang H, Yamamoto M, Martinez R, Kawagishi J, et al. Clinical outcome following cerebral AVM hemorrhage. Acta Neurochir (Wien). 2020;162:1759–66.
8. Kim H, Salman RA, McCulloch CE, Stapf C, Young WL. Untreated brain arteriovenous malformation: patient-level meta-analysis of hemorrhage predictors. Neurology. 2014;83:590–7.
9. Lasjaunias P, Chiu M, ter Brugge K, Tolia A, Hurth A, Bernstein M. Neurological manifestations of intracranial dural arteriovenous malformations. J Neurosurg. 1986;64:724–30.
10. Lawton MT, Kim H, McCulloch CE, Mikhak B, Young WL. A supplementary grading scale for selecting patients with brain arteriovenous malformations for surgery. Neurosurgery. 2010;66:702–13.
11. Li G, Zhang Y, Zhao J, Zhu X, Yu J, Hou K. Isolated subdural hematoma secondary to dural arteriovenous fistula: a case report and literature review. BMC Neurol. 2019;19:43.
12. Nikoubashman O, Rocco D, Davagnanam I, Mankad K, Zerah M, Wiesmann M. Prospective hemorrhage rates of cerebral cavernous malformations in children and adolescents based on MRI appearance. AJNR Am J Neuroradiol. 2015;36:2177–83.
13. Ondra SL, Troupp H, George ED, Schwab K. The natural history of symptomatic arteriovenous malformations of the brain: a 24-year follow-up assessment. J Neurosurg. 1990;73:387–91.
14. Parr M, Patel N, Kauffmann J, Al-Mufti F, Roychowdhury S, Narayan V, et al. Arteriovenous malformation presenting as traumatic subdural hematoma: a case report. Surg Neurol Int. 2020;11:203.
15. Reynolds MR, Lanzino G, Zipfel GJ. Intracranial dural arteriovenous fistulae. Stroke. 2017;48:1424–31.
16. Spetzler RF, Martin NA. A proposed grading system for arteriovenous malformations. J Neurosurg. 1986;65:476–83.
17. Spetzler RF, Ponce FA. A 3-tier classification of cerebral arteriovenous malformations. Clinical article. J Neurosurg. 2011;114:842–9.
18. Stapf C, Mohr JP, Pile-Spellman J, Solomon RA, Sacco RL, Connolly ES. Epidemiology and natural history of arteriovenous malformations. Neurosurg Focus. 2001;11:1–5.

19. Suzuki K, Kamezaki T, Tsuboi K, Kobayashi E. Dural cavernous angioma causing acute subdural hemorrhage—case report. Neurol Med Chir (Tokyo). 1996;36:580–2.
20. Taslimi S, Modabbernia A, Amin-Hanjani S, Barker FG 2nd, Macdonald RL. Natural history of cavernous malformation: systematic review and meta-analysis of 25 studies. Neurology. 2016;86:1984–91.
21. Zabramski JM, Wascher TM, Spetzler RF, Johnson B, Golfinos J, Drayer BP, et al. The natural history of familial cavernous malformations: results of an ongoing study. J Neurosurg. 1994;80:422–32.

Chapter 23
Chronic Subdural Hematoma and Intracranial Arachnoid Cysts

Nevin Aydın, Ceren Kızmazoğlu, Hasan Emre Aydın, and Ali Arslantaş

23.1 Introduction

Chronic subdural hematoma (CSDH) are related to trauma or rarely the rupture of an arachnoid cyst (AC). Both CSDH and AC are common diseases in neurosurgical practice when considered separately. However, CSDH and AC identified concurrently are quite rare. AC-related CSDH formation is frequently observed in young adults due to minor head traumas caused by sports and similar activities in addition to the spontaneous rupture with its related bleeding. Hypotheses on the formation mechanism have been presented although its etiology is not clear. Clinical and radiological follow-up of these cases are important in their treatment. Surgical treatment methods such as burr hole or craniotomy can be used to drain the blood based on the conditions in those cases with progressive clinical findings. Morbidity and mortality rates should be considered when determining the surgical method to be used.

23.2 Chronic Subdural Hematoma

CSDH is a neurosurgical disorder which is a type of intracranial hemorrhage that occurs spontaneously or traumatically between the dura and the pial or arachnoid layer and the surface of the brain parenchyma. CSDH may occur independently or

N. Aydın
Department of Radiology, Eskişehir Osmangazi University, Eskişehir, Turkey

C. Kızmazoğlu
Department of Neurosurgery, İzmir Dokuz Eylül University, İzmir, Turkey

H. E. Aydın (✉) · A. Arslantaş
Center of Technology Innovation, Eskişehir Osmangazi University, Eskişehir, Turkey

M. Turgut et al. (eds.), *Subdural Hematoma*,
https://doi.org/10.1007/978-3-030-79371-5_23

is due to cerebral atrophy and the increased venous fragility in elders. This collection typically develops 2–3 weeks after the inciting event and often has a poor prognosis. Although an osmotic theory or fibrinolysis theory explains its etiology and pathophysiology today, CSDH is a disease with minimal morbidity and mortality after effective treatment. The incidence of CSDH in the population ranges from 8.2 to 17.6/100,000. CSDH prevalence has increased due to an increased global population of elderly people [2]. Trauma is among the most important factors in CSDH etiology. CSDH is more common in males due to their trauma exposure [31]. Subdural hematoma occurs due to the tearing of bridging veins caused by the sudden deceleration and acceleration of brain parenchyma. Subdural hematoma develops more often due to the brain tissue atrophy seen in alcoholics and elderly patients [32].

23.2.1 Diagnosis

CT (computed tomography) is frequently used for the diagnosis and follow-up after surgery of CSDH. CSDH density can be hypodense, isodense, hyperdense, or mixed compared to brain parenchyma according to the classification described by Lanksch et al. (Fig. 23.1). Acute bleeding and membrane formation cause a hyperdense

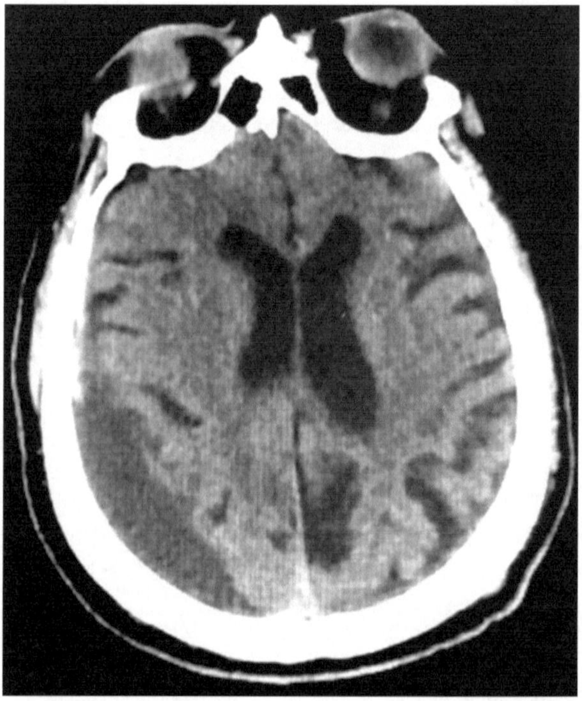

Fig. 23.1 Right-side chronic subdural hematoma. Note the low signal intensity of blood

hematoma. Follow-up clinical and radiological analyses were conducted on the first and at postoperative day 7 with brain CT. In addition, cranial magnetic resonance imaging (MRI) gives detailed information on the determination of the different subdural hematoma phases, dimensions, and age. Cranial MRI would be appropriate in a case of an isodense or bilateral lesions [10]. Although the etiology is not completely clear, chronic subdural hematoma may have calcification in up to 2.7% of cases. Large calcified CSDH cases covering a large part of the cortex are called "Armored Brain" [19]. Calcified CSDH was first detected by von Rokitansky during an autopsy and the first surgically excised CSDH case was reported by Goldhahn [12, 30].

23.2.2 Clinic

Headache, seizure, paresis, plegia, or behavioral changes are among the possible clinical symptoms of CSDH. While neurological deficit is more common in single-sided CSDH, symptoms such as a walking disorder stand out in addition to sensorial disorders such as behavioral changes and slower thinking [16]. Although nonspecific, headache is one of the most common neurological complaints [28]. The Glasgow Coma Scale (GCS), Karnofsky performance score, and the neurological grading system for CSDH were used for the preoperative and postoperative clinical evaluation of the patients [21]. While CSDH generally has an asymptomatic course, it may also present with nonspecific findings such as headache, seizure, paresis, and plegia [6]. Early diagnosis and treatment significantly lower the mortality and morbidity.

23.2.3 Treatment

The options for the treatment for CSDH were surgery, endoscopic surgery, or conservative management. The methods of surgical treatment were either single or double burr hole craniotomies and saline irrigation. The rate of success of conservative treatment was reported to reach 18% in CSDH. Follow-up can be planned especially for individuals who are old and have mild clinical symptoms or for those with randomly detected bleedings [17]. Although the methods are still controversial, CSDH treatment is surgical. Twist-drill craniostomy, burr hole craniostomy, and craniotomy are the most commonly used surgical methods. A significant decrease in mortality resulted through burr hole drainage as the surgical treatment of CSDH. Drainage through twist-drill craniostomy is known to be more advantageous compared to burr hole craniostomy and craniotomy. It's about the this treatment method. This treatment method also used for the other types like multilocated and seperated hemratomas, neuroendoscopic techniques are used rarely. Burr hole drainage is specifically used for non-septated and mostly liquefied CSDHs [25, 34].

23.2.4 Complications

Recurrent CSDH is an important postoperative problem. Recurrence rates up to 31% were reported in the literature. Lack of re-expansion of the brain that remains under pressure for a long duration is considered the most important factor in recurrent hematoma formation [31]. The neurological condition of the patient on admission is among the most important risk factors. The surgical success is decreased and the recurrence risk is increased when the neurological clinical presentation is poor. Pneumocephalus and epilepsy are potential complications. Pneumocephalus in the subdural region most often occurs after the surgery and restricts the expansion of the brain. Studies recommend the use of prophylactic antiepileptic medications for 6 months following CSDH diagnosis. Studies have reported the complication rate following craniotomy and burr hole applied surgery as 6.7% after a small craniotomy and 22.8% in the burr hole group. As a result, craniotomy was claimed to be a better surgical alternative [20]. The pathogenesis of brain atrophy, under-expansion of the brain, and perioperative hematoma volumes have been evaluated as risk factors for CSDH recurrence after surgery.

The risk of calcification formation in CSDHs following trauma is higher than in those occurring due to other causes [15]. The time that passes between the trauma and surgery was evaluated. Higher mortality and morbidity and poor prognosis were observed in cases with trauma less than 60 days before surgery.

23.3 Intracranial Arachnoid Cysts

Arachnoid cysts (ACs) are non-neoplastic, extra-axial lesions. The incidence of ACs among intracranial space occupying lesions is 1% and they are seen three times more often in males than in females. Among ACs which are defined as congenital and acquired in the pediatric period, those with a congenital structure are formed due to the deviations in brain spinal fluid pathway during the development of the arachnoid membrane. ACs form with CSF flow and these collections form towards the endomeninx which will form the pia and the arachnoid coat after the embryological formation of the subarachnoid space [3]. Acquired ACs constituting another group follow the exposure to external factors. They occur due to the brain cerebrospinal fluid collecting within the formed scar tissue especially due to trauma, bleeding, or tumoral lesion [4].

23.3.1 Clinic

Intracranial ACs are generally asymptomatic and are detected randomly. Although the clinical findings of intracranial ACs change according to lesion location, they generally occur with nonspecific symptoms such as headache, vomiting, or seizure.

23.3.2 Diagnosis

Radiological methods such as CT and MRI are used for the diagnosis of intracranial arachnoid cysts. They appear as limited, hypodense, non-enhancing, subarachnoid area located lesions on cerebral CT imaging (Fig. 23.2). Distinguishing the presence of a CSDH is important for the definitive diagnosis and CT may not be sufficient. Advanced diagnostic methods such as diffusion MR and MR spectroscopy can be used for making a definite diagnosis. On cerebral MRI, ACs look like CSF with the same appearance in all sequences (Fig. 23.3). If evaluation through specialized imaging is required, constructive interference in steady state (CISS) sequence clarifying T2 values between the neural structures and CSF and pathological structures in MRI can be used to monitor the AC wall [1].

23.3.3 Location

Intracranial ACs are most often localized in the middle cranial fossa and secondarily in the posterior fossa. Galassi classification defined by Galassi et al. in 1982 is a simple classification grouping ACs into three different types (Table 23.1). The sizes, pressure findings, and effects of middle cranial fossa cysts are evaluated in this classification. A type 1 arachnoid cyst is small and is located in the anterior middle cranial fossa and a type 2 AC lies along the sylvian fissure and has a pressure effect on the temporal lobe and a type 3 AC presses against the parietal and frontal lobe where it fills the entire middle cranial fossa and generally displaces the brain. This classification system can be used to better evaluate the clinical and radiological findings and facilitate making the diagnosis [9].

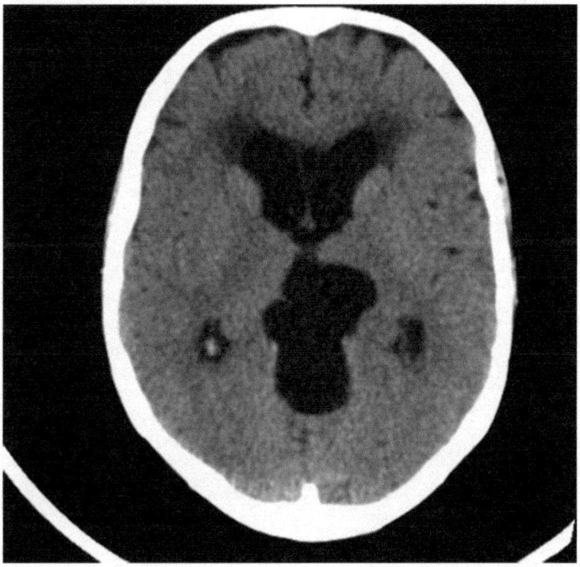

Fig. 23.2 Intracranial arachnoid cyst (AC) of the quadrigeminal system with hydrocephalus

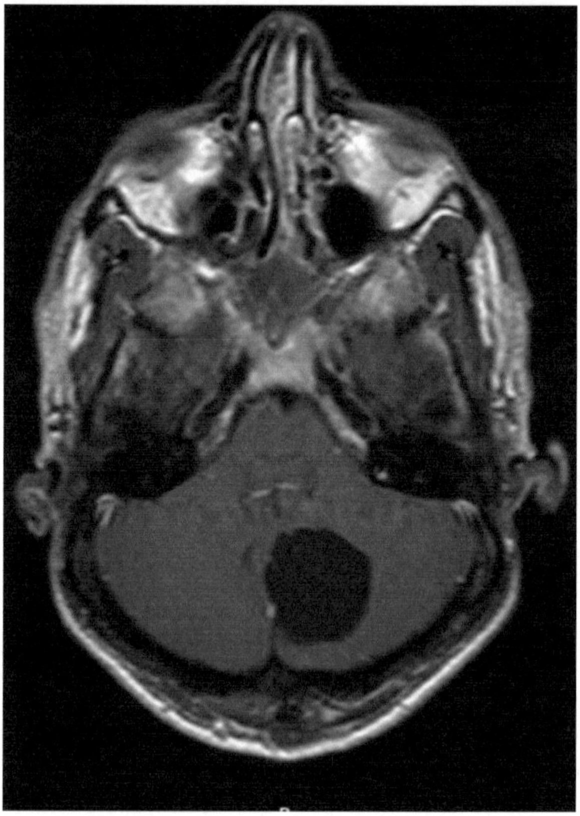

Fig. 23.3 ACs of left cerebellar hemisphere

Table 23.1 Galassi classification[a]

• **Type I**
– Small, spindle-shaped
– Limited to the anterior portion of the middle cranial fossa, below the sphenoid ridge
– Free communication of subarachnoid space
• **Type II**
– Superior extent along the Sylvian fissure
– Displacement of the temporal lobe
– Slow communication with subarachnoid space
• **Type III**
– Large
– Fills the whole middle cranial fossa
– Displacement of not only the temporal lobe but also the frontal and parietal lobes
– Often results in midline shift
– Little communication with subarachnoid space

[a]This table was taken from Galassi et al. [9]

23.3.4 Treatment

Although the treatment of ACs is still controversial, radiological follow-up is important for the lesions without clinical findings and progression on radiological follow-ups [5]. Surgical treatment can be considered when the dimensions of the lesion increase and persistent clinical findings are observed in the follow-up period of the lesion. Specific surgical indications are an intracranial pressure increase, progressive hydrocephalus, parenchymal pressure, and EEG-verified medication resistant epilepsy. Surgical treatment can be applied for treating the cyst or for hydrocephalus occurring due to the pressure effect of the cyst. Cystoperitoneal shunt, ventriculoperitoneal shunt, and endoscopic fenestration of the cyst into the ventricle or cisterna magna can be considered among the surgical treatment methods. Clinical evaluation is very important for surgical decision making. As clinical findings such as headache which represents an intracranial pressure increase are generally nonspecific, the surgery should be decided upon after verifying that the clinical findings that developed are due to the AC after eliminating other causes [13].

23.3.5 Complications

Complications such as subdural hematoma and hygroma may frequently occur after surgery in patients receiving surgical treatment. Foreign object reaction and meningitis may occur following cystoperitoneal or ventriculoperitoneal shunt placement [7]. Lower complication and higher surgical success rates were reported after surgical treatment in hydrocephalus accompanied cases.

23.4 Chronic Subdural Hematoma Associated with Arachnoid Cysts

CSDH occurring due to head traumas during sports or similar conditions was observed to be related to AC. The risk of CSDH on the same side due to congenital ACs is high especially in young patients. Different from spontaneous CSDH, it mostly affects boys, youngsters, and young adults having sport-related injuries. Although the head trauma risk of hitting a wall is unknown, the potential for CSDH formation increases in the presence of an underlying AC [21]. Based on the literature, CSDH formed with an AC due to taekwondo sports and in addition to soccer [22]. CSDH risk is higher especially in temporal fossa located ACs [11]. Clinical findings generally occur due to an intracranial pressure increase and it has nonspecific symptoms such as headache, vomiting, and hemiparesis [27].

Drainage through a burr hole is generally applied for the treatment in symptomatic cases. The surgical decision is not independent from its relationship with AC and changes according to lesion characteristics [13]. AC membrane resection is not compulsory for patients with asymptomatic AC during surgery [33].

ACs are clear, colorless, and fluid-filled cysts forming through arachnoid mater division and emerge during brain development. CSDH is generally a completely liquified old blood collection present between the dura mater and arachnoid mater. In addition to spontaneous formation, trauma also constitutes an important reason for CSDH formation.

The AC and CSDH relationship and the natural course of the disease have not been completely clarified. ACs which are generally asymptomatic may become symptomatic following cyst growth and cyst rupture related to subdural effusion or subdural bleeding. Bleeding accompanying the cyst results due to sport-related head trauma in young patients and spontaneous bleeding is quite rare. Weak leptomeningeal and bridging veins inside the cyst or on the cyst wall tear and cause subdural bleeding. Severe membranous adhesions and brain compliance decrease are the predisposing factors in subdural bleeding formation [14].

AC rupture related bleeding at a distance from the subdural may occur spontaneously due to minor head trauma or without trauma. Because of a closed system valve mechanism, the fluid cannot return inside the cyst and accumulates distant from the subdural [11]. Another hypothesis claims that CSF passes into the arachnoid space from the distant subarachnoid space after the trauma and tears the cyst wall through increasing intracystic pressure and the intracystic fluid passes into the distant subdural. Spontaneous or post-traumatic rupture of ACs distant to the subdural was reported. The clinical condition is again an important factor leading to the decision whether to wait for the spontaneous resolution of the resulting hygroma or whether to proceed surgically with drainage [13].

AC rupture may occur spontaneously. Afterwards the cyst membrane weakly bonds to the convex dura. Mechanical forces develop during head trauma that cause the separation of the cyst membrane from the dura and may cause bleeding. The parietal cyst membrane covers the region where the sylvian veins cause bleeding and form the bridging structure that enters the dural venous sinuses behind the sphenoid ridge. Even moderate manipulation of the parietal membrane may damage these veins and cause bleeding into subdural space [8, 10].

Although AC-related CSDH is quite rare, most of these patients were treated through surgery. AC rupture may cause sudden life-threatening symptoms. Thus, the risk of rupturing the cyst should be considered especially in the presence of any dimensional change [10]. Treatment method for the CSDH and intracystic bleedings that result from AC complications differ. The surgical approach is generally preferred for these complications. It was reported in the literature that the cysts following trauma or their spontaneous rupture and the cyst rupture related to bleeding resolve without any surgical intervention [13].

Different AC-related CSDH treatment methods are available. Parsch et al. treated 13 out of 16 patients with AC secondary CSDH and hygroma patients by draining the fluid at the distant subdural without any intervention on the cyst and radiologically followed up the previously asymptomatic ACs [26]. AC excision following hematoma discharge, clearing the adhesions between the subarachnoid membrane and cyst wall, cyst subarachnoid and distant subdural fenestration constitute a more commonly applied treatment method. Another treatment method is the surgical placement of a shunt. James et al. stated that the shunt is not only less invasive but also an operation allowing the cyst to constrict and parenchymal tissue expansion [18]. Lesoin et al. placed shunts in five out of seven head trauma patients with AC [23]. Kulali and von Wild treated a patient who had a head trauma a month ago and had headache, nausea, and vomiting complaints through a subdural-peritoneal shunt insertion [21]. When fenestration of an AC through opening it is compared to subdural peritoneal shunt, it was shown that this operation has high mortality (1%) and a high complication rate (morbidity 10–15%). But the repeat intervention rate is much lower than that for the shunt [13, 24, 29].

Although both lesions were anatomically septated and divided, the radiological imaging findings had similar signal intensity. CSDH can infiltrate into the AC and the fluid change can be observed through micro transitions. This mechanism may explain the reason behind CSF accumulation in the area where the hematoma is reabsorbed in the postoperative period. Since complication prevalence is higher in craniotomy performance compared to trephination among surgical methods, trephination should be the first option for the treatment of CSDH coexisting with AC [7].

23.5 Conclusion

Even though CSDH is generally observed in elderly people, it is more common in young people in the presence of AC. The importance of CT for arachnoid cyst and for CSDH diagnosis should be emphasized. Although AC-related CSDH pathogenesis has not been clearly explained, it is considered to be related to CSF collection in the distant subdural. Clinical findings change based on the bleeding and cyst location. CT is used for diagnosis regardless of AC. MR can be used for postoperative patient follow-up. Hematoma drainage through a burr hole is generally adequate for surgical treatment if the patient has clinical findings. As a result, clinical findings and surgical treatment methods are determined based on the CSDH in the patients, regardless of the etiology.

References

1. Aleman J, Jokura H, Higano S, Akabane A, Shirane R, Yoshimoto T. Value of constructive interference in steady-state three-dimensional, Fourier transformation magnetic resonance imaging for the neuroendoscopic treatment of hydrocephalus and intracranial cysts. Neurosurgery. 2001;48:1291–5.
2. Bostantjopoulou S, Katsarou Z, Michael M, Petridis A. Reversible parkinsonism due to chronic bilateral subdural hematomas. J Clin Neurosci. 2009;16(3):458–60.
3. Brackett CE, Rengachary SS. Arachnoid cysts. Youmans JR (ed), Neurological surgery, Philadelphia: WB Saunders, 1982;3(2)1436–1446.

4. Cagnoni G, Fonda C, Pancani S, Pampaloni A, Mugnaini L. Intracranial arachnoid cysts in pediatric age. Pediatr Med Chir. 1996;18:85–90.
5. Cokluk C, Senel A, Celik F, Ergur H. Spontaneous disappearance of two asymptomatic arachnoid cysts in two different locations. Minim Invasive Neurosurg. 2003;46(2):110–2.
6. Dammers R, ter Laak-Poort MP, Maas AI. Neurological picture. Armoured brain: case report of a symptomatic calcified chronic subdural haematoma. J Neurol Neurosurg Psychiatry. 2007;78:542–3.
7. Duz B, Kaya S, Daneyemez M, Gonul E. Surgical management strategies of intracranial arachnoid cysts: a single institution experience of 75 cases. Turk Neurosurg. 2012;22:591–8.
8. Fewel ME, Levy ML, McComb JG. Surgical treatment of 95 children with 102 intracranial arachnoid cysts. Pediatr Neurosurg. 1996;25:165–73.
9. Galassi E, Tognetti F, Gaist G, et al. CT scan and metrizamide CT cisternography in arachnoid cysts of the middle cranial fossa: classification and pathophysiological aspects. Surg Neurol. 1982;17(5):363–9.
10. Gelabert-González M, Iglesias-Pais M, García-Allut A, Martínez-Rumbo R. Chronic subdural haematoma: surgical treatment and outcome in 1000 cases. Clin Neurol Neurosurg. 2005;107:223–9. https://doi.org/10.1016/j.clineuro.2004.09.015.
11. Gelabert-González M, Castro-Bouzas D, Arcos-Algaba A, Santín-Amo JM, Díaz-Cabanas L, Serramito-García R, Arán-Echabe E, Prieto-González A, García-Allut A. Hematoma subdural crónico asociado a quiste aracnoideo. Presentación de 12 casos [Chronic subdural hematoma associated with arachnoid cyst. Report of 12 cases]. Neurocirugia (Astur). 2010;21(3):222–7.
12. Goldhahn R. Uber ein grosso-es, operativ entfernte s, verkaklktes, intra-kranielles Hamatom. Dtsch Z Chir. 1930;224:323–31.
13. Gregori F, Colistra D, Mancarella C, Chiarella V, Marotta N, Domenicucci M. Arachnoid cyst in young soccer players complicated by chronic subdural hematoma: personal experience and review of the literature. Acta Neurol Belg. 2020;120(2):235–46. https://doi.org/10.1007/s13760-019-01224-1.
14. Harding BN, Copp AJ. Malformations. In: Graham DI, Lantos PL, editors. Greenfield's neuropathology. 7th ed. New York: Oxford University Press; 2002. p. 451–2.
15. He XS, Zhang X. Giant calcified chronic subdural hematoma: a long term complication of shunt hydrocephalus. J Neurol Neurosurg Psychiatry. 2005;76:367.
16. Huang KT, Bi WL, Abd-El-Barr M, et al. The neurocritical and neurosurgical care of subdural hematomas. Neurocrit Care. 2016;24:294–307. https://doi.org/10.1007/s12028-015-0194-x.
17. Iorio-Morin C, Touchette C, Lévesque M, et al. Chronic subdural hematoma: toward a new management paradigm for an increasingly complex population. J Neurotrauma. 2018;35:1882–5. https://doi.org/10.1089/neu.2018.5872.
18. James HE. Encephalocele, dermoid sinus and arachnoid cyst. Pediatr Neurosurg. 1989:97–106.
19. Kavcic A, Meglic B, Meglic NP, Vodusek DB, Mesec A. Asymptomatic huge calcified subdural hematoma in a patient on oral anticoagulant therapy. Neurology. 2006;66:758.
20. Kertmen H, Gürer B, Yilmaz ER, Sekerci Z. Chronic subdural hematoma associated with an arachnoid cyst in a juvenile taekwondo athlete: a case report and review of the literature. Pediatr Neurosurg. 2012;48(1):55–8. https://doi.org/10.1159/000339354. Epub 2012 Jul 21. PMID: 22832284.
21. Kulali A, von Wild K. Post-traumatic subdural hygroma as a complication of arachnoid cysts of the middle fossa. Neurosurg Rev. 1989;12(Suppl):508–13.
22. Lee JK, Choi JH, Kim CH, Lee HK, Moon JG. Chronic subdural hematomas: a comparative study of three types of operative procedures. J Korean Neurosurg Soc. 2009;46:210–4. https://doi.org/10.3340/jkns.2009.46.3.210.
23. Lesoin F, Dhellemmes P, Rousseaux M, Jomin M. Arachnoid cysts and head injury. Acta Neurochir (Wien). 1983;69:43–51.
24. Markwalder TM. Chronic subdural haematomas: a review. J Neurosurg. 1981;54:637–45.
25. Okada Y, Akai T, Okamoto K, Iida T, Takata H, Iizuka H. A comparative study of the treatment of chronic subdural hematoma—burr hole drainage versus burr hole irrigation. Surg Neurol. 2002;57:405–9. https://doi.org/10.1016/S0090-3019(02)00720-6.

26. Parsch CS, Krauss J, Hofmann E, Meixensberger J, Roosen K. Arachnoid cysts associated with subdural hematomas and hygromas: analysis of 16 cases, long-term follow-up, and review of the literature. Neurosurgery. 1997;40:483–90. PubMed: 9055286.
27. Prabhu VC, Bailes JE. Chronic subdural hematoma complicating arachnoid cyst secondary to soccer-related head injury: case report. Neurosurgery. 2002;50(1):195–7; discussion 197–8. https://doi.org/10.1097/00006123-200201000-00029. PMID: 11844251.
28. Stanisic M, Lund-Johansen M, Mahesparan R. Treatment of chronic subdural hematoma by burr-hole craniostomy in adults: influence of some factors on postoperative recurrence. Acta Neurochir (Wien). 2005;147(12):1249–56; discussion 1256–7. https://doi.org/10.1007/s00701-005-0616-1. Epub 2005 Aug 29. PMID: 16133770.
29. Tabaddor K, Shulmon K. Definitive treatment of chronic subdural hematoma by twist-drill craniostomy and closed-system drainage. J Neurosurg. 1977;46:220–6. https://doi.org/10.3171/jns.1977.46.2.0220.
30. von Rokitansky C. Handbuch der pathologischen anatomie. Cilt:2 Vienna: Braunmuller and Scidel; 1844. p. 717.
31. Wright DW, Merck LH. Head trauma in adults and children. In: Tintinalli JE, Stapczynski JS, Ma OJ, Cline DM, Cydulka RK, Meckler GD, editors. Tintinalli's emergency medicine, vol. 7. New York: McGraw Hill; 2011. p. 1692–708.
32. Wu X, Li G, Zhao J, Zhu X, Zhang Y, Hou K. Arachnoid cyst-associated chronic subdural hematoma: report of 14 cases and a systematic literature review. World Neurosurg. 2018;109:118–30. https://doi.org/10.1016/j.wneu.2017.09.115. Epub 2017 Sep 28. PMID: 28962953.
33. Yang W, Huang J. Chronic subdural hematoma epidemiology and natural history. Neurosurg Clin N Am. 2017;28:205–10. https://doi.org/10.1016/j.nec.2016;11:002.
34. Yoshimoto Y, Kwak S. Frontal small craniostomy and irrigation for treatment of chronic subdural haematoma. Br J Neurosurg. 1997;11:150–1. https://doi.org/10.1080/02688699746519.

Chapter 24
Rare Intracranial Locations of Chronic Subdural Hematoma

Kossi Kouma Félix Segbedgi, Gbetoho Fortuné Gankpe, and Mohammed Benzagmout

24.1 Introduction

Chronic subdural hematoma (CSDH) represents an encapsulated collection of blood and fluid, encysted between the dura mater and the arachnoid. This entity develops over the course of 3 or more weeks. The membranes surrounding the hematoma were identified as a source of fluid exudation and continued hemorrhage. Indeed, angiogenic stimuli lead to the formation of fragile blood vessels within the membrane walls while fibrinolytic processes prevent clot formation [9, 30]. An abundance of inflammatory cells and markers have been identified within the hematoma membranes and subdural fluid [2, 9, 10]. They are likely to contribute to spreading the inflammatory response which stimulates further ongoing membrane growth and fluid accumulation.

CSDH is usually located supratentorially, over the cortical convexity [39]. However, uncommon locations are also reported, especially in the posterior fossa, interhemispheric space, and even in the spinal canal. The aim of this paper is to focus on the clinical and radiological features of these rare intracranial locations of CSDH, and to discuss their appropriate management.

K. K. F. Segbedgi
Department of Neurosurgery, University Hospital of Fez, Fez, Morocco

G. F. Gankpe
Neurosurgery Department, Regional University Hospital Abomey Calavi, Ouidah, Benin

M. Benzagmout (✉)
Department of Neurosurgery, University Hospital of Fez, Fez, Morocco

Clinical Neurosciences Laboratory, Sidi Mohammed Benabdellah University Fez, Fez, Morocco

M. Turgut et al. (eds.), *Subdural Hematoma*,
https://doi.org/10.1007/978-3-030-79371-5_24

24.2 Posterior Fossa CSDH

24.2.1 Etiology

Posterior fossa CSDH (pCSH) is extremely rare [6, 22, 28]. The pathogenesis of pCSH is poorly elucidated [7]. A history of head trauma is often missing [14]. However, a wall injury of occipital, sigmoid, and transverse sinuses; injury of cerebellar veins or some relatively large emissary veins; coagulation disorders, anticoagulation/antiplatelet therapy; posterior fossa surgery, arachnoid cysts, and intracranial hypotension were all suggested in the pathophysiology of this particular location [7, 32, 40, 41].

24.2.2 Clinical Manifestations

The clinical diagnosis of pCSH is challenging because the clinical manifestations are miscellaneous [7]. They include headache, nausea, vomiting, dizziness, altered consciousness, limb ataxia, and gait disturbance [42]. In some cases, the presenting symptoms may suggest posterior fossa lesions, especially cerebellar symptoms, cranial nerve dysfunction, vertigo, and nystagmus [17, 29, 40].

It is important to note that associated hydrocephalus may suddenly cause deterioration in the neurological status of the patient, leading to death by brainstem compression before a correct diagnosis is made [7, 18, 40].

24.2.3 Radiological Features

The CT scan reveals generally a low to high density area in the posterior fossa subdural space. However, this imaging modality is inappropriate for the radiological exploration of the posterior fossa space-occupying lesions because of bony artifacts, rendering difficult the evaluation for subdural hematoma and the possible underlying causes as well [6, 7, 18, 32, 40].

Magnetic resonance imaging (MRI) represents the exam of choice. This study demonstrates the subdural collection as hypo- to hyperintense on T1-weighted images, and hyperintense on T2-weighted images (Fig. 24.1). Izumihara et al. [18] have illustrated the first case of pCSH diagnosed by MRI in the literature. Preoperative cerebral angiography is not mandatory. Nevertheless, it can be an important contribution in assessing the sinuses, emissary veins, and other underlying vascular structures.

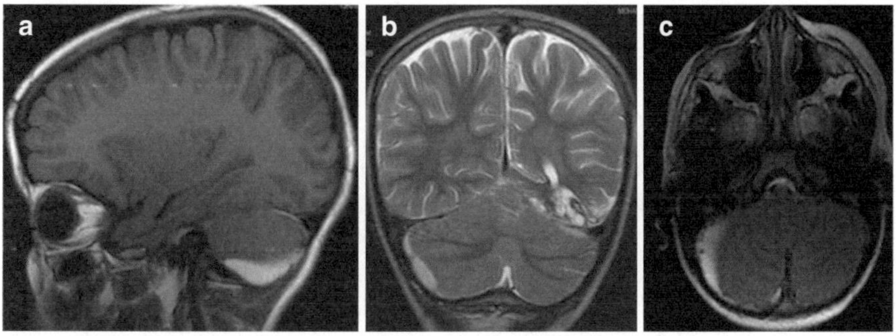

Fig. 24.1 Brain MRI on sagittal non-contrast T1 (**a**), coronal T2 (**b**) and perfusion axial sequence (**c**) demonstrating a posterior fossa CSDH over the right cerebellar hemisphere

24.2.4 Management

Symptomatic patients will usually undergo surgery. Surgical techniques include lateral subdural craniotomy, small craniectomy, and burr-hole craniostomy. The patient is generally operated on in the prone position under local or general anesthesia [14].

Since most cases of pCSH have coagulation disorders, minimally invasive burr-hole surgery under local anesthesia would be appropriate, even for the bilateral cases [14]. However, it will be difficult to manage intraoperative excessive bleeding from sinus injury through a simple burr hole [14]. Hence, the choice of craniectomy must be discussed because the allowed operative field is sufficiently large to address any encountered bleeding [42]. A subdural drain may be placed at surgery and removed within the first 48 h [42, 44].

Bilateral pCSH might be evacuated with two burr holes, one on each side, through a midline sub-occipital approach in the prone position [22, 32, 40]. Nevertheless, Inoue et al. have suggested placing a single burr hole near the transverse-sigmoid sinus junction to evacuate bilateral pCSH because of the presence of a connection between the two hematoma sides [14].

Posterior fossa CSDH associated to obstructive hydrocephalus remains a life-threatening emergency; therefore, early management is highly recommended [14]. Hematoma evacuation leads generally to the disappearance of the associated hydrocephalus [3, 4, 14, 40]; otherwise, it requires ventricular shunting [23, 32].

In cases of asymptomatic or mildly symptomatic pCSH with no associated hydrocephalus, conservative treatment can lead to a good clinical outcome [18, 23, 41]. Furthermore, conservative treatment may be a reasonable therapeutic alternative in those patients presenting with coagulation/hemostasis disturbances [41]. Surgery under the influence of anticoagulant therapy and thrombocytopenia carries high perioperative risks. For such cases, platelet infusion and discontinuation of anticoagulants are considered to be effective at least for a short period; the hematoma resolved spontaneously within a period of 2 weeks to 2 months and patients showed good neurological recovery [41].

24.3 Interhemispheric CSDH

24.3.1 Etiology

The interhemispheric location of CSDH is uncommon. First described by Aring and Evans [3], interhemispheric CSDH (ICSH) is extremely rare, representing roughly 0.4% of all chronic subdural hematomas [36]. In most cases, the ICSH is usually unilateral and the main etiology is head trauma [5]. Other causes of ICSH include coagulopathy, aneurysm rupture, and spontaneous hypertensive cerebral hemorrhage which lead to a chronic hematoma with increasing thickness [16, 25]. The origin of ICSH is variable, including the bridging veins of the interhemispheric fissure, branches of the pericallosal artery or a brain laceration in the interhemispheric fissure [43].

24.3.2 Clinical Manifestations

Neurological symptoms are reliant on several factors, including the clinical course of the disease, age of the patient, thickness of the interhemispheric collection, and the anatomic location of the lesion [33]. Generally, the clinical presentation of ICSH is characterized by headaches, epileptic seizures associated with the classic falx syndrome defined as contralateral hemiparesis most marked in the lower limb [5, 24, 31].

24.3.3 Radiological Features

The computed tomography (CT) scan represents the neuroimaging modality of choice to diagnose ICSDH. The classic description of a low-density extra-axial collection close to the brain cortex surface applies also for ICSDH (Fig. 24.2). In addition, the CT scan allows for determining the size of the hematoma, its thickness, anterior-to-posterior location, and whether there are other associated lesions. In some cases, MRI might be useful in the preoperative planning for accurate localization of the bridging veins to guide the optimal placement of the craniotomy [34].

ICSH is located in the interhemispheric fissure, just beneath the superior sagittal sinus. It is more common in the posterior part of the falx than in the anterior part due to the gravity [1]. The ICSDH can be isolated [21, 34, 37] or associated with a convexity CSDH [13, 26, 34]. This association occurs after hematoma liquefaction and migration, and might be considered as the resorption mode of the ICSDH [11, 13, 15, 31].

The hematoma is usually confined to one side of the interhemispheric fissure [34]. However, bilateral ICSDH have also been reported [8, 19, 46]. The shape of the interhemispheric hematoma is characteristic with a convex lateral and straight medial margin [46].

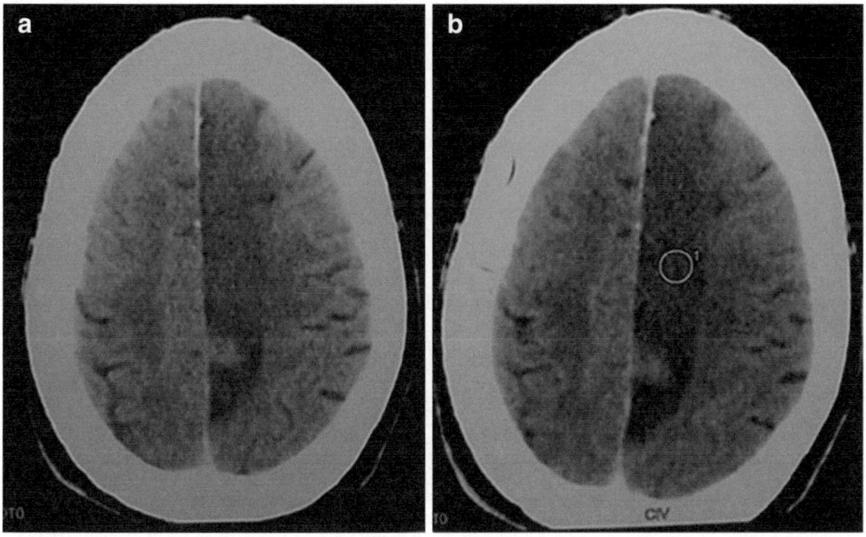

Fig. 24.2 Cerebral CT scan in the axial plane before (**a**) and after (**b**) contrast showing a left interhemispheric CSDH

24.3.4 Management

Treatment options available for ICSDH are parasagittal craniotomy, small unilateral craniotomy or trephine, burr-hole irrigation and drainage, twist-drill craniostomy, and non-surgical treatment [34].

Surgery is indicated in clinically symptomatic ICSDH that remains confined to the interhemispheric fissure [34]. ICSDH may be treated by trepanation above or near the interhemispheric fissure [12]. However, the anatomic location just beneath the superior sagittal sinus makes minor and straight forward approaches, such as burr-hole or twist-drill craniostomy, potentially hazardous.

In addition, surgical evacuation of ICSDH can be performed via craniotomy [20, 33, 38]. A well-placed paramedian bone flap or trephination is performed under general anesthesia. The medial edge of the craniotomy must be close to the midline to allow easy exploration of the interhemispheric region with minimal retraction on the inner surface of the brain cortex. A flexible catheter may be used to wash out the interhemispheric hematoma using physiologic saline [34]. In case there are significant membranes and lobulations inside the hematoma, a large anteroposterior craniotomy might be necessary. Moreover, endoscopy could be an appropriate associated technique [34]. It allows for the cutting of different septa inside the hematoma cavity, fenestrating the internal membrane, and coagulating eventual neovessels [27, 45].

Interestingly, convexity burr-hole washout procedures have been reported to indirectly decompress an ICSDH in cases where it was associated with a concomitant convexity hematoma [13].

Conservative management is recommended for patients without disturbed sensory or significant motor deficit who remain clinically stable while under close observation. This strategy was already proposed for some cases of interhemispheric CSDH with good clinical outcomes [21, 35].

24.4 Conclusion

Intracranial CSDH is usually located in the supratentorial space, over the cortical convexity. The interhemispheric and posterior fossa locations of CSDH are extremely rare. Clinical manifestations are various, and the radiological diagnosis is often made using the CT scan in ICSDH and MRI in pCSH. Currently, the optimal treatment for these unusual CSDH locations remains controversial because of the relative paucity of cases and the lack of general guidelines. Conservative management is discussed for asymptomatic or clinically stable patients provided with close follow-up. However, early surgical decompression should be indicated in patients presenting with marked neurologic compromise or neurologic deterioration, especially in their level of consciousness.

References

1. Ahn JM, Lee KS, Shim JH, Oh JS, Shim JJ, Yoon SM. Clinical features of interhemispheric subdural hematomas. Korean J Neurotrauma. 2017;13:103–7.
2. Aoyama M, Osuka K, Usuda N, Watanabe Y, Kawaguchi R, Nakura T, Takayasu M. Expression of mitogen-activated protein kinases in chronic subdural hematoma outer membranes. J Neurotrauma. 2015;32:1064–70.
3. Aring C, Evans JP. Aberrant location of subdural hematoma. Arch Neurol Psychiatr (Chicago). 1940;4:1296–306.
4. Ashkenazi E, Pomeranz S. Nystagmus as the presentation of tentorial incisure subdural haematoma. J Neurol Neurosurg Psychiatry. 1994;57:830–1.
5. Bartels RH, Verhagen WI, Prick MJ, Dalman JE. Interhemispheric subdural hematoma in adults: case reports and a review of the literature. Neurosurgery. 1995;36:1210–4.
6. Berhouma M, Houissa S, Jemel H, Khaldi M. Spontaneous chronic subdural hematoma of the posterior fossa. J Neuroradiol. 2007;34:213–5.
7. Costa LB Jr, de Andrade A, Valadão GF. Chronic subdural hematoma of the posterior fossa associated with cerebellar hemorrhage: report of rare disease with MRI findings. Arq Neuropsiquiatr. 2004;62:170–2.
8. Cronin TG, Shippey DU. Bilateral interhemispheric subdural hematoma: a case report. Am J Neuroradiol. 1987;8:909–10.
9. Edlmann E, Giorgi-Coll S, Whitfield PC, Carpenter KLH, Hutchinson PJ. Pathophysiology of chronic subdural haematoma: inflammation, angiogenesis and implications for pharmacotherapy. J Neuroinflammation. 2017;14:108.
10. Fedorko S, Walter J, Younsi A, Zweckberger K, Unterberg AW, Beynon C. Intraoperative point-of-care assessment of an inflammatory biomarker in chronic subdural hematomas: technical note. Clin Neurol Neurosurg. 2019;183:105396.
11. Fruin AH, Juhl GL, Taylon C. Interhemispheric subdural hematoma. Case report. J Neurosurg. 1984;60:1300–2.

12. Ho SU, Spehlmann R, Ho HT. CT scan in interhemispheric subdural hematoma. Clinical and pathological correlation. Neurology. 1977;27:1097–8.
13. Houtteville JP, Toumi K, Theron J, Derlon JM, Benazza A, Hubert P. Interhemispheric subdural haematomas: seven cases and review of the literature. Br J Neurosurg. 1988;2:357–67.
14. Inoue T, Hirai H, Shima A, Suzuki F, Matsuda M. Bilateral chronic subdural hematoma in the posterior fossa treated with a burr hole irrigation: a case report and review of the literature. Case Rep Neurol. 2019;11:87–93.
15. Iplikçioğlu AC, Bayar MA, Kökes F, Doğanay S, Gökçek C. Interhemispheric subdural hematomas. Br J Neurosurg. 1994;8:627–31.
16. Ishikawa E, Sugimoto K, Yanaka K, et al. Interhemispheric subdural hematoma caused by a ruptured internal carotid artery aneurysm: case report. Surg Neurol. 2000;54:82–6.
17. Isla A, Alvarez F, Manrique M, Castro A, Amaya C, Blázquez MG. Posterior fossa subdural hematoma. J Neurosurg Sci. 1987;31:67–9.
18. Izumihara A, Orita T, Kajiwara K, Tsurutani T. Simultaneous supra-and infratentorial chronic subdural hematoma. Eur J Radiol. 1993;16:183–5.
19. Kasdon DL, Magruder MR, Stevens EA, Paullus WS Jr. Bilateral interhemispheric subdural hematomas. Neurosurgery. 1979;5:57–9.
20. Koyama S, Nishimura T. A case of bilateral interhemispheric subdural hematoma. No Shinkei Geka. 1990;18:289–94.
21. Kuk-Jin L, Eun-Jeong K, Ha-Young C. Interhemispheric chronic subdural hematoma showing falx syndrome—case report. J Korean Neurosurg Soc. 2002;32:268–71.
22. Kurisu K, Kawabori M, Niiya Y, Ohta Y, Mabuchi S, Houkin K. Bilateral chronic subdural hematomas of the posterior fossa. Neurol Med Chir. 2012;52:822–5.
23. Lagares A, Domínguez J, Lobato RD, González P. Bilateral posterior fossa subdural hematomas secondary to anticoagulant therapy. Acta Neurochir. 1998;140:1097–8.
24. Lang EW, Hohenstein C, Nabavi A, Mehdorn HM. Interhemispheric subdural hematoma. Nervenarzt. 1998;69:342–5.
25. Marinelli L, Parodi RC, Renzetti P, Bandini F. Interhemispheric subdural haematoma from ruptured aneurysm: a case report. J Neurol. 2005;252:364–6.
26. Minami M, Hanakita J, Suwa H, Suzui H, Fujita K, Nakamura T. Interhemispheric chronic subdural hematoma-case report. Neurol Med Chir. 1997;37:177–80.
27. Mobbs R, Khong P. Endoscopic-assisted evacuation of subdural collections. J Clin Neurosci. 2009;16:701–4.
28. Mochizuki Y, Kobayashi T, Kawashima A, Funatsu T, Kawamata T. Chronic subdural hematoma of the posterior fossa treated by suboccipital craniotomy. Surg Neurol Int. 2018;9:20.
29. Murthy VS, Deshpande DH, Narayana-Reddy GN. Chronic subdural hematoma in the cerebellopontine angle. Surg Neurol. 1980;14:227–9.
30. Nomura S, Kashiwagi S, Fujisawa H, Ito H, Nakamura K. Characterization of local hyperfibrinolysis in chronic subdural hematomas by SDS-PAGE and immunoblot. J Neurosurg. 1994;81:910–3.
31. Ogsbury JS, Schneck SA, Lehman RA. Aspects of interhemispheric subdural haematoma, including the falx syndrome. J Neurol Neurosurg Psychiatry. 1978;41:72–5.
32. Pollo C, Meuli R, Porchet F. Spontaneous bilateral subdural hematomas in the posterior cranial fossa revealed by MRI. Neuroradiology. 2003;45:550–2.
33. Requejo PR, Vaitsman RP, Paiva MS, Machado AL, Barroso MV, Salame JM, Louzada PR. Interhemispheric chronic subdural haematoma: case report and brief review of the literature. Brain Inj. 2010;24:1039–43.
34. Sadrolhefazi A, Bloomfield SM. Interhemispheric and bilateral chronic subdural hematoma. Neurosurg Clin N Am. 2000;11:455–63.
35. Sakashita Y, Kuzuhara S, Fuse S, Yamanouchi H, Toyokura Y. Interhemispheric subdural hematoma complicated by chronic neurologic diseases: report of two cases diagnosed by CT scan. Rinsho Shinkeigaku. 1987;27:31–7.
36. Sambasivan M. An overview of chronic subdural hematoma: experience with 2300 cases. Surg Neurol. 1997;47:418–22.

37. Shankar A, Joseph M, Chandy MJ. Interhemispheric subdural hematoma: an uncommon sequel of trauma. Neurol India. 2003;51:63–4.
38. Sibayan RQ, Gurdjian ES, Thomas LM. Interhemispheric chronic subdural hematoma. Report of a case. Neurology. 1970;20:1215–8.
39. Sikahall-Meneses E, Salazar-Pérez N, Sandoval-Bonilla B. Chronic subdural hematoma: surgical management in 100 patients. Cir Cir. 2008;76:199–203.
40. Stendel R, Schulte T, Pietilä TA, Suess O, Brock M. Spontaneous bilateral chronic subdural haematoma of the posterior fossa. Case report and review of the literature. Acta Neurochir. 2002;144:497–500.
41. Takami H, Oshiro N, Hiraoka F, Murao M, Ide T. Rapid resolution of a spontaneous large chronic subdural hematoma in the posterior fossa under conservative treatment with platelet administration to aplastic anemia. Clin Neurol Neurosurg. 2013;115:2236–9.
42. Takemoto Y, Matsumoto J, Ohta K, Hasegawa S, Miura M, Kuratsu J. Bilateral posterior fossa chronic subdural hematoma treated with craniectomy: case report and review of the literature. Surg Neurol Int. 2016;7:S255–8.
43. Wang Y, Wang C, Cai S, Dong J, Yang L, Chen L, Maas A. Surgical management of traumatic interhemispheric subdural hematoma. Turk Neurosurg. 2014;24:228–33.
44. Weigel R, Krauss JK, Schmiedek P. Concepts of neurosurgical management of chronic subdural haematoma: historical perspectives. Br J Neurosurg. 2004;18:8–18.
45. Yan K, Gao H, Wang Q, et al. Endoscopic surgery to chronic subdural hematoma with neovessel septation: technical notes and literature review. Neurol Res. 2016;38:467–76.
46. Zimmerman RD, Russell EJ, Yurberg E, Leeds NE. Falx and interhemispheric fissure on axial CT: II. Recognition and differentiation of interhemispheric subarachnoid and subdural hemorrhage. Am J Neuroradiol. 1982;3:635–42.

Chapter 25
Chronic Subdural Hematoma Related to Sport Head Injury

Hassan Baallal, Hatim Belfquih, and Ali Akhaddar

25.1 Introduction

Sports activities have become very important and have a large following in modern societies, mainly due to their health benefits and the popularity of some sports. However, sports injuries are among the most common injuries in Western societies [55]. Sports-related chronic subdural hematomas are known to occur as a result of ball games, bicycle sports, snowboarding, race walking, and roller coasters. All these sports cause chronic subdural hematoma (CSDH) related to head trauma. Intracranial hemorrhage is a rare but potentially devastating condition affecting athletes. Although injuries to the upper and lower extremities are the most common in sports, head injuries can have devastating neurological consequences and are potentially fatal. Subdural hematomas develop over hours and days following impact and are a leading cause of death and morbidity in athletes [11]. Mortality rates have been reported as high as 90% when not recognized and treated promptly [69]. Nevertheless, subdural hematoma (SDH) is the most common cause of death and severe disability among sports-related head injuries [40, 50].

In general, SDH is classified by the lapse of time from the initial head trauma to when symptoms first appear as either an acute subdural hematoma if it occurs within 48–72 h, or a subacute hematoma if it occurs 3–20 days after the initial trauma, or as a chronic hematoma if it occurs three or more weeks after the initial trauma. The time interval until the first symptom appears increases as the age of the patient increases because the hematoma accumulates until the symptoms are clearly identified due to cerebral atrophy.

H. Baallal (✉) · H. Belfquih
Department of Neurosurgery, Avicenne Military Hospital of Marrakech, Marrakech, Morocco

A. Akhaddar
Avicenne Military Hospital of Marrakech, Department of Neurosurgery, Mohammed V University in Rabat, Rabat, Morocco

M. Turgut et al. (eds.), *Subdural Hematoma*,
https://doi.org/10.1007/978-3-030-79371-5_25

CSDH is a commonly encountered entity in neurosurgical practice. It is defined as a collection of blood overlying the surface of the brain which is diagnosed on cranial imaging as a predominantly hypodense or isodense collection in the subdural space on computed tomography (CT) [68].

This study analyzed the clinical features of 66 sport-related cases of CSDH across 52 studies in order to provide a quantitative analysis.

25.2 Literature Review

A comprehensive search of PubMed/MEDLINE, Google scholar EMBASE, and Cochrane Library databases was performed from the year 1950 through March 1, 2020, including all case reports, case series, images or pictures, original articles, technical notes, conference proceedings, and letters to editors reporting cases of sport players developing CSDH. Our search strategy consisted of the following key terms: CSDH in athletic, mild traumatic brain injury after sport, as well as their subject-related synonyms to examine the literature for all possible papers discussing sports and CSDH.

The aim of this study was to summarize all sport-related cases of CSDH and to provide a quantitative analysis. For each case, we analyzed age, sex, sport activity practiced, delay between sport activity and diagnosis, symptoms, brain imaging, treatment performed, the outcome, and evolution, and all data has been summarized in Table 25.1.

25.3 Epidemiology

SDHs are classified as chronic when the initial hemorrhage produces no clinical signs or symptoms for 3 weeks or longer.

CSDH is generally believed to occur in elderly patients, occasionally in pediatric or young patients with certain predisposing factors. Its overall incidence is about 5/100,000/year in the general population [68] and at least 8.2/100,000/year in the population over 70 years of age [1]. In our research we analyzed a total of 66 cases that were found across 52 studies, dating back to 1950; 53 cases (80.3%) were males and 13 cases (19.7%) were females. The mean age was 24.51 years (range, 6–75 years). The most represented sport was soccer, with 16 cases (24.2%). Other sports activities included roller-coaster riding, generic sport/physical training/activity, and bicycle riding in six cases (9%) each. Basketball and martial arts had five cases (7.5%) each. Other cases were reported in the following sport activities: water skiing, rugby, football, judo, taekwondo, breakdance, and volleyball. All data has been summarized in Table 25.2.

In our study, the male-to-female ratio was 10:1.91, suggesting that male predominance is an obvious tendency in young patients with CSDH. 13 of the 66

Table 25.1 Summary of the analyzed data of 66 cases

First author [ref]	Publication year	Age (yrs)/sex	antecedent	Sport	Interval from trauma to diagnostic	Symptoms	Imaging findings	Treatment	Outcome
Oliver [52]	1958	21/M	WA	Soccer	12 W	Headache vomiting and diplopia	Electroencephalography suggested a lesion in the left parietal lobe, but ventriculography showed displacement of the ventricles to the left	Open craniotomy	Uneventful recovery
Weinberg [83]	1973	20/M	NR	Martial arts	NR	Headache	A left carotid angiogram: presence of a subdural hematoma in the convexity regions	Burr hole; open craniotomy	NR
Lacour [38]	1978	13/F	WA	Water skiing	2 m	Bifrontal headaches with vomiting	CT scan: right isodense SDH	Burr holes	Uneventful recovery
Varma [81]	1981	17/M	WA	Rugby football	5 W	Frontal headache	Carotid angiogram showed evidence of a right-sided extracerebral collection	Temporal craniotomy	Uneventful recovery
Hara [27]	1984	13/M	WA	Bicycle	SW	Headache and nausea	CT scan: large low-density area in the right frontotemporal region,	Frontotemporal craniotomy	Uneventful recovery
McNeil [46]	1987	17/M	WA	Break dancing with basketball	3 m	Headache	CT scan: isodense SDH	Temporal craniotomy	Uneventful recovery
Page [53]	1987	57/M	WA	Equestrian	NR	Headache, nausea	CT scan: left isodense SDH	Craniotomy	NR

(continued)

Table 25.1 (continued)

First author [ref]	Publication year	Age (yrs)/ sex	antecedent	Sport	Interval from trauma to diagnostic	Symptoms	Imaging findings	Treatment	Outcome
Yokoyama [86]	1989	17/M	AC	Judo	2 m	Headache and nausea	CT scan: hypodense SDH	Two burr holes	NR
Rogers [66]	1990	11/M	WA	Bicycle	1 m	Headache, diplopia, vomiting	CT scan: right hypodense SDH	Two burr holes	NR
Rogers [66]	1990	10/F	AC	Basketball	3 W	Headache, diplopia	CT scan: Left hypodense SDH	Two burr holes	NR
Maeda [42]	1993	14/M	WA	Soccer	2 m	Headache	CT scan: left isodense SDH	Temporal craniotomy	Clinical recovery was complete
Fernandes [21]	1994	26/M	WA	Roller coaster	NR	Headache	CT scan: bilateral chronic SDH	Two burr holes	NR
Ochi [51]	1995	11/M	AC	Physical training.	3 m	Headache and vomiting	Convexity hematoma	NR	NR
Bo-abbass [6]	1995	64/M	WA	Roller coaster	10 W	Headache	CT scan: left SDH	NR	Uneventful recovery
Jacome [31]	1989	65/M	WA	Heavy lifting	2 m	Headaches and burning dysesthesias	CT scan: large right isodense SDH	Two burr holes	Uneventful recovery
Keller [35]	1998	43/M	WA	Basketball	3 W	Bifrontal throbbing headaches.	(CT) scan: bilateral frontoparietal SDH	Craniotomy	Uneventful recovery
Kawanishi [34]	1999	11/M	AC	Soccer	7 W	Headache and vomiting	Convexity hematoma	Two burr holes	Uneventful recovery
Kawanishi [34]	1999	14/M	AC	Soccer	2 m	Headache	NR	Two burr holes	Uneventful recovery

Fukutake [23]	2000	26/F	WA	Roller coaster	NR	Headache	(CT) scan: bilateral SDH	NR	Uneventful recovery
Fukutake [23]	2000	64/M	WA	Roller coaster	NR	Headache	(CT) scan: left chronic SDH	NR	Uneventful recovery
Chillala [14]	2001	21/M	WA	Soccer	3 W	Headache and vomiting	(CT) scan: Bilateral hypodense chronic SDH	Surgery, unspecified	Uneventful recovery
Fukutake [23]	2000	73/M	WA	Roller coaster	NR	Headache	(CT) scan: left SDH	NR	He died 13 days later
Mori [50]	2002	14/M	WA	Physical training	1 m	Headache and right hemiparesis	CT scan: high density subdural hematoma in the left side	Two burr holes	Uneventful recovery
Prabhu [60]	2002	15/F	WA	Soccer	2 m	Headaches	MRI: left frontotemporal convexity SDH	Temporal craniotomy	Uneventful recovery
Ulmer [80]	2002	44, M	WA	NR	4 W	Headache	NR	Open craniotomy	Uneventful recovery
Prabhu [60]	2002	16/F	WA	Soccer	1 m	Occipital headaches and numbness of the right face and body	CT scan showed isodense subdural hematoma	Two burr holes	Clinical recovery was satisfactory
Tsuzuki [79]	2003	16/F	WA	Basketball	SW	Intractable headache	MRI: left frontotemporal convexity CSDH	Two burr holes	NR
Carmont [13]	2002	65/M	WA	Competitive race walking	SW	Headaches with foot drop on his left side and weakness of his left arm	CT scan: right-sided subdural hematoma	Two burr holes	Uneventful recovery

(continued)

Table 25.1 (continued)

First author [ref]	Publication year	Age (yrs)/sex	antecedent	Sport	Interval from trauma to diagnostic	Symptoms	Imaging findings	Treatment	Outcome
Demetriades [16]	2004	24/M	WA	Soccer	6 W	Increasing headache and vomiting and mild right-sided weakness	CT scan: large subdural hematoma	Two burr holes	Clinical recovery was satisfactory
Miele [47]	2004	24/F	WA	Boxer	12 m	Headache and nausea of increasing intensity the morning	CT scan: left heterogeneous subdural hematoma	Frontal temporoparietal craniotomy	NR
Pretorius [61]	2005	11/M	WA	Activities during the trip	SW	Increasing headache and nausea	MRI: large right-sided extra-axial lesion along the convexity	Two burr holes	Uneventful recovery
Alaraj [2]	2005	24/M	WA	Weight lifter	SW	Worsening headaches	CT scan: left frontoparietal SDH	Two burr holes	NR
Miele [48]	2006	31/M	WA	Boxer	SW	Headaches memory trouble	MRI: two small SDHs that were causing no mass effect or midline shift	Craniotomy	Clinical recovery was satisfactory
Robles [64]	2006	20/M	WA	Boxer	1 m	Headaches and vomiting	Left isodense chronic SH with important mass effect	Craniotomy	Uneventful recovery
Roldan-Valadez [67]	2006	13/F	WA	Roller coaster	3 W	Hemiparesis on the right side of the body, as well as cephalea	MRI: large subacute SDH covering the left lateral convexity	NR	Uneventful recovery

Zhang [88]	2007	21/M	WA	Swimming/ water sports	NR	Headaches and vomiting	(CT) scan: left frontal-parietal-temporal chronic SDH	Craniotomy	Uneventful recovery
Zhang [88]	2007	9/F	WA	Running	3 W	Headaches and vomiting	(CT) scan: Left frontal-parietal-temporal SDH	Craniotomy	Uneventful recovery
Türkoğlu [78]	2008	25/M	WA	Martial arts	6 m	Headaches	(CT) scan: hypodensity in the left subdural area	Two burr holes	Uneventful recovery
Tsitsopoulos [76]	2008	15/M	WA	Athletic event	3 W	Headache accompanied by nausea and intermittent vomiting	CT scan: subacute SDH in the right frontotemporal region	Two burr holes	Uneventful recovery
Domenicucci [18]	2009	7/M	WA	Soccer	NR	NR	CT scan: left frontotemporal SDH	Two burr holes	Uneventful recovery
Domenicucci [18]	2009	41/M	WA	Bicycle	NR	NR	CT scan: right frontotemporal SDH	Two burr holes	Uneventful recovery
Pillai [57]	2009	23/M	AC	Bicycle	1 m	Headaches, nausea and vomiting.	CT scan: bilateral mixed density SDH	Burr hole + open craniotomy	Uneventful recovery
Pillai [57]	2009	41/M	WA	NR	12 W	Headache and nausea	CT scan: left frontotemporal hypodense SDH	Two burr holes	Uneventful recovery
Hamada [26]	2010	15/M	WA	Volleyball	SW	Headache with vomiting	MRI: SDH covering the left lateral convexity	Craniectomy	Clinical recovery was satisfactory
Zeng [87]	2011	14/M	WA	Jump training	3 W	Headache accompanied by projectile vomiting	CT scan: left frontal-parietal-hypodense temporal SDH	Craniectomy	Uneventful recovery

(continued)

Table 25.1 (continued)

First author [ref]	Publication year	Age (yrs)/sex	antecedent	Sport	Interval from trauma to diagnostic	Symptoms	Imaging findings	Treatment	Outcome
Zeng [87]	2011	16/M	AC	Football	4 W	Increasing headache and nausea	CT scan: temporal-frontal-parietal hypodense SDH	Two burr holes	Uneventful recovery
Işik [30]	2010	13/M	WA	Soccer	SW	Headache	CT scan: isodense SDH	NR	NR
Kertmen [36]	2012	12/M	WA	Taekwondo trainings.	3 W	Progressive headache	CT scan: frontoparietal isodense SDH	Two burr holes	Uneventful recovery
Park [54]	2013	75/M	Hypertension, diabetes mellitus, renal insufficiency and gout	Weight training	3 W	Headache	CT scan: isodense bilateral SDH	Two burr holes	Uneventful recovery
Blereau [5]	2013	7/F	NR	Bicycle	NR	NR	NR	Two burr holes	Uneventful recovery
Maher [43]	2013	16/M	NR	Football	3 W	Headache	NR	No surgery	Uneventful recovery
Maher [43]	2013	12/F	NR	Soccer	3 W	Headache vomiting	NR	No surgery	Uneventful recovery
Cress [15]	2013	45/M	WA	Football	2 m	Headaches memory trouble	CT scan: convexity hematoma	Craniotomy	NR
Zheng [90]	2013	16/M	WA	Sport related (not specified)	7 W	Headache and nausea	CT scan: isodense subdural hematoma	NR	Uneventful recovery
Edmondson [19]	2014	14/M	WA	Soccer	NR	Headache	CT scan: hyperdense left fronto-temporo-parietal SDH	Two burr holes	NR

Hou [29]	2014	17/M	WA	Basketball	NR	Increasing headache and nausea	CT scan: convexity hematoma	Two burr holes	Clinical recovery was satisfactory
Takizawa [74]	2015	15/M	WA	Soccer	8 W	Headaches memory trouble	CT scan: left isodense subdural hematoma	Craniotomy	Uneventful recovery
Takizawa [74]	2015	13/M	WA	Bicycle	7 W	Headaches	CT scan: left hypodense SDH	Two burr holes	NR
Takizawa [74]	2015	31/M	WA	Martial arts	4 W	Headaches	CT scan: right isodense SDH	Two burr holes	NR
Takizawa [74]	2015	35/F	WA	Ski/ snowboarding	20 W	Headaches GCS 8/15	CT scan: left hypodense SDH	Two burr holes	NR
Takizawa [74]	2015	32/M	WA	Ski/ snowboarding	16 W	Headaches	CT scan: left hypodense SDH	Craniotomy	NR
Pascoe [56]	2015	43/M	AC	Football	3 W	Nausea, vomiting and headaches	CT scan: right isodense SDH	Craniotomy	NR
Yaldiz [85]	2016	16/M	AC	Soccer	3 W	Progressive headache	CT scan: right isodense SDH	Craniotomy	Uneventful recovery
Gregori [25]	2019	18/M	WA	Soccer	1 m	Nausea and headache	MRI: left fronto-temporoparietal hyperintense SDH	Two burr holes	Uneventful recovery
Gregori [25]	2019	6/M	WA	Soccer	3 W	Headache and nausea	CT scan: hyperdense left fronto-temporo-parietal SDH	Frontotemporal craniotomy.	Uneventful recovery

AC arachnoid cyst, *SDH* subdural hematoma, *CT* computed tomography, *F* female, *NR* not reported, *M* male, *m* month, *MRI* magnetic resonance imaging, *ref* reference, *W* week, *SW* several weeks, *yrs* years, *WA* without antecedent

Table 25.2 Sporting activities in the 66 included cases

Sport	First author and year	No. of cases (%)
Soccer	Gregori 2019 (2 cases)/Yaldiz 2016 Takizawa 2015/ Edmondson 2014/ Maher 2013/Işik 2011/Domenicucci 2009/Demetriades 2004/ Prabhu 2002 (2 cases)/Chillala 2001/Kawanishi 1999 (2 cases)/Maeda 1993/ Oliver 1958	16 (24.2%)
Bicycle	Takizawa 2015/Blereau 2013/Domenicucci 2009/Pillai 2009/Rogers 1990/Hara 1984	6 (9%)
Rollercoaster	Roldan-Valadez 2006/Fukutake 2000(3 cases)/Bo-abbass 1995/Fernandes 1994	6 (9%)
Physical/weight training	Park 2013/Zeng 2011/Tsitsopoulos 2008/Zhang 2007/ / Carmont 2002/Mori 2002	6 (9%)
Basketball	Hou 2014/Tsuzuki 2003/Rogers1990/Keller 1998/McNeil 1987	5 (7.5%)
Martial arts	Takizawa 2015/Kertmen 2012/Türkoğlu 2008/Yokoyama 1989/Weinberg 1973	5(7.5)
Football	Pascoe 2015/Maher 2013/Cress 2013/	4(6%)
Swimming/water sports	Zhang 2007/Mori 1995/Rogers 1990	3 (4.5)
Boxing	Roldan-Valadez 2006/Fukutake 2000(3 cases)/Bo-abbass 1995/Fernandes 1994	3 (4.5%)
Ski/snowboarding	Takizawa 2015/Rogers 1990/Lacour 1978	3 (4.5%)
Volleyball	Hamada 2010	1 (1.5%)
Rugby	Varma 1981	1 (1.5%)
Dancing	McNeil 1987	1 (1.5%)
Equestrian	Page 1987	1 (1.5%)
Heavy lifting	Jacome 1989	1 (1.5%)

patients in our series were young males playing soccer. In our study, 38 of our 66 patients were under the age of 18, joining the data of the study reported by Fabrizio Gregori [25] where 33 patients were of 18 years of age or less, with the presence of an arachnoid cyst that included 13 in soccer. This finding clearly raises the question of whether the recent Zurich guidelines recommending that athletes under the age of 18 should not return to the same contest after a concussion should also be extended to those over the age of 18.

Because of the large number of participants in soccer and the likelihood that significant exposure yields a high risk (50% during 10 years of play) of concussion, it may be timely to consider headgear use for soccer [34]. In soccer players, the rate is approximately 0.15 concussions per 1000 athlete exposures [3, 7]. A recent analysis of ten high school sports with 23,566 injuries reported disclosed that girls' soccer was the third most common cause of concussion. Master et al. [44] recently reported that 27% of amateur soccer players had incurred one soccer-related concussion, and 23% had experienced multiple concussions during their amateur career.

25.4 Pathophysiology and Second Impact Syndrome

Direct head trauma is the most common cause of SDH that occurs by transmission of an external force to the brain; because of translational (linear) acceleration or rotational acceleration, it causes brain damage, where a static or dynamic mechanical load is delivered to the skull. In the case of noncontact head trauma, the brain injury can be explained by translation, rotation, or angular motion of the head, causing acceleration and deceleration of the brain. This loading can sometimes be so powerful that it causes very serious intracerebral hemorrhage and displaced skull fractures and occasionally just mild stretching of the veins. These stretching forces may lead to torn arachnoid or bridging veins. The effect of centrifugal force is more pronounced on the cerebral parenchyma than at the surface of the brain. It interferes with long nerve fiber tracts and fine intracerebral vessels.

In addition to injury from the mass effect of blood beneath the dura mater, there is often significant associated damage (contusion or edema) to the underlying brain due to multiple (sometimes hundreds) blows. Concern about what has been termed, "second impact syndrome" (SIS) is a major factor determining return-to-play decisions after concussion. However, SIS has been defined as occurring when an athlete who has sustained an initial head injury, most often a concussion, sustains a second head injury before symptoms associated with the first have fully cleared [9, 12].

Historically, the first clinical description of SIS was made in 1881 by Otto Bollinger who used the term "traumatischespät-apoplexie" [9]. SIS occurs when a person sustains a second brain injury before the symptoms of an initial brain injury resolve [9, 12]. Severe brain edema develops due to cerebral vasculature dysautoregulation and causes significant neurologic deficits [9, 84]. SIS is a rare condition that occurs primarily in adolescents and young adults. Severe neurologic deficits and death typically occur with SIS [9, 12]. There is little epidemiological data about SIS; therefore the exact incidence is unknown and risk factors have not yet been established. Over a decade ago, the existence of this syndrome was brought into question, and since that time, other authors have begun to raise similar concerns as to the underlying entity [4, 8].

The pathophysiology of second impact syndrome is thought to involve a loss of autoregulation in the brain's blood supply where the cerebral circulation has the capacity to maintain blood flow at a relatively constant level during changes in blood pressure. Pressure autoregulation can be disturbed by cranial surgery, trauma, and even pharmaceuticals, and yet its absence does not correlate well with head injury severity or outcomes [8]. In the absence of trauma and any predisposing conditions, subdural bleeding might instead result from a sudden increase in intravenous pressure, which can occur when forcible exhalation occurs against a closed glottis. It has been proposed that weight training could potentially cause a subdural hematoma through generation of a Valsalva maneuver during the "clean and jerk" lift, where the athlete first squats and inhales as the weight is lifted to the chest from the floor. They then exhale against a closed glottis as the weight is moved into position above their head (a Valsalva maneuver). Intracranial hypotension can also be secondary to systemic hypotension resulting from dehydration. Nevertheless, it is possible that an episode of acute and transient dehydration while exercising can result in intracranial hypotension and precipitate a SDH, the average marathon runner loses 5% body weight and 6.5% of plasma volume while racing [45].

The total volume of the brain, CSF, and the intracranial blood remains constant inside the rigid skull. Therefore, a decrease in one of these components should cause a reciprocal increase in either or both of the remaining two [49]. Downward displacement of the brain due to low CSF pressure may produce tears of the bridging veins of the dural border cell layer, causing these veins to rupture. The rupture of bridging dural veins while performing the Valsalva maneuver during heavy lifting can cause the bleed. Intracranial hypotension, another risk factor for spontaneous subdural hemorrhage, can occur following exercise, as bouts of submaximal dynamic exercise result in systemic vascular hypotension [17]. In one study, systolic blood pressure was found to be reduced by 20 mmHg at 10 min after exercise [35, 41].

25.5 Locations of Subdural Hematomas

Forty-three patients (65.2%) had unilateral hematomas and five patients (7.6%) had bilateral hematomas. The affected side was left in 33 patients (50%), while in 10 cases (15.2%), the right side was affected. Finally, in 18 cases (27.3%), the affected side was not specified. Interestingly, we found that 80.3% (53/66) of patients with CSDH had an arachnoid cyst (AC).

25.6 Clinical Features

A CSDH is defined as a hematoma present 3 weeks or more after a traumatic injury. The pathogenesis of CSDH involves an injury that results in bleeding into the subdural space. The initial hemorrhage may be a small amount that fails to generate significant brain compression. However, bleeding or oozing of blood into the subdural space may continue [33].

The time interval between trauma and clinical manifestation increases with age, as brain atrophy in the elderly allows the hematoma to accumulate before symptoms become obvious. It is important to understand that CSDH in athletes are dissimilar to those commonly seen in the elderly and in many non-athletes who are trauma victims. The athlete usually does not have the large potential subdural space that an elderly patient possesses, and therefore mass effect and increases in intracranial pressure can occur with greater rapidity. In addition to injury from the mass effect of blood beneath the dura mater, there is often significant associated parenchymal damage (contusion or edema). In the present series, the most common symptoms of patients were headache. It is more common in young patients because they tend to suffer from increased intracranial pressure caused by CSDH.

Based on our review, headache was present in 96% of patients, vomiting and/or nausea in nearly 40%, and diplopia in 10%. In our investigation, younger CSDH patients had shorter symptom duration before seeking clinical attention, caused by having less space due to a pre-existing atrophied brain that is present in elderly patients (Table 25.1). The longer duration is explained by the insidious onset of symptoms in patients with CSDH that is related to the intracranial components accommodating the progressive accumulation of this hematoma in the subarachnoid space.

Older patients can endure a larger volume of hematoma collecting in the subdural space before experiencing clinical manifestation. All these symptoms may be referred to pre-existing atrophied brain in the elderly patients. As seen in our review according to Fogelholm et al. [22], older CSDH patients tend to show more hemiparesis and mental deterioration, whereas younger patients are more likely to complain of headache and demonstrate papilledema on physical examination. Elderly patients can endure a larger volume of hematoma collecting in the subdural space before experiencing clinical manifestation.

It is inviting to hypothesize about the imaging semblance between sport players and the typical victims of non-accidental trauma (NAT) that develop CSDH. Both types of victims have likely suffered repetitive head injury. It has been shown that there is an increased incidence of hypoxic-ischemic injury in infants and children who are victims of NAT in comparison to accidental head trauma. There is also animal study evidence of the increased vulnerability of the younger brain to repeated mild traumatic brain injury [62].

25.7 Imaging Findings

SDH can occur in acute and chronic forms. It is usually caused by high speed injury, the accumulated blood leaking from bridging veins on the surface of the brain, damaged by the sheering forces of the head injury or from contused brain. The imaging exam of choice for the diagnosis remains the CT scan, mainly because it is faster and less costly compared to MRI, and also can be used in patients with metallic implants and a cardiac pacemaker.

CSDH has a variety of imaging characteristics on CT; low, intermediate, or high density relative to brain parenchyma where isodensity was the most common density of CSDH [70]. There are some reports that the hypodensity was the most common type of CSDH seen on CT scanning. However, isodense CSDH were often reported as more common than the hypodense lesions [89]. It may depend on the patient population, resolution of the CT scan, and methods of density classification. In the present series the density of CSDH was isodense in 17 patients (25.8%), hypodense in 17 patients (25.8%), mixed in 3 cases 4.5%, and in 29 cases (43.9%) the density was not specified in the paper.

Although CSDH are usually concavo-convex in shape, rarely they may mimic acute epidural hematomas. Magnetic resonance imaging (MRI) is more sensitive than CT for determining the size and internal structures of CSDH, such as multiple locations and intrahematoma membranes. Fresh bleeding, hemolysis, and hemoglobin changes can also be observed on MRI. The diffusion tensor imaging can examine anisotropic changes of the pyramidal tracts displaced by CSDH [89].

25.8 Treatment

The main therapeutic goal should be the interruption of the vicious cycle of rebreeding and fibrinolysis by removing of fibrin degradation products from the subdural space. Multiple standard surgical techniques exist for the evacuation of CSDH and it is a controversial topic, ranging from percutaneous subdural tapping [20] to large craniotomy with removal of the hematoma membranes [73, 79]. However, burr hole craniotomy and closed-system drainage are the most widely accepted methods for evacuation of the hematoma [82]. Many other surgical techniques have been reported, such as twist drill craniostomy, craniotomy and excision of the subdural membranes, reservoir shunting for continuous irrigation and drainage, percutaneous needle trephination and open system drainage with repeated saline rinsing, etc.

Sixty-four patients with a CSDH related to sport injury underwent surgery, after the execution of a brain image due to their clinical conditions. In 29 cases (43.9%), the surgical strategy used was a burr hole. In 24 cases (36.4%), it was a craniotomy. In eight cases (12.1%), the authors chose a combination of burr hole and craniotomy. In three patients (4.5%), the surgical strategy adopted was not clearly specified.

25.9 Prognosis

A good clinical outcome was reported in 46 patients (69.6%) where preoperative clinical symptoms completely resolved within 48 h from surgery, while in 19 cases (28.78%), the outcome was not reported, although postoperative clinical follow-up did not reveal any recurrence. Regrettably, in a 73-year-old patient who died after 13 days, the circumstances of death were not detailed in the paper reported by Fukutake et al. [23].

There is little in the medical literature to guide us regarding the return of athletes to their sport after a CSDH. It is important to point out that the types of capacity of individuals and the way they are affected by illness, traumatisms, or even aging differ. The term intrinsic capacity is used to deal with the set of physical and mental capacities, while functional capacity refers to the capacity for performing activities. Considering intrinsic capacity added to the possibilities that the environment provides and/or access to the use of auxiliary devices, it concerns the person's intrinsic capacity to interact with the organization; rules and production procedures, rhythm and goals, content, division of labor, and hierarchical levels [28].

We need to assess return-to-play strategies prospectively on the basis of symptom resolution and cognitive recovery and determine that the outcomes of this approach are safe for the player concerned and appropriate for the sport played [10]. Until such studies are performed, the management should follow the experience of most team physicians who safely treat these athletes with a combination of good common sense and clinical judgment. There is general agreement that players should be free of the residual effects before returning to competition in order to avoid the dangerous potential consequences of premature return to play.

The critical questions are how can we prevent the onset of cerebral swelling and can we predict which children or athletes are at risk of developing this condition and treat them aggressively to reduce the morbidity and mortality? To date, we do not have the answers to these questions. To successfully care for head injuries, both players and coaches need to understand the risks of multiple head injuries and how return-to-play guidelines guide decision-making. Players often decide to return to play after a head injury without seeking medical attention. This action is at times motivated by the fear of ridicule from the coaching staff and fellow players. Also, players often are ignorant of the possible life-threatening consequences of returning to play without proper medical attention [24]. Although these athletes who have returned to competition have not suffered a recurrence of intracranial hemorrhage, much less is known about the long-term effects of their injuries.

25.10 Conclusion

With the increased level of participation in sports in virtually all countries, the number of cases of development of SDH in patients with sports has increased. The real incidence of sports complicated by CSDH is not clear. This study will be of interest to all neurosurgeons and other physicians who treat patients with sports-related CSDH. The outcome is generally excellent but in people who are involved in contact or collision sports, the presence of an arachnoid cyst is thought to be a relative contraindication to participation because of the risk of bleeding into the cyst. Nevertheless, we should inform these patients and their families of the possibility of a complication with CSDH and advise care to avoid head injury in sport regardless of the size and location of the cyst.

References

1. Adhiyaman V, Asghar M, Ganeshram K, Bhowmick B. Chronic subdural haematoma in the elderly. Postgrad Med J. 2002;78:71–5.
2. Alaraj AM, Chamoun RB, Dahdaleh NS, Haddad GF, Comair YG. Spontaneous subdural haematoma in anabolic steroids dependent weight lifters: reports of two cases and review of literature. Acta Neurochir. 2005;147:85–7.

3. Barnes B, Cooper L, Kirkendall D, McDermott T, Jordan B, Garrett W. Concussion history in elite male and female soccer players. Am J Sports Med. 1998;26:433–8.
4. Bey T, Ostick B. Second impact syndrome. West J Emerg Med. 2009;10:6–10.
5. Blereau RP, Haley TJ. Arachnoid cyst. Consultant. 2013;53:540–1.
6. Bo-abbass Y, Bolton CF. Roller coaster headache. N Engl J Med. 1995;332:1585.
7. Boden B, Kirkendall D, Garrett W. Concussion incidence in elite college soccer players. Am J Sports Med. 1998;26:238–41.
8. Byard R, Vink R. The second impact syndrome. Forensic Sci Med Pathol. 2009;5:36–8.
9. Cantu R. Second-impact syndrome. Clin Sports Med. 1998;17:37–44.
10. Cantu R. Athletic concussion: current understanding as of 2007. Neurosurgery. 2007;60:963–4.
11. Cantu R, Mueller F. Brain injury-related fatalities in American football, 1945–1999. Neurosurgery. 2003;52:846–52.
12. Cantu R, Gean A. Second-impact syndrome and a small subdural hematoma: an uncommon catastrophic result of repetitive head injury with a characteristic imaging appearance. J Neurotrauma. 2010;27:1557–64.
13. Carmont M, Mahattanakul W, Pigott T. Acquisition of a chronic subdural haematoma during training for competitive race walking. Br J Sports Med. 2002;36:306–7.
14. Chillala S, Read C, Evans PA. An unusual case of subdural haematoma presenting to the accident and emergency department. Emerg Med J. 2001;18:308–9.
15. Cress M, Kestle JRW, Holubkov R, Riva-Cambrin J. Risk factors for pediatric arachnoid cyst rupture/hemorrhage: a case control study. Neurosurgery. 2013;72:716–22.
16. Demetriades AK, McEvoy AW, Kitchen ND. Subdural haematoma associated with an arachnoid cyst after repetitive minor heading injury in ball games. Br J Sports Med. 2004;38:E8.
17. Denoronha R, Sharrack B, Hadjivassiliou M, Romanowski C. Subdural haematoma: a potentially serious consequence of spontaneous intracranial hypotension. J Neurol Neurosurg Psychiatry. 2003;74:752–5.
18. Domenicucci M, Russo N, Giugni E, Pierallini A. Relationship between supratentorial arachnoid cyst and chronic subdural hematoma: neuroradiological evidence and surgical treatment. J Neurosurg. 2009;110:1250–5.
19. Edmondson L, Upshaw J, Tuuri R. A 14-year-old male with a 10-week history of headaches. Pediatr Ann. 2014;43:220–3.
20. Ernestus R, Beldzinski P, Lanfermann H, Klug N. Chronic subdural hematoma: surgical treatment and outcome in 104 patients. Surg Neurol. 1997;48:220–5.
21. Fernandes CMB, Daya MR. A roller-coaster headache: case report. J Trauma. 1994;37:1007–10.
22. Fogelholm R, Heiskanen O, Waltimo O. Chronic subdural hematoma in adults. Influence of patient's age on symptoms, signs, and thickness of hematoma. J Neurosurg. 1975;42:43–6.
23. Fukutake T, Mine S, Yamakami I. Roller coaster headache and subdural hematoma. Neurology. 2000;54:264.
24. Gerberich SG, Priest JD, Boen JR, Straub CP, Maxwell RE. Concussion incidences and severity in secondary school varsity football players. Am J Public Health. 1983;73:1370–5.
25. Gregori F, Colistra D, Mancarella C, Chiarella V, Marotta N, Domenicucci M. Arachnoid cyst in young soccer players complicated by chronic subdural hematoma: personal experience and review of the literature. Acta Neurol Belg. 2020;120:235–46.
26. Hamada H, Hayashi N, Umemura K. Middle cranial fossa arachnoid cyst presenting with subdural effusion and endoscopic detection of tear of the cyst. Neurol Med Chir (Tokyo). 2010;50:512–4.
27. Hara H, Inoue T, Matsuo K. Unusual computed tomographic findings in a case of arachnoid cyst in the middle cranial fossa. Surg Neurol. 1984;22:79–82.
28. Hilleshein E, Souza L, Lautert L, Paz A, Catalan VM, Teixeira M, et al. Capacidade para o trabalho de enfermeiros de umhospitaluniversitário. Rev Gaúcha Enf. 2011;32:509–15.
29. Hou K, Li CG, Zhang Y, Zhu BX. The surgical treatment of three young chronic subdural hematoma patients with different causes. J Korean Neurosurg Soc. 2014;55:218–21.

30. Işik SH, Yildiz Ö, Ceylan Y. Chronic subdural hematoma caused by soccer ball trauma associated with arachnoid cyst in childhood: case report. Neurol Sci Neurophysiol. 2011;28:398–401.
31. Jacome DE, Yanez GF. Subdural haematoma upon straining. J Neurol Neurosurg Psychiatry. 1989;52:134.
32. Jones N, Blumbergs P, North J. Acute subdural haematomas: aetiology, pathology and outcome. Aust N Z J Surg. 1986;56:907–13.
33. Kaste M, Waltimo O, Heiskanen O. Chronic bilateral subdural haematoma in adults. Acta Neurochir (Wien). 1979;48:231–6.
34. Kawanishi A, Nakayama M, Kadota K. Heading injury precipitating subdural hematoma associated with arachnoid cysts: two case reports. Neurol Med Chir (Tokyo). 1999;39:231–3.
35. Keller T, Holland M. Chronic subdural haematoma: an unusual injury from playing basketball. Br J Sports Med. 1998;32:338–9.
36. Kersey RD. Acute subdural hematoma after a reported mild concussion: a case report. J Athl Train. 1998;33:264–8.
37. Kertmen H, Gürer B, Yilmaz ER, Sekerci Z. Chronic subdural hematoma associated with an arachnoid cyst in a juvenile taekwondo athlete: a case report and review of the literature. Pediatr Neurosurg. 2012;48:55–8.
38. Lacour F, Trevor R, Carey M. Arachnoid cyst and associated subdural hematoma. Observations on conventional roentgenographic and computerized tomographic diagnosis. Arch Neurol. 1978;35:84–9.
39. Lindsay KW, McLatchie G, Jennett B. Serious head injury in sport. BMJ. 1980;281:789–91.
40. Logan S, Bell G, Leonard J. Acute subdural hematoma in a high school football player after 2 unreported episodes of head trauma: a case report. J Athl Train. 2001;36:433–6.
41. MacDonald JR, MacDougall JD, Interisano SA, Smith KM, McCartney N, Moroz JS, et al. Hypotension following mild bouts of resistance exercise and submaximal dynamic exercise. Eur J Appl Physiol Occup Physiol. 1999;79:148–54.
42. Maeda M, Kawamura Y, Handa Y. Value of MR imaging in middle fossa arachnoid cyst with intracystic and subdural hematoma. Eur J Radiol. 1993;17:145–7.
43. Maher CO, Garton HJ, Al-Holou WN, Trobe JD, Muraszko KM, Jackson EM. Management of subdural hygromas associated with arachnoid cysts. J Neurosurg Pediatr. 2013;12:434–43.
44. Matser E, Kessels A, Lefak M, Jordan B, Troost J. Neuropsychological impairment in amateur soccer players. JAMA. 1999;282:971–3.
45. Maughan R, Whiting P, Davidson R. Estimation of plasma volume changes during marathon running. Br J Sports Med. 1985;19:138–41.
46. McNeil SL, Austin Spruill W, Langley RL. Multiple subdural hematomas associated with breakdancing. Ann Emerg Med. 1987;16:114–6.
47. Miele VJ, Carson L, Carr A. Acute on chronic subdural hematoma in a female boxer: a case report. Med Sci Sports Exerc. 2004;36:1852–5.
48. Miele VJ, Bailes JE, Cantu RC, Rabb CH. Subdural hematomas in boxing: the spectrum of consequences. Neurosurg Focus. 2006;21:E10.
49. Mokri B. The Monro-Kellie hypothesis: applications in CSF volume depletion. Neurology. 2001;56:1746–8.
50. Mori T, Katayama Y, Kawamata T. Acute hemispheric swelling associated with thin subdural hematomas: pathophysiology of repetitive head injury in sports. Acta Neurochir Suppl. 2006;96:40–3.
51. Ochi M, Morikawa M, Ogino A. Supratentorial arachnoid cyst and associated subdural hematoma: neuroradiologic studies. Eur Radiol. 1996;6:640–4.
52. Oliver LC. Primary arachnoid cysts: report of two cases. BMJ. 1958;1:1147–9.
53. Page A, Paxton RM, Mohan D. A reappraisal of the relationship between arachnoid cysts of the middle fossa and chronic subdural haematoma. J Neurol Neurosurg Psychiatry. 1987;50:1001–7.
54. Park HR, Lee KS, Bae HG. Chronic subdural hematoma after eccentric exercise using a vibrating belt machine. J Korean Neurosurg Soc. 2013;54:265–7.

55. Parkkari J, Kujala M, Kannus P. Is it possible to prevent sports injuries? Sports Med. 2001;31:985–95.
56. Pascoe HM, Phal PM, King JA. Progressive post traumatic tearing of an arachnoid cyst membrane resulting in intracystic and subdural haemorrhage. J Clin Neurosci. 2015;22:897–9.
57. Pillai P, Menon SK, Manjooran RP, Kariyattil R, Pillai AB, Panikar D. Temporal fossa arachnoid cyst presenting with bilateral subdural hematoma following trauma: two case reports. J Med Case Rep. 2009;3:53.
58. Pothe H. Chronic subdural haematoma in prize fighters (In German). Beitr Neurochir. 1964;8:232–7.
59. Powell J, Barber-Foss K. Traumatic brain injury in high school athletes. JAMA. 1999;282:958–63.
60. Prabhu VC, Bailes JE. Chronic subdural hematoma complicating arachnoid cyst secondary to soccer-related head injury: case report. Neurosurgery. 2002;50:195–7.
61. Pretorius PM, McAuley DJ. Something old, something new? Br J Radiol. 2005;78:1063–4.
62. Raghupathi R, Mehr M, Heflaer M, Margulies S. Traumatic axonal injury is exacerbated following repetitive closed head injury in the neonatal pig. J Neurotrauma. 2004;21:307–16.
63. Rashid S, Watson C, Agarwal R. Episodic headache and arachnoid cyst related subdural hematoma. Headache. 2016;56:1354–5.
64. Robles LA, Hernandez V. Subdural and intracystic hematomas in an arachnoid cyst secondary to a boxing injury. Inj Extra. 2006;37:375–8.
65. Rogers MA, Klug GL, Siu KH. Middle fossa arachnoid cysts in association with subdural hematomas. A review and recommendations for management. Br J Neurosurg. 1990;4:497–502.
66. Roldan-Valadez E, Facha MT, Martinez-Lopez M, Herrera-Mora P. Subdural hematoma in a teenager related to roller-coaster ride. Eur J Paediatr Neurol. 2006;10:194–6.
67. Ross R, Oschner M. Acute intracranial boxing related injuries in US Marine Corps recruits: report of two cases. Mil Med. 1999;164:68–70.
68. Santarius T, Hutchinson P. Chronic subdural haematoma: time to rationalize treatment. Br J Neurosurg. 2004;18:328–32.
69. Seelig J, Becker D, Miller D, Greenberg R, Ward J, Choi S. Traumatic acute subdural hematoma: major mortality reduction in comatose patients treated within four hours. N Engl J Med. 1981;304:1511–8.
70. Senturk S, Guzel A, Bilici A, Takmaz I, Guzel E, Aluclu MU, et al. CT and MR imaging of chronic subdural hematomas: a comparative study. Swiss Med Wkly. 2010;140:335–40.
71. Shell D, Carico G, Patton R. Can subdural hematoma result from repeated minor head trauma? Phys Sportsmed. 1993;21:74–84.
72. Strahle J, Selzer B, Geh N. Sports participation with arachnoid cysts. J Neurosurg Pediatr. 2016;17:410–7.
73. Svien HJ, Gelety JE. On the surgical management of encapsulated subdural hematoma. A comparison of the results of membranectomy and simple evacuation. J Neurosurg. 1964;21:172–7.
74. Takizawa K, Sorimachi T, Honda Y, Ishizaka H, Baba T, Osada T. Chronic subdural hematomas associated with arachnoid cysts: significance in young patients with chronic subdural hematomas. Neurol Med Chir (Tokyo). 2015;55:727–34.
75. Torg JS, Vegso JJ, Sennelt B. The national football head and neck injury registry: 14-year report on cervical quadriplegia, 1971 through 1984. JAMA. 1985;254:3439–43.
76. Tsitsopoulos PP, Pantazis GC, Syrmou EC, Tsitsopoulos PD. Intracranial arachnoid cyst associated with traumatic intracystic hemorrhage and subdural haematoma. Hippokratia. 2008;12:53–5.
77. Tsuzuki N, Katoh H, Ohtani N. Chronic subdural hematoma complicating arachnoid cyst secondary to soccer-related head injury: case report. Neurosurgery. 2003;53:242–3.
78. Türkoğlu E, Serbes G, Sanli M, Sari O, Sekerci Z. Chronic subdural hematoma in capoeira sport. Turk Neurosurg. 2008;18:39–41.
79. Tyson G, Strachan WE, Newman P, Winn HR, Butler A, Jane J. The role of craniectomy in the treatment of chronic subdural hematomas. J Neurosurg. 1980;52:776–81.

80. Ulmer S, Engellandt K, Stiller U, Nabavi A, Jansen O, Mehdorn MH. Chronic subdural hemorrhage into a giant arachnoidal cyst (Galassi classification type III). J Comput Assist Tomogr. 2002;26:647–53.
81. Varma TRK, Sedzimir CB, Miles JB. Post-traumatic complications of arachnoid cysts and temporal lobe agenesis. J Neurol Neurosurg Psychiatry. 1981;44:29–34.
82. Wakai S, Hashimoto K, Watanabe N, Lnoh S, Ochiai C, Nagai M. Efficacy of closed-system drainage in treating chronic subdural hematoma: a prospective comparative study. Neurosurgery. 1990;26:7713.
83. Weinberg PE, Flom RA. Intracranial subarachnoid cysts. Radiology. 1973;106:329–33.
84. Wetjen N, Pichelmann M, Atkinson J. Second impact syndrome: concussion and second injury brain complications. J Am Coll Surg. 2010;211:553–7.
85. Yaldiz C, Kacira T, Ceylan D, Asil K. Chronic subdural hemorrhage associated with an arachnoid cyst after sports injury in childhood. Neurosurg Q. 2016;26:361–4.
86. Yokoyama K, Tonami N, Kimura M. Scintigraphic demonstration of intracranial communication between arachnoid cyst and associated subdural hematoma. Clin Nucl Med. 1989;14:350–3.
87. Zeng T, Shi S, Lin Y. Chronic subdural hematoma associated with sylvian arachnoid cyst in juvenile athletes: report of two cases and literature review. Chin J Traumatol. 2011;14:174–7.
88. Zhang H, Zhang JM, Chen G. Chronic subdural hematoma associated with arachnoid cyst: report of two cases. Chin Med J (Engl). 2007;120:2339–40.
89. Zhao KJ, Zhang RY, Sun QF, Wang XQ, Gu XY, Qiang Q, et al. Comparisons of 2/3Sh estimation technique to computer-assisted planimetric analysis in epidural, subdural and intracerebral hematomas. Neurol Res. 2010;32:910–7.
90. Zheng S-P, Li G, You C. Chronic subdural hematoma associated with arachnoid cysts in young people. Neurosurg Q. 2013;23:258–61.

Chapter 26
Neuroimaging Differential Diagnosis (Imaging Mimicking Conditions) of Cranial Chronic Subdural Hematoma

Ali Akhaddar

26.1 Introduction

Cranial chronic subdural hematoma (CSDH) is usually diagnosed by computed tomography scan (CT-scan). This hematoma classically appears as a concavo-convex pericerebral fluid collection along the cranial convexity. Most commonly the density of the collection is low; however, isodense, mixed, or heterogeneous density lesions are also seen (Fig. 26.1a–d). Often unilateral with a significant mass effect and midline shift, CSDH can be bilateral, interhemispheric but rarely in the posterior fossa or adjacent to the skull base. Although rare, some hematoma may be organized, calcified or even ossified (Fig. 26.1e, f) [44, 55]. Therefore, diagnosis of CSDH can be challenging due to the variable clinical presentation of the disease and potentially subtle neuroimaging appearances. For that reason, a high index of suspicion needs to be kept in mind to avoid mismanagement and possible complications.

In addition to medical history, clinical information and biologic data are essential for the radiologist to achieve an appropriate analysis and to fine the list of differential diagnoses.

Intracranially, a wide variety of normal appearances and different etiologies may mimic a CSDH on CT-scan and/or on magnetic resonance imaging (MRI), ranging from traumatic, infectious, inflammatory, and tumoral lesions. Furthermore, some forms of subdural hematomas can be difficult to diagnose on CT-scan (Table 26.1). On the other hand, the coexistence of CSDH with other conditions has been previously reported in the literature and is important to be taken into consideration in the management of any appearance of subdural hematomas [11, 20, 25, 28, 29, 50, 59]. To mention all of these diagnostic difficulties is beyond the scope of this chapter. A

A. Akhaddar (✉)
Avicenne Military Hospital of Marrakech, Department of Neurosurgery,
Mohammed V University in Rabat, Rabat, Morocco

M. Turgut et al. (eds.), *Subdural Hematoma*,
https://doi.org/10.1007/978-3-030-79371-5_26

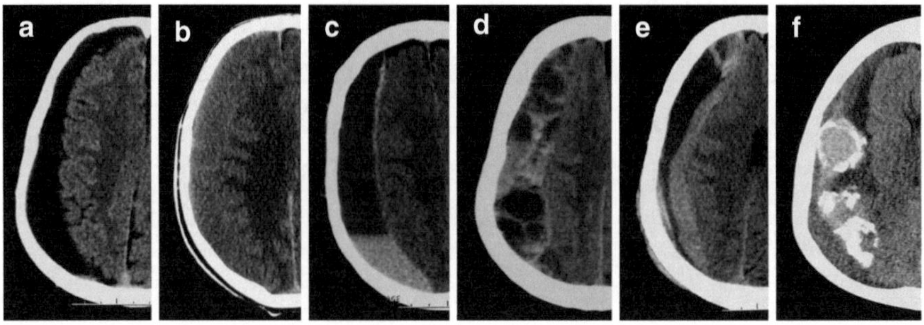

Fig. 26.1 Computed tomography appearance of various types of intracranial chronic subdural hematomas. (**a**) Low density. (**b**) Isodensity. (**c**) Acute on chronic SDH. (**d**) Mixed density with multilayer loculations. (**e**) Organized SDH. (**f**) Calcified/ossified SDH

Table 26.1 Main differential diagnosis of intracranial chronic subdural hematomas

– Subdural empyema
– Epidural empyema
– Acute/subacute subdural hematoma
– Subarachnoid hemorrhage
– Ischemic stroke
– Tumor/sarcoma/metastasis (dural and/or subdural)
– Subdural hygroma (hydroma)
– Arachnoid cyst
– Extracerebral fluid collections in children:
Chronic extra-axial fluid collection
Cerebral atrophy
External hydrocephalus
Normal variant: Enlarged subarachnoid spaces and interhemispheric fissure
Craniocerebral disproportion
– Hypertrophic cranial pachymeningitis
– Leptomeningeal lesions (Rosai-Dorfman)
– Normal intracranial anatomic variants
– "*Undiagnosed CSDH on CT-scan*"
– Artifacts

summary of the most frequent imaging differential diagnoses of CSDH is given according to the origin and pathogenesis of the lesions.

26.2 Subdural Empyema

Intracranial subdural empyema is a pyogenic collection developed between the dura and the leptomeninges. Paranasal sinusitis, otitis media, or odontogenic infections are the most common contiguous sources of subdural empyema. However, other causes are meningitis, cranial osteomyelitis, postoperative complications (including surgery for CSDH), post-traumatic infections, or hematogenous dissemination from a remote source of infection [3, 12, 14].

On CT-scan, subdural empyema generally appears as an iso or hypodensity crescent-shape fluid collection with or without loculations. Brain shift is caused more by the edema (encephalitis) than by the empyema itself. The borders are better demarcated after contrast injection especially along the inner (cortical) margin of the suppuration (Fig. 26.2). Associated paranasal sinusitis or mastoiditis is common. On MRI, restricted diffusion on diffusion-weighted imaging (DWI), hypointensity on apparent diffusion coefficient (ADC) images (hypointensity), and elevated lactate on spectroscopy (elevated lactate) help to confirm the diagnosis [3]. The thickened dura appears markedly enhanced after gadolinium administration. Extensive cerebral edema, encephalitis, thrombophlebitis, and venous infarction are encountered in serious forms. Sometimes, cranial extradural/epidural empyema must also be considered (Fig. 26.3).

A large range of bacterial pathogens may be responsible for the subdural empyema; however, two previous publications reported two cases of subdural neurocysticercosis (parasitic infection) in which multiple free cysticercal cysts present in the subdural space mimicked a chronic subdural hematoma [13, 21].

26.3 Acute/Subacute Subdural Hematoma

Acute and subacute subdural hematomas are often secondary to a head injury with commonly underlying brain damages such as contusions and intracerebral hematomas, brain swelling, and diffuse axonal injuries. There are two common causes of traumatic acute and subacute subdural hematomas:

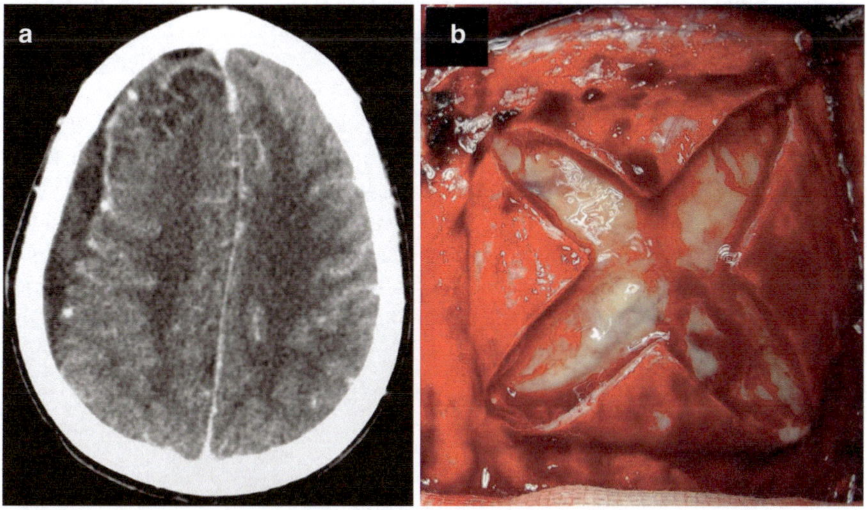

Fig. 26.2 Axial cranial post-contrast CT-scan showing frontal subdural empyema on the right side (**a**). Operative view of the frontal subdural empyema following dural opening (**b**)

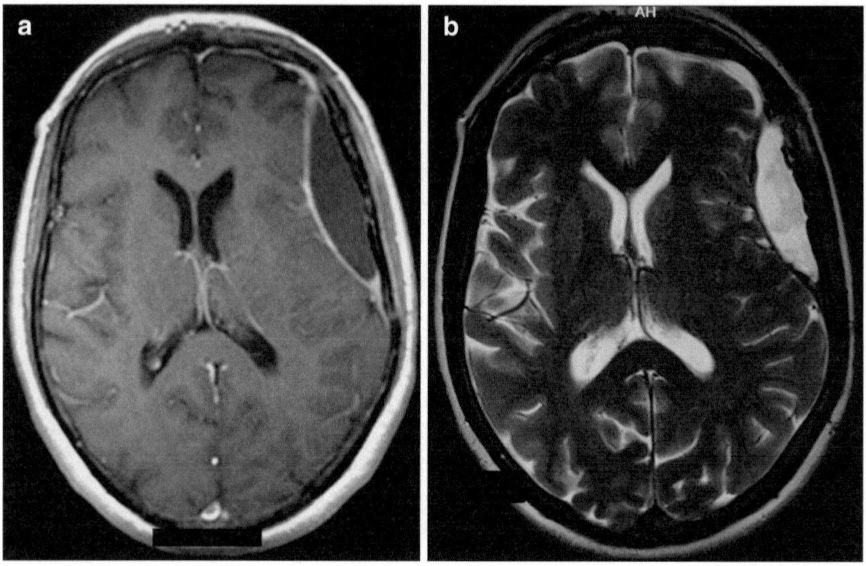

Fig. 26.3 Axial cranial T1-weighted MRI after gadolinium administration (**a**) and on T2-weighted MRI (**b**) revealing a frontal extradural empyema on the left side

- Accumulation of bleeding around parenchymal laceration.
- Cortical and/or bridging vessels torn secondary to the inertial forces (acceleration/deceleration) during brutal head movement.

Also, some acute/subacute subdural hematomas may occur in patients who did not have a history of trauma but suffer from bleeding disorders (receiving anticoagulant therapies or having coagulation diseases) or other unusual secondary etiologies as neoplasms or vascular malformations. In addition, a few cases have been described following cranial or spinal surgery. For further details, please refer to Chap. 2 of the present book.

On CT-scan, there is a hyperdense (acute hematoma) (Figs. 26.4 and 26.5) or isodense (subacute hematoma) (Fig. 26.6) crescentic mass adjacent to the inner cranial table, usually with associated edema, mass effect, and midline shift. Severe presentations are accompanied by cerebral contusions, intraparenchymal hematomas, uncal herniation, effacement of basal cisterns, and dilatation of the contralateral temporal horn. Acute and subacute subdural hematomas can be sometimes confused with CSDH especially when there are acute/subacute clots mixed to the chronic hypodense collection (Fig. 26.1c–e).

26.4 Subarachnoid Hemorrhage

In Japan, some publications have described that CSDH can be mistaken for acute or delayed subarachnoid hemorrhage [42, 51, 54]. On CT-scan, iso or hyperdensity fluid collection in the basal cisterns and subarachnoid spaces do not always indicate

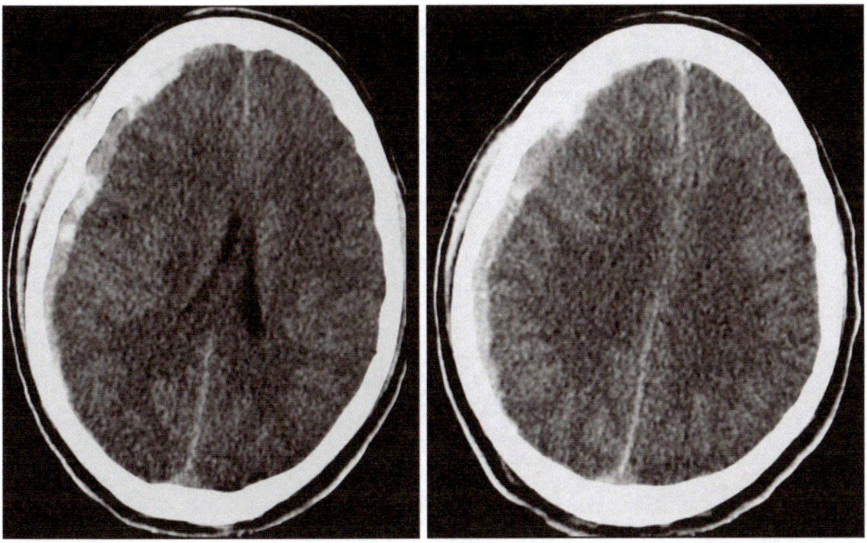

Fig. 26.4 Axial CT-scan revealing a post-traumatic acute subdural hematoma on the right side

Fig. 26.5 Axial CT-scan: spontaneous right acute subdural hematoma with subarachnoid bleeding (arrows) in a patient receiving anticoagulant drugs

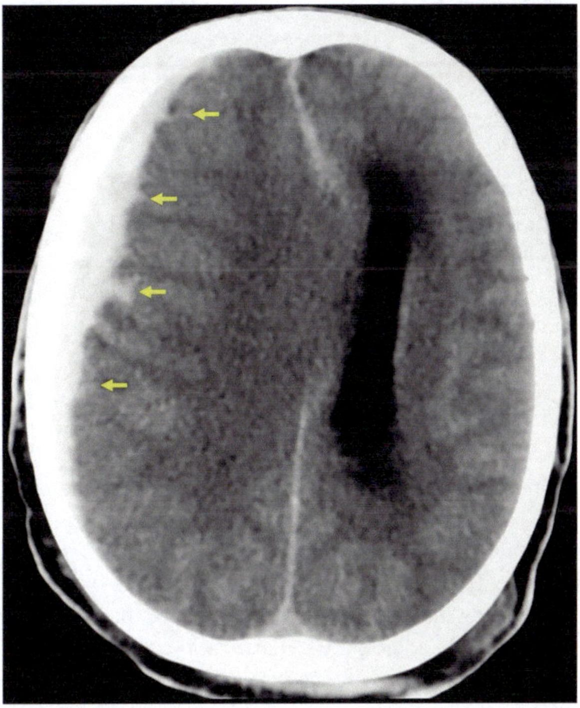

subarachnoid bleeding (Fig. 26.5). For Ohno et al., MRI is useful in differentiating subarachnoid hemorrhage from CSDH especially using fluid-attenuated inversion recovery (FLAIR) sequences [42].

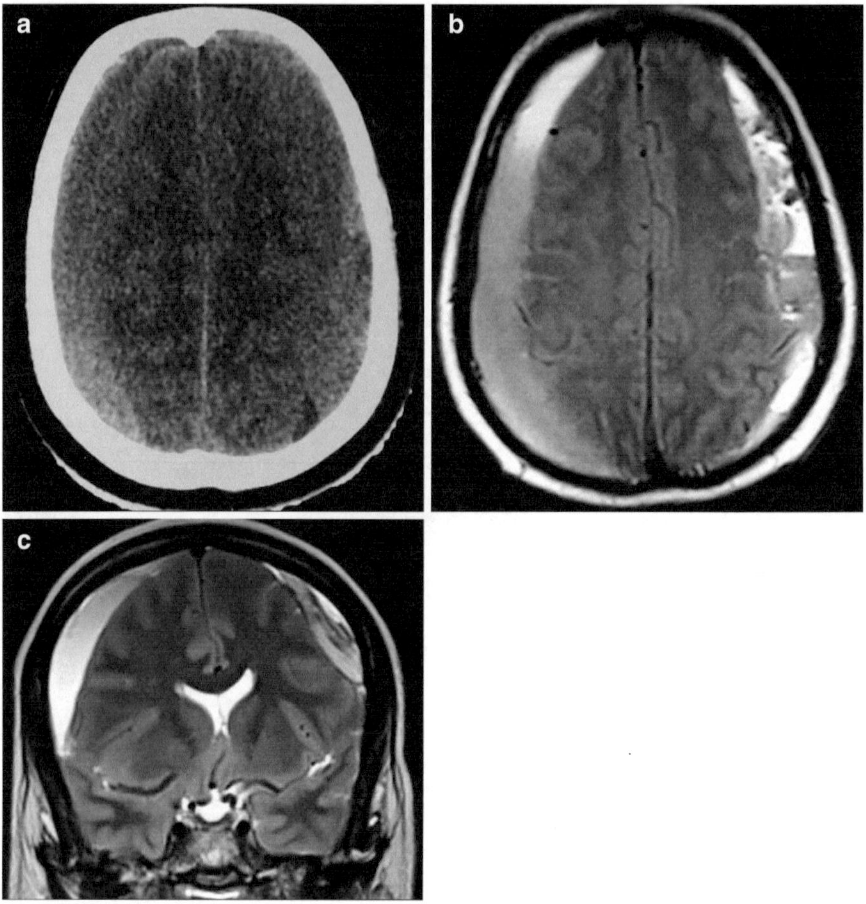

Fig. 26.6 Bilateral intracranial isodense chronic subdural hematoma on CT-scan (**a**). Better distinction of the SDH on MRI: axial (**b**) and coronal (**c**) T2-weighted images

26.5 Extradural Hematoma

An intracranial extradural hematoma (EDH) is characterized by the accumulation of blood between the skull and the dura mater. The most common development is a temporal bone fracture causing a bleeding in the middle meningeal artery in the epidural space. An EDH typically appears as a hyperdense biconvex extraparenchymal brain lesion on CT-scan and does not have the crescentic tail seen in a classic CSDH (Fig. 26.7). In addition, EDH does not cross suture lines unless sutural diastasis or a bony fracture is present. In rare cases, CSDH can appear lentiform/biconvex shape on CT-scan, mimicking the extradural hematoma [1, 2]. Only 15 cases of this atypical form were reported in the literature between 1987 and 2017 [45]. Retrospectively, a crescentic tail, at the margin of CSDH, was seen in 7 of those 15 patients. The

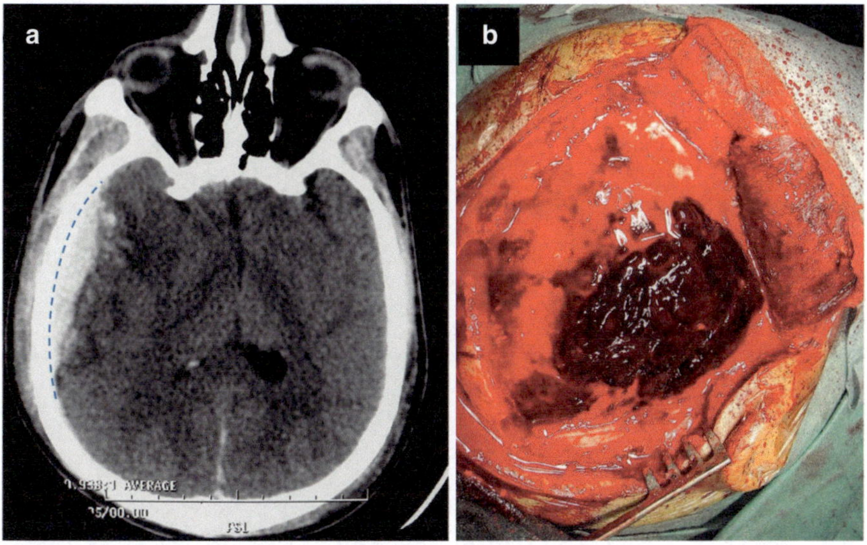

Fig. 26.7 Axial CT-scan: post-traumatic acute temporal extradural hematoma on the right side (**a**). Operative view after removing the bone flap: the acute hematoma (blood clots) was revealed on the epidural (**b**)

cause of the biconvex shape of the CSDH remains ambiguous but may result from the obstruction of the subdural space by some adhesions. Interestingly, all the published cases had operated on with craniotomy and evacuation of hematoma [45].

Some intracranial hematomas are described as "interdural." In this rare condition, a bleeding splits the periosteal dura mater from the meningeal dura mater. Diagnosis of this distinct entity is not easy and requires confirmation by surgical and/or histopathologic results [9, 46].

26.6 Ischemic Stroke

Although some clinical forms of CSDH may appear as ischemic attack, there is no difficulty in differentiating ischemic stroke from subdural hematoma on CT-scan. In one of our patients, a right temporo-occipital chronic heterogeneous subdural hematoma was highly suspected on cranial CT-scan but the correct diagnosis of "brain ischemia" was obtained following MRI features (Fig. 26.8). Retrospectively, CT-scan images had shown brain edema, loss of gray-white differentiation, and no brain shift. As reported by Shimizu et al., the distribution of the low density region did not correspond exactly to the area of the brain arteries and the well-separated margins were not characteristic of classic brain ischemic infarction [49]. The definitive diagnosis will be based on MRI features. This atypical presentation should be considered in elderly with a history of cerebro-vascular diseases.

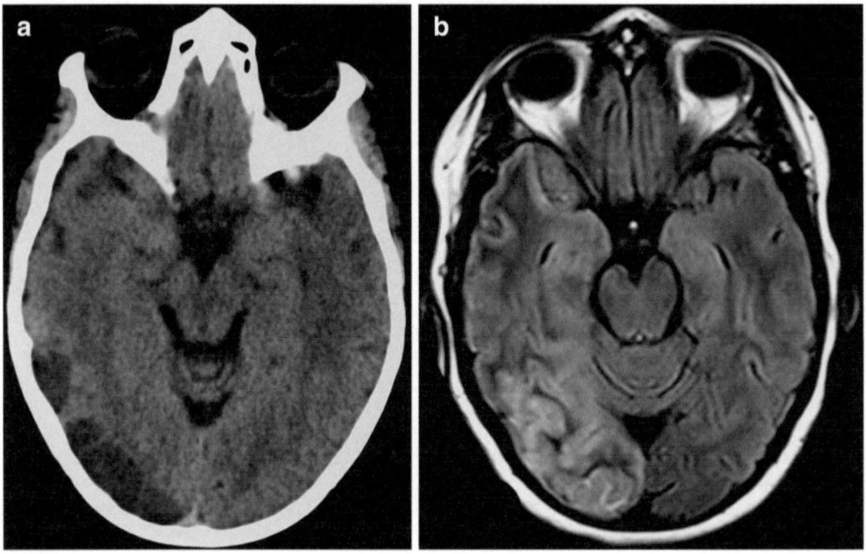

Fig. 26.8 Cranial axial CT-scan: suspicion of "chronic heterogeneous subdural hematoma" on the right side (**a**). Axial MRI on FLAIR sequences showing brain area of ischemia (**b**). Note the brain edema, loss of gray-white differentiation, and no brain shift

26.7 Traumatic Subdural Hygroma (Hydroma)

CSDH and subdural hygroma occur in the subdural space usually after trauma; however, CSDH differs from subdural hygroma in many aspects such as the content of subdural fluid collection, neuroimaging appearance, and clinical manifestations [34]. In some cases, distinction between these two entities is not easy because the subdural content within subdural hygroma is habitually a mixture of blood and cerebrospinal fluid [30]. In addition, it is not uncommon that subdural hygroma becomes a CSDH [See Chap. 16 about CSDH following Traumatic Subdural Hygroma].

Subdural hygroma are considered to occur as a result of the separation of the dura/arachnoid interface after trauma, presenting as small subdural fluid collections. A leptomeningeal (arachnoid membrane) tear and flap valve hypothesis are generally accepted as the pathogenic mechanism [22]. Furthermore, a sufficient potential subdural space (especially cerebral atrophy in the elderly) represents a crucial condition for the expansion of the subdural hygroma [22, 30]. Most hygromas occur around the Sylvian fissure and the frontal lobe convexities.

On both CT-scan and MRI, simple subdural hygromas manifest as subdural collections with density and signal similar to cerebrospinal fluid (Fig. 26.9). However, there have been publications mentioning the development of the increased density within hygroma on CT-scan as well as some heterogeneous signal on MRI related to the CSF admixed with some bleeding [30]. Note that cortical veins should not traverse the fluid collections in subdural hygromas [36].

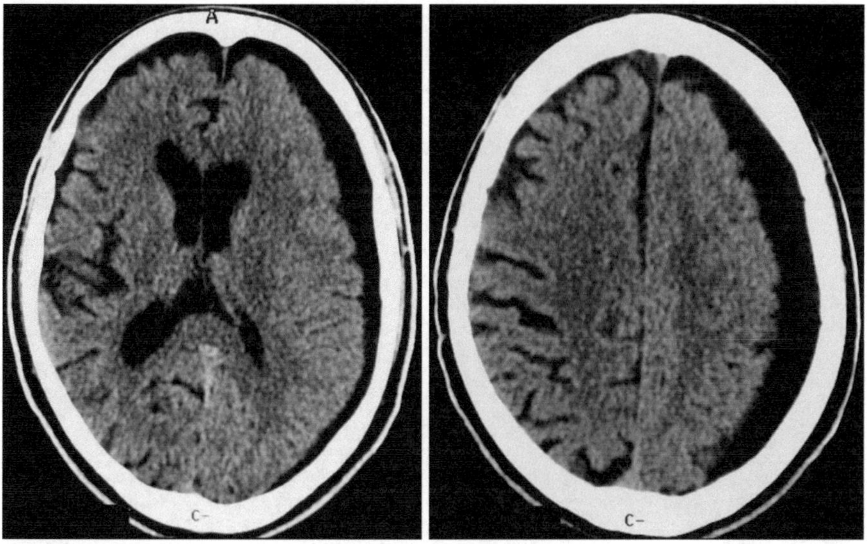

Fig. 26.9 Axial cranial CT-scan showing a left hemispheric subdural hygroma with parenchymal brain compression

26.8 Tumor

A large variety of dural and subdural tumors, primary or metastasis, can be disguised as a CSDH on neuroimaging including lymphoma, metastasis, sarcoma, glioblastoma, meningioma, and solitary fibrous tumor [8, 10, 18–20, 23, 31, 32, 37, 39, 41, 48, 53]. Also, such lesions could be either the cause or the recurrence of CSDH [11, 29, 38]. Taking into account the clinical history, a neoplasm must be suspected in the absence of a head trauma, presence of a nodular appearance of the subdural mass, and enlargement of the lesion on follow-up imaging (Fig. 26.9). In 2016, a systematic review of subdural hematoma mimickers had found that the most common mimicker was lymphoma (29%), followed by metastasis (21%) and sarcoma (15%) [8]. In several reported cases, diagnosis was only made during or after surgery [20, 41, 53]. Non-contrast CT-scan is usually inadequate to differentiate a tumoral lesion from CSDH. However, some appearances can help detecting CSDH on CT-scan including bony change (hyperostosis with meningioma and bony erosion with dural metastasis), nodular and lobular borders, multifocal lesions, and heterogeneous appearance incoherent with different age bleeding [11, 57]. Associated brain edema and cortical extension are also evocative of a malignant neoplasm (Fig. 26.10a). Although post-contrast CT-scan will be useful for identifying the presence of a tumor, gadolinium-enhanced MRI may provide a better resolution including multiplanar imaging (Fig. 26.10b) [32]. Unlike CSDH, sarcoma enhances homogeneously following the gadolinium administration on MRI [23]. Dural metastasis appears as a thickening pachymeningitis with a homogeneous

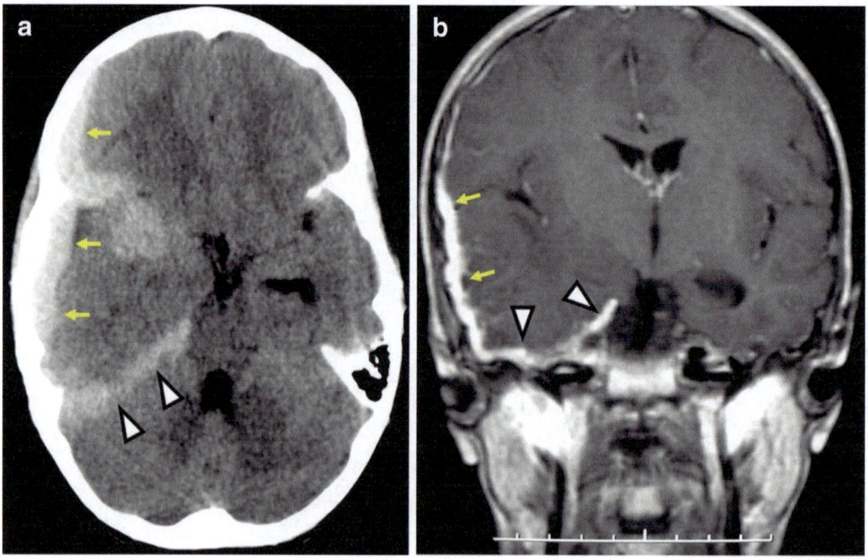

Fig. 26.10 Axial non-enhanced cranial CT-scan (**a**) and coronal post-gadolinium T1-weighted MRI (**b**) revealing an extensive dural lymphoma on the right fronto-temporal convexity (arrows) with tentorial and skull base extension (head-arrows)

gadolinium enhancement [18]. MRI is also valuable to detect small brain parenchymal metastatic extension [29].

26.9 Extracerebral Fluid Collections in Children

Extracerebral or extra-axial fluid collection is a term widely used in pediatric population with intracranial extra-axial fluid collections. Different names have been found in the literature for the same or similar conditions such as benign subdural collection, symptomatic chronic extra-axial fluid collection, external hydrocephalus, subdural hygroma, subdural hematohygromas, pseudohydrocephalus, benign communicating hydrocephalus, and extraventricular obstructive hydrocephalus [17, 26, 33, 40, 59]. This condition can be sometimes confused with CSDH [30]. However, with modern MRI technology, it has become easier to diagnose extracerebral fluid collections in infancy and to differentiate this condition from CSDH [17]. On CT-scan, extracerebral fluid collections appear as peripheral hypodensities over the frontal lobes with dilatation of the interhemispheric fissure, cortical sulci, and sylvian fissure [19, 30]. Ventricles are often normal or slightly distended without transventricular absorption. Many etiologies have been suspected including perinatal trauma, post-infection (e.g., meningitis), shunt revision, post-asphyxia, and defect hemostasis [27, 33].

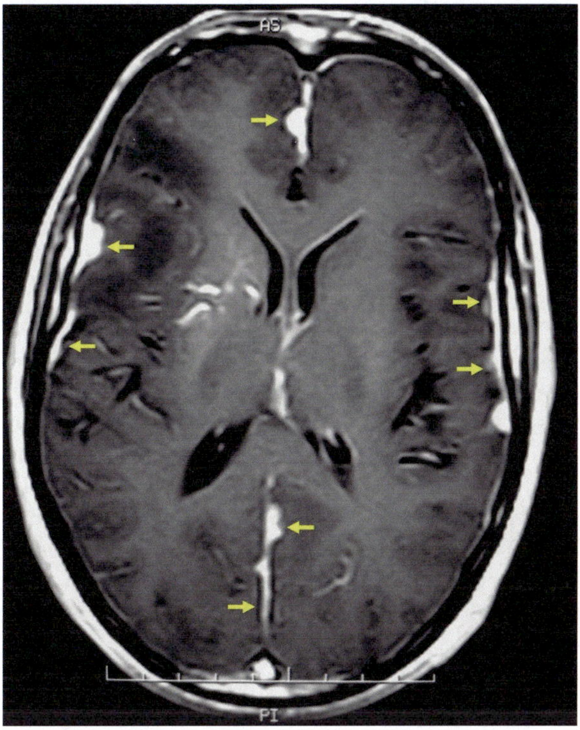

Fig. 26.11 Axial cranial T1-weighted MRI after gadolinium injection showing features of diffuse hypertrophic pachymeningitis with adjacent brain edema. Note the thickened dural enhancement (arrows)

26.10 Hypertrophic Cranial Pachymeningitis

It is known that some forms of CSDH had peripheral membranes that may enhance following post-gadolinium administration on MRI. This is related to fibro-collagenous change but without any coexisting diseases such as infection or malignancy [6]. In contrast, hypertrophic pachymeningitis is a rare variety of diffuse inflammatory pathologies that appears as a thickened of the dura mater usually along the tentorium and the skull base. In addition, some nodular components can be seen in the underlying and neighboring leptomeninges (Fig. 26.11). Several causes of hypertrophic pachymeningitis have been recognized including inflammations, autoimmune disorders, infections, and neoplasms [4, 6, 16, 43, 47]. Appropriate clinical history and extensive radiological, biological, and pathological investigations of extracerebral organs are important for the etiologic diagnosis. However, the exact cause remains unknown in some cases and in this situation the hypertrophic pachymeningitis is called "idiopathic." On CT-scan, the thickened dura appears hyperdense and can easily mimic a subdural hematoma. The hypertrophic dura appears hypointense on T1-weighted and T2-weighted images on MRI. Pachymeninges become enhanced on post-contrast images. Moreover, the "dural tail sign" which is a characteristic of meningiomas may also be encountered on post-gadolinium MRI [43]. Further, leptomeningeal enhancement can be associated with adjacent brain edema (Fig. 26.11).

More rarely, other autoimmune diseases as granulomatosis with polyangiitis (formerly called Wegener's) and Rosai-Dorfman disease may have leptomeningeal intracranial lesions mimicking a CSDH [27, 32, 52, 58].

26.11 Normal Anatomy

Various normal brain and venous structures can mimic CSDH on both CT-scan and MRI. Among them, prominent venous sinuses and cortical veins may be misdiagnosed as subdural hematoma. When these happen, a contrast-enhanced examination will be performed showing homogeneous central enhancement [24, 32].

Also, some lobar parenchymal structures (e.g., frontal lobes and cerebellar flocculus that extend, respectively, into the middle cranial fossa and the posterior fossa) may be a diagnostic challenge to both surgeons and radiologists. The presence of gray and white matter differentiation within the suspected lesion and the careful inspection of adjacent image sections will help in avoiding this error [32].

26.12 Undiagnosed Chronic Subdural Hematoma

Sometimes bilateral or unilateral isodense CSDH may cause a significant difficulty in their diagnosis by CT-scan (Fig. 26.12) [1, 7, 15]; this is due to:

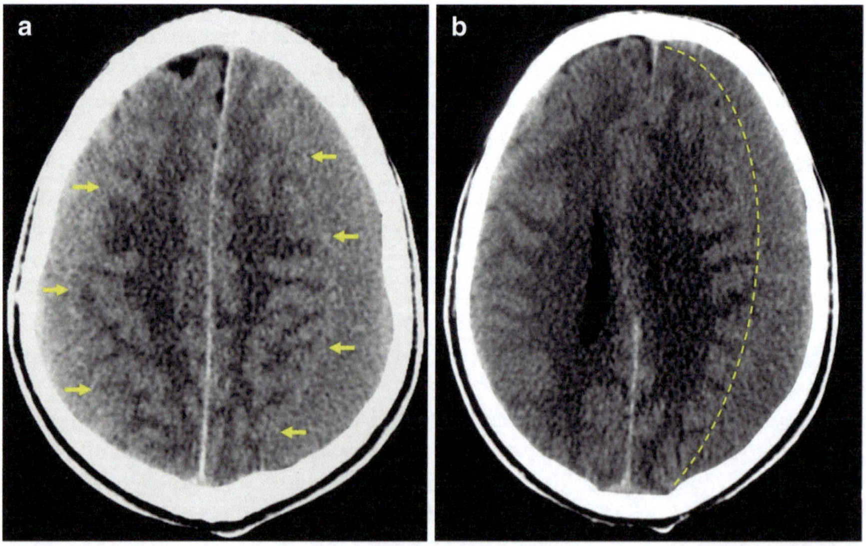

Fig. 26.12 Axial non-enhanced CT-scan. Bilateral isodense CSDH hardly distinguished from the adjacent normal brain parenchyma (arrows) (**a**). Unilateral left isodense subdural hematoma: the internal limit is difficult to differentiate from the adjacent brain parenchyma (dotted line) (**b**)

1. Both subdural collections are difficult to distinguish from the adjacent normal brain parenchyma (despite sulcal effacement).
2. Symmetrical (equivalent) lateral compression of both cerebral hemispheres and lateral ventricles. Consequently, there is no midline shift.

However, the diagnosis is frequently suspected with the so-called "rabbit ears sign" or "squeezed ventricles": medial compression of both ventricles resulting in a narrow and slit-like elongated ventricle (the anterior frontal horns sharply pointed and get closer to each other) [35]. If further confusion persists, a contrast-enhanced CT-scan may show displacement of cortical vessels. In all cases, MRI could help in making the correct diagnosis of such atypical form of CSDH (Fig. 26.6) [7, 56].

26.13 Artifacts on CT-Scan Imaging

Some artifacts can degrade the quality of CT-scan images [5]. Line artifacts along the deep surface of the frontal cranial vault may mimic subdural hematoma [32]. In addition, patient movements can cause shading, blurring, or streaking in the reconstructed CT-scan images. Radiologists must optimize image quality and prevent or suppress both scanner and patient-based artifacts.

26.14 Conclusion

Although unusual, many diagnostic pitfalls and pathologic lesions can be misdiagnosed with CSDH on CT-scan. Moreover, the coexistence of CSDH and other adjacent cranial and/or intracranial pathologies is a possible condition. In case of diagnostic doubt or atypical scanographic features, additional post-contrast CT-scan and even better post-gadolinium MRI should be requested whenever possible. This may specify the topography of the collections and their internal structures, delineating the exact margins of the lesions, and determining the relationship with adjacent anatomic formations. Such information, as well as the clinical presentation and biologic data, will be crucial for the decision-making process. Both radiologists and neurosurgeons must be prepared to identify all these possible situations in preoperative images as well as during medical and/or surgical planning, and even throughout the patient's care.

References

1. Agrawal A. Bilateral biconvex frontal chronic subdural hematoma mimicking extradural hematoma. J Surg Tech Case Rep. 2010;2:90–1. https://doi.org/10.4103/2006-8808.73625.
2. Akhaddar A. The yin-yang shaped image following head injury. Pan Afr Med J. 2013;16:133. https://doi.org/10.11604/pamj.2013.16.133.3555.
3. Akhaddar A. Cranial subdural empyemas. In: Akhaddar A, editor. Atlas of infections in neurosurgery and spinal surgery. Cham: Springer International Publishing; 2017. p. 51–64.

4. Akhaddar A, Rharrassi I. Hypertrophic cranial pachymeningitis coinfection with tuberculosis and actinomycosis. Surg Neurol Int. 2020;11:201. https://doi.org/10.25259/SNI_383_2020.
5. Barrett JF, Keat N. Artifacts in CT: recognition and avoidance. Radiographics. 2004;24:1679–91. https://doi.org/10.1148/rg.246045065.
6. Blitshteyn S, Mechtler LL, Bakshi R. Diffuse dural gadolinium MRI enhancement associated with bilateral chronic subdural hematomas. Clin Imaging. 2004;28:90–2. https://doi.org/10.1016/S0899-7071(03)00205-5.
7. Boviatsis EJ, Kouyialis AT, Sakas DE. Misdiagnosis of bilateral isodense chronic subdural haematomas. Hosp Med. 2003;64:374–5. https://doi.org/10.12968/hosp.2003.64.6.374.
8. Catana D, Koziarz A, Cenic A, Nath S, Singh S, Almenawer SA, et al. Subdural hematoma mimickers: a systematic review. World Neurosurg. 2016;93:73–80. https://doi.org/10.1016/j.wneu.2016.05.084.
9. Chen KT, Huang HC, Lin YJ, Chen MH, Hsieh TC. The relationship between hematoma and pachymeninges in an interdural hematoma: diagnosis and surgical strategy. World Neurosurg. 2018;110:492–8.e3. https://doi.org/10.1016/j.wneu.2017.11.040.
10. Cheng YK, Wang TC, Yang JT, Lee MH, Su CH. Dural metastasis from prostatic adenocarcinoma mimicking chronic subdural hematoma. J Clin Neurosci. 2009;16:1084–6. https://doi.org/10.1016/j.jocn.2008.08.008.
11. Cherif El Asri A, El Mostarchid B, Akhaddar A, Boucetta M. Chronic subdural hematoma revealing skull metastasis. Intern Med. 2011;50:791. https://doi.org/10.2169/internalmedicine.50.4654.
12. Doan N, Patel M, Nguyen HS, Mountoure A, Shabani S, Gelsomino M, et al. Intracranial subdural empyema mimicking a recurrent chronic subdural hematoma. J Surg Case Rep. 2016;2016(9):rjw158. https://doi.org/10.1093/jscr/rjw158.
13. Feinberg WM, Valdivia FR. Cysticercosis presenting as a subdural hematoma. Neurology. 1984;34:1112–3. https://doi.org/10.1212/wnl.34.8.1112.
14. French H, Schaefer N, Keijzers G, Barison D, Olson S. Intracranial subdural empyema: a 10-year case series. Ochsner J. 2014;14:188–94.
15. Guénot M. Chronic subdural hematoma: diagnostic imaging studies. Neurochirurgie. 2001;47:473–8.
16. He Z, Ding F, Rong J, Gan Y. A case of idiopathic hypertrophic cranial pachymeningitis presenting as chronic subdural hematoma. Zhejiang Da Xue Xue Bao Yi Xue Ban. 2016;45:540–3.
17. Hellbusch LC. Benign extracerebral fluid collections in infancy: clinical presentation and long-term follow-up. J Neurosurg. 2007;107(2 Suppl):119–25. https://doi.org/10.3171/PED-07/08/119.
18. Houssem A, Helene C, Francois P, Salvatore C. "The subdural collection" a great simulator: case report and literature review. Asian J Neurosurg. 2018;13:851–3. https://doi.org/10.4103/ajns.AJNS_325_16.
19. Hussain ZB, Hussain AB, Mitchell P. Extra-axial cerebrospinal fluid spaces in children with benign external hydrocephalus: a case-control study. Neuroradiol J. 2017;30:410–7. https://doi.org/10.1177/1971400917719298.
20. Ichinose T, Ueno M, Watanabe T, Murakami KI, Minato H, Hayashi Y. A rare case of chronic subdural hematoma coexisting with metastatic tumor. World Neurosurg. 2020;139:196–9. https://doi.org/10.1016/j.wneu.2020.04.029.
21. Im SH, Park SH, Oh DH, Kang BS, Kwon OK, Oh CW. Subdural cysticercosis mimicking a chronic subdural hematoma. Case illustration. J Neurosurg. 2005;102:389. https://doi.org/10.3171/jns.2005.102.2.0389.
22. Kamezaki T, Yanaka K, Fujita K, Nakamura K, Nagatomo Y, Nose T. Traumatic acute subdural hygroma mimicking acute subdural hematoma. J Clin Neurosci. 2004;11:311–3. https://doi.org/10.1016/j.jocn.2003.10.013.
23. Kanazawa T, Miwa T, Akiyama T, Ohara K, Kosugi K, Nishimoto M, et al. A case of aggressive recurrent intracranial subdural hematoma associated with angiosarcoma originating from the skull. World Neurosurg. 2019;126:120–3. https://doi.org/10.1016/j.wneu.2019.02.168.

24. Kiliç T, Akakin A. Anatomy of cerebral veins and sinuses. Front Neurol Neurosci. 2008;23:4–15. https://doi.org/10.1159/000111256.
25. Komiyama M, Yasui T, Tamura K, Nagata Y, Fu Y, Yagura H. Chronic subdural hematoma associated with middle meningeal arteriovenous fistula treated by a combination of embolization and burr hole drainage. Surg Neurol. 1994;42:316–9. https://doi.org/10.1016/0090-3019(94)90400-6.
26. Kozubek D. Widening of the pericerebral space in infants—consultative problems. Arch Med Sadowej Kryminol. 2019;69:70–81. https://doi.org/10.5114/amsik.2019.89237.
27. Kumar KK, Menon G, Nair S, Radhakrishnan VV. Rosai-Dorfman disease mimicking chronic subdural hematoma. J Clin Neurosci. 2008;15:1293–5. https://doi.org/10.1016/j.jocn.2007.09.010.
28. Kwak YS, Hwang SK, Park SH, Park JY. Chronic subdural hematoma associated with the middle fossa arachnoid cyst: pathogenesis and review of its management. Childs Nerv Syst. 2013;29:77–82. https://doi.org/10.1007/s00381-012-1896-4.
29. Lecouvet FE, Annet L, Duprez TP, Cosnard G, Scordidis V, Malghem J. Uncommon magnetic resonance imaging observation of lumbar subdural hematoma with cranial origin. J Comput Assist Tomogr. 2003;27:530–3. https://doi.org/10.1097/00004728-200307000-00013.
30. Lee HC, Chong S, Lee JY, Cheon JE, Phi JH, Kim SK, et al. Benign extracerebral fluid collection complicated by subdural hematoma and fluid collection: clinical characteristics and management. Childs Nerv Syst. 2018;34:235–45. https://doi.org/10.1007/s00381-017-3583-y.
31. Lee J, Kim MS, Kim YZ. Extensive pachymeningeal dissemination of glioblastoma mimicking chronic subdural hematoma: a case report. Brain Tumor Res Treat. 2019;7:39–43. https://doi.org/10.14791/btrt.2019.7.e24.
32. Lim M, Kheok SW, Lim KC, Venkatanarasimha N, Small JE, Chen RC. Subdural haematoma mimics. Clin Radiol. 2019;74:663–75. https://doi.org/10.1016/j.crad.2019.04.013.
33. Litofsky NS, Raffel C, McComb JG. Management of symptomatic chronic extra-axial fluid collections in pediatric patients. Neurosurgery. 1992;31:445–50. https://doi.org/10.1227/00006123-199209000-00009.
34. Liu Y, Gong J, Li F, Wang H, Zhu S, Wu C. Traumatic subdural hydroma: clinical characteristics and classification. Injury. 2009;40:968–72. https://doi.org/10.1016/j.injury.2009.01.006.
35. Marcu H, Becker H. Computed-tomography of bilateral isodense chronic subdural hematomas. Neuroradiology. 1977;14:81–3. https://doi.org/10.1007/BF00339964.
36. McCluney KW, Yeakley JW, Fenstermacher MJ, Baird SH, Bonmati CM. Subdural hygroma versus atrophy on MR brain scans: "the cortical vein sign". AJNR Am J Neuroradiol. 1992;13:1335–9.
37. Miki K, Kai Y, Hiraki Y, Kamano H, Oka K, Natori Y. Malignant meningioma mimicking chronic subdural hematoma. World Neurosurg. 2019:S1878-8750(18)32952-8. https://doi.org/10.1016/j.wneu.2018.12.129.
38. Mirsadeghi SM, Habibi Z, Meybodi KT, Nejat F, Tabatabai SA. Malignant subdural effusion associated with disseminated adenocarcinoma: a case report. Cases J. 2008;1:328. https://doi.org/10.1186/1757-1626-1-328.
39. Neeley OJ, Al-Hreish KM, Aoun SG, El Ahmadieh TY, Plitt A, Vance AZ, et al. Tumoral mimics of subdural hematomas: case report and review of diagnostic and management strategies in primary B-cell lymphoma of the subdural space. World Neurosurg. 2020;133:49–54. https://doi.org/10.1016/j.wneu.2019.09.091.
40. Nguyen VN, Wallace D, Ajmera S, Akinduro O, Smith LJ, Giles K, et al. Management of subdural hematohygromas in abusive head trauma. Neurosurgery. 2020;86:281–7. https://doi.org/10.1093/neuros/nyz076.
41. O'Brien CE, Saratsis AM, Voyadzis JM. Granulocytic sarcoma in a patient with blast crisis mimicking a chronic subdural hematoma. J Clin Oncol. 2011;29:e569–71. https://doi.org/10.1200/JCO.2010.33.1272.
42. Ohno S, Ikeda Y, Onitsuka T, Nakajima S, Haraoka J. Bilateral chronic subdural hematoma in a young adult mimicking subarachnoid hemorrhage. No To Shinkei. 2004;56:701–4.

43. Park IS, Kim H, Chung EY, Cho KW. Idiopathic hypertrophic cranial pachymeningitis misdiagnosed as acute subtentorial hematoma. J Korean Neurosurg Soc. 2010;48:181–4. https://doi.org/10.3340/jkns.2010.48.2.181.
44. Per H, Gümüş H, Tucer B, Akgün H, Kurtsoy A, Kumandaş S. Calcified chronic subdural hematoma mimicking calvarial mass: a case report. Brain Dev. 2006;28:607–9. https://doi.org/10.1016/j.braindev.2006.03.012.
45. Prasad GL, Menon GR. Lentiform subdural hematoma-a rare mimicker of extradural hematoma. World Neurosurg. 2017;97:738–41. https://doi.org/10.1016/j.wneu.2016.08.109.
46. Prieto R, Pascual JM, Subhi-Issa I, Yus M. Acute epidural-like appearance of an encapsulated solid non-organized chronic subdural hematoma. Neurol Med Chir (Tokyo). 2010;50:990–4. https://doi.org/10.2176/nmc.50.990.
47. Rossi S, Giannini F, Cerase A, Bartalini S, Tripodi S, Volpi N, et al. Uncommon findings in idiopathic hypertrophic cranial pachymeningitis. J Neurol. 2004;251:548–55. https://doi.org/10.1007/s00415-004-0362-y.
48. Semonche A, Gomez P, Kolcun JPG, Perez-Roman RJ, Starke RM. Primary central nervous system lymphoma presenting as chronic subdural hematoma: case report and review of the literature. Cureus. 2020;12:e7043. https://doi.org/10.7759/cureus.7043.
49. Shimizu S, Ozawa T, Irikura K, Sagiuchi T, Kan S, Fujii K. Huge chronic subdural hematoma mimicking cerebral infarction on computed tomography—case report. Neurol Med Chir (Tokyo). 2002;42:380–2. https://doi.org/10.2176/nmc.42.380.
50. Shrestha R, You C. Spontaneous chronic subdural hematoma associated with arachnoid cyst in children and young adults. Asian J Neurosurg. 2014;9:168–72. https://doi.org/10.4103/1793-5482.142739.
51. Son D, Kim Y, Kim C, Lee S. Pseudo-subarachnoid hemorrhage; chronic subdural hematoma with an unruptured aneurysm mistaken for subarachnoid hemorrhage. Korean J Neurotrauma. 2019;15:28–33. https://doi.org/10.13004/kjnt.2019.15.e11.
52. Song JS, Lim MK, Park BH, Park W. Acute pachymeningitis mimicking subdural hematoma in a patient with polyarteritis nodosa. Rheumatol Int. 2005;25:637–40. https://doi.org/10.1007/s00296-005-0615-9.
53. Tan LQ, Loh DD, Qiu L, Ng YP, Hwang PYK. When hoofbeats mean zebras not horses: tumour mimics of subdural haematoma—case series and literature review. J Clin Neurosci. 2019;67:244–8. https://doi.org/10.1016/j.jocn.2019.06.035.
54. Tokuno T, Sato S, Kawakami Y, Yamamoto T. Bilateral chronic subdural hematomas presented with subarachnoid hemorrhage: report of two cases. No Shinkei Geka. 1996;24:573–6.
55. Turgut M, Akhaddar A, Turgut AT. Calcified or ossified chronic subdural hematoma: a systematic review of 114 cases reported during last century with a demonstrative case report. World Neurosurg. 2020;134:240–63. https://doi.org/10.1016/j.wneu.2019.10.153.
56. Williams VL, Hogg JP. Magnetic resonance imaging of chronic subdural hematoma. Neurosurg Clin N Am. 2000;11:491–8.
57. Wu C, Liu J, Yang C. Meningioma mimics chronic subdural hematoma: a case report and discussion of differential diagnosis. Neurol India. 2012;60:549–50. https://doi.org/10.4103/0028-3886.103222.
58. Yagita K, Shinde A, Suenaga T. Rheumatoid meningitis can present MRI findings that mimic chronic subdural haematoma. BMJ Case Rep. 2019;12:e229642. https://doi.org/10.1136/bcr-2019-229642.
59. Zahl SM, Wester K, Gabaeff S. Examining perinatal subdural haematoma as an aetiology of extra-axial hygroma and chronic subdural haematoma. Acta Paediatr. 2020;109:659–66. https://doi.org/10.1111/apa.15072.

Chapter 27
Nonsurgical Treatment of Chronic Subdural Hematoma

Abad Cherif El Asri, Ali Akhaddar, and Miloudi Gazzaz

27.1 Introduction

CSDH is expected to be increasingly common with our aging population. The average incidence is approximately 13.1 per 100,000 people, but reaches 58 per 100,000 among those who are 70 years of age or older [7, 36]. While not common, CSDH can also occur in children. Since surgery is effective for removing CSDH and reducing the associated neurological deficits, its application is limited by contraindications, the old age of patients, preexisting comorbidities and there is also the high risk of recurrence. However, based on pathophysiologic mechanisms, animal experiments, and clinical studies, other more conservative options for the treatment of CSDH are worth investigating and are demonstrating promising results in well selected patients [10, 15, 16].

27.1.1 Rational for Nonsurgical Treatment: Why Surgical Treatment Is to Be Discussed?

While there is no consensus on the best treatment for the individual patient diagnosed with a CSDH, two therapeutic modes are generally chosen: observation for asymptomatic patients and hematoma drainage for symptomatic patients. A few

A. C. El Asri (✉) · M. Gazzaz
Department of Neurosurgery, Mohamed V Military Hospital, Mohamed V, University Mohammed V of Rabat, Rabat, Morocco

A. Akhaddar
Avicenne Military Hospital of Marrakech, Department of Neurosurgery, Mohammed V University in Rabat, Rabat, Morocco

M. Turgut et al. (eds.), *Subdural Hematoma*,
https://doi.org/10.1007/978-3-030-79371-5_27

studies have described spontaneous resolution of CSDH. In their meta-analysis, Horikoshi et al. reported that 2.4–18.0% of cases of CSDH resolved spontaneously without surgical or medical intervention [13, 16, 26]. Otherwise, surgery has been classically considered as the first line of treatment for CSDH and overall surgical techniques have been convincingly demonstrated as effective treatment in the current literature for CSDH patients [10]. While surgery is effective in eliminating or reducing hematoma size, 27–33% of the patients develop recurrent hematoma and the overall mortality is as high as 24–32% among surgically treated patients with CSDH [35, 38]. Surgery is also associated with infection, bleeding, and seizures. Furthermore, surgery is contraindicated in patients with severe cardiac and pulmonary diseases (heart failure and recent myocardial infarction), hereditary bleeding disorders, and intracranial or systemic infections. Because of these limitations for surgery, the safe and effective nonsurgical treatment based on stimulation of vessel maturation and anti-inflammatory pathways may contribute to the resolution of CSDH and may induce neurologic recovery [3, 7, 35].

27.1.2 Rational of Drug Use in the Treatment of CSDH

27.1.2.1 Pathophysiological Support: Fig. 27.1

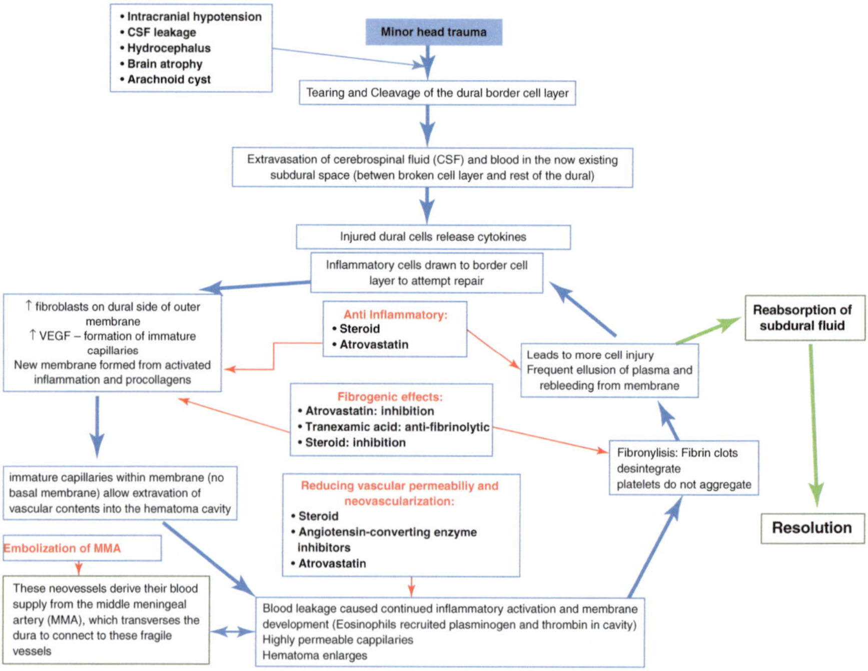

Fig. 27.1 Schematic representation of pathophysiological support of the nonsurgical treatment in CSDH

27.1.2.2 Corticosteroids: Dexamethasone (DXM)

The use of steroids in the treatment of CSDH has recently gained popularity as a therapeutic alternative [40]. It has been established that VEGF and ACE, as well as other inflammatory and angiogenic mediators, play a crucial role in the pathogenesis and maintenance of CSDH [49]. Therefore, it is postulated that corticosteroids reduce or even disrupt the inflammation-induced angiogenic reaction in CSDH through the inhibition of these inflammatory and angiogenetic factors [38, 42]. In view of this pathogenesis underlying CSDH, the efficacy of steroids has been evaluated in observational studies as a monotherapy or as an adjunct to surgical drainage [4, 7, 36, 44, 45, 52]. Most authors conclude that corticosteroids might be a valid alternative for patients with CSDH not suitable for surgical treatment. In their prospective cohort study of 112 patients comparing outcomes between patients treated with corticosteroids (DXM 4 mg four times a day for 21 days), patients treated with burr hole drainage and postoperative corticosteroids, patients with surgical drainage alone, and patients receiving neither surgery nor corticosteroids, Sun et al. observed that hospitalization time, outcome, and mortality were comparable in all groups without significant steroid-related complications [13]. Also, Delgado-Lopez et al. compared, in a retrospectively manner, conservative treatment with corticosteroids versus surgical treatment and reported that surgery was avoided in 2/3 of the cases in the corticosteroid group and that 96% showed a favorable outcome, compared to 93% in the surgical group. The authors concluded that corticosteroids were effective in 67% of the cases and are therefore a safe and feasible conservative treatment for patients presenting with CSDH with mild or moderate neurological symptoms [8].

As an adjunct to surgery, a retrospective study concluded that the use of DXM after burr hole trephination reduces disease recurrence and complication risk [4, 36]. Lastly, a recent meta-analysis by Yao et al. which involved a total of 523 patients indicated that steroid therapy, used alone or as an adjuvant, may be associated with lower recurrence rates of CSDH, but individual study results were highly heterogeneous [52].

Furthermore, Thotakura and Marabathina identified several variables (female sex, limited midline shift and hematoma thickness, and lower CT attenuation values) that are associated with a good outcome after conservative treatment with dexamethasone [44, 45]. The authors then proposed a radiological grading scale (Table 27.1) that can help predict the chance of successful treatment with corticosteroids. They concluded that in patients with low grades (0–2) corticosteroid treatment might be more successful than in the high grades (4 and 5).

On the other hand, Berghauser et al. showed that longer periods of preoperative DXM before burr hole craniotomy were independently associated with lower CSDH recurrence rates [4]. Recently, Miah et al. conducted a study to compare the clinical outcomes of patients with CSDH treated with dexamethasone as monotherapy versus primary surgical management [26]. They found no difference in good functional outcome after initial DXM therapy compared to primary surgery for symptomatic CSDH. Although surgery was prevented in 17% after initial DXM treatment, this

Table 27.1 Proposed Amit-Rao radiological grading of chronic subdural hematoma[a]

Size based on midline shift	
Small (no midline shift)	0
Medium (less than 5 mm)	1
Large (5–10 mm)	2
Massive (more than 10 mm)	3
[a]In bilateral CSDH one extra point to be added	
Density based on HU in CT scan	
Less than 30	0
31–40	1
More than 40	2

[a]This table was taken from Thotakura and Marabathina [44]

strategy is still associated with a high rate of crossover to surgery, a significantly longer overall hospital stay, and more complications.

Similar observations were reported recently by Almenawer et al. in their systematic review and meta-analysis. They found that studies describing corticosteroids use as adjuvant therapy to surgical management demonstrated significantly higher morbidities with no added benefits in recurrence and cure rates and they postulated that more evidence is needed to further investigate the role of steroids as a sole treatment for milder presentations [1].

The downside of DXM use is a higher complication rate such as diabetes, infections, and (temporary) mental changes that also resulted into a longer length of hospitalization than primary burr hole surgery. The mortality in studies using DXM for treatment of CSDH varies between 0.8 and 4% [7, 16, 26].

Given these disparate results, several trials evaluating the use of steroids in CSDH treatment are underway, such as the SUCRE, DESCA, and Dex-CSDH trials [11, 19, 25].

In summary, corticosteroids appear to play a role in the conservative treatment of CSDH despite their side effects. Moreover, the ideal dosage and duration of treatment is still unclear, and the ideal patient group for this particular treatment is still to be determined. Although the few existing studies show promising results, the rational for using corticosteroids as a medical treatment is still based on theory, and obviously needs to be ascertained through large prospective randomized studies [53].

27.1.2.3 Atorvastatin

Besides its well-known role in decreasing the levels of low-density lipoprotein cholesterol through inhibiting 3-hydroxy-3-methyl glutaryl coenzyme A reductase, atorvastatin as a statin has also demonstrated other useful proprieties by suppressing local inflammation and promoting angiogenesis in an experimental model [10, 12, 15].

In mice models of subdural hematoma, a low dose of atorvastatin (3 mg/kg/day) improves the level of peripheral blood endothelial progenitor cells and angiogenic factors and promotes angiogenesis and the formation of functional blood vessels. A higher dose of atorvastatin (8 mg/kg/day) led to a significantly increased and persistently high level of VEGF and increased levels of inflammatory factor matrix metalloprotease 9 [2, 5, 22].

As a conservative treatment method, it is also expected to suppress inflammation at the site of the hematoma. The inflammation has been widely reported to disrupt the endothelial cell barrier, leading to the formation of "leaky vessels." By reducing inflammation-induced vascular leakage and promoting angiogenesis, atorvastatin prevents the formation and accelerates the absorption of the hematoma to improve the neurological function of patients with CSDH [43, 48].

Through these mechanisms, atorvastatin could be of merit in the management of patients with CSDH and in decreasing the need for surgery [33]. In fact, several recent studies showed the role of atorvastatin in reducing the volume of hematoma and decreasing the rate of recurrent CSDH requiring surgery.

Wang et al. conducted a prospective study including 23 patients who were treated conservatively for CSDH with atorvastatin (oral dose of 20 mg once a day for 1–6 months) [49]. Among patients included in the study, a significant reduction in hematoma volume was seen within the first month of treatment in 22 patients without relapse or significant adverse events during the 36 months of follow-up, and only one patient underwent surgery because of neurological deterioration after 4 weeks of conservative treatment [49].

Jiang et al. evaluated the safety and efficacy of atorvastatin in the nonsurgical treatment of CSDH through a double-blind, randomized, placebo-controlled clinical trial and showed that the atorvastatin group had significantly higher hematoma volume reduction and clinical improvement with better quality of life, and reduced the need for surgery in patients with CSDH after 8 weeks with the absence of significant adverse events. Atorvastatin appears to be more effective for older patients with relatively larger hematomas. As 11.2% of patients in this trial failed to respond, the same authors conducted a phase II randomized trial that demonstrated the superiority of combined dexamethasone and atorvastatin compared to atorvastatin alone in reducing hematoma volume and improving neurological function [15, 49]. Some studies even suggest that atorvastatin is as effective as surgery in patients with mild CSDH [39, 41].

Therefore, the use of atorvastatin could be an effective addition to the treatment of CSDH with and without surgery [21]. In a pooled meta-analysis of six studies comprising 756 patients with CSDH, He et al. revealed that atorvastatin is effective in both conservative and surgical treatment of CSDH patients by decreasing rate of recurrence requiring surgery and improving neurological function recovery [10]. In our experience, the use of atorvastatin demonstrated its efficacy in resolving small to moderate CSDH in 5 of 6 treated patients in our ongoing prospective study (example in Fig. 27.2).

To conclude, it appears that atorvastatin is a valid and safe option for the conservative treatment of asymptomatic or mildly symptomatic CSDH patients (type C

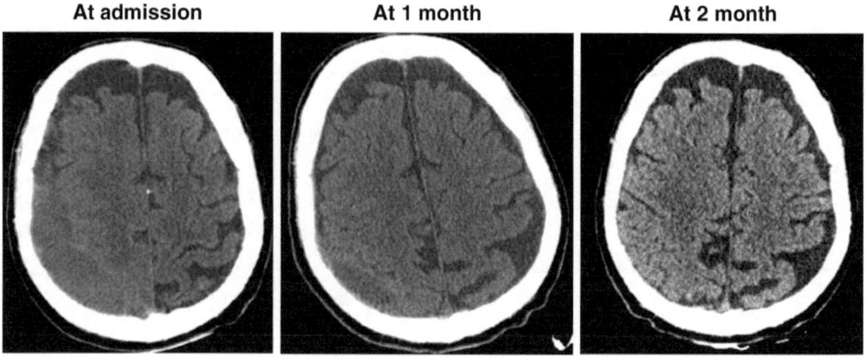

Fig. 27.2 Serial CT scan showing the progressive resorption of CSDH in a 73-year-old man, who experienced hemiparesis and headache and memory disturbance 3 weeks after a benign head trauma, treated with atorvastatin for 8 weeks

recommendation) [27, 47]. Further prospective studies with bigger cohorts are needed in order to determine the true value of statins in the conservative treatment of CSDH [41].

27.1.2.4 Tranexamic Acid

Tranexamic acid (Txa) has been used as a medication to reduce bleeding events in various types of surgeries, and the effectiveness has been demonstrated. There is recent interest in the role of tranexamic acid as a conservative treatment for chronic subdural hematoma [7]. Fibrinolytic and coagulative hyperactivity seem to play a role in the liquefaction and progression of CSDH [27]. In fact, tranexamic acid decreases plasmin activity by reversibly binding to lysine sites on plasminogen, thereby reducing both fibrinolysis and inflammation. Theoretically, tranexamic acid breaks the cycle of neomembrane formation, re-hemorrhage, inflammation, and elevated vascular permeability, thus allowing gradual reabsorption of hematoma fluid within the neomembranes [36]. Based on these assumptions, a retrospective study conducted by Kageyama et al. analyzed the influence of tranexamic acid on 21 patients with CSDH managed conservatively. They showed, in 18 patients treated with 750 mg of tranexamic acid once a day as monotreatment, a complete resorption of all hematomas without adverse events [16]. Another study comprising 232 patients with CSDH were examined to compare the recurrent rates and residual hematomas between Txa and Chinese Kampo medicine Gorie-san after burr hole surgery. The authors concluded that though there was no significant difference in recurrence rates between the two, the size of the residual hematomas was much smaller in the Txa group [51]. Recently Kutty et al. conducted a prospective observational study about treatment of CSDH with Txa (750 mg/day in divided doses) in 27 patients who were mildly symptomatic and willing to have conservative management. All patients had good resolution of the hematomas, and none of the hematomas progressed during conservative treatment without any complications. They concluded that the conservative management of CSDH with Txa is both a safe and effective alternative in the absence of life-threatening symptoms [20].

Despite these promising results from observational studies, the real role of tranexamic acid in the treatment of CSDH is still uncertain, in particular, its effect on the resorption of CSDH and the adverse event rate, especially in patients at risk for thromboembolic events. The author of the most extensive series of primary Txa for CSDH has not found any adverse effects related to Txa in the form of venous thromboembolism. The results of two large randomized trials CRASH225 and CRASH which used Txa for extracranial and intracranial head injuries, respectively, also did not find any significant difference between thromboembolic episodes between Txa and placebo [6, 37]. Tranexamic acid (Txa) might be one such drug in the armamentarium for conservative management of CSDH, but because of its primary use as a hemostatic agent and the concerns regarding thromboembolic/ischemic infarcts, its safety still needs to be evaluated in larger studies and therefore recommendations cannot be made [45, 51].

27.1.2.5 Angiotensin-Converting Enzyme Inhibitors (ACE Inhibitors)

On the basis of the angiogenic hypothesis of CSDH, it is assumed that ACE inhibitors might lower the risk for developing a CSDH and for its recurrence [34, 41]. ACE inhibitors decrease VEGF production, possibly resulting in a reduction of new and immature vascularization, a decrease in extravasation of fluid into the subdural space, and a reduction in recurrence of CSDH. Only a few studies were carried out on the usage of ACE inhibitors in patients of CSDH with variable results. Weigel et al. showed a lower recurrence rate of CSDH after surgical drainage in patients treated with ACE inhibitors for hypertension. They concluded that ACE inhibitors lower the recurrence rate and might even lower the risk of developing a CSDH through their antiangiogenic mechanism [50]. However, contrary data have been presented, since ACE inhibitors are known to increase the levels of bradykinin, which is a vasoactive peptide, inducing both permeability and vasodilatation, and leading to blood extravasation from the neomembranes in CSDH, and consequently to an enlargement of the hematoma [30]. This was demonstrated by Poulsen et al. in a randomized trial on the use of perindopril on residual CSDH volume; they suggested that perindopril does not diminish the size of residual CSDH 6 weeks after burr hole surgery and that ACE inhibitors do not decrease the risk of CSDH recurrence [34, 45].

To the best of our knowledge, there are no further publications studying the role of ACE inhibitors in the treatment of CSDH, or comparing them to surgical treatment. Based on the available data, the benefit of ACE inhibitors as an adjuvant treatment to the surgical evacuation of CSDH is ambiguous. ACE inhibitors do not seem to reduce the recurrence rate of CSDH and cannot be recommended at this point [40].

27.1.2.6 Traditional Herbal Treatment "Gorei-San"

Some authors from Japan studied the usage of Gorei-san, a herbal medicine that exhibits a hydragogue effect by inhibiting the expression of aquaporins, in patients with CSDH. Okamura et al. suggested the potential role of preoperative use of Gorei-san in preventing postoperative recurrence of CSDH in their retrospective study of 125 patients [31]. Similar results in its role in minimizing the recurrence of CSDH were described recently by Katayama et al., in their randomized multicentric study in 2018, for patient treated with Gorei-san after surgery [17].

27.1.3 Who Are More Suitable for Nonsurgical Treatment?

The treatment modality could be determined according to the patient's symptoms, comorbidities and imaging features and also preference of the patient and the neurosurgeon. Some authors advocate that patients who have minimal neurological deficits and lesions of small size have a greater chance for spontaneous resolution of their hematoma [41]. Otherwise, large hematomas with moderate or severe neurological symptoms usually are recommended to have surgical evacuation. The more challenging cases are patients with moderate symptoms and or large hematoma, and which highlight the need for an early diagnosis of CSDH before the Glasgow Coma Score deteriorates and which will allow for a conservative approach and improve the outcome of patients. Furthermore, there are some factors which might influence the outcome of medical treatment in chronic subdural hematoma like the age, sex, neurological status, size, and thickness of hematoma.

27.1.3.1 Age

It is a well-known fact that CSDH incidence increases with age. The atrophy of the brain increases with the age and there will be more space available in the cranial cavity to accommodate more blood without many symptoms. Some authors suggested that age over 70 years, worsening mental function, the presence of brain atrophy, and absence of clinical and radiological symptoms due to increased intracranial pressure are clinical and radiological findings that allow one to choose conservative therapy [18, 33]. Even in surgical series, age was also reported as a risk factor, that satisfactory outcomes were achieved in only 24% of patients who are 90 years or older, regardless of the types of surgery performed [4, 8]. So, early diagnosis of CSDH in this aging population even with few symptoms might be the rule, because surgery is more likely to be contraindicated in these patients and they can have worse surgical outcomes due to preexisting comorbidities. The conservative treatment might be a valuable option.

27.1.3.2 Neurological Status

The neurological status of the patient is the most important clinical factor that decides whether medical treatment can or cannot be tried. As already shown by some authors, the medical treatment will show an initial response within 3 days to 1 week time generally and will take up to 8–12 weeks of time to resolve or decrease the size of the CSDH [7, 16, 31, 45]. Whereas, the patients who are comatose or of poor neurological grade should not be treated medically. The authors who tried different nonsurgical medical treatments included patients with a better neurological status [2, 7, 41]. The symptoms of patients who had spontaneous resolution of CSDH were reported to have mild headache and a minimal decrease in cognitive level. Although some authors recorded that the presence of hemiparesis was associated with the requirement for surgery, in our experience two patients experienced recovery of their hemiparesis when treated with atorvastatin for 2–3 months (Fig. 27.2) [7, 13, 16]. However, it is important to classify CSDH to find the subgroups of patients who will improve with medical treatment and those who are resistant to treatment. According to Markwalder, patients of CSDH can be classified into five grades (Grades 0–4) based on their neurological status [24]. Some authors modified the Markwalder neurological grading by using the Glasgow Coma Scale in the grading [23, 24, 28, 45]. Hence, only good neurological grade patients (0–2) can be treated medically.

27.1.3.3 Gender

The incidence of CSDH is much less in the female population compared to the male population [16, 36, 45]. Though reasons could not be proved, suggested theories include trauma, morphological causes, and hormonal factors. Thotakura and Marabathina noted more successful results with steroid treatment in female patients compared to male patients. Five out of 6 female patients (83.3%) were treated successfully, when only 6 of the 20 male patients (30%) could be treated successfully with steroids [26]. Giuffrè et al. observed a higher incidence of estrogen receptors and progesterone receptors in men rather than in women in their study of the hematoma external membrane [9]. According to the investigators, in men, whose tissues are not usually adapted to the estrogen action, the effect of estrogen on responsive tissue, such as a newly vascularized hematoma external membrane, could lead to increased formation of tissue plasminogen activator, which could maintain local hyperfibrinolysis [35, 36, 44, 45, 47]. The factors that help the female population in preventing the formation of chronic SDH, mostly hormonal factors, might also help them to achieve good outcomes with steroid treatment [44].

27.1.3.4 Size of the Lesion

Size of the chronic subdural hematoma, represented by the volume, is an important factor that is responsible for the degree of mass effect and the symptoms of the patient. The size of the CSDH is classified into small, medium, large, and massive hematoma based on the amount of midline shift. In bilateral chronic subdural hematomas, one additional point to add is there will be more mass effect and a lower incidence of midline shift [46]. Minimum possible grade is 0 and maximum possible grade is 5. Low grades include 0 to 2, high grades include 4 and 5, and the remaining one, grade 3 is termed intermediate grade [44]. Some authors noted that small-sized CSDH responds better with medical treatment. Horikoshi et al. stated that asymptomatic SDHs localized in the frontal region with minimal signs of mass effect can be expected to disappear spontaneously without deterioration [13]. Delgado-Lopez et al. noted in their study that large- to massive-sized lesions cause more mass effect, some of them have poor clinical grades and most of them require surgery [7].

On the other hand, midline shift can also be given more importance as it represents the overall mass effect on the brain and is easy to measure on imaging. The midline shift is correlated with the neurological status of the patient and consequently it must be considered in the choice and decision to treat the CSDH.

27.1.3.5 Density of the Hematoma

CSDH has been classified, according to its density on computed tomography (CT), into high, mixed, iso, and low density hematomas. Park et al. added layered type to the existing types [32]. A radiological classification of the internal architecture of the hematoma, corresponding to various stages in the natural history of CSDH, was suggested by Nakaguchi et al. in 2001, and they categorized the stages as distinct homogeneous type, Laminar type, Separated type, and Trabecular type [29]. Ito et al. demonstrated that the amount of hemoglobin is correlated with the density (HU) in the subdural hematomas. The high density collections are richer in hemoglobin and consequently require more time to resolve by natural means or by medical management. The less dense hematomas will be absorbed more easily and respond better with steroids [14]. Similar conclusions were made by Thotakura and Marabathina in their further work [44]. Nakamura et al. stated that the decreased fibrinolytic activity of the hematoma capsule and the fluid might have caused spontaneous resolution. They also noted that the resolving hematoma appeared as a low-density area or an area of decreasing density, from mixed to low, on successive CT scans [18].

27.2 Conclusion

It can be thought that the CSDH is a spectrum of disease. The small lesions cause less mass effect with fewer symptoms and may resolve spontaneously. Surgical treatment is still considered the gold standard for symptomatic CSDH, but may become complex because most of the patients are advanced in age and/or are being treated with anticoagulation. Furthermore, conservative treatment may be highly valuable in some situations. Clinical and radiological classifications are more important and useful for medical treatment protocols as the patient can be classified on admission and appropriate treatment can be planned. Once the conservative option is chosen, the remaining issue appears to be which of the medications to use, its dosage, the duration of treatment, and also the method to measure the drug's efficacy.

In our point of view and through our ongoing experience, atorvastatin appears to be of more convincing benefit by its proven efficacy with few side effects compared to other nonsurgical options. Further prospective studies with larger patient cohorts are needed in order to determine the true value of each drug in the conservative treatment of CSDH.

References

1. Almenawer SA, Farrokhyar F, Hong C, Alhazzani W, Manoranjan B, Yarascavitch B, et al. Chronic subdural hematoma management: a systematic review and meta-analysis of 34,829 patients. Ann Surg. 2014;259(3):449–57.
2. Araujo FA, Rocha MA, Mendes JB, Andrade SP. Atorvastatin inhibits inflammatory angiogenesis in mice through down regulation of VEGF, TNF-alpha and TGF-beta1. Biomed Pharmacother. 2010;64:29–34.
3. Bender MB, Christoff N. Nonsurgical treatment of subdural hematomas. Arch Neurol. 1974;31:73–9.
4. Berghauser Pont LM, Dirven CM, Dippel DW, Verweij BH, Dammers R. The role of corticosteroids in the management of chronic subdural hematoma: a systematic review. Eur J Neurol. 2012;19(11):1397–403.
5. Chan DYC, Chan DTM, Sun TFD, et al. The use of atorvastatin for chronic subdural haematoma: a retrospective cohort comparison study. Br J Neurosurg. 2017;31(1):72–7.
6. Collaborators Crash-3. Effects of tranexamic acid on death, disability, vascular occlusive events and other morbidities in patients with acute traumatic brain injury (CRASH-3): a randomised, placebo-controlled trial. Lancet. 2019;394:1713–23.
7. Delgado-Lopez PD, Martin-Velasco V, Castilla-Diez JM, Rodriguez-Salazar A, Galacho-Harriero AM, Fernandez-Arconada O. Dexamethasone treatment in chronic subdural haematoma. Neurocirugia (Astur). 2009;20(4):346–59.
8. Dran G, Berthier F, Fontaine D, Rasenrarijao D, Paquis P. Effectiveness of adjuvant corticosteroid therapy for chronic subdural hematoma: a retrospective study of 198 cases. Neurochirurgie. 2007;53:477–82.
9. Giuffrè R, Palma E, Liccardo G, Sciarra F, Pastore FS, Concolino G. Sex steroid hormones in the pathogenesis of chronic subdural haematoma. Neurochirurgia (Stuttg). 1992;35:103–7.
10. He C, Xia P, Xu J, Chen L, Zhang Q. Evaluation of the efficacy of atorvastatin in the treatment for chronic subdural hematoma: a meta-analysis. Neurosurg Rev. 2021;44(1):479–84. https://doi.org/10.1007/s10143-019-01218-w.
11. Henaux P-L, Le Reste P-J, Laviolle B, Morandi X. Steroids in chronic subdural hematomas (SUCRE trial): study protocol for a randomized controlled trial. Trials. 2017;18(1):252.
12. Holl DC, Volovici V, Dirven CMF, Peul WC, Jellema K, van der Gaag NA, et al. Pathophysiology and targets for non-surgical therapy of chronic subdural haematoma: evolution from past to present to future. World Neurosurg. 2018;116:402–11.
13. Horikoshi T, Naganuma H, Fukasawa I, Uchida M, Nukui H. Computed tomography characteristics suggestive of spontaneous resolution of chronic subdural hematoma. Neurol Med Chir (Tokyo). 1998;38:527–33.

14. Ito H, Maeda M, Uehara T, Yamamoto S, Tamura M, Takashima T. Attenuation values of chronic subdural hematoma and subdural effusion in CT scans. Acta Neurochir. 1984;72:211–7.
15. Jiang R, Zhao S, Wang R, Feng H, Zhang J, et al. Safety and efficacy of atorvastatin for chronic subdural hematoma in chinese patients: a randomized ClinicalTrial. JAMA Neurol. 2018;75(11):1338–46.
16. Kageyama H, Toyooka T, Tsuzuki N, Oka K. Nonsurgical treatment of chronic subdural hematoma with tranexamic acid. J Neurosurg. 2013;119(2):332–7.
17. Katayama K, Matsuda N, Kakuta K, Naraoka M, Takemura A, Hasegawa S, Akasaka K, Shimamura N, Itoh K, Asano K, Konno H, Ohkuma H. The effect of Goreisan on the prevention of chronic subdural hematoma recurrence: multi-center randomized controlled study. J Neurotrauma. 2018;35(13):1537–42.
18. Kim HC, Ko JH, Yoo DS, Lee SK. Spontaneous resolution of chronic subdural hematoma: close observation as a treatment strategy. J Korean Neurosurg Soc. 2016;59(6):628–36.
19. Kolias AG, Edlmann E, Thelin EP, et al. Dexamethasone for adult patients with a symptomatic chronic subdural haematoma (Dex-CSDH) trial: study protocol for a randomised controlled trial. Trials. 2018;19(1):670.
20. Kutty RK, Leela SK, Sreemathyamma SB, Sivanandapanicker JL, Asher P, Peethambaran A, Prabhakar RB. The outcome of medical management of chronic subdural hematoma with tranexamic acid—a prospective observational study. J Stroke Cerebrovasc Dis. 2020;29(11):105273.
21. Laldjisinga ERA, Cornelissenb FMG, Gadjradj PS. Practice variation in the conservative and surgical treatment of chronic subdural hematoma. Clin Neurol Neurosurg. 2020;195:105899.
22. Li T, Wang D, Tian Y, Yu H, Wang Y, Quan W, et al. Effects of atorvastatin on the inflammation regulation and elimination of subdural hematoma in rats. J Neurol Sci. 2014;341:88–96.
23. Marcikic M, Hreckovski B, Samardzic J, Martinovic M, Rotim K. Spontaneous resolution of post-traumatic chronic subdural hematoma: case report. Acta Clin Croat. 2010;49:331–4.
24. Markwalder TM. Chronic subdural hematomas: a review. J Neurosurg. 1981;54:637–45.
25. Miah IP, Holl DC, Peul WC, et al. Dexamethasone therapy versus surgery for chronic subdural haematoma (DECSA trial): study protocol for a randomised controlled trial. Trials. 2018;19(1):575.
26. Miah IP, Herklots M, Roks G, Peul WC, Walchenbach R, Dammers R, Lingsma HF, den Hertog HM, Jellema K, Van der Gaag NA. Dexamethasone therapy in symptomatic chronic subdural hematoma (DECSA-R): a retrospective evaluation of initial corticosteroid therapy versus primary surgery. J Neurotrauma. 2020;37:366–72.
27. Min X, Pin C, Xun Z, Cun-Zu W, Xue-Qiang S, Bo Y. Effects of atorvastatin on conservative and surgical treatments of chronic subdural hematoma in patients. World Neurosurg. 2016;91:23–8.
28. Naganuma H, Fukamachi A, Kawakami M, Misumi S, Nakajima H, Wakao T. Spontaneous resolution of chronic subdural hematomas. Neurosurgery. 1986;19:794–8.
29. Nakaguchi H, Tanishima T, Yoshimasu N. Factors in the natural history of chronic subdural hematomas that influence their postoperative recurrence. J Neurosurg. 2001;95:256–62.
30. Neidert MC, Schmidt T, Mitova T, Fierstra J, Bellut D, Regli L, et al. Preoperative angiotensin converting enzyme inhibitor usage in patients with chronic subdural hematoma: associations with initial presentation and clinical outcome. J Clin Neurosci. 2016;28:82–6.
31. Okamura A, Kawamoto Y, Sakoda E, Murakami T, Hara T. Evaluation of recurrence factors and Gorei-san administration for chronic subdural hematoma after percutaneous subdural tapping. Hiroshima J Med Sci. 2013;62:77–82.
32. Park HR, Lee KS, Shim JJ, Yoon SM, Bae HG, Doh JW. Multiple densities of the chronic subdural hematoma in CT scans. J Korean Neurosurg Soc. 2013;54:38–41.
33. Parlato C, Guarracino A, Moraci A. Spontaneous resolution of chronic subdural hematoma. Surg Neurol. 2000;53(4):312–5; discussion 315–7.
34. Poulsen FR, Munthe S, Søe M, Halle B. Perindopril and residual chronic subdural hematoma volumes six weeks after burr hole surgery: a randomized trial. Clin Neurol Neurosurg. 2014;123:4–8.

35. Prud'homme M, Mathieu F, Marcotte N, Cottin S. A **pilot** placebo controlled randomized trial of dexamethasone for chronic subdural hematoma. Can J Neurol Sci. 2016;43:284–90.
36. Qian Z, Yang D, Sun F, Sun Z. Risk factors for recurrence of chronic subdural hematoma after burr hole surgery: potential protective role of dexamethasone. Br J Neurosurg. 2017;31:84–8.
37. Roberts I, Shakur H, Coats T, Hunt B, Balogun E, Barnetson L, et al. The CRASH-2 trial: a randomised controlled trial and economic evaluation of the effects of tranexamic acid on death, vascular occlusive events and transfusion requirement in bleeding trauma patients. Health Technol Assess. 2013;17:1–79.
38. Santarius T, Lawton R, Kirkpatrick PJ, Hutchinson PJ. The management of primary chronic subdural haematoma: a questionnaire survey of practice in the United Kingdom and the Republic of Ireland. Br J Neurosurg. 2008;22:529–34.
39. Shofty B, Grossman R. Treatment options for chronic subdural hematoma. World Neurosurg. 2016;87:529–30.
40. Soleman J, Taussky P, Fandino J, Muroi C. Chapter 12: Evidence-based treatment of chronic subdural hematoma. Traumatic brain injury. In: Sadaka F. IntechOpen; 2014. https://doi.org/10.5772/57336.
41. Soleman J, Nocera F, Mariani L. The conservative and pharmacological management of chronic subdural haematoma. Swiss Med Wkly. 2017;147:w14398.
42. Sun TF, Boet R, Poon WS. Non-surgical primary treatment of chronic subdural haematoma: preliminary results of using dexamethasone. Br J Neurosurg. 2005;19(4):327–33.
43. Tang R, Shi J, Li X, et al. Effects of atorvastatin on surgical treatments of chronic subdural hematoma. World Neurosurg. 2018;117:e425–9.
44. Thotakura AK, Marabathina NR. Nonsurgical treatment of chronic subdural hematoma with steroids. World Neurosurg. 2015;84:1968–72.
45. Thotakura AK, Marabathina NR. The role of medical treatment in chronic subdural hematoma. Asian J Neurosurg. 2018;13(4):976–83.
46. Tsai TH, Lieu AS, Hwang SL, Huang TY, Hwang YFA. Comparative study of the patients with bilateral or unilateral chronic subdural hematoma: precipitating factors and postoperative outcomes. J Trauma. 2010;68:571–5.
47. Wang D, Li T, Tian Y, Wang S, Jin C, Wei H, et al. Effects of atorvastatin on chronic subdural hematoma: a preliminary report from three medical centers. J Neurol Sci. 2014;336(1–2):237–42.
48. Wang D, Li T, Wei H, et al. Atorvastatin enhances angiogenesis to reduce subdural hematoma in a rat model. J Neurol Sci. 2016;362:91–9.
49. Wang D, Gao C, Xu X, et al. Treatment of chronic subdural hematoma with atorvastatin combined with low-dose dexamethasone: phase II randomized proof-of-concept clinical trial. J Neurosurg. 2020:1–9.
50. Weigel R, Hohenstein A, Schlickum L, Weiss C, Schilling L. Angio-tensin converting enzyme inhibition for arterial hypertension reduces the risk of recurrence in patients with chronic subdural hematoma possibly by an antiangiogenic mechanism. Neurosurgery. 2007;61(4):788–92; discussion 792–3.
51. Yamada T, Natori Y. Prospective study on the efficacy of orally administered tranexamic acid and Goreisan for the prevention of recurrence after chronic subdural hematoma burr hole surgery. World Neurosurg. 2020;134:e549–53.
52. Yao Z, Hu X, Ma L, You C. Dexamethasone for chronic subdural haematoma: a 449 systematic review and meta-analysis. Acta Neurochir (Wien). 2017;159(11):2037–44.
53. Zarkou S, Aguilar MI, Patel NP, Wellik KE, Wingerchuk DM, Demaerschalk BM. The role of corticosteroids in the management of chronic subdural hematomas: a critically appraised topic. Neurologist. 2009;15(5):299–302.

Chapter 28
Anesthesia for Chronic Subdural Hematoma

Kathryn Rosenblatt, Ji Yoon Baek, Fenghua Li, and Reza Gorji

28.1 Anesthesia for Chronic Subdural Hematoma

28.1.1 General Consideration and Effect of Chronic Subdural Hematoma on Cerebral Physiology

Chronic subdural hematoma (CSDH) is one of the most frequently encountered neurosurgical conditions especially in elderly patients. CSDH is an encapsulated collection of fluid, blood, and blood degradation products layered between the arachnoid and dura mater coverings on the brain's surface. The incidence of CSDH is estimated to be 17 per 100,000 people per year and increases with age [99]. Patients with CSDH may present to the hospital with altered mental status, focal neurological deficits, headache, falls, seizures, and transient neurological deficits. Risk factors for CSDH include older age, use of anticoagulants, male sex, alcoholism, and history of direct or indirect head trauma [1]. Although small size and asymptomatic CSDH can be managed conservatively, surgical treatment remains the first choice for management of CSDH [65]. Surgical modality differs depending on patient characteristics and surgeons' experiences, but bur-hole craniotomy is the most preferred performed [17, 65]. Both local anesthesia and general anesthesia are utilized during surgical procedures. Numbers of studies have shown the advantages of local anesthesia over general anesthesia [13, 63, 78], but there was no difference

K. Rosenblatt
Department of Anesthesiology and Critical Care Medicine, Johns Hopkins University, Baltimore, MD, USA
e-mail: krosenb3@jhmi.edu

J. Y. Baek · F. Li · R. Gorji (✉)
Department of Anesthesiology, Upstate Medical University, Syracuse, NY, USA
e-mail: BaekJ@upstate.edu; Lif@upstate.edu

M. Turgut et al. (eds.), *Subdural Hematoma*,
https://doi.org/10.1007/978-3-030-79371-5_28

in outcome found between the types of anesthesia in a large retrospective study [44]. Ninety-three percent of bur-hole craniotomies were performed under general anesthesia in a recent prospective study [17]. Type of anesthesia must be based on the patient's conditions in consultation with the neurosurgeon.

The effect of CSDH on cerebral physiology mainly depends on the size of the subdural hematoma and its compression on brain tissue. Patients with growing CSDH have increased intracranial pressure (ICP) and reduced cerebral blood flow (CBF) in the whole brain [57]. Marked increase in ICP is not common due to the slow expanding nature of CSDH. Untreated CSDH can lead to an increase in ICP and brain herniation. Regional and remote areas of CBF are reduced in CSDH, but CBF reduction in the thalamus and putamen is worse than that in the cortical areas [111]. It is postulated that CSDH induces neurological dysfunction primarily through a mechanical distortion of central brain regions [67, 111]. Thus, the effect of CSDH on ICP and CBF is not the major cause of neurologic dysfunction; distortion of the remote brain structures plays a more significant role than local compression of brain structures in causing a reduction in regional CBF [59, 67, 111]. Reduction in CBF in the hemisphere may also be related to a decrease in cerebral metabolism in a dysfunctional brain [122]. Studies suggest that cerebral oxygen metabolism is maintained in cortical area by means of increased regional oxygen extraction fraction (rOEF), but oxygen metabolism is reduced in the thalamus, striatum, and cingulate gyrus [67].Despite changes in CBF, cerebral autoregulation (the ability to maintain constant microvascular perfusion under fluctuating arterial blood pressure and ICP) is typically preserved in patients with CSDH [106, 113]. Anesthetic goals are to avoid further increases in ICP, to maintain cerebral perfusion by keeping cerebral perfusion pressure between 60 and 80 mmHg, and to prevent secondary brain injury. Anesthetics choice should be tailored to individual patient needs to optimize cerebral physiology.

28.1.2 Preoperative Evaluation of Patients for Planned Neurosurgical Intervention for Chronic Subdural Hematoma

The anesthesia preoperative evaluation is the cornerstone of perioperative management whose fundamental purpose is to obtain a thorough knowledge of the patient's pertinent medical history and to formulate an assessment of the intraoperative risk and requisite perioperative optimization. Preoperative patient education and discussions with the patient and the patient's family or advocates can reduce patient and family anxiety and fears of the anesthesia process and the perioperative neurosurgical experience [64, 108]. This conversation, a comprehensive and thoughtful preoperative evaluation, and a discussion with the neurosurgeon about the patient and the planned procedure can reduce operative morbidity and enhance patient outcomes.

Although some patients are first assessed by the anesthesiologist on the day of surgery, increasingly patients are evaluated and prepared for surgery in a preoperative program or clinic before the surgical date. This is recommended prior to the neurosurgical intervention of CSDH given the typically older age distribution of these patients and the concomitant increased medical risks and comorbid conditions. The preoperative assessment for a non-emergent neurosurgical intervention involves the holistic integration of the neurologic state of the patient, the general health of the patient, and the planned operative intervention.

28.1.3 Assessment of Current Neurologic Status and Pre-existing Neurologic Conditions Affecting Anesthesia Management with Most Intracranial Masses

The effects of subdural hematomas on neurologic status and perioperative management depend on the speed with which they grow. Ascertaining the history of the subdural hemorrhage and the timeline of associated neurologic symptoms will help guide anesthesia management. CSDHs may present with subtle and often prolonged symptoms that typically indicate adequate intracranial compensation. However, new findings or worsening symptoms suggest decreased intracranial compliance and autoregulation and that the limits of homeostasis are approaching and may be met with any additional change in the ICP-volume curve. Indications of raised intracranial pressure in the neurologic history include new or worsening headache, nausea, vomiting, blurred vision, increased somnolence, or a decrease in level of consciousness.

History of past neurologic diseases and injuries, both related and unrelated to the CSDH, is meaningful information and records of previous investigations and therapies are important. History of stroke or symptoms of cerebrovascular insufficiency such as transient neurologic deficits are strong predictors of perioperative stroke [69]. The etiology and treatment of ischemic stroke are often intimately related to CSDH and risks associated with antithrombotic medication cessation for management of CSDH and in preparation of surgery increase the chance of perioperative stroke from atrial fibrillation, mechanical heart valves, carotid disease, or left atrial or ventricular thrombus. Currently, there is a lack of high-quality data regarding how soon anesthesia and surgery are safe after stroke. Prevention of reperfusion injury and maintenance of collateral circulation require tight blood pressure monitoring and control if surgery for CSDH is required soon after an acute ischemic stroke.

Seizure disorder may be a sequela of and a risk factor for CSDH. If pre-existing or new onset seizure disorder is present, the type, frequency, and symptomatology of seizures should be ascertained and the timing and dose of antiepileptic drugs (and the patient's compliance to the regimen) should be documented during the preoperative evaluation. Medications to control seizures have multiple side effects including leukopenia, thrombocytopenia, hyponatremia, macrocytic anemia, PR prolongation, and bone marrow suppression. Preoperative testing should be directed at suspected abnormalities based on history and physical exam findings. An electrocardiogram, CBC, platelet count, and electrolyte levels are commonly obtained. Routine testing of serum drug levels of antiepileptic drugs (AEDs) is not indicated unless toxicity is a concern since patients with adequate seizure control may have levels outside the therapeutic range. Many AEDs have wide ranging drug interactions with anesthetic agents and other AEDs due to induction (phenytoin, phenobarbital, carbamazepine) or inhibition (valproic acid) of cytochrome P450 isoenzyme activity or competition for protein-binding sites (phenytoin, benzodiazepines, valproic acid) which affect hepatic metabolism and free drug levels of several anesthetic agents.

28.1.4 Importance of Neurologic Examination During the Preoperative Anesthesia Evaluation

A basic preoperative physical examination should involve a focused neurologic assessment documenting deficits (and absence of deficits) in mental status, speech, cranial nerves, motor and sensory function, and gait. Although it is tempting to focus the evaluation on only the previously documented or predicted abnormality, the exam should be performed in a uniform manner each time and proceed from higher to lower levels of integration so that new findings are not missed. The neurologic examination involves evaluation of both peripheral and central nervous system function and much of the exam may be accomplished while taking the patient's history. The physical examination of other organ systems such as the cardiac and pulmonary exams may be performed before or after the neurologic exam. However, integration of systemic physical findings with presenting neurological abnormalities is necessary to appropriately differentiate neurologic symptoms related to CSDH from manifestations of another organ or musculoskeletal dysfunction. Assessment of level of consciousness with the Glasgow Coma Scale is quick, easy, reproducible, and has diagnostic, therapeutic, and prognostic utility. Lower Glasgow Coma Scale (GCS) scores indicate to the anesthesiologist that hypnotic/sedative agents may have an exaggerated or more rapid effect during induction of anesthesia with an associated early loss of airway protection. Baseline neurocognitive testing of geriatric patients using the Mini-Mental State Exam (MMSE) is a routine component of preoperative anesthesia assessments in some centers. Patients with perioperative MMSE-determined cognitive impairment have higher rates of postoperative delirium, in-hospital mortality, and mortality within 1 year than patients without cognitive impairment [20]. Detailed testing of all 12 cranial nerves can be performed succinctly with adequate practice. Anosmia has recently gained attention with its association to SARS-CoV-2 infection. Olfactory nerve dysfunction, however, also suggests increased intracranial pressure, frontal lobe or pituitary lesions, meningitis, hydrocephalus, preclinical neurodegenerative diseases such as Alzheimer and Parkinson, or an anterior fossa skull fracture and can be assessed by asking the patient to identify some common odors. Additional physical exam signs of increased ICP include decreased alertness, papilledema, unilateral pupillary dilation, abducens (cranial nerve VI) or oculomotor (cranial nerve III) palsy, and neck rigidity. Assessing for papilledema requires fundoscopic examination with an ophthalmoscope which is typically performed by an ophthalmologist. Assessing pupil size, reactivity, and reaction time are equally important in determining relative intracranial pressure and obvious findings such as anisocoria and diminished reactivity can be seen with a bright light. A pupillometer may be used to provide a Neurological Pupil index (NPi) and to detect subtle oculomotor nerve findings [21]. The NPi combines variables of pupil size, latency, constriction velocity, and dilation velocity to provide a scaled value that is based on a model of normal pupilometer values [105]. Oculomotor nerve dysfunction prevents the patient from looking down, up, or medially. Binocular horizontal diplopia may indicate cranial nerve VI palsy secondary to increased ICP and testing will reveal an inability to look laterally with the involved eye. Muscle strength, tone, and size should be evaluated for asymmetry as well as increased resistance to passive muscle stretching. Reflex testing and evaluation of the peripheral sensory system are also important to detect and document baseline pathology. CSDH has been referred to as the "great neurologic imitator" as it can mimic dementia, ischemic stroke, Parkinson's disease, or spinal cord injury. This is because the most frequently occurring signs and symptoms are hemiparesis and headaches followed by mental status changes, decreased consciousness, papilledema, seizures, and expressive aphasia. Resolution of symptoms occurs in a majority of patients undergoing surgery for CSDH. Yet, baseline documentation of neurologic findings allows comparison of new deficits postoperatively.

28.1.5 Detecting Pre-existing Comorbidities Affecting General Health Status

Cardiovascular, respiratory, renal, endocrine, and gastrointestinal systems interact with neuroanesthesia and require thorough preoperative evaluation. Establishing the severity of organ- or systemic-disease, current or recent exacerbations, stability, and previous treatments or planned interventions are equally important to identifying the presence of disease. The degree of control of disease, its extent, and any limitations in activity caused by the condition are likewise important. Dosage and frequency of prescription and over-the-counter medications, including supplements and herbs, should be noted as well as recent cessation of medications. Inquiring about allergic reactions and the specific response of exposure to drugs and substances such as latex or radiographic dye is necessary as well as documentation of use of tobacco, alcohol, or illicit substances. Special emphasis during a review of systems should be placed on airway abnormalities, personal or family history of adverse events related to anesthesia, snoring and daytime somnolence if sleep apnea is not already diagnosed, and history of significant heartburn associated with reflux. A personal or family history of malignant hyperthermia or pseudocholinesterase deficiency should be identified preoperatively to allow appropriate arrangements to be made before surgery. Records from previous anesthesia are always useful and may clarify uncertain elements of the history.

28.1.5.1 Preoperative Assessment of Cardiovascular Health

Cardiovascular risk stratification is an important part of preoperative evaluation, shared surgical decision-making, and optimization. A focused history and physical examination are required to identify signs and symptoms of ischemic heart disease, severe valvular disease, severe hypertension, pulmonary hypertension, arrhythmias, and heart failure. Patients should be asked whether they can perform workloads of four or greater metabolic equivalent tasks (METs) such as climbing up two or more flights of stairs or walking up a hill without symptomatic limitation. The Goldman Index of Cardiac Risk developed over 40 years ago, followed by the Revised Cardiac Risk Index (RCRI) proposed by Lee et al., and modified by the American College of Cardiology and American Heart Association (ACC/AHA) Task Force uses a six-point scale to identify individuals with low risk (<1%) and higher risk (≥1%) for perioperative major adverse cardiovascular events (MACE) within 30 days of surgery [42, 50, 70]. However, the 21-component American College of Surgeons National Surgical Quality Improvement Program (ACS NSQIP) universal surgical risk calculators and the new Cardiovascular Risk Index may provide superior predictive discrimination [4, 11, 28, 52, 116, 117] (see Table 28.1). While cardiovascular testing such as exercise electrocardiographic stress testing, stress testing (exercise or pharmacological) with imaging such as echocardiography, nuclear perfusion, or cardiac magnetic resonance imaging are rarely indicated in patients at low risk for MACE, if the results from testing would change the perioperative medical, anesthesia, or surgical management, stress testing may be considered in patients at higher risk (determined by <4 METs) [107] (see Fig. 28.1). Brain perfusion and oxygenation depend on cardiovascular health and inversely intracranial pathology such as vasogenic edema and intracranial hypertension seen with CSDH may alter cardiovascular function.

28.1.5.2 Preoperative Assessment of Pulmonary Health

The preoperative medical history, symptoms, and physical examination of patients with chronic obstructive pulmonary disease such as bronchitis and emphysema, asthma, and pulmonary and extrapulmonary restrictive lung diseases prompt further directed evaluations and diagnostic tests if any. When taking a history, questions should focus on shortness of breath, chest tightness, cough, change in amount of

Table 28.1 Risk scores and calculators[a]

			National surgical quality improvement program			
			Risk calculators			
	Goldman index of cardiac risk [21], 1977	Revised cardiac risk index [78], 1999	Perioperative MI and cardiac arrest [105], 2011	Universal surgical [50], 2013	Geriatric-sensitive perioperative cardiac risk index [70], 2017	Cardiovascular risk index [42], 2019
Criteria	• Aged >70 years (5 points)	• Ischemic heart disease (1 point)	• Age	• Age group	• Age	• Age ≥ 75 years (1 point)
	• Had an MI within 6 months (10 points)	• Cerebrovascular disease (1 point)	• ASA class	• Sex	• Sex	• History of heart disease (1 point)
	• Jugular venous distention or a third heart sound on auscultation (11 points)	• History of congestive heart failure (1 point)	• Preoperative function	• ASA class	• ASA class	• Symptoms of angina or dyspnea (1 point)
	• ≥5 PVCs/min (7 points)	• Insulin therapy for diabetes (1 point)	• Creatinine level	• Functional status	• High-risk surgery	• Hemoglobin level <12 mg/dL (1 point)
	• Nonsinus rhythm or PAC on preoperative ECG (7 points)	• Serum creatinine level ≥2.0 mg/dL (1 point)	• Procedure type: anorectal: aortic; bariatric; brain; breast; cardiac; ear, nose, or throat; foregut or hepatopancreatobiliary; gallbladder, appendix, adrenal, or spleen; intestinal; neck; obstetric or gynecologic; orthopedic; other abdomen; peripheral vascular; skin; spine; thoracic; urological; or vein	• Emergency case	• History of heart failure	• Vascular surgery (1 point)

(continued)

Table 28.1 (continued)

			National surgical quality improvement program			
			Risk calculators			
	Goldman index of cardiac risk [21], 1977	Revised cardiac risk index [78], 1999	Perioperative MI and cardiac arrest [105], 2011	Universal surgical [50], 2013	Geriatric-sensitive perioperative cardiac risk index [70], 2017	Cardiovascular risk index [42], 2019
	• Aortic stenosis (3 points)	• Planned high-risk procedure (intra-peritoneal, intrathoracic, or vascular surgery) (1 point)		• Steroid use for chronic condition	• Stroke	• Emergency surgery (1 point)
	• Intraperitoneal, intrathoracic, or aortic surgery (3 points)			• Ascites within 30 days preoperatively	• Required insulin	
	• Any emergency surgery (4 points)			• System sepsis within 48 h preoperatively	• Diabetes	
				• Required ventilator	• Dialysis	
				• Disseminated cancer	• Medications for hypertension	
				• Diabetes	• Current tobacco use	
				• Hypertension requiring medication	• History of COPD	

			National surgical quality improvement program			
			Risk calculators			
	Goldman index of cardiac risk [21], 1977	Revised cardiac risk index [78], 1999	Perioperative MI and cardiac arrest [105], 2011	Universal surgical [50], 2013	Geriatric-sensitive perioperative cardiac risk index [70], 2017	Cardiovascular risk index [42], 2019
				• Prior cardiac event	• Functional status (partially vs totally dependent)	
				• Congestive heart failure within 30 days preoperatively	• Creatinine level	
				• Dyspnea	• Surgical category	
				• Current smoker within 1 years	• Dyspnea	
				• History of COPD	• BUN level	
				• Dialysis	• Laparoscopic surgery	
				• Acute kidney failure		
				• BMI		

(continued)

Table 28.1 (continued)

			National surgical quality improvement program			
			Risk calculators			
	Goldman index of cardiac risk [21], 1977	Revised cardiac risk index [78], 1999	Perioperative MI and cardiac arrest [105], 2011	Universal surgical [50], 2013	Geriatric-sensitive perioperative cardiac risk index [70], 2017	Cardiovascular risk index [42], 2019
				• *CPT*-specific linear risk		
Score range	• Class I: 0–5 points (lowest risk)	• Class I: 0 points (lowest risk)	0–100% (0%, lowest risk; 100%, highest risk)	0–100% (0%, lowest risk; 100%, highest risk)	0–100% (0%, lowest risk; 100%, highest risk)	• 0 points (lowest risk)
	• Class II: 6–12 points	• Class II: 1 point				• 1 point
	• Class III: 13–25 points	• Class III: 2 points				• 2 points
	• Class IV: ≥26 points (highest risk)	• Class IV: ≥3 points (highest risk)				• 3 points
						• >3 points (highest risk)
Threshold denoting elevated risk	≥Class II (≥6 points)	>1 point	>1%	>1%	>1%	≥2 points
Outcome	Intraoperative or postoperative MI, pulmonary edema, VT, cardiac death	MI, pulmonary edema, ventricular fibrillation, complete heart block, cardiac death	Intraoperative or postoperative MI or cardiac arrest within 30 days	Cardiac arrest, MI, all-cause mortality within 30 days	Cardiac arrest, MI, all-cause mortality within 30 days	Death, MI, or stroke at 30 days

			National surgical quality improvement program			
			Risk calculators			
	Goldman index of cardiac risk [21], 1977	Revised cardiac risk index [78], 1999	Perioperative MI and cardiac arrest [105], 2011	Universal surgical [50], 2013	Geriatric-sensitive perioperative cardiac risk index [70], 2017	Cardiovascular risk index [42], 2019
Derivation population	1001	1422	211,410	1,414,006	584,931	3284
Set ROC						
Derivation	0.61	0.76	0.88	0.90 (cardiac arrest or MI); 0.94 (mortality)		0.90
Validation	0.70	0.81; 0.75[b]	0.87[c]	0.88 (cardiac arrest or MI); 0.94 (mortality)[c]	0.83 (0.76 in adults aged ≥65 years)[c]	0.82[c]

Abbreviations: *ASA* American Society of Anesthesiologists, *BMI* body mass index, *BUN* blood (serum) urea nitrogen, *COPD* chronic obstructive pulmonary disease, *CPT* current procedural terminology, *EDG* electrocardiogram, *MI* myocardial infarction, *PAC* premature atrial contraction, *PVC* premature ventricular contraction, *ROC* receiver operating characteristic curve, *VT* ventricular tachycardia

[a]This table was reproduced with permission from JAMA. 2020;324(3):279–290. See source article doi: https://doi.org/10.1001/jama.2020.7840 for citation links and references

[b]Pooled validation studies assessing the performance in mixed noncardiac surgery [116]

[c]Validated using the National Surgical Quality Improvement Program database. The risk calculators are available at https://riskcalculator.facs.org/RiskCalculator/PatientInfo.jsp

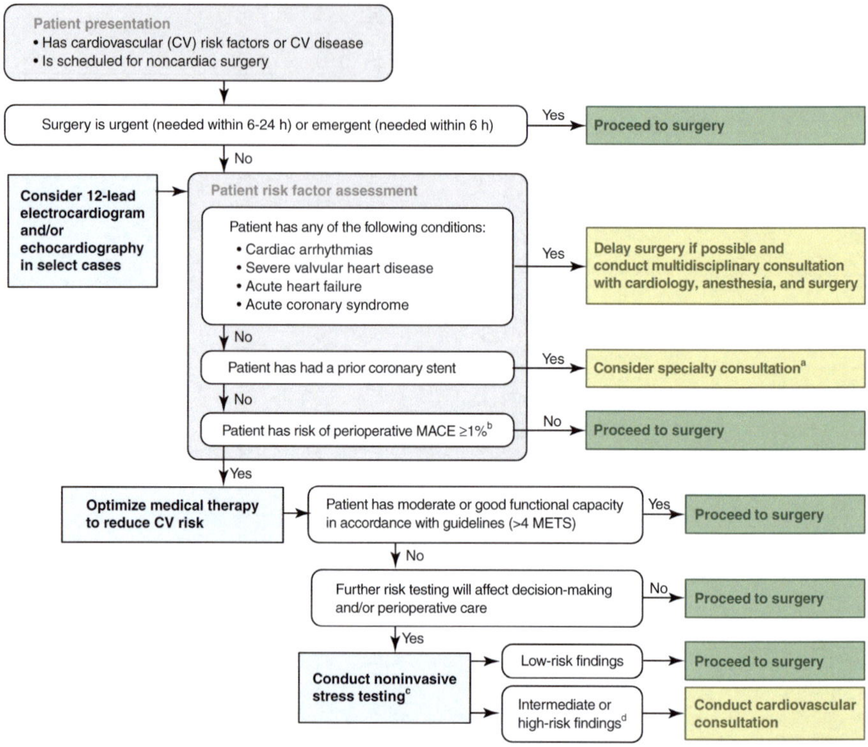

Fig. 28.1 A proposed algorithm for perioperative cardiovascular risk assessment. The algorithm has not been validated. MACE indicates major adverse cardiovascular events; METs metabolic equivalent tasks. (Reproduced with permission from JAMA. 2020;324 (3):279–290. Copyright©2020 American Medical Association. All rights reserved). [a]Perioperative considerations during consultation shown in Fig. 2 (see source article doi:https://doi.org/10.1001/jama.2020.7840). [b]Risk of perioperative MACE as determined by a clinical risk calculator. [c]Testing options include: (1) exercise electrocardiographic stress testing without myocardial imaging; or (2) stress testing (exercise or pharmacological) with imaging such as echocardiography, nuclear perfusion via single-photon emission computed tomography, positron emission tomography, or cardiac magnetic resonance imaging. [d]Intermediate or high-risk findings by stress testing may include moderate to severe myocardial ischemia, ischemia provoked at a low workload, a hypotensive response to exercise, transient ischemic dilatation, and ventricular arrhythmias during stress testing

sputum, sputum color, recent exacerbations, therapy or oxygen use, hospitalizations, intubations, previous exacerbations with anesthesia, and best exercise level. Quality of breath sounds, degree of wheezing, and quantity of air movement should be assessed with simple auscultation. Determination of oxygen saturation by pulse oximetry is useful to establish a baseline but arterial blood gas analysis, chest radiograph, and pulmonary function tests are not necessary except when establishing an initial diagnosis or evaluating acute or progressive worsening, infection, or pneumothorax [41]. Risk factors for pulmonary complications include cigarette use for greater than 40 pack years, American Society of Anesthesiologists Physical Status score greater than 2, age greater than 70 years, COPD, neurologic, aortic, upper abdominal, thoracic, or neck surgery, anticipated procedures greater than 2 h, hypoalbuminemia, BMI greater than 30 and less than 4 METS [7]. While as many as one in four deaths occurring within a week of surgery are related to pulmonary complications, studies indicate that preoperative arterial blood gas analysis, PFTs, and chest radiograph findings do not predict risk for complications after non-thoracic and noncardiac surgery [7, 85, 121]. Instead, PFTs and chest scans may be indicated to help differentiate dyspnea caused by lung disease versus heart failure or to assess need for antibiotics, bronchodilators, or steroids. Tobacco exposure increases the risk for many perioperative complications; however the greatest benefit of smoking abstinence is realized only after several months of cessation.

28.1.5.3 Preoperative Assessment of Endocrine Dysfunction and Diabetes

Patients with diabetes are at risk for multiorgan dysfunction, including renal insufficiency, peripheral neuropathy, stroke, autonomic dysfunction, cardiovascular disease, gastroparesis, and retinopathy and patients with diabetes is considered an intermediate risk factor for perioperative cardiac complications similar to angina or a previous myocardial infarction. Assessing organ damage and optimizing perioperative glucose control should be the focus of the preoperative anesthesia evaluation. It is well established that hyperglycemia before or during cerebral ischemia worsens neurologic outcome. An increased preischemic serum glucose level may accelerate the detrimental effect of lactic acidosis by providing additional substrate for anaerobic glycolysis. Conversely, intensive glucose control carries risk of hypoglycemia with its consequent net movement of glucose out of the brain along its concentration gradient. Based on the American Association of Clinical Endocrinologists and the American Diabetes Association recommendations and the currently available evidence, maintaining perioperative blood glucose levels between 140 and 180 mg/L (7.8–10.0 mmol/L) is a reasonable target at least until additional prospective studies address glucose management targets for specific neurologic injuries or neurosurgical procedures [49, 88].

28.1.5.4 Perioperative Assessment of Coagulopathy

Patients with any degree or type of coagulopathy (both inherited or acquired disorders) may develop CSDH spontaneously or with seemingly trivial trauma. Nevertheless, antithrombotic medications may appear on the preoperative medication list of patients presenting for elective neurosurgical intervention of their CSDH especially in cases of stable CSDH where the benefit of continuing therapy outweighs the bleeding risk. Preoperative cessation and/or reversal of antithrombotic agents, however, is necessary given the potential for hematoma expansion during surgical intervention and in order to prevent perioperative complications and cSDH recurrence postoperatively. In the elective, non-acute setting, time will allow for renal and hepatic clearance of many medications. Prior to surgical intervention, the activated prothrombin time (aPTT) should be normalized, and the international normalized ratio (INR) should be below 1.4. Holding vitamin K antagonists for several days (typically >5 days for those taking warfarin) will reduce the anticoagulant effect and checking an INR level the morning of surgery is recommended to confirm the reversal.

In patients with significant hypercoagulability or existing clot burden requiring anticoagulation, the risks and benefits of "bridging" with a shorter-acting agent such as unfractionated heparin or low molecular weight heparin in the perioperative period are unclear and typically require careful calculations and comparisons of the thromboembolic and bleeding risks [110]. Major factors that increase thromboembolic risk are atrial fibrillation, prosthetic heart valves, and venous or arterial thromboembolism in the preceding 3 months. Patients with these risk factors are composed of heterogenous groups and scores like the CHA3DS2-VASc and HAS-BLED incorporate additional important clinical variables for thromboembolic and bleeding risk stratification [95]. However, use of risk scores have not been prospectively validated in the perioperative setting and no scoring system can substitute clinical judgment. For patients with very high risk of thromboembolism, such as ischemic stroke within the previous 3 months, or in patients with nonvalvular atrial fibrillation who have had inadequate anticoagulation in the preceding month, attempts should be made to delay elective surgery, if possible, until risk has returned to baseline. If delaying is not possible or in patients with chronically elevated thromboembolic risk who are receiving warfarin, anticoagulation should be stopped as close to surgery as possible, with the use of a bridging agent for those on warfarin and a temporary inferior vena cava for selected individuals. The heparin bridge is typically prescribed to begin 3 days before the planned procedure (i.e., 2 days after stopping warfarin), when the INR has started to drop below the therapeutic range. Low molecular weight heparin may be discontinued 24 h before the planned surgery, based on an elimination half-life of approximately 3–5 h, and an infusion of therapeutic unfractionated heparin may be continued up until 4–6 h before the procedure, based on its elimination half-life of approximately 45 min.

Increasingly, patients with thromboembolic risk are prescribed direct oral anticoagulants (DOACs) and parenteral direct-acting anticoagulants such as dabigatran, apixaban, edoxaban, and rivaroxaban. Unlike warfarin and other vitamin K antagonists (e.g., acenocoumarol, phenprocoumon, and fluindione), which work indirectly by blocking the function of vitamin K epoxide reductase complex in the liver, leading to depletion of the reduced form of vitamin K that serves as a cofactor for gamma γ-carboxylation of vitamin-K-dependent coagulation factors II, VII, IX, and X, these direct thrombin (factor II) and direct factor Xa inhibitors block major procoagulant activities involved in the generation of a fibrin clot [6]. Direct thrombin inhibitors such as bivalirudin, argatroban, desirudin, and dabigatran prevent thrombin from cleaving fibrinogen to fibrin and bind directly to thrombin, rather than by enhancing the activity of antithrombin, as heparin does. Direct factor Xa inhibitors including rivaroxaban, apixaban, edoxaban, and betrixaban prevent factor Xa from cleaving prothrombin to thrombin and bind directly to factor Xa. Given the high bleeding risk involved with surgical intervention of CSDH, omitting direct factor Xa inhibitors for 2 days prior to surgery regardless of kidney function and direct thrombin inhibitors for 2 days in patients with normal kidney function is recommended based on elimination half-lives of 9–14 h for DOACs39. For patients with creatinine clearance 30–50 mL/min receiving dabigatran, the same pharmacokinetic approach recommends omission to begin 4 days prior to CSDH intervention based on an elimination half-life of 18–24 h in patients with impaired renal function [48]. Unlike cessation of vitamin K antagonists in patients with high thromboembolic risk, bridging is not necessary for the direct-acting anticoagulants.

Patients with CSDH and history of percutaneous coronary intervention (PCI) within the prior 12 months may be taking antiplatelet agents such as aspirin and platelet P2Y12 receptor blocking therapy to prevent coronary stent thrombosis. Based on the results of the large POISE-2 trial, it is recommended that in patients treated with aspirin monotherapy for primary or secondary prevention of cardiovascular disease events hold such therapy for 5–7 days before surgery [33]. For patients taking dual antiplatelet therapy (DAPT) after PCI with stenting, cessation prior to the recommended duration of its use (at least 6 months after either bare metal stenting or drug-eluting stenting and 14 days after PCI using balloon angioplasty without stenting) is associated with increased risk of adverse cardiovascular events such as myocardial infarction, stent thrombosis, and death [74]. Deferring elective noncardiac surgery for 6 months after PCI with stenting to prevent interruption of DAPT is recommended, but with surgical interventions that cannot wait 6 months, the minimal duration of DAPT is 4–6 weeks after PCI with stenting and 48 h after balloon angioplasty if possible [38, 56, 114]. Patients with CSDH may require even more immediate intervention. Moreover, the risk of bleeding attributable to DAPT with neurosurgical intervention for CSDH is likely greater than the risk of adverse cardiovascular events from cessation, and therefore these therapies should be held perioperatively. For patients taking clopidogrel, ticagrelor, and prasugrel, it is recommended to hold therapy 5 days, 3–5 days, and 7 days before surgery, respectively, based on the manufacturer's package insert for each drug.

28.1.6 Physical Examination During the Preoperative Anesthesia Evaluation

28.1.6.1 Airway Examination

Inspection of the airway may be the single most important component of the preoperative physical examination. Although it occupies the least amount of preoperative time, specialized training and experience in airway evaluation and management is required to perform an adequate airway assessment. The main purpose of the airway evaluation is to examine the patient for specific physical and physiological attributes that predict the likelihood of difficulty in performing any of the major procedures in airway management. Components of the airway exam include the Mallampati classification, inspection of teeth, range of motion of the neck, neck circumference, thyromental distance, body habitus, and pertinent deformities, and chest auscultation. These physical attribute variables have been incorporated into mnemonics coined by researchers and experts based on validated studies of difficult airway management. Two such validated tools are the LEMON evaluation adopted by the American College of Surgeons' Advanced Trauma Life Support (ATLS) course and the ROMAN mnemonic, which assess for difficult laryngoscopic intubation and difficult bag-valve-mask ventilation, respectively [5, 68, 103]. When challenging airways are identified, it is important to prepare patients for possible awake fiberoptic intubation when applicable and advance planning is necessary to ensure requisite equipment and skilled personnel are available.

28.1.6.2 General Physical Examination

Auscultation of the heart, including third or fourth heart sounds, murmurs, rhythm disturbances, and rales, inspection of pulses, peripheral and central veins, and for the presence of edema in the extremities may aid in developing a perioperative plan. Physical findings should focus on signs of volume overload, jugular venous distention, ascites, and hepatomegaly as well as auscultation of the neck for bruits. Auscultation for wheezing, rhonchi, or course, diminished, or other abnormal breath sounds will also aid in preoperative planning. Effort of breathing, cyanosis, clubbing, and use of accessory muscles should be noted. A large neck circumference, hypertension, and obesity predict an increased incidence of obstructive sleep apnea (OSA). Data suggest that there is an increased incidence of postoperative complications and death among patients suspected of having OSA, and untreated OSA patients are known to have a higher incidence of difficult intubation, admission to the intensive care unit, postoperative complications, and a greater duration of hospital stay [15]. OSA detection using tools such as the STOP-Bang questionnaire, Berlin questionnaire, and ASA (American Society of Anesthesiologists) checklist have been developed to identify patients at risk of OSA [24–26]. If patients receive early treatment for their OSA because of screening in a preoperative clinic, there may be a reduction in OSA-related perioperative adverse events and long-term health benefits for the patient. While overnight-attended polysomnography is the standard in diagnosis of OSA, it is expensive and inconvenient and there is typically little time for a sleep medicine referral in the preoperative timeline of surgical intervention for CSDH. Instead, practicing perioperative precautions such as using short-acting anesthesia agents, preparing for possible difficult mask ventilation and difficult intubation, adequate neuromuscular blocking agent reversal, use of CPAP postoperatively, and continuous pulse oximetry monitoring postoperatively may help prevent adverse outcomes in patients classified as high risk of OSA by the STOP-Bang questionnaire [97].

28.1.7 Estimating Anesthesia Risks

While evidence-based guidelines published by multiple medical specialties have led to evaluation protocols for preparing patients for anesthesia and surgery, the anesthesiologist is the only preoperative physician who can truly assess the risks associated with anesthesia, discuss these risks with the patient and the surgical team, and manage them intraoperatively. Regarding risk-benefit ratio disclosures and informed consent, anesthesia is unique in the preoperative discourse. It confers risk to the patient without direct benefit. The benefits of anesthesia are reaped by allowing others to do things that may potentially benefit the patient. As neurosurgery for CSDH has evolved with innovations in minimally invasive, endoscopic, and endovascular techniques, a general anesthetic requiring potent medications, instrumentation of the airway, and mechanical ventilation with associated physiologic perturbations may pose a significant and greater risk than the surgery itself to some patient groups. The American Society of Anesthesiologists (ASA) Physical Status Classification System was developed 80 years ago and is still in use today [84]. The purpose of the ASA Physical Status Classification System is to subjectively assess and communicate a patient's pre-anesthesia medical comorbidities without consideration for type of anesthesia or surgical procedure. Several studies have shown a correlation between ASA Physical Status and adverse cardiopulmonary outcomes, longer hospital stays, and unanticipated intensive care unit admissions. While the ASA Physical Status Classification System does not by itself quantify risk, the system was incorporated in both the ACS NSQI and the RCRI. Combined patient and surgical risk tools like these offer perioperative clinicians, and ultimately patients, a comprehensive risk assessment that allows some estimation of the chance of complications occurring and assists in deciding if surgery should be postponed until interventions improve risk such as poorly controlled hypertension or unstable ischemic heart disease.

28.2 Intraoperative Management of Chronic Subdural Hematoma

28.2.1 Choice of Anesthesia

Anesthesia choice is dictated by patient and surgeon preference with consideration of any clinical and psychological limitations of the affected patient.

28.2.1.1 Local Anesthesia

Mini-craniotomy for CSDH is associated with lower rate of recurrence. Mahmood and colleagues found that mini-craniotomy for CSDH, when done with local anesthesia, is equally effective to general anesthesia [79]. In a prospective-randomized study comparing dexmedetomidine sedation versus general anesthesia for surgical treatment of CSDH, dexmedetomidine combined with a local anesthesia was found to be effective when evacuating a CSDH via a burr hole. The technique was associated with shorter operative time and fewer hemodynamic changes and postoperative complications. An added benefit was a shorter hospital stay [109]. The use of dexmedetomidine for monitored anesthesia care (MAC) was associated with less intraoperative patient movement, faster recovery time, and better surgeon and patient satisfaction score when compared with midazolam-fentanyl combination [12]. A further study comparing combinations of dexmedetomidine and ketamine (DK) and dexmedetomidine-midazolam-fentanyl (DMF) drug cocktails found both groups to have comparable recovery time, onset time, cardiorespiratory variables, and analgesia. However, the DMF group showed better sedation quality and satisfaction scores despite lower dose of dexmedetomidine and a higher incidence of bispectral index <60 than the DK group [23].

28.2.1.2 Local Versus General Anesthesia

A large study with 1029 patients found postoperative complications much higher in patients receiving general anesthesia than patients treated with local anesthesia. With multivariable analysis, patients who received general anesthesia were 1.8 times more likely to develop postoperative problems (aOR 1.8, 95%, CI: 1.0–3.3). Interestingly enough, the association decreased when adjusted for the hospital that the surgery was performed. The same study found shorter hospital stay in local anesthesia cases [13].

It is difficult to truly differentiate the benefits of one technique over another in CSDH since the literature offers limited resources. Poor study designs do not help, and this is seen when reviewing the literature. Furthermore, general anesthesia is sometimes implicated in postoperative cognitive issues which may in fact not be related to anesthesia used but to other factors such as inflammatory responses and increase in cytokines and surgical stress [14, 102]. Other factors like patient movement due to discomfort can increase surgical discomfort [62].

28.2.2 Intraoperative General Anesthesia Management

When a liquefied CSDH fails to resorb spontaneously, a burr hole placed with subsequent drainage of the hematoma is an effective treatment [83]. A drain is effective in preventing recurrence and it also reduces morbidity and mortality associated with surgery [101]. A craniotomy to evacuate the clot and associated membranes around the clot is effective in reaccumulation of a CSDH [71, 90, 118].

In most cases, patients with CSDH have increased ICP. As such, preparation for brain relaxation is needed. These include administration of diuretics, osmotherapy, and glucocorticoids as well as management of partial pressure of carbon dioxide ($PaCO_2$), anesthetics drugs, and cerebrospinal fluid (CSF) drainage.

28.2.2.1 Monitoring

In procedures where small CSDHs are being evacuated, monitoring needs can be met with American Society of Anesthesiologists (ASA) monitors. The monitors include electrocardiogram (ECG), blood pressure (BP), pulse oximetry, temperature, oxygen analyzer, and end-tidal carbon dioxide ($ETCO_2$). A similar set of monitors can be employed when a mini-craniotomy is performed. In most cases though, more invasive monitoring will be needed.

Continuous arterial BP (ABP) monitoring with an intra-arterial catheter is indicated in cases where a craniotomy is expected. A continuous ABP helps optimize cerebral perfusion pressure (CPP), assessment of volume status and allowing blood sampling for electrolyte and glucose measurement.

Monitoring for air embolism is a concern if the operative site is above the level of the heart. In a sitting craniotomy, air embolism is a common and serious complication [80]. However it can also occur during skull opening along venous sinuses. It also has occurred where the pins are placed on the skull [51]. Monitoring of $ETCO_2$ is mandatory for all patients receiving general anesthesia. In context of detecting a venous air embolism, $ETCO_2$ is very sensitive, detecting as little as 0.25 mg/kg [39].

Patients may have an extraventricular drain (EVD) prior to arriving in the operating room. Patient may present with an extraventricular drain device (EVD) to the operating room. The EVD may be used for ICP monitoring or for CSF drainage or to monitor ICP.

The EVD may also be used to drain CSF and further reduce ICP. EVD monitoring is most helpful until the point when the dura is opened, at which time, the ICP becomes equal to the environment's pressure.

Some cases of CSDH may need neurophysiologic monitoring. The use of electroencephalography (EEG) and evoked potentials will dictate the choice of anesthesia. For example, motor evoked potentials (transcranial) monitoring is usually accompanied by the use of total intravenous anesthesia.

28.2.2.2 Intravenous Access Is a Must

Adequate intravenous access is needed for evacuation of CSDHs. The authors all place two peripheral intravenous catheters in patients unless there is central access, in which case, one should suffice.

Central venous access may be needed in these patients. Administration of vasoactive drugs and volume resuscitation are reasons for placement of a central venous catheter. If a central line is placed, then a chest X-ray should be performed to rule out a pneumothorax. If VAE is likely, a multi-orificed single lumen central line needs to be placed if none was placed preoperatively. Confirmation of placement at 2 cm below the superior vena cava and slightly above the right atrium can be done easily by fluoroscopy and is shown to allow for good air aspiration [18].

28.2.2.3 Induction of General Anesthesia

Induction of general anesthesia aims to reduce the cerebral metabolic rate (CMR), cerebral blood flow, and intracranial pressure (or no change in latter). There is a multitude of agents that can be used. Commonly a combination of agents is used to induce anesthesia.

Propofol will reduce CMR, CBF (cerebral blood flow), and ICP (intracranial pressure) [96, 115]. Autoregulation and carbon dioxide (CO_2) responsiveness are maintained [43].

Barbiturates are rarely used in the United States to induce anesthesia due to unavailability. Thiopental and methohexital were agents previously used to induce anesthesia since similarly to propofol, they reduce CMR, CBF, and ICP while maintaining autoregulation and CO_2 responsiveness.

Etomidate can be used to induce anesthesia in patients with CSDH. However, there is a problem with significant postoperative nausea [19] and vomiting as well as adrenal corticosteroid production suppression [32]. Etomidate maintains CPP and reduces ICP and CBF [27]. Etomidate preserves CO_2 responsiveness [27].

Ketamine use in neuroanesthesia and specifically during a craniotomy is controversial. Its effect on CBF, CMR, and ICP is controversial with some studies showing increases in these parameters and others showing no change [3, 29, 58]. It is our opinion to use ketamine with caution in patients with CSDH. There is no literature to a position of use or not in patients with CSDH.

Opioids are used not only to induce anesthesia but to maintain anesthesia as well. Multiple agents are available such as fentanyl, sufentanil, and remifentanil. These agents' effect on CBF, ICP, and CMR are minimal [72].

28.2.2.4 Maintenance of General Anesthesia

Following induction of anesthesia, the anesthesiologist works on placing additional IV access and an arterial line.

Following placement of the Mayfield clamp, there might be a variable time prior to incision as other surgical issues are addressed (navigation setup, prepping skin). During this time period, it is usually necessary to reduce the amount of anesthesia given to allow for optimal hemodynamic variables (avoiding hypotension).

During the placement of a Mayfield clamp, there is usually a brief period of painful stimulus that can lead to hypertension and tachycardia. A variety of medication could be used to attenuate these responses. Fentanyl (50–150 mcg IV), remifentanil (25–50 mcg IV), propofol (20–50 mg IV), lidocaine (1 mg/kg IV), and esmolol

(10–30 mg IV) can be titrated to effect. Local anesthesia may help to attenuate the responses to skull pinning [47, 104].

Patients with CSDH may have increased intracranial pressure, but unlike cases of acute SDH, there has been time for compensatory mechanisms. Use of anesthetic drugs takes into account degree of intracranial pathology as well as other comorbidities. Furthermore, neurophysiologic monitoring will have an influence on the type of anesthesia used.

In patients who may have significant increases in ICP, a technique may comprise volatile agents and narcotics (infusion or boluses). The use of nitrous oxide (N_2O) is controversial in craniotomies. There is no clear agreement among anesthesiologist on the optimal type of anesthesia (TIVA versus inhalation anesthesia). In a large study looking at various anesthesia techniques, propofol-based anesthesia technique (TIVA) and the use of volatile agents had similar brain relaxation scores. In propofol maintained anesthesia, ICP and CPP were better optimized but a definitive conclusion as to neurological morbidity and mortality could not be reached [22].

All volatile agents (sevoflurane, isoflurane, desflurane, and halothane) are cerebral vasodilators [76, 112]. Specifically, sevoflurane causes vasodilation of large vessels but vasoconstriction at the arteriole level probably caused by decreased CMR [89]. CMR is reduced and autoregulation is decreased, thus causing an uncoupling of CBF and metabolism (luxury perfusion) [31]. This effect is dose dependent with major uncoupling occurring above 1 MAC [77].

Total intravenous anesthesia (TIVA) can be used as the sole anesthetic in patients with CSDH. This could be a propofol infusion which reduces CMR, CBF, CBV, and ICP. CO_2 responsiveness is maintained. Opioid use is common during craniotomies. They have minimal effect on CBF and ICP. Sometimes as part of TIVA, dexmedetomidine can be used as an adjunct. Dexmedetomidine is an alpha 2 agonist that has sedative and analgesic properties. It causes a reduction of CBF and CMR [35]. Dexmedetomidine will cause cerebral vasoconstriction. There is no evidence to suggest cerebral ischemia in patients with compromised cerebral vasculature [119].

Hemodynamic management during evacuation of CSDH must take into account patient factors and the size and effect of the CSDH. The aim is to maintain CPP, avoid a cerebral ischemia, stroke, more brain injury, and hypertension. The management is similar to patients undergoing a craniotomy for mass lesions.

The intraoperative use of antiepileptic drugs occurs at some institutions. In many cases, patient's preoperative seizure medications are continued. Even in cases with no prior epilepsy, epilepsy can occur although the incidence is low (5.3%) [120]. In patients with acute subdural hematomas, post-traumatic seizure is a common malady. It is our opinion that the prophylactic use of anti-seizure medication is justified to avoid this serious complication.

Near isotonic crystalloid solutions should be administered during evacuation of CSDHs. Hypotonic saline fluids can cause interstitial edema. Hypertonic saline solutions will cause an increase in the brain volume in cases of damaged blood-brain barrier [73]. Colloid solution use in craniotomies is controversial but if the patient is hypovolemic, albumin can be used.

Hyperventilation to help with brain relaxation is often useful. Aim is to get improved surgical conditions by having the $PaCO_2$ of 25–30 mmHg [45]. Frequent use of arterial blood gases can help guide the clinician. Hyperventilation is commonly used in patients with intracranial hemorrhage to reduce ICP and relax a tight brain. Improved patient outcomes have not been proven in the literature [123].

28.3 General Postoperative Care

After a craniotomy for subdural hematoma evacuation, patients may recover in the PACU (postoperative care unit) or be transported directly to an intensive care setting. In either location, the patient is monitored closely, with the goals of early detection of serious postoperative complications and to facilitate intervention [100]. In order to optimize recovery, it is crucial to control blood pressure, treat pain, and prevent and treat delirium and postoperative nausea and vomiting. Careful consideration should be given as to when would be an optimal time to re-institute anticoagulants in these patients.

28.3.1 Postoperative Neurological Assessment

It is mandatory to perform post-procedural neurological evaluations in the immediate postoperative period, in order to detect any postoperative cerebral complication in a timely manner [40]. Glasgow coma score analysis, cranial nerve exam, and sensory, motor, language, and cerebellar function exploration are generally implemented. When there is a new neurological deficit, a brain CT scan should be performed immediately to rule out a neurosurgical complication. It is mandatory to perform post-procedural neurological evaluation in the immediate postoperative period, in order to detect any postoperative cerebral complications in a timely manner [40].

28.3.2 Postoperative Nausea and Vomiting

Postoperative nausea and vomiting is one of the most frequently reported side effects of general anesthesia. Retching or vomiting can raise the patient's blood pressure, intra-abdominal and intrathoracic pressure, which may lead to high intracranial pressure and cause postoperative intracranial bleeding [37]. Additionally, the patients can have compromised swallowing reflex post-craniotomy and hence can be at elevated risk for aspiration after vomiting [37].

Therefore, it is recommended to take a multimodal approach to treat nausea in post-craniotomy patients. Most commonly used pharmacological agents for this purpose include intravenous metoclopramide and ondansetron [37].

28.3.3 Pain Control

Although post-craniotomy patients are assumed to experience lower degree of pain than other surgical patients, about 60% of the patients report moderate-to severe pain postoperatively [30]. Under-treated pain can lead to sympathetic stimulation that results in hypertension with potential to precipitate secondary intracranial hemorrhage [9]. However, excessive pain medication can lead to sedation, which can mask new onset neurological deficits. Also, the depressed respiratory effect from excessive doses of opioid pain medication can cause hypercarbia and can consequently raise intracranial pressure. Therefore, it is imperative to maintain an appropriate neurological state, at the same time providing adequate analgesia in these patients.

Multimodal analgesia may be implemented on post-craniotomy patients in effort to achieve this delicate balance [9]. The first-line drugs frequently used in the immediate postoperative are opioids and intravenous acetaminophen. Fentanyl boluses are commonly used due to its advantage in high potency, although it is limited by its short duration of action. Intravenous morphine is an alternative to fentanyl as it has longer duration of action, and, as long as it is carefully titrated with close monitoring of the patients, serious side effects such as sedation and respiratory depression, can be avoided [36]. Once the patient is awake, extubated, and able to tolerate oral feeding, they can be transitioned to oral medications including tramadol, oxycodone, and oral acetaminophen.

28.3.4 Blood Pressure Control

Blood pressure higher than 160/90 mmHg has shown to significantly predispose to post-craniotomy intracranial hematoma formation [9]. When the blood pressure exceeds the upper limit of cerebral autoregulation, this will result in increased cerebral blood flow, which in turn can break down the blood brain barrier, and transudation of intravascular fluid and hemorrhage may ensue. Intracranial hematoma can cause increased intracranial pressure, exacerbate cerebral edema, and result in local and global cerebral ischemia, which may subsequently lead to life-threatening cerebral herniation [61].

Vasodilators (i.e., nitroprusside, nitroglycerin, and hydralazine), calcium channel blockers (i.e., nicardipine), and beta blockers (i.e., labetalol and esmolol) have been used to treat hypertension postoperatively in post-craniotomy patients.

Out of these agents, intravenous nicardipine and labetalol are most commonly administered. Labetalol is considered as an ideal antihypertensive for post-craniotomy patients because it does not influence cerebral blood flow or cerebral blood flow autoregulation [94, 98]. Esmolol (which has a short half-life of approximately 9 min) can be used safely while titrating the long-acting labetalol to achieve the safe range of blood pressure without inducing hypotension.

However, in those patients who do not respond well to these agents, or those with pulmonary conditions (i.e., asthma and chronic obstructive pulmonary disease) in whom the use of beta blockers is contraindicated, intravenous calcium channel blockers (i.e., nicardipine) are used alternatively. There are reported cases of bradycardia, tachycardia, and hypotension that resulted from intravenous boluses of nicardipine. Also, there are concerns for dose-dependent cerebral vasodilation and cerebral autoregulation inhibition with nicardipine [66]. These effects can lead to decreases in regional cerebral blood flow [2]. However, many studies have demonstrated that, when administered as a continuous infusion, nicardipine has high efficacy in rapidly decreasing blood pressure with minimal occurrence of side effects [93].

Postoperative hypotension (decrease in mean blood pressure by more than 30% from baseline) should also be avoided, as it may lead to cerebral hypo-perfusion and therefore result in perioperative cerebral ischemia [10].

Norepinephrine and phenylephrine are commonly used pressors in hypotensive patients postoperatively. However, it is important to note that norepinephrine increases arterial pressure but does not increase the cerebral perfusion pressure and, with higher doses, it has a negative effect on cerebral oxygenation [16, 91]. Phenylephrine has been found to decrease cerebral oxygen saturation, probably through a reduction in cardiac output [86]. Maintaining normocapnia was found to prevent this effect of phenylephrine [87].

28.3.5 Delirium Prevention

Delirium is a common and significant postoperative complication that is difficult to recognize, prevent, and treat. Risk factors for delirium include sleep disturbance, sensory impairment, pain social isolation, daylight depression, infections, withdrawal syndrome, dehydration, anemia, blood transfusion, electrolyte abnormalities, acid-base abnormalities, hypoxemia, temperature derangements, seizures, and endocrine dysfunction [46, 81, 82]. Some of the ways to prevent and treat delirium are early discontinuation of limb restraints, bladder catheters, invasive lines, tracheal tube, and surgical drains, as these may cause unnecessary discomfort and agitation in patients [60]. Antipsychotic medications are frequently administered to treat agitation in delirious patients, but their impact on outcome is still unknown [53, 54, 75]. Postoperative pain control is another factor in treating delirium but it is challenging because, although pain can lead to delirium, opioid pain medications can also precipitate delirium. Non-sedating analgesics should be considered in patients vulnerable to delirium. However, in patients with severe postoperative pain, opioid analgesics have been shown to alleviate both pain and delirium [34].

Early recognition of delirium and instituting non-pharmacological and pharmacological interventions as mentioned above are key to decreasing the incidence of postoperative delirium.

28.3.6 Re-institution of Anticoagulant

CSDH is often associated with long-term anticoagulant use for treatment of thromboembolic and cardiovascular disorders. Additionally, pre-injury anticoagulant usage is associated with an increased risk of CSDH recurrence after evacuation [92].

The risk of hematoma recurrence must be balanced against the risk of thromboembolic events.

Patients with atrial fibrillation are at high risk of early thromboembolic events within the first 90 days of interruptions in anticoagulation [8]. In fact, the estimated risk of stroke within the first 7 days is 2.5–5% [55]. Early resumption of anticoagulation therapy can lower this risk, but may also increase risk of possible CSDH recurrence [92]. Few studies have examined the optimal timing for anticoagulation re-institution in patients with CSDH, and they are limited by small sample sizes and poor methodology.

For this reason, there is considerable variation in practice patterns and perceived risk of hemorrhage and embolic complications with early versus late anticoagulant reintroduction after CSDH evacuation. However, there are two commonly used approaches to restarting anticoagulation therapy: early restarting at approximately 1 week after surgery versus delayed restarting at approximately 4 weeks after surgery [92].

Additionally, an individual patient condition needs to be taken into consideration before deciding when to re-institute anticoagulation therapy. For instance, patient's baseline risk of stroke measured by CHADS score may impact the perceived risk of stroke when holding anticoagulation therapy [92]. Conversely, high-risk bleeding features such as coagulopathies may sway the clinician from re-instituting the anticoagulant early [92].

References

1. Adhiyaman V, Asghar M, Ganeshram Bhowmick KNBK. Chronic subdural haematoma in the elderly. Postgrad Med J. 2002;78:71–5. https://doi.org/10.1136/pmj.78.916.71.
2. Akopov S, et al. Regional cerebral blood flow in patients with internal carotid artery stenosis: effects of nifedipine and nimodipine. Int J Angiol. 2011;2(01):16–21. https://doi.org/10.1007/bf02651556.
3. Albanèse J, Arnaud S, Rey M, et al. Ketamine decreases intracranial pressure and electroencephalographic activity in traumatic brain injury patients during propofol sedation. Anesthesiology. 1997;87:1328.
4. Alrezk R, Jackson N, Al Rezk M, et al. Derivation and validation of a geriatric-sensitive perioperative cardiac risk index. J Am Heart Assoc. 2017;6(11):e006648. https://doi.org/10.1161/JAHA.117.006648.
5. American College of Surgeons, Committee on Trauma. Advanced trauma life support: student course manual. American College of Surgeons; 2018.
6. Ansell J, Hirsh J, Hylek E, Jacobson A, Crowther M, Palareti G. Pharmacology and management of the vitamin K antagonists: American College of Chest Physicians evidence-based clinical practice guidelines (8th edition). Chest. 2008;133(6 Suppl):160S–98S. https://doi.org/10.1378/chest.08-0670.

7. Arozullah AM, Daley J, Henderson WG, Khuri SF. Multifactorial risk index for predicting postoperative respiratory failure in men after major noncardiac surgery. The National Veterans Administration Surgical Quality Improvement Program. Ann Surg. 2000;232(2):242–53. https://doi.org/10.1097/00000658-200008000-00015.
8. Baechli H, et al. Demographics and prevalent risk factors of chronic subdural haematoma: results of a large single-center cohort study. Neurosurg Rev. 2004;27(4):263–6. https://doi.org/10.1007/s10143-004-0337-6.
9. Basali A, et al. Relation between perioperative hypertension and intracranial hemorrhage after craniotomy. Anesthesiology. 2000;93(1):48–54. https://doi.org/10.1097/00000542-200007000-00012.
10. Bijker JB, Gelb AW. Review article: the role of hypotension in perioperative stroke. Can J Anaesth. 2012;60(2):159–67. https://doi.org/10.1007/s12630-012-9857-7.
11. Bilimoria KY, Liu Y, Paruch JL, Zhou L, Kmiecik TE, Ko CY. Development and evaluation of the universal ACS NSQIP surgical risk calculator: a decision aid and informed consent tool for patients and surgeons. J Am Coll Surg. 2013;217(5):833-42.e1–3.
12. Bishnoi V, Kumar B, Bhagat H, Salunke P, Bishnoi S. Comparison of dexmedetomidine versus midazolam-fentanyl combination for monitored anesthesia care during Burr-hole surgery for chronic subdural hematoma. J Neurosurg Anesthesiol. 2016;28(2):141–6. https://doi.org/10.1097/ANA.0000000000000194. PMID: 26018670.
13. Blaauw J, Jacobs B, den Hertog HM, van der Gaag NA, Jellema K, Dammers R, Lingsma HF, van der Naalt J, Kho KH, Groen RJM. Neurosurgical and perioperative management of chronic subdural hematoma. Front Neurol. 2020;11:550. https://doi.org/10.3389/fneur.2020.00550. eCollection 2020. PMID: 32636797; PMCID: PMC7317017.
14. Bodenham AR, Howell SJ. General anaesthesia vs local anaesthesia: an ongoing story. Br J Anaesth. 2009;103:785–9. https://doi.org/10.1093/bja/aep310.
15. Bolden N, Posner KL, Domino KB, et al. Postoperative critical events associated with obstructive sleep apnea: results from the Society of Anesthesia and Sleep Medicine Obstructive Sleep Apnea Registry. Anesth Analg. 2020;131(4):1032–41. https://doi.org/10.1213/ANE.0000000000005005.
16. Brassard P, et al. Is cerebral oxygenation negatively affected by infusion of norepinephrine in healthy subjects? Br J Anaesth. 2009;102(6):800–5. https://doi.org/10.1093/bja/aep065.
17. Brennan PM, Kolias AG, Joannides AJ, Shapey J, Marcus HJ, Gregson BA, et al. The management and outcome for patients with chronic subdural hematoma: a prospective, multicenter, observational cohort study in the United Kingdom. J Neurosurg. 2017;127:732–9. https://doi.org/10.3171/2016.8.JNS16134.
18. Bunegin L, Albin MS, Helsel PE, Hoffman A, Hung TK. Positioning the right atrial catheter: a model for reappraisal. Anesthesiology. 1981;55(4):343–8. https://doi.org/10.1097/00000542-198110000-00003. PMID: 7294368.
19. Camu F, Lauwers MH, Verbessem D. Incidence and aetiology of postoperative nausea and vomiting. Eur J Anaesthesiol Suppl. 1992;6:25.
20. Cao S, Chen D, Yang L, Zhu T. Effects of an abnormal mini-mental state examination score on postoperative outcomes in geriatric surgical patients: a meta-analysis. BMC Anesthesiol. 2019;19(1):74. https://doi.org/10.1186/s12871-019-0735-5.
21. Chen JW, Gombart ZJ, Rogers S, Gardiner SK, Cecil S, Bullock RM. Pupillary reactivity as an early indicator of increased intracranial pressure: the introduction of the Neurological Pupil index. Surg Neurol Int. 2011;2:82. https://doi.org/10.4103/2152-7806.82248.
22. Chui J, Mariappan R, Mehta J, Manninen P, Venkatraghavan L. Comparison of propofol and volatile agents for maintenance of anesthesia during elective craniotomy procedures: systematic review and meta-analysis. Can J Anaesth. 2014;61(4):347–56. https://doi.org/10.1007/s12630-014-0118-9. Epub 2014 Jan 31. PMID: 24482247.
23. Chun EH, Han MJ, Baik HJ, Park HS, Chung RK, Han JI, Lee HJ, Kim JH. Dexmedetomidine-ketamine versus dexmedetomidine-midazolam-fentanyl for monitored anesthesia care dur-

ing chemoport insertion: a prospective randomized study. BMC Anesthesiol. 2016;16(1):49. https://doi.org/10.1186/s12871-016-0211-4. PMID: 27484227; PMCID: PMC4970235.
24. Chung F, Yegneswaran B, Liao P, et al. STOP questionnaire: a tool to screen patients for obstructive sleep apnea. Anesthesiology. 2008;108(5):812–21. https://doi.org/10.1097/ALN.0b013e31816d83e4.
25. Chung F, Yegneswaran B, Liao P, et al. Validation of the Berlin questionnaire and American Society of Anesthesiologists checklist as screening tools for obstructive sleep apnea in surgical patients. Anesthesiology. 2008;108(5):822–30. https://doi.org/10.1097/ALN.0b013e31816d91b5.
26. Chung F, Subramanyam R, Liao P, Sasaki E, Shapiro C, Sun Y. High STOP-Bang score indicates a high probability of obstructive sleep apnoea. Br J Anaesth. 2012;108(5):768–75. https://doi.org/10.1093/bja/aes022.
27. Cold GE, Eskesen V, Eriksen H, et al. CBF and CMRO2 during continuous etomidate infusion supplemented with N2O and fentanyl in patients with supratentorial cerebral tumour. A dose-response study. Acta Anaesthesiol Scand. 1985;29:490.
28. Dakik HA, Chehab O, Eldirani M, et al. A new index for pre-operative cardiovascular evaluation. J Am Coll Cardiol. 2019;73(24):3067–78. https://doi.org/10.1016/j.jacc.2019.04.023.
29. Dawson B, Michenfelder JD, Theye RA. Effects of ketamine on canine cerebral blood flow and metabolism: modification by prior administration of thiopental. Anesth Analg. 1971;50:443.
30. De Benedittis G, et al. Postoperative pain in neurosurgery: a pilot study in brain surgery. Neurosurgery. 1996;38(3):466–70. https://doi.org/10.1097/00006123-199603000-00008.
31. De Deyne C, Joly LM, Ravussin P. Les nouveaux agents volatils halogénés en neuroanesthésie: quelle place pour le sévoflurane ou le desflurane? [Newer inhalation anaesthetics and neuro-anaesthesia: what is the place for sevoflurane or desflurane?]. Ann Fr Anesth Reanim. 2004;23(4):367–74. https://doi.org/10.1016/j.annfar.2004.01.012. French. PMID: 15120783.
32. de Jong FH, Mallios C, Jansen C, et al. Etomidate suppresses adrenocortical function by inhibition of 11 beta-hydroxylation. J Clin Endocrinol Metab. 1984;59:1143.
33. Devereaux PJ, Mrkobrada M, Sessler DI, et al. Aspirin in patients undergoing noncardiac surgery. https://doi.org/10.1056/NEJMoa1401105.
34. Dhallu MS, et al. Perioperative management of neurological conditions. Health Serv Insights. 2017;10:117863291771194. https://doi.org/10.1177/1178632917711942.
35. Drummond JC, Dao AV, Roth DM, et al. Effect of dexmedetomidine on cerebral blood flow velocity, cerebral metabolic rate, and carbon dioxide response in normal humans. Anesthesiology. 2008;108:225.
36. Durieux ME, Himmelseher S. Pain control after craniotomy: off balance on the tightrope? J Neurosurg. 2007;106(2):207–8. https://doi.org/10.3171/jns.2007.106.2.207.
37. Eberhart LHJ, et al. Prevention and control of postoperative nausea and vomiting in postcraniotomy patients. Best Pract Res Clin Anaesthesiol. 2007;21(4):575–93. https://doi.org/10.1016/j.bpa.2007.06.007.
38. Egholm G, Kristensen SD, Thim T, et al. Risk associated with surgery within 12 months after coronary drug-eluting stent implantation. J Am Coll Cardiol. 2016;68(24):2622–32. https://doi.org/10.1016/j.jacc.2016.09.967.
39. English JB, Westenskow D, Hodges MR, Stanley TH. Comparison of venous air embolism monitoring methods in supine dogs. Anesthesiology. 1978;48(6):425–9. https://doi.org/10.1097/00000542-197806000-00009. PMID: 666025.
40. Fàbregas N, Bruder N. Recovery and neurological evaluation. Best Pract Res Clin Anaesthesiol. 2007;21(4):431–47. https://doi.org/10.1016/j.bpa.2007.06.006.
41. Feely MA, Collins CS, Daniels PR, Kebede EB, Jatoi A, Mauck KF. Preoperative testing before noncardiac surgery: guidelines and recommendations. Am Fam Physician. 2013;87(6):414–8.

42. Fleisher LA, Fleischmann KE, Auerbach AD, et al. 2014 ACC/AHA guideline on perioperative cardiovascular evaluation and management of patients undergoing noncardiac surgery: executive summary: a report of the American College of Cardiology/American Heart Association Task Force on Practice Guidelines. Circulation. 2014;130(24):2215–45. https://doi.org/10.1161/CIR.0000000000000105.
43. Fox J, Gelb AW, Enns J, et al. The responsiveness of cerebral blood flow to changes in arterial carbon dioxide is maintained during propofol-nitrous oxide anesthesia in humans. Anesthesiology. 1992;77:453.
44. Gelabert-González M, Iglesias-Pais M, García-Allut Martínez-Rumbo AR. Chronic subdural haematoma: surgical treatment and outcome in 1000 cases. Clin Neurol Neurosurg. 2005;107:223–9. https://doi.org/10.1016/j.clineuro.2004.09.015.
45. Gelb AW, Craen RA, Rao GS, et al. Does hyperventilation improve operating condition during supratentorial craniotomy? A multicenter randomized crossover trial. Anesth Analg. 2008;106:585.
46. George J, et al. Causes and prognosis of delirium in elderly patients admitted to a district general hospital. Age Ageing. 1997;26(6):423–7. https://doi.org/10.1093/ageing/26.6.423.
47. Geze S, Yilmaz AA, Tuzuner F. The effect of scalp block and local infiltration on the haemodynamic and stress response to skull-pin placement for craniotomy. Eur J Anaesthesiol. 2009;26(4):298–303. https://doi.org/10.1097/EJA.0b013e32831aedb2. PMID: 19262392.
48. Godier A, Dincq A-S, Martin A-C, et al. Predictors of pre-procedural concentrations of direct oral anticoagulants: a prospective multicentre study. Eur Heart J. 2017;38(31):2431–9. https://doi.org/10.1093/eurheartj/ehx403.
49. Godoy DA, Di Napoli M, Biestro A, Lenhardt R. Perioperative glucose control in neurosurgical patients. Anesthesiol Res Pract. 2012;2012:690362. https://doi.org/10.1155/2012/690362.
50. Goldman L, Caldera DL, Nussbaum SR, et al. Multifactorial index of cardiac risk in noncardiac surgical procedures. N Engl J Med. 1977;297(16):845–50. https://doi.org/10.1056/NEJM197710202971601.
51. Grinberg F, Slaughter TF, McGrath BJ. Probable venous air embolism associated with removal of the Mayfield skull clamp. Anesth Analg. 1995;80(5):1049–50. https://doi.org/10.1097/00000539-199505000-00036. PMID: 7726406.
52. Gupta PK, Gupta H, Sundaram A, et al. Development and validation of a risk calculator for prediction of cardiac risk after surgery. Circulation. 2011;124(4):381–7. https://doi.org/10.1161/CIRCULATIONAHA.110.015701.
53. Hatta K, et al. Antipsychotics for delirium in the general hospital setting in consecutive 2453 inpatients: a prospective observational study. Int J Geriatr Psychiatry. 2013;29(3):253–62. https://doi.org/10.1002/gps.3999.
54. Hawkins SB, et al. Quetiapine for the treatment of delirium. J Hosp Med. 2013;8(4):215–20. https://doi.org/10.1002/jhm.2019.
55. Hohnloser SH, Eikelboom JW. The hazards of interrupting anticoagulation therapy in atrial fibrillation. Eur Heart J. 2012;33(15):1864–6. https://doi.org/10.1093/eurheartj/ehs032.
56. Holcomb CN, Graham LA, Richman JS, Itani KMF, Maddox TM, Hawn MT. The incremental risk of coronary stents on postoperative adverse events: a matched cohort study. Ann Surg. 2016;263(5):924–30. https://doi.org/10.1097/SLA.0000000000001246.
57. Horinaka N, Yasumoto Y, Kumami K, Matsumura K. Evaluation of regional cerebral blood flow in chronic subdural hamatoma. Keio J Med. 2000;49(Suppl 1):A156–8.
58. Hougaard K, Hansen A, Brodersen P. The effect of ketamine on regional cerebral blood flow in man. Anesthesiology. 1974;41:562.
59. Inao S, Kawai T, Kabeya R, Sugimoto T, Yamamoto M, Hata N, Isobe T, Yoshida J. Relation between brain displacement and local cerebral blood flow in patients with chronic subdural hematoma. J Neurol Neurosurg Psychiatry. 2001;71:741–6.
60. Inouye SK. Precipitating factors for delirium in hospitalized elderly persons. JAMA. 1996;275(11):852. https://doi.org/10.1001/jama.1996.03530350034031.
61. Jian M, et al. Flurbiprofen and hypertension but not hydroxyethyl starch are associated with post-craniotomy intracranial haematoma requiring surgery. Br J Anaesth. 2014;113(5):832–9. https://doi.org/10.1093/bja/aeu185.

62. Kim SE, Kim E. Local anesthesia with monitored anesthesia care for patients undergoing thyroidectomy—a case series. Korean J Anesthesiol. 2016;69:635–9. https://doi.org/10.4097/kjae.2016.69.6.635.
63. Kim SO, Jung Il S, Won YS, Choi Yang CSJY. A comparative study of local versus general anesthesia for chronic subdural hematoma in elderly patients over 60 years. Korean J Neurotrauma. 2013;9:47–51. https://doi.org/10.13004/kjnt.2013.9.2.47.
64. Klopfenstein CE, Forster A, Van Gessel E. Anesthetic assessment in an outpatient consultation clinic reduces preoperative anxiety. Can J Anesth. 2000;47(6):511. https://doi.org/10.1007/BF030189.
65. Kolias AG, Chari A, Santarius Hutchinson TPJ. Chronic subdural haematoma: modern management and emerging therapies. Nat Rev Neurol. 2014;10:570–8. https://doi.org/10.1038/nrneurol.2014.163.
66. Kross RA, et al. A comparative study between a calcium channel blocker (nicardipine) and a combined α-β-blocker (labetalol) for the control of emergence hypertension during craniotomy for tumor surgery. Anesth Analg. 2000;91(4):904–9. https://doi.org/10.1097/00000539-200010000-00024.
67. Kuwabara H. Regional cerebral blood flow and metabolism in chronic subdural hematoma. Neurosurg Clin N Am. 2000;11:499–502.
68. Langeron O, Masso E, Huraux C, et al. Prediction of difficult mask ventilation. Anesthesiology. 2000;92(5):1229–36.
69. Leary MC, Varade P. Perioperative stroke. Curr Neurol Neurosci Rep. 2020;20(5):12. https://doi.org/10.1007/s11910-020-01033-7.
70. Lee TH, Marcantonio ER, Mangione CM, et al. Derivation and prospective validation of a simple index for prediction of cardiac risk of major noncardiac surgery. Circulation. 1999;100(10):1043–9. https://doi.org/10.1161/01.cir.100.10.1043.
71. Lee JY, Ebel H, Ernestus RI, Klug N. Various surgical treatments of chronic subdural hematoma and outcome in 172 patients: is membranectomy necessary? Surg Neurol. 2004;61(6):523–7; discussion 527–8. https://doi.org/10.1016/j.surneu.2003.10.026. PMID: 15165784.
72. Leone M, Albanèse J, Viviand X, et al. The effects of remifentanil on endotracheal suctioning-induced increases in intracranial pressure in head-injured patients. Anesth Analg. 2004;99:1193.
73. Lescot T, Degos V, Zouaoui A, et al. Opposed effects of hypertonic saline on contusions and noncontused brain tissue in patients with severe traumatic brain injury. Crit Care Med. 2006;34:3029.
74. Levine GN, Bates ER, Bittl JA, et al. 2016 ACC/AHA guideline focused update on duration of dual antiplatelet therapy in patients with coronary artery disease: a report of the American College of Cardiology/American Heart Association task force on clinical practice guidelines. J Am Coll Cardiol. 2016;68(10):1082–115. https://doi.org/10.1016/j.jacc.2016.03.513.
75. Liu C-Y, et al. Efficacy of risperidone in treating the hyperactive symptoms of delirium. Int Clin Psychopharmacol. 2004;19(3):165–8. https://doi.org/10.1097/00004850-200405000-00008.
76. Lutz LJ, Milde JH, Milde LN. The cerebral functional, metabolic, and hemodynamic effects of desflurane in dogs. Anesthesiology. 1990;73:125.
77. Madsen JB, Cold GE, Hansen ES, Bardrum B. The effect of isoflurane on cerebral blood flow and metabolism in humans during craniotomy for small supratentorial cerebral tumors. Anesthesiology. 1987;66:332.
78. Mahmood SD, Waqas M, Baig Darbar MZA. Mini-craniotomy under local anesthesia for chronic subdural hematoma: an effective choice for elderly patients and for patients in a resource-strained environment. World Neurosurg. 2017;106:676–9. https://doi.org/10.1016/j.wneu.2017.07.057.
79. Mahmood SD, Waqas M, Baig MZ, Darbar A. Mini-craniotomy under local anesthesia for chronic subdural hematoma: an effective choice for elderly patients and for patients in a resource-strained environment. World Neurosurg. 2017;106:676–9. https://doi.org/10.1016/j.wneu.2017.07.057. Epub 2017 Jul 19. PMID: 28735131.
80. Mammoto T, Hayashi Y, Ohnishi Y, Kuro M. Incidence of venous and paradoxical air embolism in neurosurgical patients in the sitting position: detection by transesophageal echocardiogra-

phy. Acta Anaesthesiol Scand. 1998;42(6):643–7. https://doi.org/10.1111/j.1399-6576.1998.tb05295.x. PMID: 9689268.
81. Marcantonio ER. A clinical prediction rule for delirium after elective noncardiac surgery. JAMA. 1994;271(2):134–9. https://doi.org/10.1001/jama.271.2.134.
82. Marcantonio ER, et al. The association of intraoperative factors with the development of postoperative delirium. Am J Med. 1998;105(5):380–4. https://doi.org/10.1016/s0002-9343(98)00292-7.
83. Mayer S, Rowland L. Head injury. In: Rowland L, editor. Merritt's neurology. Philadelphia: Lippincott Williams & Wilkins; 2000. p. 401.
84. Mayhew D, Mendonca V, Murthy BVS. A review of ASA physical status—historical perspectives and modern developments. Anaesthesia. 2019;74(3):373–9. https://doi.org/10.1111/anae.14569.
85. McAlister FA, Bertsch K, Man J, Bradley J, Jacka M. Incidence of and risk factors for pulmonary complications after nonthoracic surgery. Am J Respir Crit Care Med. 2005;171(5):514–7. https://doi.org/10.1164/rccm.200408-1069OC.
86. Meng L, et al. Effect of phenylephrine and ephedrine bolus treatment on cerebral oxygenation in anaesthetized patients. Br J Anaesth. 2011;107(2):209–17. https://doi.org/10.1093/bja/aer150.
87. Meng L, et al. Impact of phenylephrine administration on cerebral tissue oxygen saturation and blood volume is modulated by carbon dioxide in anaesthetized patients †. Br J Anaesth. 2012;108(5):815–22. https://doi.org/10.1093/bja/aes023.
88. Moghissi ES, Korytkowski MT, DiNardo M, et al. American Association of Clinical Endocrinologists and American Diabetes Association Consensus Statement on inpatient glycemic control. Diabetes Care. 2009;32(6):1119–31. https://doi.org/10.2337/dc09-9029.
89. Molnár C, Settakis G, Sárkány P, Kálmán S, Szabó S, Fülesdi B. Effect of sevoflurane on cerebral blood flow and cerebrovascular resistance at surgical level of anaesthesia: a transcranial Doppler study. Eur J Anaesthesiol. 2007;24(2):179–84. https://doi.org/10.1017/S0265021506001335. Epub 2006 Sep 14. PMID: 16970835.
90. Moon HG, Shin HS, Kim TH, Hwang YS, Park SK. Ossified chronic subdural hematoma. Yonsei Med J. 2003;44(5):915–8. https://doi.org/10.3349/ymj.2003.44.5.915. PMID: 14584111.
91. Moppett IK. Sympathetic activity and cerebral oxygenation. Br J Anaesth. 2009;103(5):769–70. https://doi.org/10.1093/bja/aep281.
92. Nassiri F, et al. Reinitiation of anticoagulation after surgical evacuation of subdural hematomas. World Neurosurg. 2020;135:e616–22. https://doi.org/10.1016/j.wneu.2019.12.080.
93. Neutel JM, et al. A comparison of intravenous nicardipine and sodium nitroprusside in the immediate treatment of severe hypertension. Am J Hypertens. 1994;7(7 Pt 1):623–8. https://doi.org/10.1093/ajh/7.7.623.
94. Olsen KS, et al. Effect of labetalol on cerebral blood flow, oxygen metabolism and autoregulation in healthy humans. Br J Anaesth. 1995;75(1):51–4. https://doi.org/10.1093/bja/75.1.51.
95. Omran H, Bauersachs R, Rübenacker S, Goss F, Hammerstingl C. The HAS-BLED score predicts bleedings during bridging of chronic oral anticoagulation. Thromb Haemost. 2012;108(07):65–73. https://doi.org/10.1160/TH11-12-0827.
96. Petersen KD, Landsfeldt U, Cold GE, et al. Intracranial pressure and cerebral hemodynamic in patients with cerebral tumors: a randomized prospective study of patients subjected to craniotomy in propofol-fentanyl, isoflurane-fentanyl, or sevoflurane-fentanyl anesthesia. Anesthesiology. 2003;98:329.
97. Practice guidelines for the perioperative management of patients with obstructive sleep apnea: a report by the American Society of Anesthesiologists Task Force on perioperative management of patients with obstructive sleep apnea. Anesthesiology. 2006;104(5):1081–93. https://doi.org/10.1097/00000542-200605000-00026.
98. Qureshi AI, et al. Pharmacologic reduction of mean arterial pressure does not adversely affect regional cerebral blood flow and intracranial pressure in experimental intracerebral hemorrhage. Crit Care Med. 1999;27(5):965–71. https://doi.org/10.1097/00003246-199905000-00036.

99. Rauhala M, Luoto TM, Huhtala H, Iverson GL, Niskakangas T, Öhman J, et al. The incidence of chronic subdural hematomas from 1990 to 2015 in a defined Finnish population. J Neurosurg. 2019;22:1–11. https://doi.org/10.3171/2018.12.JNS183035.
100. Rhondali O, et al. Do patients still require admission to an intensive care unit after elective craniotomy for brain surgery? J Neurosurg Anesthesiol. 2011;23(2):118–23. https://doi.org/10.1097/ana.0b013e318206d5f8.
101. Santarius T, Kirkpatrick PJ, Ganesan D, Chia HL, Jalloh I, Smielewski P, Richards HK, Marcus H, Parker RA, Price SJ, Kirollos RW, Pickard JD, Hutchinson PJ. Use of drains versus no drains after burr-hole evacuation of chronic subdural haematoma: a randomised controlled trial. Lancet. 2009;374(9695):1067–73. https://doi.org/10.1016/S0140-6736(09)61115-6. PMID: 19782872.
102. Shapira-Lichter I, Beilin B, Ofek K, Bessler H, Gruberger M, Shavit Y, et al. Cytokines and cholinergic signals co-modulate surgical stress-induced changes in mood and memory. Brain Behav Immun. 2008;22:388–98. https://doi.org/10.1016/j.bbi.2007.09.006.
103. Sharrock MF, Rosenblatt K. Acute airway management and ventilation in the neurocritical care unit. In: Nelson SE, Nyquist PA, editors. Neurointensive care unit: clinical practice and organization. Cham: Springer International Publishing; 2020. p. 31–47. https://doi.org/10.1007/978-3-030-36548-6_3.
104. Shiau JM, Chen TY, Tseng CC, Chang PJ, Tsai YC, Chang CL, Lee CG. Combination of bupivacaine scalp circuit infiltration with general anesthesia to control the hemodynamic response in craniotomy patients. Acta Anaesthesiol Sin. 1998;36(4):215–20. PMID: 10399517.
105. Shoyombo I, Aiyagari V, Stutzman SE, et al. Understanding the relationship between the neurologic pupil index and constriction velocity values. Sci Rep. 2018;8(1):6992. https://doi.org/10.1038/s41598-018-25477-7.
106. Slotty PJ, Kamp MA, Steiger HJS, Cornelius JF, Macht S, Stumer W, Turowski B. Cerebral perfusion changes in chronic subdural hematoma. J Neurotrauma. 2013;30:347–51.
107. Smilowitz NR, Berger JS. Perioperative cardiovascular risk assessment and management for noncardiac surgery: a review. JAMA. 2020;324(3):279. https://doi.org/10.1001/jama.2020.7840.
108. Stamenkovic DM, Rancic NK, Latas MB, et al. Preoperative anxiety and implications on postoperative recovery: what can we do to change our history. Minerva Anestesiol. 2018;84(11):1307–17. https://doi.org/10.23736/S0375-9393.18.12520-X.
109. Surve RM, Bansal S, Reddy M, Philip M. Use of dexmedetomidine along with local infiltration versus general anesthesia for Burr hole and evacuation of chronic subdural hematoma (CSDH). J Neurosurg Anesthesiol. 2017;29(3):274–80. https://doi.org/10.1097/ANA.0000000000000305. PMID: 27100913.
110. Tafur A, Douketis J. Perioperative management of anticoagulant and antiplatelet therapy. Heart. 2018;104(17):1461–7. https://doi.org/10.1136/heartjnl-2016-310581.
111. Tanaka A, Nakayama Y, Yoshinaga S. Cerebral blood flow and intracranial pressure in chronic subdural hematoma. Surg Neurol. 1997;47:346–52.
112. Todd MM, Drummond JC. A comparison of the cerebrovascular and metabolic effects of halothane and isoflurane in the cat. Anesthesiology. 1984;60:276.
113. Trofimova AO, Kalentiev G, Voennov O, Yuriev M, Agarkova D, Trofimov S, Bragin DE. Comparison of two algorithms for analysis of perfusion computed tomography (PCT) data for evaluation of cerebral microcirculation in chronic subdural hematoma. Adv Exp Med Biol. 2016;923:407–12.
114. Valgimigli M, Bueno H, Byrne RA, et al. 2017 ESC focused update on dual antiplatelet therapy in coronary artery disease developed in collaboration with EACTS: the Task Force for dual antiplatelet therapy in coronary artery disease of the European Society of Cardiology (ESC) and of the European Association for Cardio-Thoracic Surgery (EACTS). Eur Heart J. 2018;39(3):213–60. https://doi.org/10.1093/eurheartj/ehx419.
115. Vandesteene A, Trempont V, Engelman E, et al. Effect of propofol on cerebral blood flow and metabolism in man. Anaesthesia. 1988;43(Suppl):42–3.

116. Vaziri S, Wilson J, Abbatematteo J, et al. Predictive performance of the American College of Surgeons universal risk calculator in neurosurgical patients. J Neurosurg. 2018;128(3):942–7. https://doi.org/10.3171/2016.11.JNS161377.
117. Vaziri S, Abbatematteo JM, Fleisher MS, et al. Correlation of perioperative risk scores with hospital costs in neurosurgical patients. J Neurosurg. 2019;132(3):818–24. https://doi.org/10.3171/2018.10.JNS182041.
118. Victor M, Ropper A. Craniocerebral trauma. In: Victor M, Ropper A, editors. Adams and Victor's principles of neurology. 7th ed. New York: McGraw-Hill; 2001. p. 925.
119. Wang X, Ji J, Fen L, Wang A. Effects of dexmedetomidine on cerebral blood flow in critically ill patients with or without traumatic brain injury: a prospective controlled trial. Brain Inj. 2013;27(13–14):1617–22. https://doi.org/10.3109/02699052.2013.831130. Epub 2013 Oct 8. PMID: 24102571.
120. Won SY, Konczalla J, Dubinski D, Cattani A, Cuca C, Seifert V, Rosenow F, Strzelczyk A, Freiman TM. A systematic review of epileptic seizures in adults with subdural haematomas. Seizure. 2017;45:28–35. https://doi.org/10.1016/j.seizure.2016.11.017. Epub 2016 Nov 25. PMID: 27914224.
121. Wong DH, Weber EC, Schell MJ, Wong AB, Anderson CT, Barker SJ. Factors associated with postoperative pulmonary complications in patients with severe chronic obstructive pulmonary disease. Anesth Analg. 1995;80(2):276–84. https://doi.org/10.1097/00000539-199502000-00013.
122. Yoshida K, Furuse M, Izawa A, Lizima N, Hirano T, Kuchiwaki H, Inao S, Sugita K. Dynamics of cerebral metabolism in patients with chronic subdural hematoma evaluated with phosphorus 31MR spectroscopy before and after surgery. AJNR Am J Neuroradiol. 1994;15:1681–6.
123. Zhang Z, Guo Q, Wang E. Hyperventilation in neurological patients: from physiology to outcome evidence. Curr Opin Anaesthesiol. 2019;32(5):568–73. https://doi.org/10.1097/ACO.0000000000000764. PMID: 31211719; PMCID: PMC6735527.

Chapter 29
Surgical Treatment of Chronic Subdural Hematoma

Kemal Ertilav, Ümit Kocaman, and Arif Önder

29.1 Introduction

Subdural hematoma (SDH) usually occurs as a result of the rupture of bridging cortical veins into the potential space between the pia-arachnoid membrane and the dura mater. Injury of a dural sinus, an arachnoid granulation, or a small cortical artery can also cause a SDH [1]. Because of the low resistance in the subdural space, the hemorrhage spreads in the form of a crescent over the hemispheric surface within this space. In addition, excessive bleeding in this space can appear thinner than it actually is since it can spread along the falx and tentorium [6]. Hemorrhage is usually due to tears in the bridging veins with the acceleration-deceleration mechanism during trauma [28]. This disorder is common in late-advanced and advanced ages since the capacity of the brain to move increases and the flexibility of the parenchyma decreases with cerebral atrophy. Hemorrhages are classified as acute before 4 days, subacute between 4 and 21 days, and chronic after 21 days [28]. Chronic subdural hematomas (CSDHs) most likely begin as an acute SDH. The existing clot triggers an inflammatory response. Then, fibroblasts enter the clot and cover the inner surface of the dura in the first 24 h. Fibroblasts are responsible for membrane formation and gradually completely surround the clot. A parietal

K. Ertilav (✉)
Department of Neurosurgery, Suleyman Demirel University Faculty of Medicine, Isparta, Turkey

Department of Internal Medicine, Suleyman Demirel University Faculty of Medicine, Isparta, Turkey

Ü. Kocaman
Department of Neurosurgery, Bakircay University Faculty of Medicine, Izmir, Turkey

A. Önder
Department of Health Sciences, Istanbul Gelisim University, Istanbul, Turkey

M. Turgut et al. (eds.), *Subdural Hematoma*,
https://doi.org/10.1007/978-3-030-79371-5_29

membrane is formed within 7 days and visceral membrane within 21 days. Membrane formation is followed by neovascularization. The lysis of the existing clot increases fibrin degradation products and this prevents hemostasis. The weak neovascular sinusoidal structures formed in the CSDH capsule are prone to bleeding. Recurrent hemorrhages decrease the pressure inside the SDH to below that of the venous and capillary pressure and increase the passage of plasma first into the neovascularized structure and then into the capsule. Hemorrhage originating from the neovascularized structure cannot be completely prevented due to impaired hemostasis. In addition, the hemorrhage from the weak neovascularized structures, and the fibrin degradation products formed after their lysis, also create a vicious cycle and disrupt hemostasis. Thus, the CSDH receives plasma and expands progressively due to the effect of the newly formed bleeding foci as well as the low internal pressure [1, 4, 6, 28].

29.2 Surgical Principles

The most commonly used method for SDH treatment was craniotomy until the 1970s. After the 1980s, burr-hole craniostomy became the most common method. Twist drill craniostomy was introduced in 1977. Closed system drainage is still in use as the most commonly used method after craniotomies. Surgical drainage provides a rapid improvement in the symptoms [16]. A neurological deficit was found in 67.8% of the patients in a series of 208 cases [20]. Surgery eliminates the risk of herniation. Surgery is also indicated in symptomatic CSDH as this condition is a neurosurgical emergency. Surgical treatment is the fundamental basis of the approach to symptomatic CSDHs [8, 22]. It is more appropriate to make a joint decision when it is difficult to decide between surgical and nonsurgical treatment [16].

The main principles of the treatment are lowering the intracranial pressure and maintaining the balance between re-bleeding and fluid absorption. These two entities create the distinction between surgical and conservative treatment. The balance between re-bleeding and fluid absorption is deemed to be disrupted and thus progressive in CSDH with a thickness of 1 cm or more. In this case, the surgical option is indicated even if the patient is asymptomatic [8]. Symptoms develop when the intracranial pressure is increased. The patient may present with a broad spectrum of symptoms such as headaches, disorientation, epileptic seizure, focal deficits, lethargy, confusion, or coma [8, 28]. Surgical treatment is also indicated for CSDHs smaller than 1 cm if a focal deficit, mental status changes, or epileptic seizures are present with no other explanation [8]. A conservative approach can be adopted by keeping the follow-up interval short in CSDHs thinner than 1 cm without any other signs or symptoms. There is no surgical treatment indication for a CSDH thinner than 1 cm that is not increasing in size during follow-up and has no symptoms or physical findings [8].

29.3 Two Burr-Hole Craniostomy

A frontal burr-hole 1 cm in front of the coronal suture on the superior temporal line and a posterior parietal burr-hole are opened [15, 21]. We recommend that the burr-hole diameter is 12 mm. This diameter allows the appropriate angle for advancement of the subdural drain. The dura is opened and adhered to the internal tabula with bipolar cautery. Four-way irrigation is performed through the frontal and parietal burr-holes using warm saline and a drain with a soft and blunt tip. Saline is used for continuing irrigation, which is continued until the fluid becomes clear [8, 15, 21]. A soft, blunt-tipped subdural drain is then inserted carefully through the frontal and parietal burr-holes. The parietal burr-hole is closed first to prevent pneumocephalus; the subdural area is filled with saline through the frontal burr-hole to allow the air to come out with the saline [15]. Meanwhile, the Valsalva maneuver can be performed according to the surgeon's preference. The frontal burr-hole is then also closed and a dual closed free drainage system is used. The drains are withdrawn after 48 h on average.

29.4 Single Wide Burr-Hole Craniostomy

A temporo-parietal burr-hole widened to 20–25 mm is opened on the superior temporal line [8, 15]. The dura is opened and adhered to the internal tabula with the help of bipolar cautery. The parietal membrane is coagulated first if observed; it is then incised and the subdural hematoma drained. Four-way irrigation is performed by using warm saline and a drain with a soft and blunt tip. Saline irrigation is continued until the fluid becomes clear [8, 15]. A soft-tipped subdural drain is placed in the dorsal to antero-basal direction, and the burr-hole is closed after gelfoam of the same diameter is placed on it. The subdural area is filled with saline and placed in closed free drainage. The drain is withdrawn after 48 h.

29.5 Twist Drill Craniostomy

Twist drill craniostomy drainage is indicated in patients with a high risk of surgery in CSDH without septation. The advantage and main feature of the procedure is that it can be performed at the bedside under local anesthesia. A point 10 mm anterior to the coronal suture and on the superior temporal line is marked for the entry [8, 17, 34]. The most important requirement for using this method is for the SDH to have a thickness of at least twice the bone thickness on brain computed tomography. If this condition is met, 2% lidocaine solution is administered after the scalp is prepared with alcohol and povidone-iodine solution. An incision approximately 5 mm long is made at the entry point with a no. 15 scalpel. The bone and dura are drilled perpendicularly with a twist-drill [8, 17]. This perpendicular movement at this stage prevents the drill from sliding and therefore separates the dura from the inner tabula. The inner tabula is then shaved at a 45-degree angle to the entrance surface with a twist drill to prevent the permanent catheter from penetrating the cortex [8, 17]. The drain is advanced 50 mm in a postero-inferior direction, towards the ear. A standard ventriculostomy catheter is used. Irrigation and aspiration are not performed. A closed drainage system is applied. The catheter is withdrawn after 48 h [8, 17].

29.6 Wide Craniotomy

Craniotomy is indicated for CSDH, multiloculated, organized and calcified or ossified CSDH. This procedure is also a good surgical option for CSDH with significant membranes. Via craniotomy, ossified membranes can be safely addressed with a wider field of view [32]. Craniotomy is performed according to the location of the CSDH. The conventional method is by fronto-temporo-parieto-occipital craniotomy for SDHs that spread over the entire hemispheric surface. Following the opening of the dura, the intermembranous SDH is drained with a parietal membranotomy [21] (Figs. 29.1 and 29.2). The aim of this membranotomy is not to excise the membranes but to make an opening in the membranous structure, similar to a dural opening. For example, the membranotomy can be performed by incising in the form of an envelope or a flap. It would be appropriate to coagulate any membrane that is weak and prone to bleeding due to neovascularization before the incision is made. Irrigation should again be performed with warm saline and four-way irrigation, as explained for the previous methods [8, 21]. The visceral membrane must be differentiated from the arachnoid before performing the incision. This membrane is thinner than the parietal membrane and usually has a yellowish color. It is very

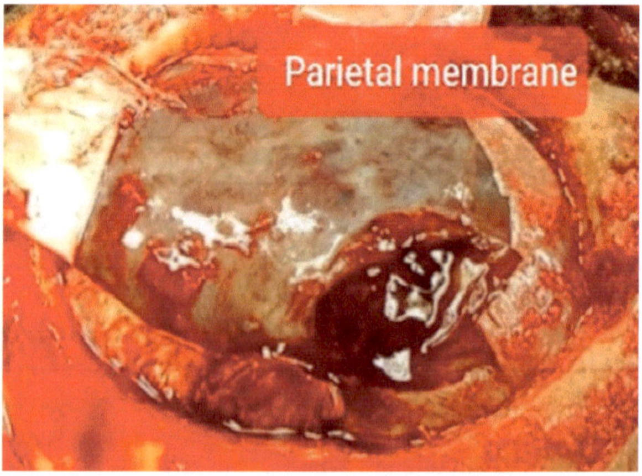

Fig. 29.1 The picture shows the parietal membrane surrounding the hematoma from above under the dura in a 77-year-old female patient treated with wide craniotomy

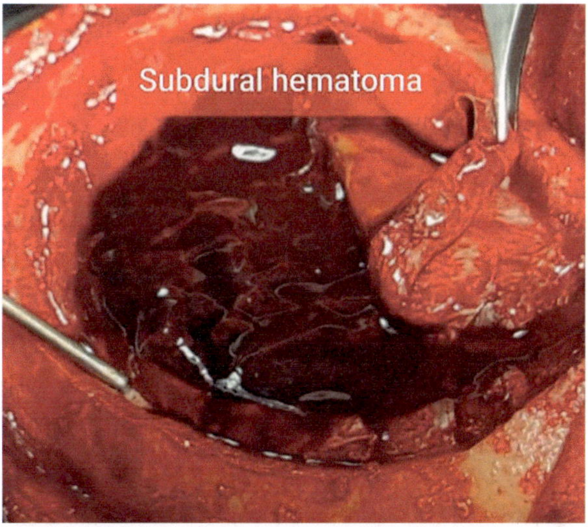

Fig. 29.2 The picture shows chronic subdural hematoma in the form of a clot in a 77-year-old female patient after parietal membranectomy

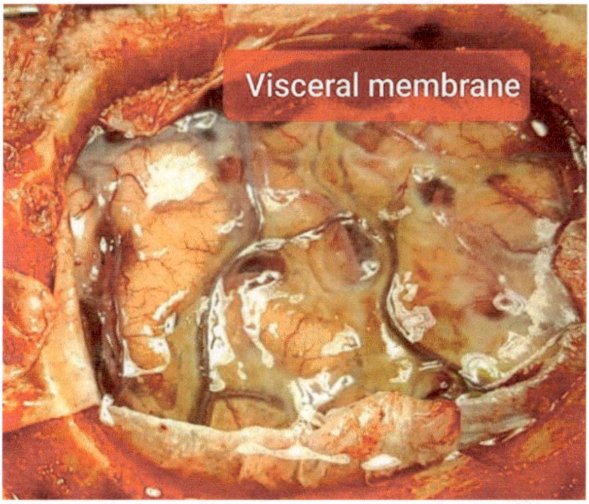

Fig. 29.3 The picture shows the dirty yellow visceral membrane partially adhered to the arachnoid and cortex after subdural clot excision in a 77-year-old woman

similar to the arachnoid membrane in thickness and appearance (Fig. 29.3). This tissue can be elevated and cut with a no. 15 scalpel at an area without vascularization with the help of a dissector and through a small incision. Forceful maneuvers should be avoided during the cutting of the visceral membrane [8, 21]. We have found visceral membranotomy to be the most effective maneuver to ensure the closure of the subdural distance by increasing cerebral expansion and thus preventing recurrence [13]. Following bleeding control, a drain is placed in the subdural space. The dura is closed and the bone flap is fixed back into place. The drain is withdrawn after 48 h.

29.7 Endoscopic Technique

Endoscopic surgery is indicated for the removal of solid clots under direct vision in organized and multiloculated CSDH. Endoscopic therapy can make the procedure safer with improved intraoperative visualization. This technique can allow neo-membranes to be identified and removed [34]. For endoscopic drainage of the CSDH, a 40 mm skin incision is made in the parietal region, the most curved part of the cranium, according to the location of the hematoma. A 30 mm mini-craniotomy is preferably performed. The inner and outer tabula are drilled with the endoscope to provide a straight view of the hematoma [2, 9, 35]. The dura is opened in the form of an envelope and held back. After the parietal membrane is differentiated and the membranotomy is performed, the endoscope is advanced through the parietal and visceral membranes to provide visibility. Hematoma drainage is ensured with the help of an aspirator. The septations are opened with the help of an endoscope and hematoma drainage is performed in the different compartments. Four-way irrigation is performed with a soft drain using warm saline solution. A drain is placed in the distant subdural space, the dura is closed, and the cavity is filled with saline. The bone flap is fixed in place. The drain is withdrawn after 48 h [31, 34].

29.8 Middle Meningeal Artery Embolization

We can define middle meningeal artery (MMA) embolization as a "subdural devascularization procedure." This procedure helps to break the vicious circle favoring continued exudation and blood product accumulation, by shifting the balance to reabsorption. The middle meningeal artery is a branch of the maxillary artery originating from the carotid artery. It enters the cranium through the foramen spinosum at the base of the skull and then vascularizes the dura with its frontal and parietal branches. The MMA supplies the meninges with the anterior meningeal artery and posterior meningeal artery. In other words, the MMA feeds the complex structure of a CSDH located on the mid-anterior and mid-posterior cerebral convexity. Its distal branches anastomose with the ophthalmic artery through the recurrent meningeal artery. The MMA also anastomoses with the posterior auricular artery. Accidental infiltration of embolizing particles into these anastomoses can cause ophthalmic nerve and facial nerve injuries. The origin of the ophthalmic artery is the MMA in 13% of subjects. In this case, performing MMA embolization for the treatment of CSDH is contraindicated [5]. This treatment can be performed in three ways: (1) as a single treatment; (2) as a preoperative additional treatment; and (3) as a postoperative additional treatment [26]. The classic method used for embolization is particle embolization with polyvinyl alcohol (PVA). Another method is to use liquid embolizing agents. The advantage of PVA embolization is that it has more distal penetration. This is a good method to block the vascular supply of the organized hematoma structure from collaterals consisting of arteries other than the MMA. The disadvantage is that PVA is not an opaque substance and is therefore difficult to follow visually. While microcatheters can provide only limited dispersion of PVA particles, large amounts of liquid embolic agents can be distributed [5].

29.9 Mini-Craniotomy and Basal (Visceral) Membranotomy

This technique is a modification of the wide craniotomy and single burr-hole techniques. However, the diameter is set at 40 mm [13]. The dura is opened and held open in a horseshoe shape. After the parietal membrane is opened, the intermembranous SDH is drained. The compartments are opened and the confined hematoma areas are drained. The visceral membranous structure has a dirty yellow appearance and the thickness of an onion membrane. This structure differs from the arachnoid by its color and being slightly thicker. The visceral membrane is carefully opened [13, 21]. Irrigation is performed with warm saline by advancing the soft drain in four directions through the cleavage between the visceral membrane and the arachnoid. The biggest advantage of visceral membranotomy is that it helps to close the subdural space by contributing to cerebral expansion. This decreases recurrence significantly. Then, a drain is placed in the subdural space, and the dura is closed. The bone flap is fixed in place. The drain is withdrawn after 48 h [13].

29.10 Recurrent Subdural Hematoma, Surgical Technique Decision, Drain Issue, Young and Pediatric Patients, Other Issues: Discussion

Recurrence of CSDH is not rare. Failure of surgical drainage is possible at a rate of 9.4–30%. This rate is usually around 18% in burr-hole drainage series [20]. Once the primary surgical treatment is unsuccessful, the recurrence rate can go up to 46% in repeated surgical treatment. The Oslo recurrence detection and grading system for recurrence that will require surgery after CSDH burr-hole drainage can guide the surgeon in this regard [27] (Table 29.1). According to this prediction system, no CSDH requiring repeat surgery developed in any patient with a total score of 0. CSDH requiring repeat surgery developed in 6% of those with 1 or 2 points, 30% of those with 3 or 4 points, and 63% of those with 5 points.

The depressed cerebral volume on the seventh day after burr-hole craniostomy was considered to be the most important factor in determining recurrence in a study on 291 patients. The cutoff volume value was found to be 51.6 cm^3 with a sensitivity and specificity of 79.3% and 67.9%, respectively [11].

A study including 461 patients determined that the factors that increased the risk of recurrence were a midline shift over 10 mm, severe brain atrophy, severe postoperative pneumocephalus, and drainage of more than 100 mL of hematoma [24].

Table 29.1 Oslo recurrence detection and grading system for recurrence that will require surgery after CSDH burr-hole drainage[a]

– CT density based	
Isodense/hyperdense subtypes and laminar/septate types	2
Hypodense/gradation subtypes and trabecular type	0
– Preoperative volume	
Larger than 130 mL	1
Smaller than 130 mL	0
– The volume of postoperative residual cavity	
Larger than 200 mL	2
80–200 mL	1
Smaller than 80 mL	0
– Total score	0–5

[a]This table was taken from Stanišic and Pripp [27]

Contralateral SDH that requires surgery may develop after SDH drainage procedures. Some studies point to the contralateral hematoma volume after the first surgery as a risk factor in these patients. The cutoff volume value has been reported to be 37.84 cm^3 [23].

Subdural-peritoneal shunt use or placing an Ommaya reservoir and performing repetitive punctures are among the surgical treatment options for CSDHs with multiple recurrences.

One of the general conclusions to be drawn from these studies is that any cerebral tissue that does not expand in the postoperative period provides a basis for the development of CSDH recurrence.

Deciding on the appropriate surgical technique requires evaluating many factors together. The patient's age, Karnofsky performance score, additional underlying diseases, use of anti-platelet or anticoagulant treatment, and radiological characteristics of the hematoma will be important in determining the surgical technique chosen. Methods where any septations and membranes can be opened should be preferred for those with 5 points from the "Oslo recurrence detection and grading system for recurrence that will require surgery after CSDH burr-hole drainage" scoring. Our recommendations for treatment are the "single wide burr-hole technique," "mini-craniotomy and basal membranotomy technique," "craniotomy technique," and the "endoscopic method." The surgeon decides which method will be used by considering all of the factors listed above. For example, if the patient is at an advanced age and has additional underlying diseases, methods that require a shorter surgical duration and less anesthesia and create a lower surgical burden may be preferred. Another important issue is the use of anticoagulants and this factor was present in approximately 50% of the patients in some series. Major surgery may not be appropriate in patients using anticoagulants and less invasive surgical techniques should be preferred [14, 20]. The "two burr-hole technique" is a traditional and less invasive method and may be the first option for those with a grading score of less than 5. The single wide burr-hole technique could also be a potential alternative. No significant difference was found between one burr-hole and two burr-holes in terms of recurrence rate, complication rate, morbidity, and mortality in a meta-analysis [32]. Twist-drill craniostomy, which is again a less invasive method, can be used as an alternative. The application of the twist-drill craniostomy technique under local anesthesia was compared with burr-hole drainage under local and general anesthesia in a different study. No significant difference was identified regarding hematoma evacuation, recurrence rate, and hospitalization duration in this comparison. Any pre-existing neurological disorders of the patients such as Parkinson's and Alzheimer's disease were affected less by the local anesthetic approaches [3].

We have investigated the nuances of "recurrence" and "deciding on the surgical technique" until this stage of the discussion section. It is now also necessary to evaluate the surgical details. The two most common methods used for CSDH treatment are burr-hole drainage and craniotomy. The method the surgeon prefers is the most important factor in deciding on which one to use. A study has found craniotomy to be advantageous with a recurrence rate of 15.7% compared to 7.5% for the alternative. Advanced age and a low GCS score were associated with a poor prognosis in both groups. It was also found that the use of aspirin increased the 30-day mortality in patients who underwent craniotomy, while the use of coumadin also increased 30-day mortality in patients who underwent burr-hole drainage [19]. Studies where burr-hole drainage was compared with a mini-craniotomy have emphasized that no significant difference was found between the two techniques in terms of mortality and recurrence rates while other studies have reported that a mini-craniotomy based on cerebral expansion decreases the recurrence rate significantly [10, 13]. We also believe in the second option where mini-craniotomy allows for visceral membranotomy. It is also a proven method that can be used to avoid the complications of a wide craniotomy.

The mean surgical duration for endoscopic methods is 45 min with very little invasiveness when used by experienced surgeons. These methods are also effective in preventing recurrence since they allow performing septostomy and membranotomy [2, 9, 35]. Endoscopic approaches may decrease recurrence in elderly patients, especially those over the age of 85, as they allow septostomy. The patient is therefore protected from the risks of recurrent surgery [19].

MMA embolization can be used as an additional treatment before or after surgical drainage, or as a standalone treatment method in cases where surgery cannot be performed. While the recurrence rate of CSDH with this technique was found to be significantly low in some studies, there was no significant difference in the complication rate [26]. From a neurosurgical point of view, a CSDH with a surgical indication is a neurosurgical emergency and decompression should be rapid and effective. It may be more appropriate to consider MMA embolization as an additional treatment in such cases, especially in CSDHs with a high risk of recurrence.

The drain is placed in the subdural space in the usual manner when conventional methods are used. We prefer the subdural drain to be soft and have a blunt tip. We recommend the drain to be advanced approximately 3–4 cm over the brain surface. If the burr-hole drainage is performed with two holes, a subdural drain should be placed in both holes. Hard drains with a sharp tip create a risk of drain malposition. Advancing the drain more than 4 cm may also create a risk in terms of cerebral cortex penetration. In addition, there is evidence that a significant recurrence rate is possible as the depth of the drain increases [33]. The smallest recurrence rate was observed at a subdural drain depth less than 4.3 cm in the same study [33]. Another important point in avoiding cortex penetration when advancing the drain is to have a burr-hole diameter of at least 12 mm to ensure a proper drain advancing angle. Burr-hole drainage was performed and a subdural drain was used in 290 patients in a study that reported drain malposition in 73 (15.8%) patients, iatrogenic bleeding in 5 (6.9%) patients, and neurological symptoms in 9 (12.3%) patients [12]. The high rates of malposition have resulted in promoting the advantages of using a subperiosteal drain in some studies. The superiority of a subperiosteal drain over a subdural drain regarding the recurrence rate, infection rate, and iatrogenic drain injuries was also emphasized [25]. A multicentered study on drain position (frontal burr-hole/parietal burr-hole), duration, and localization (subperiosteal/subdural) also produced interesting result. The study compared the recurrence rate for these three factors and concluded that drain position, duration, and location did not affect CSDH recurrence [7].

Although CSDH is common at advanced ages, it can also be seen under the age of 40. It needs to be emphasized that head trauma is a risk factor for the development of CSDH in young patients with a ventriculo-peritoneal shunt or arachnoid cyst. Most of these patients present with headache and dizziness. However, head trauma is not a risk factor for the development of CSDH in young patients without a shunt or arachnoid cyst [18].

The skin depression into burr-holes after healing is also worth mentioning. This development causes significant patient dissatisfaction but burr-hole caps are still not used by the majority of neurosurgeons. We believe that they will be used routinely in the future [30].

A calcified SDH is a very rare diagnosis and constitutes 0.3–2.7% of all CSDHs. This process is slow and may be asymptomatic for years. Surgery is the main treatment for symptomatic cases. A database review has revealed that 72.8% of calcified SDHs required surgery. Resection of the calcified mass via craniotomy is recommended. It is important to carefully dissect the inner and outer membranes at the same time [29].

A subdural-peritoneal shunt can be used in the treatment of SDH in children. The shunt pump should be of low pressure. Subdural tap is another option. A shunt should be used in hematomas that persist following three taps [28].

29.11 Conclusion

Despite the described and employed surgical methods, the physician will make the final decision as to which method will be used. The patient's age, performance score, medical comorbidities, drugs used, additional risk factors, and the surgeon's experience all influence the surgical decision. The issue we want to emphasize is the relationship between septations and recurrence. Avoiding repetitive surgery should be the most important goal in the elderly population with comorbid diseases. We think that exposing the patient to repeated surgical interventions by using less invasive methods initially is also not appropriate. The physician should make the most accurate surgical decision for the patient by considering all the factors. Making a joint decision with the other neurosurgeons in the department will be the most appropriate method in the selection of surgical or conservative treatment as well as in cases where there is some difficulty in selecting the best surgical method.

References

1. Akpınar E, Cila A. Radiology in a head injury patient (in Turkish). In: Ozgen T, Ziyal I, editors. Emergency neurosurgery. Ankara; 2009. p. 64–6.
2. Ca Q, Guo Q, Zhang F, Sun D, Zhang W, Ji B, Chen Z, Mao S. Evacuation of chronic and subacute subdural hematoma via transcranial neuroendoscopic approach. Neuropsychiatr Dis Treat. 2019;15:385–90.
3. Certo F, Maione M, Altieri R, Garozzo M, Toccaceli G, Peschillo S, Barbagallo GMV. Pros and cons of a minimally invasive percutaneous subdural drainage system for evacuation of chronic subdural hematoma under local anesthesia. Clin Neurol Neurosurg. 2019;187:105559.
4. Feghali J, Yang W, Huang J. Updates in chronic subdural hematoma: epidemiology, etiology, pathogenesis, treatment and outcome. World Neurosurg. 2020;141:339–45.
5. Fiorella D, Arthur AS. Middle meningeal artery embolization for the management of chronic subdural hematoma. J Neurointerv Surg. 2019;11(9):912–5.
6. Gentry LR. Imaging of closed head Injury. Radiology. 1994;191(1):1–17.
7. Glancz LJ, Poon MTC, Coulter JC, Hutchinson PJ, Kolias AG, Brennan PM, British Neurosurgical Trainnee Research Collaborative (BNTRC). Does drain position and duration influence outcomes in patients undergoing burr-hole evacuation of chronic subdural hematoma? Lessons from a UK multicenter prospective cohort study. Neurosurgery. 2019;85(4):486–93.
8. Greenberg Mark S. In: Hakan OH, editor. Handbook of neurosurgery (Turkish translation). Ankara; 2013. p. 674–6.
9. Guan F, Peng WC, Huang H, Dai B, Zhu GT, Mao BB, Xiao ZY, Lin ZY, Hu ZQ. Efficacy analysis of soft neuroendoscopic techniques in the treatment of chronic subdural hematoma. Zhonghua Yi Xue Za Zhi. 2019;99(9):695–9.
10. Haron S, Bogduk N, Hansen M. A retrospective analysis of chronic subdural haematoma recurrence rates following burr hole trephination versus minicraniotomy. J Clin Neurosci. 2019;59:47–50.
11. Jang KM, Choi HH, Mun HY, Nam TK, Park YS, Kwon JT. Critical depressed brain volume influences the recurrence of chronic subdural hematoma after surgical evacuation. Sci Rep. 2020;10(1):1–8.
12. Kamenova M, Wanderer S, Lipps P, Marbacher S, Mariani L, Soleman J. When the drain hits the brain. World Neurosurg. 2020;138:e426–36.
13. Kocaman U, Yilmaz H. Description of a modified technique (mini craniotomy-basal membranotomy) for chronic subdural hematoma surgery and evaluation of the contribution of basal membranotomy performed as part of this technique to cerebral expansion. World Neurosurg. 2019;122:e1002–6.
14. Kotwica Z, Saracen A, Dziuba I. Chronic subdural hematoma (CSH) is still an important clinical problem. Analysis of 700 consecutive patients. Tranl Neurosci. 2019;10:260–3.

15. Kutty SA, Jony M. Chronic subdural hematoma: a comparison of recurrence rates following burr-hole craniostomy with and without Drains. Turk Neurosurg. 2014;24:494–7.
16. Lee KS. How to treat chronic subdural hematoma? Past and now. J Korean Neurosurg Soc. 2019;62(2):144–52.
17. Lee SJ, Hwang SC, Im SB. Twist-drill or burr hole craniostomy for draining chronic subdural hematomas: how to choose it for chronic subdural hematoma drainage. Korean J Neurotrauma. 2016;12(2):107–11.
18. Ou Y, Dong J, Wu L, Xu L, Wang L, Liu B, Li J, Liu W. The clinical characteristics, treatment, and outcomes of chronic subdural hematoma in young patients. World Neurosurg. 2019;125:e1241–6.
19. Raghavan A, Smith G, Onyewadume L, Peck MR, Herring E, Pace J, Rogers M, Momotaz H, Hoffer SA, Hu Y, Liu H, Tatsuoka C, Sajatovic M, Sioan AE. Morbidity and mortality after burr hole craniostomy versus craniotomy for chronic subdural hematoma evacuation: a single-center experience. World Neurosurg. 2020;134:e196–203.
20. Ridwan S, Bohrer AM, Grote A, Simon M. Surgical treatment of chronic subdural hematoma: predicting recurrence and cure. World Neurosurg. 2019;128:e1010–23.
21. Salcman M, Heros RC, Laws ER Jr, Volker K, Sonntag H. Subdural hematoma. Chapter 15: Kempe's Operative Neurosurgery. Springer-Verlag New York, Inc. 2004. p. 155–8.
22. Scerrati A, Visani J, Ricciardi L, Dones F, Rustemi O, Cavallo MA, Bonis PD. To drill or not to drill, that is the question: nonsurgical treatment of chronic subdural hematoma in the elderly. A systematic review. Neurosurg Focus. 2020;49(4):E7.
23. Shen J, Shao X, Gao Y, Li Q, Ge R, Wang Q, Zhou W, Jiang X. Risk factors for contralateral hematoma progression after unilateral evacuation of bilateral chronic subdural hematomas. World Neurosurg. 2019;126:e773–8.
24. Shen J, Yuan L, Ge R, Wang Q, Zhou W, Jiang XC, Shao X. Clinical and radiological factors predicting recurrence of chronic subdural hematoma: a retrospective cohort study. Injury. 2019;50(10):1634–40.
25. Soleman J, Lutz K, Schaedelin S, Kamenova M, Guzman R, Mariani L, Fanding J. Subperiosteal vs subdural drain after burr-hole drainage of chronic subdural hematoma: a randomized clinical trial (cSDH-Drain-Trial). Neurosurgery. 2019;85(5):E825–34.
26. Srivatsan A, Mohanty A, Nascimento FA, Hafeez MU, Srinivasan VM, Thomas A, Chen SR, Johnson JN, Kan P. Middle meningeal artery embolization for chronic subdural hematoma: meta-analysis and systematic review. World Neurosurg. 2019;122:613–9.
27. Stanišic M, Pripp AH. A reliable grading system for prediction of chronic subdural hematoma recurrence requiring reoperation after initial burr-hole surgery. Neurosurgery. 2017;81(5):752–60.
28. Tahta K. Traumatic intracranial hematomas (in Turkish). In: Aksoy K, editor. Basic neurosurgery. Ankara; 2005. p. 328–30.
29. Turgut M, Akhaddar A, Turgut AT. Calcified or ossified chronic subdural hematoma: a systematic reviewof 114 cases reported during last century with a demonstrative case report. World Neurosurg. 2020;134:240–63.
30. Velz J, Vasella F, Akeret K, Dias S, Jehli E, Bosinov O, Regli L, Germans MR, Stienen MN. Patterns of care: Burr-hole cover application for chronic subdural hematoma trepanation. Neurosurg Focus. 2019;47(5):E14.
31. Wakuta N, Abe H, Fukuda K, Nonaka M, Morishita T, Arima H, Inoue T. Feasibility and safety of endoscopic procedure in burr-hole surgery for chronic subdural hematoma in patients of very advanced age. World Neurosurg. 2020;134:e1037–46.
32. Wan Y, Xie D, Xue Z, Xie J, Song Z, Wang Y, Yang S. Single versus double burr hole craniostomy in surgical treatment of chronic subdural hematoma: a meta-analysis. World Neurosurg. 2019;131:e149–54.
33. Weng W, Li H, Zhao X, Yang C, Wang S, Hui J, Mao Q, Gao G, Feng J. The depth of catheter in chronic subdural haematoma: does it matter? Brain Inj. 2019;33(6):717–22.
34. Yadav YR, Parihar V, Namdev H, Bejaj J. Chronic subdural hematoma. Asian J Neurosurg. 2020;11(4):330–42.
35. Yadav YR, Ratre S, Parihar V, Bajaj J, Sinha M, Kumar A. Endoscopic management of chronic subdural hematoma. J Neurol A Cent Eur Neurosurg. 2020;81(4):330–41.

Chapter 30
Role of Endoscopy in Surgical Treatment of Chronic Subdural Hematoma

Ali Hazama, Said Shukri, Fakhri Awawdeh, and Walter A. Hall

30.1 Incidence of Chronic Subdural Hematoma

The annual incidence of chronic subdural hematoma (CSDH) is about 1–5.3 cases per 100,000 persons [10]. Risk factors that increase the rate of subdural hematomas are advanced age, male gender, and use of anticoagulants [17]. In a study from Finland documenting the incidence of CSDH between 1990 and 2015, it was established that the rate of CSDH had increased significantly from 8.2 in 1990 to 17.6 per 100,000 people in 2015 [9]. This change was due to the increasing use of anticoagulants as well as the increased survival of the world population into advanced age [9]. In the same study, the median age of patients with CSDHs was between 73 and 79 years, where they were more prevalent among the population >80 years of age.

30.2 Risk Factors for Chronic Subdural Hematoma

The most prevalent risk factors for CSDH are old age, male gender, and head injury [15]. Other known risk factors for subdural hematomas include epilepsy, chronic alcoholism, coagulopathy, anticoagulant therapy, arachnoid cysts, diabetes mellitus,

---

A. Hazama (✉)
Department of Neurosurgery, SUNY Upstate Medical University, Syracuse, NY, USA
e-mail: HazamaA@Upstate.edu

S. Shukri
Jacobs School of Medicine, University at Buffalo, Buffalo, NY, USA
e-mail: saidshuk@buffalo.edu

F. Awawdeh
College of Arts and Sciences, Syracuse University, Syracuse, NY, USA
e-mail: fbawawda@syr.edu

W. A. Hall
Department of Neurosurgery, SUNY Upstate Medical University,
Syracuse, New York, USA
e-mail: hallw@upstate.edu

M. Turgut et al. (eds.), *Subdural Hematoma*,
https://doi.org/10.1007/978-3-030-79371-5_30

thrombocytopenia, and cardiovascular disease [11]. However, conditions such as chronic kidney disease and heart disease were protective against developing a CSDH because they restricted mobility, decreasing the likelihood of patients sustaining a head injury or trauma [15].

30.3 Role of Endoscopy in the Treatment of Chronic Subdural Hematoma

Endoscopy involves the insertion of a long, thin instrument with a camera at the tip directly into the body through a small incision. This approach allows for the direct visualization and evaluation of an internal organ or other tissue in detail. This technique enables surgeons to perform minor surgeries, tissue resections, and drainage of unwanted collections with minimal disruption to normal structures. Endoscopic procedures are beneficial for the management of CSDH. Classically, treatment of CSDH requires procedures such as craniotomy, mini-craniotomy, burr hole drainage, and twist drill evacuation in combination with the placement of subdural drains. Recently, endoscopy has demonstrated usefulness in the treatment of CSDH [4]. Compared to other techniques, endoscopy offers direct visualization and inspection of the entire cavity containing the CSDH. Moreover, endoscopy has been used to successfully evacuate a subdural hematoma [15]. In a study conducted by Yadav et al., the endoscopic technique helped remove CSDH within 35–80 min [15]. This result can be compared to a craniotomy, which can take anywhere from 3 to 5+ h [16].

Other studies examining endoscopy in this area determined that angiogenesis was one of the main reasons responsible for recurrence of CSDH [2]. While some of the traditional surgical techniques do not usually allow for a complete removal of this neovasculature, endoscopy will allow—for direct visualization and resection of these abnormal findings, further minimizing the risks of CSDH recurrence. Studies evaluating endoscopy as a treatment for CSDH have not revealed significant negative results related to endoscopy [2, 15]. In the Yadav study, there were no reported subdural recurrences, acute hemorrhages, injury to the brain, or any infections in the 68 patients who underwent endoscopic evacuation of a CSDH [15]. Nonetheless, common risks associated with cranial surgery remain a risk for endoscopy such as infection and re-bleeding.

The safety and efficacy of endoscopic evacuation of CSDH was demonstrated by Guo et al. This study established that endoscopy significantly decreased the hematoma recurrence and complication rates in patients significantly and was thereby considered a safer approach to CSDH treatment [1]. The study concluded that endoscope-assisted surgery is highly effective and safe in treating CSDH. Mini-craniotomies and burr hole aspiration are known to have limited visualization of the entire CSDH cavity. This diminished view restricts the evaluation of the subdural cavity and adds to the potential for incomplete evacuation of subdural collections. Furthermore, the mean operative time in the endoscopic-assisted procedures were

37.4 min which was significantly shorter than in non-endoscopic procedures that required 43.1 min [5]. In addition to a more complete evacuation of the subdural collection, the optimal tissue visualization afforded by the endoscope created a conducive environment for protecting the brain surface and the bridging veins [5].

30.4 Endoscopic Technique

Craniotomy for CSDH evacuation is commonly performed under general anesthesia. However, the use of a small incision and a single burr hole allows for endoscopic evacuation to be performed under local anesthesia in a subset of patients [3]. Increasing age and increased comorbid burden can render invasive treatment strategies to be of high risk [8]. This subgroup may benefit from less invasive, endoscopic techniques avoiding the risks associated with endotracheal intubation and general anesthesia. As for the surgical technique, a 4 cm incision is sufficient for placing a burr hole in the skull. The dura is then opened whereby there is usually an initial gush spontaneously of chronic subdural fluid. A flexible endoscope is then introduced into the subdural space and the hematoma is drained. Further coagulation and removal of neo-membranes can be performed through the working channel of the scope. The cavity is then inspected and any discernable bleeding is coagulated under direct visualization. After complete hemostasis and satisfactory evacuation of the CSDH, a drain can be placed in the subdural space followed by closure of the incision [13]. A postoperative CT is used to confirm the adequacy of the reduction of the hematoma [3].

30.5 Costs of Endoscopy

The cost of conducting endoscopic procedures varies widely between countries. In the United States, the national average cost is approximated to be $2750 [7]. The national range is between $1250 and $4800 [2]. In other parts of the world, such as India, endoscopy is relatively less expensive. For instance, in India, the procedure can cost anywhere between $15 and $100, depending on the facility where a patient receives treatment. More importantly, various factors can affect the cost of endoscopy in the United States that include the facility setting, type of insurance, and the state in which the procedure is performed. In terms of facility setting, performing the procedure in an inpatient facility is costlier when compared to an outpatient center. In contrast with other treatment options for CSDH evacuation, endoscopy is significantly lower in cost. In the United States, a craniotomy costs between $20,936 and $50,090 [14]. On the other hand, burr hole aspiration procedures are less costly than craniotomies but remain about twice as expensive as endoscopy, costing roughly $7588 [6]. Evacuation of CSDH under sedation and local anesthesia is not only safer compared to general anesthesia but it is also more cost effective.

30.6 Survival Outcomes of Surgical Interventions

According to a study completed by Lee et al., patients who underwent surgical interventions for CSDH had a statistically significant survival rate. At follow-up, 92.9% and 81.4% of the patients in the surgical group survived for at least 30 days and 6 months, respectively. This outcome can be compared to 58.1% and 41.9% survival rate in the conservative group, respectively, using the same time frames [12]. Furthermore, compared with burr hole craniotomy surgery, endoscope-assisted surgery showed a significantly lower recurrence rate and complication rate for CSDH; however the mortality rate did not demonstrate a significant difference between the two groups [1]. When comparing the use of endoscopy and craniotomy as treatment options for cerebral hemorrhage, Sun et al. reported that the endoscopy group in their study exhibited a decrease in mean blood loss, blood transfusion, and surgical duration. Furthermore, the endoscopy group had an increase in the average hematoma clearance rate and postoperative activity of daily living scores [18]. The overall length of hospital stay was also shorter in patients treated with endoscope-assisted burr hole craniotomy when compared to standard burr hole craniotomy [18]. Depending on the amount of cerebral damage caused by the hematoma, patients can fully recover anywhere from 2 weeks to a few months after endoscopic intervention [15].

30.7 Conclusion

Endoscopy is an effective technique for the treatment of CSDH. The technique provides better visualization and subdural cavity assessment. Endoscopy allows for a more complete hematoma evacuation and resection of neovasculature, decreasing the likelihood for CSDH recurrence. In some cases, general anesthesia and endotracheal intubation are not required, and the comorbidities inherent with these interventions can therefore be avoided. The endoscopic technique should be added to the armamentarium of those surgical treatment options available for CSDH.

References

1. Guan F, Peng W, Huang H, Dai B, Zhu G, Xiao Z, Hu Z. Efficacy analysis of flexible neuroendoscopy combined with dry-field techniques in the treatment of chronic subdural hematoma. Chin Med J. 2019;132(11):1359–62.
2. Guo S, Gao W, Cheng W, Liang C, Wu A. Endoscope-assisted surgery vs. burr-hole craniostomy for the treatment of chronic subdural hematoma: a systematic review and meta-analysis. Front Neurol. 2020;11(3):1–6.
3. Kawasaki T, Kurosaki Y, Fukuda H, et al. Flexible endoscopically assisted evacuation of acute and subacute subdural hematoma through a small craniotomy: preliminary results. Acta Neurochir. 2018;160:241–8.

4. Kim D-J, et al. Continuous monitoring of the Monro-Kellie doctrine: is it possible? J Neurotrauma. 2012;29(7):1354–63.
5. Kon H, et al. Endoscopic surgery for traumatic acute subdural hematoma. Case Rep Neurol. 2014;5(3):208–13.
6. Lee L, et al. Outcomes of chronic subdural hematoma drainage in nonagenarians and centenarians: a multicenter study. J Neurosurg. 2016;124(2):546–51.
7. Leuthardt EC, Voigt J, Kim AH, Sylvester P. A single-center cost analysis of treating primary and metastatic brain cancers with either brain laser interstitial thermal therapy (LITT) or craniotomy. Pharmacoecon Open. 2017;1(1):53–63.
8. Maryua J. Endoscopic hematoma evacuation following emergent Burr hole surgery for acute subdural hematoma in critical conditions: technical note. Interdiscip Neurosurg. 2018;12:48–51.
9. Rauhala M, Luoto TM, Huhtala H, Iverson GL, Niskakangas T, Ohman J, Helen P. The incidence of chronic subdural hematomas from 1990 to 2015 in a defined Finnish population. J Neurosurg. 2019;22(3):1–11.
10. Sahyouni R, Goshtasbi K, Mahmoodi A, Tran D, Chen J. Chronic subdural hematoma: a historical and clinical perspective. World Neurosurg. 2017;108:948–53.
11. Sim Y, Min K, Lee M, Kim Y, Kim D. Recent changes in risk factors of chronic subdural hematoma. J Korean Neurosurg Soc. 2012;52(3):234–9.
12. Sun G, et al. Comparison of keyhole endoscopy and craniotomy for the treatment of patients with hypertensive cerebral hemorrhage. Medicine. 2019;98(2):e14123.
13. Vanvuren C. What is the cost of an endoscopy? New Choice Health; 2020. https://www.newchoicehealth.com/endoscopy/cost#:~:text=The%20average%20cost%20of%20an,or%20an%20outpatient%20surgery%20center. Accessed 15 Dec 2020.
14. Wick JY. The true cost of chronic subdural hematoma. HCPLive; 2015. www.hcplive.com/view/the-true-cost-of-chronic-subdural-hematoma. Accessed 20 Dec 2020.
15. Yadav YR, Ratre S, Parihar V, Bajaj J, Sinha M, Kumar A. Endoscopic management of chronic subdural hematoma. J Neurol Surg. 2020;81(4):330–41.
16. Yan K, Gao H, Wang Q, Xu X, Wu W, Zhou X. Endoscopic surgery to chronic subdural hematoma with neovessel septation: technical notes and literature review. Neurol Res. 2016;38(5):467–76.
17. Yang W, Huang J. Chronic subdural hematoma: epidemiology and natural history. Neurosurg Clin N Am. 2017;28(2):205–10.
18. Zhang J, et al. The use of endoscopic-assisted burr-hole craniostomy for septated chronic subdural haematoma: a retrospective cohort comparison study. Brain Res. 2018;1678:245–53.

Chapter 31
Middle Meningeal Artery Embolization for Chronic Subdural Hematomas

Stephanie Zyck and Harish Babu

31.1 Rationale and Physiologic Basis for Endovascular Treatment

Chronic subdural hematomas (CSDH) are classically treated surgically with craniotomy and drainage or burr hole drainage and irrigation. However, recurrence rates for this pathology are notoriously high. Reported recurrence rates in the literature vary widely, but on an average range from 10 to 30% [3]. Advanced age, medical comorbidities, and antithrombotic medication use that are commonly seen in this patient population further complicate the surgical decision-making process when hematomas recur.

The pathophysiology behind CSDH recurrence has important implications for the way in which this condition is treated. After an initial hemorrhagic event into the subdural space, such as the rupture of a bridging vein from minor head trauma, a proinflammatory cascade is triggered. This event leads to migration of inflammatory cells and fibroblasts from the dura, leading to an encapsulation of the subdural collection by a membrane. This membrane results in subsequent angiogenesis and formation of neovascularized membranes [13]. Studies have demonstrated that these neovascularized outer membranes contain fragile sinusoidal channels and microcapillaries with absent basement membranes or endothelial cell junctions. These new blood vessels are also devoid of smooth muscle cells or pericytes, permitting continuous leakage of plasma and red blood cells into the subdural space [13, 14, 20]. This results in further inflammation in a vicious cycle.

S. Zyck · H. Babu (✉)
Department of Neurosurgery, SUNY Upstate Medical University, Syracuse, NY, USA
e-mail: zycks@upstate.edu; babuh@upstate.edu

M. Turgut et al. (eds.), *Subdural Hematoma*,
https://doi.org/10.1007/978-3-030-79371-5_31

The middle meningeal artery (MMA), which arises from the internal maxillary artery off of the external carotid artery, supplies the dura via its frontal and parietal branches. Histologic and radiographic studies have supplied evidence that the MMA provides blood flow to the outer CSDH membranes [17, 18]. One study demonstrated an increased size of the MMA on the ipsilateral side of a CSDH compared with the contralateral side [16]. MMA embolization has been explored as a treatment for CSDH by eliminating the blood supply from the MMA and halting the microhemorrhages from immature blood vessels. Thus, the underlying pathophysiology is described.

31.2 Current Indications

The first description of MMA embolization for the treatment of recurrent CSDH was published by Komiyama in 1994 [11]. Since then, multiple single institution and multicenter studies have reported their experience performing MMA embolization either as a primary or rescue treatment for CSDH over the cerebral convexity. General indications that are commonly cited include clinical symptoms related to the hematoma, midline shift greater than 5 mm, or recurrence after prior surgical intervention. Embolization of the MMA is a particularly attractive option for patients who are poor candidates for surgery, such as those with advanced age, underlying coagulopathy, or significant medical comorbidities that are commonly seen in the patient population who present with CSDHs. MMA embolization has been performed both on its own and as an adjunct to surgical hematoma evacuation, burr hole drainage, and bedside placement of a surgical evacuating port system [7, 9]. Because MMA embolization works by preventing continued bleeding from the hematoma membranes while the hematoma is resorbed over time, the treatment effect is not immediate. When clinical symptoms such as contralateral weakness from hematoma mass effect are present, our institution favors either craniotomy or bedside subdural evacuating port system placement with adjunctive MMA embolization over embolization alone in order to relieve the mass effect.

Patients who are not typically considered for endovascular treatment include those with an underlying neoplasm, severe renal failure, and nonconvexity subdural hematoma (SDH) in which the MMA vascular territory would not supply the hematoma membranes. While preoperative computed tomography (CT) angiography of the head and neck is useful for planning access and technical considerations, it is also useful for ruling out anatomic contraindications to embolization. One important example of this is an ophthalmic origin of the MMA, in which case embolization can inadvertently lead to vision loss. Finally, althrough vascular malformations such as dural arteriovenous fistulas that involve the MMA can be associated with SDHs and may be appropriate for embolization in some cases, such cases are generally treated as a separate entity other than as a CSDH.

31.3 Endovascular Techniques

MMA embolization is performed in the neurointerventional suite in an inpatient setting. This may be performed under either moderate sedation or general anesthesia, depending on the patient's ability to tolerate the procedure under sedation and their overall medical status. Transradial or transfemoral access may be used to secure access with a five or six French sheath. A guide catheter is then used to select the proximal external carotid artery. A selective angiogram is performed to verify that the MMA does arise off of the internal maxillary artery. A microcatheter is then advanced into the MMA under fluoroscopic roadmap guidance, where superselective angiography is then performed to identify dangerous anastomoses such as the petrosal or lacrimal branches that can be seen in approximately 10% of cases [9]. These anastomotic vessels must be carefully protected during embolization in order to prevent a postoperative neurologic deficit.

Embolization may then be performed either at the trunk of the MMA or selectively in the proximal frontal and parietal branches. The location of the hematoma in relation to the MMA branches, as well as the relationship of important collateral branches to the take-off points of MMA branches from the main trunk, may dictate the part of the vessel chosen for embolization. When the ophthalmic and petrosal branches are identified, the microcatheter should be advanced for targeted treatment distal to those collaterals so as not to cause blindness or a facial nerve palsy. Materials chosen for embolization may include liquid embolics such as Onyx™ or *N*-butyl cyanoacrylate, coils, or particles such as polyvinyl alcohol or microspheres. The presence of clinically significant collateral blood vessels nearby may favor the use of coils over embolic materials. Embolization is continued under fluoroscopic roadmap until stasis of flow is seen in the target branches. A vascular blush that is sometimes observed within the hematoma may no longer be visible following treatment (Fig. 31.1).

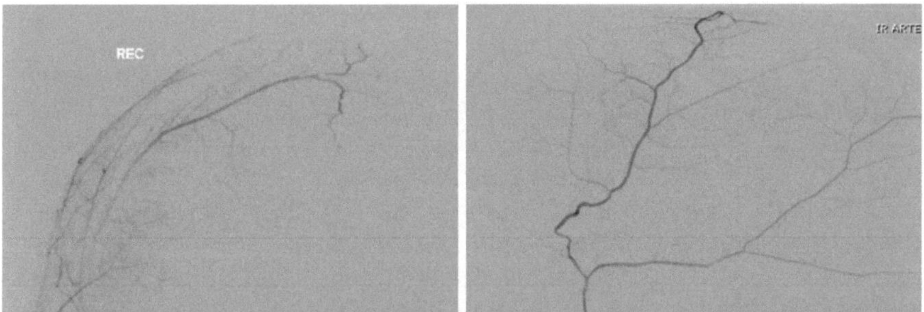

Fig. 31.1 Anteroposterior (left) and lateral (right) views of superselective right middle meningeal artery (MMA) angiogram demonstrate a faint vascular blush arising from the MMA that is associated with an underlying chronic subdural hematoma (CSDH)

31.4 Clinical and Radiologic Outcomes

Several meta-analyses of clinical studies have been performed to evaluate the safety and efficacy of MMA embolization for CSDHs. One meta-analysis by Srivatsan and colleagues evaluated hematoma recurrence, complications, and modified Rankin Scale score in three double-arm studies comparing MMA embolization (with or without adjunct surgery) and conventional surgical treatment [15]. Two studies included burr hole drainage as part of the treatment protocol for the cohort undergoing MMA embolization, while the third study utilized burr hole drainage in addition to MMA embolization only for symptomatic patients in the endovascular cohort [1, 10, 12]. In the meta-analysis, hematoma recurrence rate was found to be significantly less in the embolization group at 2.1% versus 27.7% in the conventional treatment group. There was no statistically significant difference between complications or modified Rankin Scale scores when pooling the data from the three double-arm studies [15]. Another meta-analysis by Jumah and colleagues incorporated 11 studies, including small case series and single-arm studies. With regard to hematoma recurrence, the need for surgical rescue, and complications, all three endpoints were found to be significantly less in the embolization group [8]. This data suggests that MMA embolization, with or without adjunctive burr hole drainage, increases the efficacy of CSDH treatment compared with burr hole drainage alone without a significant increase in complication rates.

A third meta-analysis by Haldrup and colleagues included 18 papers with a total of 191 patients who underwent MMA embolization for either primary or recurrent CSDH. One hundred and nineteen patients underwent MMA embolization for primary CSDH, while 72 patients underwent MMA embolization for recurrent SDH. There was no significant difference of recurrence rates between these two groups, which supports the notion that MMA embolization is a reasonable primary or rescue treatment option for CSDHs [6]. In the studies included in the meta-analyses, no complications directly related to the endovascular procedures were reported.

However, known risks of any endovascular procedure include access site complications, renal injury from contrast administration, and stroke. Risks of blindness and facial nerve palsy related to embolic material reflux into the ophthalmic and petrosal branches, respectively, must also be considered and carefully avoided. In one series of 154 patients who underwent MMA embolization for CSDH, there was one symptomatic rupture of the MMA during the procedure, one postoperative seizure, and one facial droop that was reported [9]. Other complications reported in the literature have been related to medical comorbidities unrelated to endovascular embolization or to the open surgical aspect of the treatment, such as wound complications or postoperative hematomas. In the same series, 90.3% of patients had improvement in hematoma thickness while 70.8% of cases achieved a specific primary outcome of 50% or greater reduction in hematoma thickness at follow-up [10]. Improvement in modified Rankin Scale and National Institute of Health Scale scores was 44% and 30%, respectively, at variable follow-up times [9]. For the same measures of clinical outcome, no significant difference was noted in 79% and 46% of cases, respectively [9].

Overall, current evidence demonstrates overall safety and efficacy of MMA embolization for both primary and recurrent CSDH, either with or without adjunctive surgical drainage.

31.5 Case Illustration

An 80-year-old man with a history of hypertension, diabetes mellitus, and recent left-sided stroke for which he was taking aspirin and clopidogrel presented with several weeks of dizziness and frequent falls. His right-sided weakness from his prior stroke had initially resolved, but then worsened since his recent fall episodes. A CT scan of his head revealed a mixed density left convexity SDH with predominantly subacute and chronic components. The greatest diameter of the hematoma was approximately 24 mm and 7 mm of midline shift were present. His antiplatelet medications were held and he was referred for neurosurgical evaluation. On neurological assessment, a right-sided pronator drift and leg lag were noted that the patient reported had increased from his baseline. Due to his age and comorbidities, he was determined to be a good candidate for a left-sided subdural evacuating port system placement. He underwent the procedure and tolerated it well. His postoperative CT scan showed some residual extra-axial blood but significant improvement in the midline shift and size of the hematoma. His pronator drift and leg lag also improved with only the trace residual right arm weakness that was known to be his baseline.

Two weeks after being discharged to a rehabilitation center, he returned to the emergency department after having multiple additional falls and increasing right-sided weakness. A new CT scan of his head found that the left-sided SDH had re-accumulated. The patient agreed to undergo repeat subdural bolt evacuating port system due to the symptoms from the mass effect of the hematoma. The CT scans before and after each subdural bolt procedure are shown in Fig. 31.2.

Because of the recurrent nature of the SDH, a MMA embolization was also offered to the patient. A prior CT angiogram had been obtained which did not reveal any anatomic contraindications to endovascular treatment, such as an ophthalmic origin of the MMA. Thus, the patient was taken for endovascular embolization.

Left external carotid artery angiography was performed and a microcatheter was advanced into the middle meningeal artery (Fig. 31.3). Because of contrast reflux into a petrosal branch in close proximity to the parietal branch, coil embolization was chosen for the parietal branch in order to prevent inadvertent liquid embolic reflux into the petrosal artery. Onyx™ embolization was then utilized for the frontal branch due to the ability of the liquid embolic material to precisely occlude the frontal branch. This was completed without any complication (Fig. 31.4).

The patient did well post-procedurally, and at 1 month follow-up, the hematoma was noted to be diminishing in size. A CT scan obtained at follow-up 2 months post-procedurally demonstrated near resolution of the SDH (Fig. 31.5).

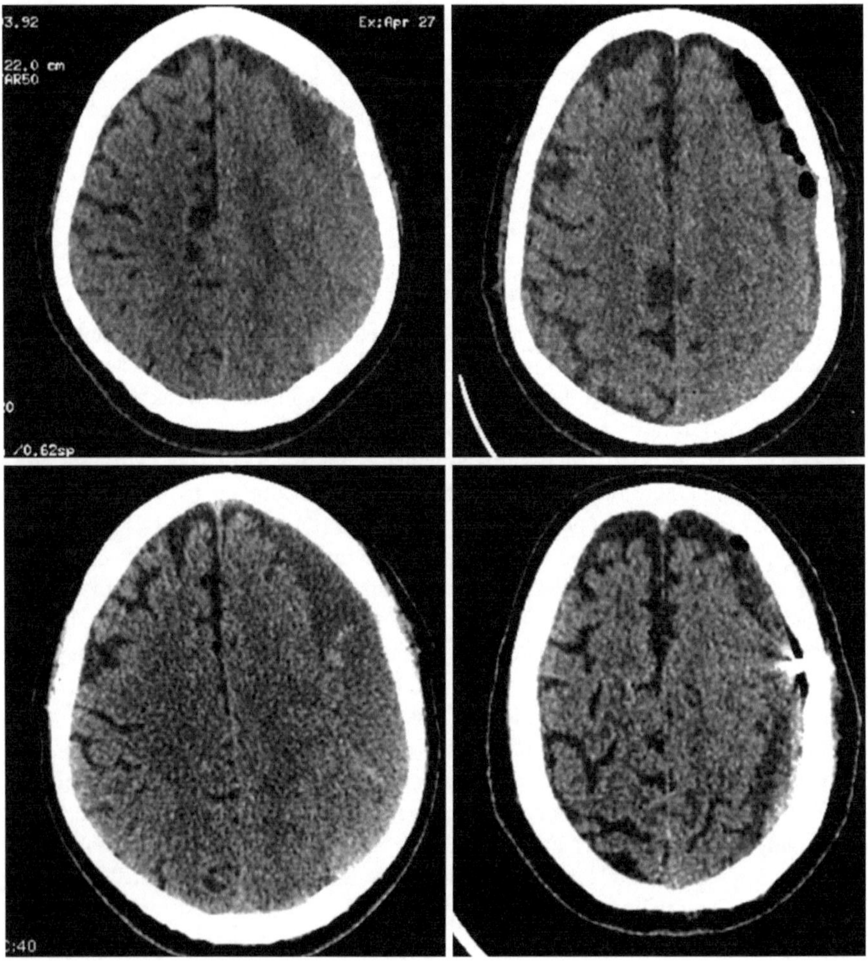

Fig. 31.2 Computed tomography (CT) of the head on initial presentation showed a mixed density subacute and chronic left convexity subdural hematoma (SDH) (top left). Decreased size of the hematoma is seen after subdural bolt placement (top right). Recurrence occurred after 2 weeks (bottom left), which again improved after a repeat bolt drainage procedure (bottom right)

31.6 Future Directions

Several randomized controlled trials are currently underway to compare clinical outcomes between MMA embolization and surgical evacuation [2, 4, 5, 19]. Future studies should also further compare endovascular treatment for primary

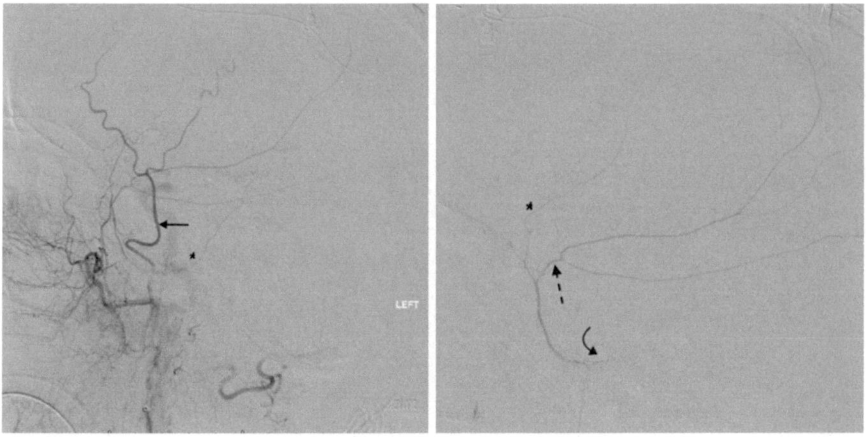

Fig. 31.3 Left external carotid artery angiography (left) demonstrates normal appearing external carotid circulation with MMA (asterisk) and superficial temporal artery (arrow) being seen. Superselective angiography of the MMA angiography is shown on the right panel with frontal (asterisk) and parietal (dotted arrow) branches. A petrosal branch is faintly seen (curved arrow)

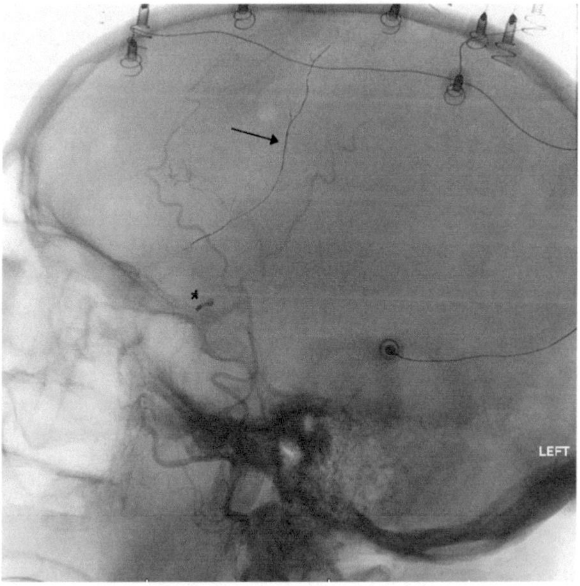

Fig. 31.4 The final angiographic run of the external carotid artery demonstrates complete occlusion of the MMA with no contrast filling. The frontal branch is occluded with an Onyx™cast (arrow). The parietal branch was coil embolized (asterisk). The superficial temporal artery is seen filling with contrast adjacent to the now embolized MMA

and recurrent SDH, MMA embolization alone compared with being in addition to various surgical treatments, and which embolic agents produce the best clinical outcomes.

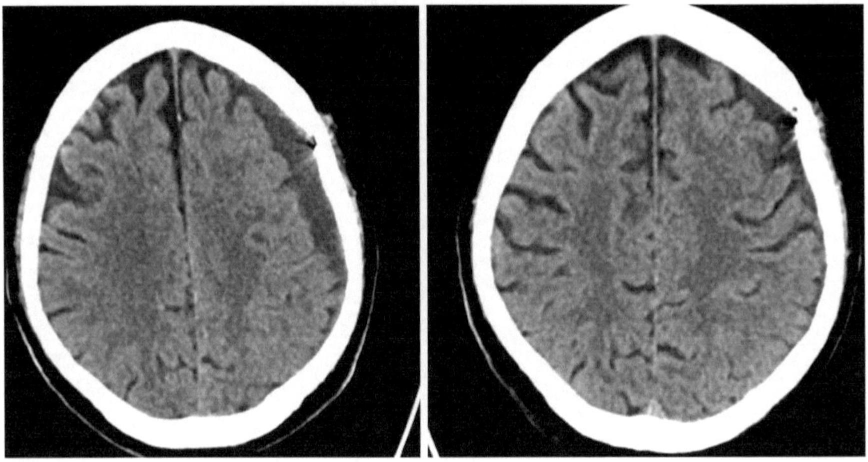

Fig. 31.5 CT scans obtained at 1 month (left) and 2 months (right) post MMA embolization demonstrate progressive resolution of the hematoma over time

References

1. Ban SP, et al. Middle meningeal artery embolization for chronic subdural hematoma. Radiology. 2018;286(3):992–9.
2. Dartmouth Middle Meningeal Embolization Trial (DaMMET). ClinicalTrials.gov Identifier: NCT04270955.
3. Ducruet AF, et al. The surgical management of chronic subdural hematoma. Neurosurg Rev. 2012;35(2):155–69.
4. Embolization of the Middle Meningeal Artery for the Prevention of Chronic Subdural Hematoma Recurrence in High Risk Patients (EMPROTECT). ClinicalTrials.gov Identifier: NCT04372147.
5. Embolization of the Middle Meningeal Artery With ONYX™ Liquid Embolic System for Subacute and Chronic Subdural Hematoma. ClinicalTrials.gov Identifier: NCT04402632.
6. Haldrup M, et al. Embolization of the middle meningeal artery in patients with chronic subdural hematoma-a systematic review and meta-analysis. Acta Neurochir (Wien). 2020;162(4):777–84.
7. Joyce E, et al. Middle meningeal artery embolization treatment of nonacute subdural hematomas in the elderly: a multiinstitutional experience of 151 cases. Neurosurg Focus. 2020;49(4):E5.
8. Jumah F, et al. Efficacy and safety of middle meningeal artery embolization in the management of refractory or chronic subdural hematomas: a systematic review and meta-analysis. Acta Neurochir (Wien). 2020;162(3):499–507.
9. Kan P, et al. Middle meningeal artery embolization for chronic subdural hematoma: a multicenter experience of 154 consecutive embolizations. Neurosurgery. 2021;88(2):268–77.
10. Kim E. Embolization therapy for refractory hemorrhage in patients with chronic subdural hematomas. World Neurosurg. 2017;101:520–7.
11. Komiyama M, et al. Chronic subdural hematoma associated with middle meningeal arteriovenous fistula treated by a combination of embolization and burr hole drainage. Surg Neurol. 1994;42(4):316–9.

12. Matsumoto H, et al. Which surgical procedure is effective for refractory chronic subdural hematoma? Analysis of our surgical procedures and literature review. J Clin Neurosci. 2018;49:40–7.
13. Moshayedi P, Liebeskind DS. Middle meningeal artery embolization in chronic subdural hematoma: implications of pathophysiology in trial design. Front Neurol. 2020;11:923.
14. Sato S, Suzuki J. Ultrastructural observations of the capsule of chronic subdural hematoma in various clinical stages. J Neurosurg. 1975;43(5):569–78.
15. Srivatsan A, et al. Middle meningeal artery embolization for chronic subdural hematoma: meta-analysis and systematic review. World Neurosurg. 2019;122:613–9.
16. Takizawa K, et al. Enlargement of the middle meningeal artery on MR angiography in chronic subdural hematoma. J Neurosurg. 2016;124(6):1679–83.
17. Tanaka T, et al. [Superselective angiographic findings of ipsilateral middle meningeal artery of chronic subdural hematoma in adults]. No Shinkei Geka. 1998;26(4):339–47.
18. Tanaka T, Kaimori M. [Histological study of vascular structure between the dura mater and the outer membrane in chronic subdural hematoma in an adult]. No Shinkei Geka. 1999;27(5):431–6.
19. The SQUID Trial for the Embolization of the Middle Meningeal Artery for Treatment of Chronic Subdural Hematoma (STEM). ClinicalTrials.gov Identifier: NCT04410146.
20. Weigel R, Hohenstein A, Schilling L. Vascular endothelial growth factor concentration in chronic subdural hematoma fluid is related to computed tomography appearance and exudation rate. J Neurotrauma. 2014;31(7):670–3.

Chapter 32
Perioperative Medical Management of Chronic Subdural Hematoma

Mohammed Benzagmout, Tokpo Armel Junior, and Said Boujraf

32.1 Introduction

Chronic subdural hematoma (CSDH) refers to a pathological blood collection in the subdural space with insidious onset and progression [15]. The incidence of CSDH is increasing with age while it primarily affects elderly. CSDH could be managed medically; however, the surgical evacuation becomes mandatory in some conditions and profiles of patients. Indeed, surgery is indicated for symptomatic lesions especially when the hematoma thickness is measuring more than 10 mm on CT scan evaluation, and after unsuccessful primary conservative treatment [65].

Despite the large prevalence of CSDH, various surgical strategies are used to deal with CSDH. This state of varying approaches is due to the lack of level 1 evidence for establishing therapeutic guidelines in order to optimize the perioperative management of this critical disease [65].

In this chapter, we are highlighting the medical strategies that have been used before, during, and after surgical treatment of CSDH, and we discuss their limitations and validities.

M. Benzagmout (✉) · S. Boujraf
Department of Neurosurgery, University Hospital of Fez, Fez, Morocco

Clinical Neurosciences Laboratory, Sidi Mohammed Benabdellah University Fez, Fez, Morocco

T. A. Junior
Department of Neurosurgery, University Hospital of Fez, Fez, Morocco

M. Turgut et al. (eds.), *Subdural Hematoma*,
https://doi.org/10.1007/978-3-030-79371-5_32

32.2 Preoperative Medical Management

32.2.1 Correction of Coagulopathy

Coagulopathy is one of major risk factors inducing CSDH growth and recurrence. Therefore, coagulopathy control is essential before surgical evacuation to avoid any immediate life-threatening event. Since CSDH affects mostly elderly people with simultaneous comorbidities, iatrogenous bleeding disorder is frequently encountered.

32.2.1.1 Iatrogenous Coagulopathy

Preoperatively, the management of patients under anticoagulation therapy requires a multidisciplinary approach including neurosurgeon, cardiologist, hematologist, and anesthesiologist. The main goal is to discontinue the anticoagulation treatment during enough periods to make surgery safe without generating an embolic event. Indeed, the medical treatment strategy used depends of the emergency profile of patients and benefit-risk ratio.

Regarding the use of vitamin K antagonist (VKA), in case of elective surgery, an oral administration of vitamin K is completed until obtaining correct International Normalized Ratio (INR). However, fresh frozen plasma (FFP), prothrombin complex concentrate (PCC), or recombinant activated factor VII (rfVIIa) could be used for critical situations. Besides, FFP could be an issue in patients with cardiac dysfunction and PCC becomes a valuable option [65].

In 2017, a revised guideline has been proposed for direct oral anticoagulants (DOA) by the French working group on perioperative hemostasis. According to their recommendations and considering that surgical evacuation of CSDH is an intracranial procedure, the last intake of xaban drug should be 3 days before surgery. However, Dabigatran use depends on the creatinine clearance; hence, 5 days free-period intake are needed if clearance ranged between 30 and 50 mL/mn and only 4 days if above 50 mL/mn. Nonetheless, the use of PCC or FFP remains effective in case emergency [1, 73]. In addition, Andexanet alfa is a specific antidote to xaban drugs; it is recommended safely in critical situation [14] and should be preceded by measuring anticoagulation plasma level [73].

Besides, another strategy has been used. It consists of bridging therapy with Heparin either Low Weight Molecular Heparin (LWMH) or Unfractionated Heparin (UFH). This strategy remains controversial but widespread. It had been proposed to reduce the risk of thromboembolic events during the perioperative period in patients with non-valvular atrial fibrillation or mechanical valves.

Both, the European Society of cardiology (ESC) and the American College of Cardiology (ACC) have suggested some interesting guidelines, respectively, in 2016 and 2017 [72].

Regarding the mechanical valves prothesis, ESC recommends the UFH use after INR falls under therapeutic range. Then, UFH has to be stopped 4–6 h before surgery. On the other hand, the ACC suggested a detailed guideline for managing anticoagulation in patients with non-valvular atrial fibrillation. This involved approach using CHAD2-DS2-VASc score to establish the annual risk of thromboembolic events and HAS-BLED score to evaluate the risk of bleeding [19, 81]. Tables 32.1 and 32.2 are reporting respective score details. These scores are the most reliable and practical scoring system recommended so far. The ACC recommendations are summarized in Fig. 32.1.

32.2.1.2 Pathological Coagulopathy

Cases of CSDH associated with congenital bleeding disorders have been reported in the literature. Commonly, the management of these cases required a concerted approach between neurosurgeons, anesthesiologists, and hematologists to address the primary deficit by specific and/or general measures.

Table 32.1 CHAD2-DS2-VASc scoring. Low risk (total score = 0); Intermediate risk (total score = 1); High risk (total score > 1) [19]

	CHA2-DS2-VASc acronym	Score
C	Congestive heart failure/left ventricle dysfunction (ejection fraction under 35%)	1
H	Hypertension	1
A2	Age > or = 75 years	2
D	Diabetes mellitus	1
S2	Stroke/transient ischemic attack (TIA)/systemic thromboembolism	2
V	Vascular disease	1
A	Age 65–74 years	1
Sc	Sex (female)	1

Table 32.2 HAS-BLED score [**HAS-BLED: H**ypertension, **A**bnormal Renal/Liver Function, **S**troke, **B**leeding History or Predisposition, **L**abile INR, **E**lderly, **D**rugs/Alcohol Concomitantly]. Low risk (maximum score = 0); Moderate risk (maximum score = 1–2); High risk (maximum score > or = 3) [81]. (Abbreviations: *AST* aspartate-transaminase, *ALT* alanine-transaminase, *Cr* creatinine, *INR* International Normalized Ratio, *NSAIDs* non steroidal anti-inflammatory drugs)

HAS-BLED acronym	Points
Hypertension	1
Renal disease (Dialysis, transplant, Cr >2.26 mg/dL or >200 μmol/L)	1
Liver disease (Cirrhosis or bilirubin >2× normal with AST/ALT >3× normal)	1
Stroke history	1
Bleeding history (prior major bleeding or predisposition to bleeding)	1
Labile INR (unstable/high INRs)	1
Age > 65 years	1
Medication usage predisposing to bleeding Aspirin, clopidogrel, NSAIDs	1
Alcohol use	1
Maximum score	9 points

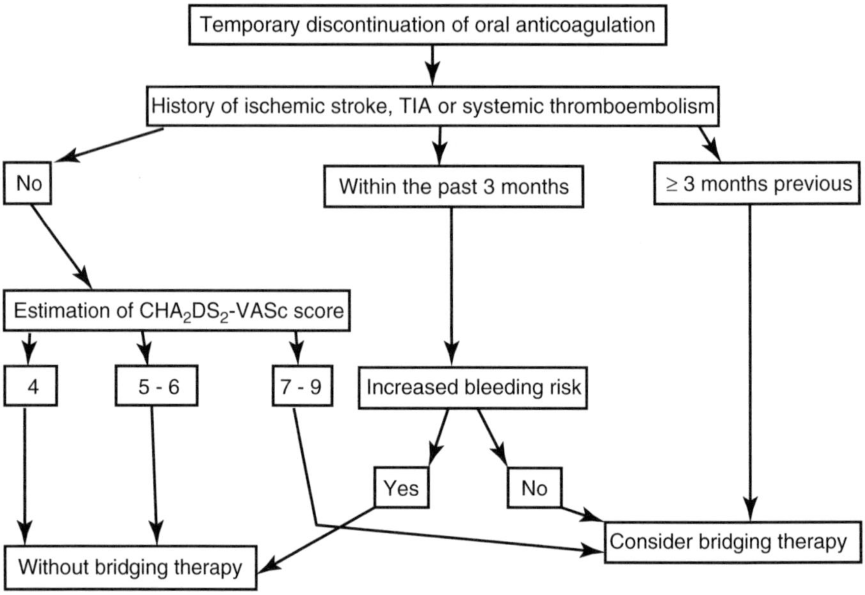

Fig. 32.1 Bridging therapy before a surgical procedure on patients with non-valvular atrial fibrillation according to the American College of Cardiology [72]

In 2017, a reported study was conducted on 16 young adults (27–59 years old) suffering from spontaneous CSDH. Complete screening of coagulation factors revealed that one patient exhibited von Willebrand alteration while six others presented alteration of factor VII. Recurrence was associated with four patients with unknown factor VII deficiency [12]. Previously, the neurosurgical team of "San carlo" hospital (Potenza, Italy) reported three cases of CSDH on young patients "O positive" blood type with von Willebrand disease [39, 40]. Therefore, they recommended a systematic screening of coagulation factors before performing surgery in young adults with unexplained CSDH.

In 2019, a CSDH has been associated with severe deficit in factor V. The case was successfully managed with administration of FFP [43]. In another case, CSDH occurrence was linked to low factor XIII activity [66].

32.2.2 Correction of Thrombopathy

32.2.2.1 Iatrogenous Thrombopathy

Despite being controversial, it is well known that continuation of antiplatelet drugs during the perisurgical period is associated with an increased risk of bleeding [30]. On the other hand, discontinuation of that treatment exposes the patient to high risk of myocardial infarction, stent thrombosis, or even death. Therefore, the management of antiplatelet therapy during the perioperative period is a multidisciplinary decision and different strategies have emerged. They are taking into account both risks bleeding and thrombosis. Also, other factors should be considered especially if antiplatelet drugs have been initiated for primary or secondary prevention of cardiovascular event, whether or not the patient is on single or dual antithrombotic drugs, and whether or not the CSDH surgery is required urgently or could be postponed.

Indeed, discontinuation of aspirin for 7–10 days is considered to be safe when used as a primary or secondary prevention before CSDH evacuation [52, 64]. The same period is usually suggested for clopidogrel before surgery [52].

In contrast, the management of dual antiplatelet therapy (DAPT) is more complex. In fact, the combination of aspirin and adenosine diphosphate receptors antagonists (Clopidogrel, Prasugrel, Ticagrelor, etc.) inferred a hypercoagulable state [52]. After stenting procedures, premature interruption of DAPT before complete endothelialization of the stent might have severe consequences. Indeed, thrombotic risk is higher after the first month and is then gradually reduced at 2–6 months, 6–12 months, and over 1 year [30, 64]. For these high-risk situations, delaying surgery when affordable to a least threatening moment is highly recommended. If not, surgery should be performed 5 days after discontinuation of both drugs and instauration of a bridging therapy even if data about bridging in this setting are scarce [30, 52]. In addition, bridging therapy with heparin agents is not effective and intravenous short-acting glycoprotein IIb/IIIa inhibitors such as Cangrelor, Eptifibatide, and Tirofiban are generally used [33, 38, 56, 62]. Both Tirofiban and Eptifibatide can be used and then stopped 3–6 h and 4–12 h, respectively, before surgery.

For urgent situations, when cessation of one or both antiplatelets is impossible, platelets transfusion is recommended 2 h after the last aspirin intake, and 12–24 h after latest dose of clopidogrel [30, 52]. However, it is critical to remind that platelets transfusion can increase the risk of stent thrombosis.

32.2.2.2 Pathological Thrombopathy

Inherit platelet function disorders (IPFD) are rare cases [2, 28] and we did not find any cases associated with CSDH in our literature review. Hemostasis achievement in this setting requires close collaboration with hematologists, particularly in the preoperative stage. Management options will depend on whether or not criteria of emergency procedure are met [2]. According to the disorder's type, platelets transfusion, recombinant activated factor VII, desmopressin, or antifibrinolytics could be variably used.

32.2.3 Adjuvant Treatment

32.2.3.1 Antiepileptic Agents

Based on cortical irritation and/or increased intracranial pressure, some neurosurgeons prefer initiating seizures prophylaxis. However, this practice is not supported by level 1 evidence proof because randomized controlled trials are lacking. Indeed, a literature review conducted in 2013 did not find any randomized controlled trial about this topic [42]. Moreover, published data are quite heterogeneous. Some authors recommended preoperative antiepileptic drugs (AEDs) because they decreased postoperative seizures risk [21] and had no impact on patient discharge outcomes. While others did not find any benefits with prophylactic AEDs [37, 59], and are clearly against this strategy given the potential side effects of AEDs on neurocognition of elderly [16].

Recently, an interesting case report has established a clear and solid relationship between epileptic focus and sulcal flair hyperintensity on MRI images [53]. Afterwards, the authors implied that a prophylactic seizure control may be required for CSDH patients with sulcal flair hyperintensity. Other risk factors have been postulated. Preoperative midline shift, pneumocephalus, open craniotomy, and membranectomy were all considered as important risk factors for postoperative seizures [20]. Furthermore, alcohol abuse, left-sided and mixed CSDH have also been incriminated in postoperative seizures occurrence [11, 63].

On the contrary, a literature review of patients diagnosed with CSDH between 2010 and 2017 did not identify hematoma volume, midline shift, surgical strategy, and postoperative pneumocephalus as significant predictors of acute seizures/status epilepticus. Nevertheless, remote stroke, Glasgow Coma Scale of 13 or under, and hematoma recurrence within 14 days were at risk of seizures development [78]. It was also reported that levetiracetam is the most appropriate AED used in this setting [78].

With all these opposing available data, we believe that Electro-encephalography prior and after surgery is a good option to decide starting AEDs adequately [78].

32.2.3.2 Corticotherapy

Because of inflammatory processes underlying CSDH formation, steroids drugs have been proposed as either a part of medical conservative treatment or an adjunct to surgical evacuation.

Steroids were firstly used in 1962 to successfully treat three patients with CSDH [3]. Since then, various steroids have been used without clear guidelines. Indeed, indications, dosage, and duration of the treatment depend on medical team involved within the same country [5].

Steroids have been widely used in common practice without any high-level evidence proof [15]. Dexamethasone is reported to have good efficacy on CSDH as primary treatment [7, 70]. Besides, multiple studies have reported benefits of steroids on CSDH regression and even in preventing recurrence [6, 8, 47, 60]. This beneficial effect on recurrence could explain the steroids choice as adjunct to surgery but once again there is no standardized protocol.

Recently, two double-blind, randomized controlled trials were instigated to answer the questions regarding indications, dosage, and duration of corticotherapy. The first is the SUCRE trial that compared the efficacy of methylprednisolone on CSDH without clinical or radiological signs of severity [22]. The second study is the dex-CSDH trial that targeted dexamethasone in symptomatic CSDH adult patients [35]. Results of the last trial have indicated that treatment with dexamethasone resulted in fewer favorable outcomes and more adverse events than placebo at 6 months. However, fewer reoperations were performed in the dexamethasone group [24].

32.2.3.3 Other Drugs

Based on angiogenesis and vessels hyperpermeability within CSDH membranes, several drugs have been proposed for their supposed effects in hematoma resorption and decreased recurrence rate after surgical evacuation.

In fact, Angiotensin-Converting Enzyme Inhibitors (ACEI) had been evaluated through different studies and results are controversial [4, 49, 77]. Theoretically, ACEI are reducing vascular endothelial growth factor, inhibiting the development of immature and new blood vessels in the neomembrane of hematoma, and then are decreasing the permeability of vessels [77]. ACEI are also involved in the control of the arterial hypertension; hence they might also reduce microbleeding from fragile vessels resulting in resorption of the hematoma [4, 65].

Statins are drugs used for treatment of coronary heart disease and high blood cholesterol levels. The most used is Atorvastatin and it has a well-known effect in elderly people. Statins demonstrate an anti-inflammatory capacity and facilitate blood vessels repair [51]. Atorvastatin whether used solely or combined with surgery is associated with CSDH volume reduction and improvement of prognosis [10, 74, 79]. The reported observations have been confirmed by a double-blind randomized placebo-controlled clinical trial [27]. Currently, two other randomized controlled trials for evaluation of safety and efficacy of Atorvastatin are in progress including both REACH and ATOCH2 [15]. Once upcoming results are delivered, disclosures about indications, dosage, and therapy duration could be highly helpful in clinical practice for further improving the prognosis.

Another drug of interest is tranexamic acid, an antifibrinolytic which is acting as inhibitor of the kinin-kallikrein inflammatory system resulting in hematoma regression. Retrospective studies with small patient samples reported good results. Complete hematoma resolution was observed in the first case without surgery [29]. The second one showed residual hematoma shrinking within the postoperative cavity [69]. In 2020, Raja et al. have conducted a prospective observational study on 27 patients and found that tranexamic acid is a safe and effective alternative in medical management of CSDH [36]. However, this drug is currently studied in five ongoing trials to better establish its benefits and risks for further optimizing their use [15].

32.3 Peroperative Management

32.3.1 Choice of Anesthesia

Based on surgical procedure and comorbidities, anesthesia has always been an issue in elderly people. Decision regarding the anesthesia modality should be taken after discussion between surgeon, anesthesiologist, and patient family while considering the health profile and background of the patient.

Currently, there are limited results on anesthesia and CSDH surgery and these studies are suffering of methodological and interpretation biases including sample size and groups heterogeneity [65]. Even if general anesthesia (GA) and monitored anesthesia care (MAC) are used in daily practice, the prevalence of cardiac complications in elderly patients is still high with general anesthesia [31].

In 2017, a study reported a comparison of outcome after mini-craniotomy performed on two groups of CSDH patients operated with GA or under local anesthesia; fewer risks in the local anesthesia group were noticed [41]. Besides, there was no need for postoperative intensive care unit transit with minimal operative time and hospital stay compared to the GA group. This anesthetic procedure is more suitable since compatible in healthcare structures with limited resources [41].

In 2020, Blaauw et al. have examined 923 patients surgically treated for CSDH. They reported more postoperative complications with GA with no significant differences in mortality rate within 3 months [9]. This retrospective study has included three centers, and each center has had his own criteria regarding the selection of anesthesia mode. Finally, in this trial local anesthesia found that the use of dexmedetomidine (1 μg/kg) in MAC is safer than sufentanyl and showed better patient's comfort during surgery, fewer rescue maneuvers, less postoperative hospital stay, and better surgeon satisfaction [75]. Therefore, this technique could be a good alternative to general anesthesia whenever being unsuitable.

32.3.2 Oxygen Therapy

Preanesthetic evaluation allows to study the medical history of the patient and to evaluate his respiratory and cardiovascular function. During CSDH surgery, maintaining a good oxygenation is fundamental because hypoxemia is very harmful to the brain and represents a major cause of postoperative morbidity and potential permanent squeals. Hence, oxygen supplementation by nasal canula or through a facial mask using medium to high concentration should be completed systematically during surgery, especially when performed under local anesthesia.

Indeed, hypoxemia is due to the combined effects of anesthesia and postoperative diaphragmatic dysfunction, leading to pulmonary condensation and intrapulmonary shunting [4]. Besides, episodes of obstructive apnea may result from a residual anesthetic drug effect or from sleep disturbances especially in elderly people [4]. Therefore, patients should be systematically monitored by pulse oximetry during and soon after surgery.

32.3.3 Analgesic Treatment

After cranial surgery, adequate pain management is critical for ensuring patient comfort and promoting rapid recovery [44]. Current analgesic strategies lead to optimize pain control and limit potential adverse effects. Indeed, pain management starts in the perioperative stage and continues after surgery. Adequate postoperative pain control might be led by appropriate preoperative risk assessment, good patient's information about the surgical procedure, and premedication especially in elderly people [50].

It is well known that infiltration of scalp incision(s) with local anesthetic agent before CSDH surgery reduces postoperative pain by reducing scalp inflammation and pain signals [46].

Different drugs are used depending on the pain severity, patient's morbidities, and possible side effects and complications. Paracetamol or acetaminophen are generally used solely or in association to treat mild to moderate pain, while moderate to severe pain is most often treated by opioids drugs [50, 55].

32.4 Postoperative Medical Care

32.4.1 Rehydration

Intravenous fluid administration (IVFA) is considered to induce brain expansion and has been widely used postoperatively in CSDH to prevent recurrence. Indeed, CSDH patients encountered in common practice are often dehydrated and evidences have been gathered that brain volume can be reduced by dehydration [25, 26].

The role of IVFA on postoperative course of patients with CSDH was previously investigated by Janowski et al. [26]. In this study, they found that IVFA 2000 mL per day of crystalloids along 3 days after the surgery was associated to a lower hematoma recurrence and better clinical outcome. This report has also emphasized the double benefits of this attitude including promotion of bed rest during fluid administration instigate good effect on brain expansion and mobilization between drips allowing to prevent position-related complications [26].

In 2017, Montano et al. have demonstrated that adequate postoperative hydration increases brain volume and reduces significantly residual postoperative SDH; this allows ensuring therefore good clinical and radiological outcome [45]. Indeed, fluid therapy protocol consisting in postoperative administration of intravenous saline solution followed by an adequate oral hydration represents a safe and effective adjunctive treatment for residual SDH. The main advantage of fluid therapy consists of a complete absence of side effects. However, special attention should be demonstrated in older patients with a history of heart diseases and health fragility.

32.4.2 Thromboembolism Prophylaxis

The prevention of venous thromboembolism is a part of CSDH management especially in older patients with various comorbidities. In the other hand, medical thrombosis prophylaxis raised the question of rebleeding risk and hematoma recurrence in the postoperative stage.

The use of sequential leg compression devices when possible is a valuable option; besides heparin administration within 24–72 h in the postoperative stage is generally considered safe [34]. Since 2003, LWMH has been recommended for at least 12 h before and after surgery whenever needed [18, 32]. However, some authors reported an increased rate of hematoma recurrence with heparin [48, 68], while paradoxically others have noticed that early administration of preventive dose of LWMH reduces the risk of reoperation [57].

In 2017, Fornebo et al. [17] observed that preoperative morbidity was the same in patients receiving antithrombotic therapy or not. Authors showed also that early administration of antithrombotic therapy along 30 days after CSDH surgery is associated with lower thromboembolic events. In 2020, an observational prospective French multicenter study revealed that non-resumption of antithrombotic agents is associated with a significantly high risk of thromboembolism [71]. Conversely, their resumption in the first postoperative month increased the risk of hematoma recurrence [71]. Consequently, they recommended 1 month delay in antithrombotic restart after surgery.

Given the lack of consensus, the issue of thromboembolism prophylaxis should be discussed on a case-by-case basis taking into consideration the patient background and the clinical and radiological assessment particularities.

32.4.3 Anticoagulation and Antiplatelet Medication Resumption

In 2016, a meta-analysis showed that both anticoagulants and antiplatelets have been identified as risk factors of hematoma recurrence but treatment resumption reduce thromboembolism events [76]. In 2018, a systematic review and meta-analysis has addressed the question of resumption of antithrombotic agents in CSDH after surgery [55]. The authors stated that early antithrombotic recommencement can be achieved whenever required without any additional hemorrhagic or thromboembolic risk. Nonetheless, they qualified the process as a highly individual and patient profile dependent.

Later on, Zanaty et al. reported a prospectively collected database of 596 patients; they performed a retrospective multivariate analysis and identified that the optimal period to restart an oral anticoagulation ranges between 2 and 21 days after surgery. They concluded that this interval is characterized by a lower risk of both hematoma recurrence and stroke [80].

Resumption of antithrombotic agents after intracranial surgery is usually considered as a multidisciplinary decision. Specific guidelines after CSDH evacuation are lacking [71]; however, HAS-BLED and the CHA2DS2-VASc risk scores might help to determine the ideal time and strategy for anticoagulation treatment.

Regarding VKA previously discussed, to restart the anticoagulation treatment depends on the bleeding risk and VKA could be introduced at the earliest by day 1 postoperatively since VKA would become effective only after 4–7 days. During this period of time, it is recommended to run a thromboembolism prophylaxis or a bridging therapy [73]. This last therapy should be restarted as soon as possible after surgery especially for patients with mechanical valve prosthesis [72].

DOA can be restarted within 48–72 h postoperatively, and if venous thromboprophylaxis is needed, heparin should be used [73]. The first therapeutic dose of DOA should be taken at least 12 h after the last heparin administration [1].

For antiplatelets, there are no guidelines for the optimal timing of resumption and clinical trials are required [65]. To date, there is no link established between antiplatelets use and rebleeding risk in older adults [48].

32.4.4 Antiepileptic Treatment

In order to prevent epileptic seizures, postoperative use of AEDs had been evaluated in a randomized controlled trial [59]. Results were published in 2019, and showed that there is not any significant effect on seizures occurrence. Moreover, 8% of patients experienced adverse effects with AEDs [59].

Although predicted risk factors have been alleged by different studies [3, 11, 63, 78], there is no strong relationship between such risk factors and seizures occurrence. Besides, results of the reported studies are quite paradoxical.

After a burr-hole evacuation of CSDH, postoperative seizures demonstrated a low incidence of 2.3% and therefore prophylactic AEDs should not be systematically indicated considering the significant risks of side effects [16]. Finally, we found that recommending an EEG assessment before initiating any AED treatment is very relevant [3, 20].

32.4.5 Corticotherapy

As we said before, steroids are known to induce spontaneous regression of CSDH and to decrease the recurrence rate after surgical evacuation [6, 47]. However, they are still somehow undergoing blind-used and future studies might better clarify indications, doses, and effects of the treatment. This might yield a future consensus on this therapeutical approach.

Indeed, corticosteroids are recommended either preoperatively or in the postoperative stage of CSDH. Berghauser et al. have described that the adjunction of a longer period of preoperative dexamethasone administration in surgical treatment of CSDH is associated with a lower recurrence rate [6]. Furthermore, Drapkin recommended systematic postoperative corticotherapy for patients with persistent or recurrent symptoms [13].

32.4.5.1 Other Treatments

Several drugs were suggested as adjunctive therapies in the postoperative stage of CSDH to prevent recurrence. Indeed, angiotensin-converting enzyme inhibitors, tranexamic acid, and atorvastatin were all reported in the literature [61, 67, 77, 79]. Oral tranexamic acid [69] and oral etizolam [23] were associated to a significant reduction of SDH volume at follow-up. However, oral perindopril administration [58] and oral streptokinase-streptodornase [54] were not associated with a significant effect on the residual SDH.

32.5 Conclusion

CSDH is a benign pathological condition; it is most frequently encountered in elderly people. Although CSDH is the most common disorder encountered in daily neurosurgical practice, several aspects of its management are still subject of controversies.

The perioperative medical management of CSDH could be tricky with currently associated comorbidities, especially with antithrombotics withdrawal and resumption. There are few data in the literature on this topic while guidelines and general recommendations are lacking.

Besides, various treatments including corticotherapy, statins or tranexamic acid have emerged to prevent recurrence after surgical evacuation. However, proof level is still required. Currently, many prospective randomized trials are running to assess the efficiency of common empiric used strategies such as corticotherapy and novel promising drugs such as atorvastatin and tranexamic acid.

References

1. Albaladejo P, Bonhomme F, Blais N, et al. Management of direct oral anticoagulants in patients undergoing elective surgeries and invasive procedures: updated guidelines from the French Working Group on Perioperative Hemostasis (GIHP)—September 2015. Anaesth Crit Care Pain Med. 2017;36(1):73–6.
2. Al-Huniti A, Kahr WH. Inherited platelet disorders: diagnosis and management. Transfus Med Rev. 2020;34(4):277–85.
3. Ambrosetto C. Post-traumatic subdural hematoma. Further observations on nonsurgical treatment. Arch Neurol. 1962;6:287–92.
4. Baillard C. Oxygen supplementation in the postoperative period: when and how? Le Praticien en Anesthésie Réanimation. 2011;15(5):310–4.
5. Bartek J Jr, Sjåvik K, Schaible S, et al. The role of angiotensin-converting enzyme inhibitors in patients with chronic subdural hematoma: a Scandinavian population-based multicenter study. World Neurosurg. 2018;113:e555–60.
6. Baschera D, Tosic L, Westermann L, Oberle J, Alfieri A. Treatment standards for chronic subdural hematoma: results from a survey in Austrian, German, and Swiss neurosurgical units. World Neurosurg. 2018;116:e983–95.

7. Berghauser Pont LM, Dammers R, Schouten JW, Lingsma HF, Dirven CM. Clinical factors associated with outcome in chronic subdural hematoma: a retrospective cohort study of patients on pre-operative corticosteroid therapy. Neurosurgery. 2012;70(4):873–80.
8. Berghauser Pont LM, Dirven CM, Dippel DW, Verweij BH, Dammers R. The role of corticosteroids in the management of chronic subdural hematoma: a systematic review. Eur J Neurol. 2012;19(11):1397–403.
9. Blaauw J, Jacobs B, den Hertog HM, et al. Neurosurgical and perioperative management of chronic subdural hematoma. Front Neurol. 2020;11:550.
10. Chan DY, Chan DT, Sun TF, et al. The use of atorvastatin for chronic subdural hematoma: a retrospective cohort comparison study. Br J Neurosurg. 2016;31(1):72–7.
11. Chen CW, Kuo JR, Lin HJ, et al. Early post-operative seizures after burr-hole drainage for chronic subdural hematoma: correlation with brain CT findings. J Clin Neurosci. 2004;11:706–9.
12. Dobran M, Iacoangeli M, Scortichini AR, et al. Spontaneous chronic subdural hematoma in young adult: the role of missing coagulation factors. G Chir. 2017;38(2):66–70.
13. Drapkin AJ. Chronic subdural hematoma: pathophysiological basis for treatment. Br J Neurosurg. 1991;5:467–73.
14. Enriquez A, Lip GY, Baranchuk A. Anticoagulation reversal in the era of the non-vitamin K oral anticoagulants. Europace. 2016;18(7):955–64.
15. Feghali J, Yang W, Huang J. Updates in chronic subdural hematoma: epidemiology, etiology, pathogenesis, treatment, and outcome. World Neurosurg. 2020;141:339–45.
16. Flores G, Vicenty JC, Pastrana EA. Post-operative seizures after burr hole evacuation of chronic subdural hematomas: is prophylactic anti-epileptic medication needed? Acta Neurochir (Wien). 2017;159:2033–6.
17. Fornebo I, Sjåvik K, Alibeck M, et al. Role of antithrombotic therapy in the risk of hematoma recurrence and thromboembolism after chronic subdural hematoma evacuation: a population-based consecutive cohort study. Acta Neurochir (Wien). 2017;159(11):2045–52.
18. Gerlach R, Scheuer T, Beck J, Woszczyk A, Seifert V, Raabe A. Risk of postoperative hemorrhage after intracranial surgery after early nadroparin administration: results of a prospective study. Neurosurgery. 2003;53:1028–34.
19. Giralt-Steinhauer E, Cuadrado-Godia E, Ois A, et al. Comparison between $CHADS_2$ and CHA_2DS_2-VASc score in a stroke cohort with atrial fibrillation. Eur J Neurol. 2013;20(4):623–8.
20. Goertz L, Speier J, Schulte AP, et al. Independent risk factors for postoperative seizures in chronic subdural hematoma identified by multiple logistic regression analysis. World Neurosurg. 2019;132:e716–21.
21. Grobelny BT, Ducruet AF, Zacharia BE, et al. Preoperative antiepileptic drug administration and the incidence of postoperative seizures following bur hole-treated chronic subdural hematoma. J Neurosurg. 2009;111(6):1257–62.
22. Henaux PL, Le Reste PJ, Laviolle B, Morandi X. Steroids in chronic subdural hematomas (SUCRE trial): study protocol for a randomized controlled trial. Trials. 2017;18(1):252.
23. Hirashima Y, Kuwayama N, Hamada H, Hayashi N, Endo S. Etizolam, an antianxiety agent, attenuates recurrence of chronic subdural hematoma. Evaluation by computed tomography. Neurol Med Chir (Tokyo). 2002;42:53–5.
24. Hutchinson PJ, Edlmann E, Bulters D, et al. Trial of dexamethasone for chronic subdural hematoma. N Engl J Med. 2020;383(27):2616–27.
25. Jack A, O'Kelly C, McDougall C, Findlay JM. Predicting recurrence after chronic subdural haematoma drainage. Can J Neurol Sci. 2015;42:34–9.
26. Janowski M, Kunert P. Intravenous fluid administration may improve post-operative course of patients with chronic subdural hematoma: a retrospective study. PLoS One. 2012;7(4):e35634.
27. Jiang R, Zhao S, Wang R, et al. Safety and efficacy of atorvastatin for chronic subdural hematoma in Chinese patients: a randomized clinical trial. JAMA Neurol. 2018;75(11):1338–46.
28. Jung N, Shim YJ. Current knowledge on inherited platelet function disorders. Clin Pediatr Hematol Oncol. 2020;27(1):1–13.

29. Kageyama H, Toyooka T, Tsuzuki N, et al. Nonsurgical treatment of chronic subdural hematoma with tranexamic acid. J Neurosurg. 2013;119:332–7.
30. Keeling D, Tait RC, Watson H, British Committee of Standards for Haematology. Peri-operative management of anticoagulation and antiplatelet therapy. Br J Haematol. 2016;175(4):602–13.
31. Kim SO, Jung SI, Won YS, Choi CSYJ. A comparative study of local versus general anesthesia for chronic subdural hematoma in elderly patients over 60 years. Korean J Neurotrauma. 2013;9(2):47–51.
32. Kleindienst A, Harvey HB, Mater E, et al. Early antithrombotic prophylaxis with low molecular weight heparin in neurosurgery. Acta Neurochir (Wien). 2003;145:1085–90.
33. Koenig-Oberhuber V, Filipovic M. New antiplatelet drugs and new oral anticoagulants. Br J Anaesth. 2016;117(S2):ii74–84.
34. Kolias AG, Chari A, Santarius T, Hutchinson PJ. Chronic subdural haematoma: modern management and emerging therapies. Nat Rev Neurol. 2014;10:570–8.
35. Kolias AG, Edlmann E, Thelin EP, et al. Dexamethasone for adult patients with a symptomatic chronic subdural haematoma (Dex-CSDH) trial: study protocol for a randomised controlled trial. Trials. 2018;19(1):670.
36. Kutty RK, Leela SK, Sreemathyamma SB, et al. The outcome of medical management of chronic subdural hematoma with tranexamic acid—a prospective observational study. J Stroke Cerebrovasc Dis. 2020;29(11):10527372.
37. Lavergne P, Labidi M, Brunet MC, et al. Efficacy of anti-seizure prophylaxis in chronic subdural hematoma: a cohort study on routinely collected health data. J Neurosurg. 2019;1:1–5.
38. Lizza BD, Kauflin MJ. Extended-infusion eptifibatide to prevent stent thrombosis in a patient undergoing orthopedic surgery. Ann Pharmacother. 2011;45(5):e28.
39. Luongo M, Pizzuti M, Godano U. Bilateral chronic subdural non-traumatic hematoma associated with von Willebrand's type I disease: a case report. Acta Neurochir (Wien). 2012;154(6):1087–8.
40. Luongo M, Pizzuti M, Godano U. Chronic subdural non traumatic hematoma associated with von Willebrand's disease: a real clinical association or just a mere coincidence? Clin Neurol Neurosurg. 2013;115(8):1569–70.
41. Mahmood SD, Waqas M, Baig MZ, Darbar A. Mini-craniotomy under local anesthesia for chronic subdural hematoma: an effective choice for elderly patients and for patients in a resource-strained environment. World Neurosurg. 2017;106:676–9.
42. Mehta V, Harward SC, Sankey EW, Nayar G, Codd PJ. Evidence based diagnosis and management of chronic subdural hematoma: a review of the literature. J Clin Neurosci. 2018;50:7–15.
43. Meidert AS, Kinzinger J, Möhnle P, et al. Perioperative management of a patient with severe factor V deficiency presenting with chronic subdural hematoma: a clinical report. World Neurosurg. 2019;127:409–13.
44. Merrill SA, Khan D, Richards AE, Kalani MA, Patel NP, Neal MT. Functional recovery following surgery for chronic subdural hematoma. Surg Neurol Int. 2020;11:450.
45. Montano N, Stifano V, Skrap B, Mazzucchi E. Management of residual subdural hematoma after burr-hole evacuation. The role of fluid therapy and review of the literature. J Clin Neurosci. 2017;46:26–9.
46. Mulligan P, Raore B, Liu S, Olson JJ. Neurological and functional outcomes of subdural hematoma evacuation in patients over 70 years of age. J Neurosci Rural Pract. 2013;4(3):250–6.
47. Nagatani K, Wada K, Takeuchi S, Nawashiro H. Corticosteroid suppression of vascular endothelial growth factor and recurrence of chronic subdural hematoma. Neurosurgery. 2012;70(5):E1334.
48. Nathan S, Goodarzi Z, Jette N, Gallagher C, Holroyd-Leduc J. Anticoagulant and antiplatelet use in seniors with chronic subdural hematoma: systematic review. Neurology. 2017;88(20):1889–93.
49. Neidert MC, Schmidt T, Mitova T, et al. Preoperative angiotensin converting enzyme inhibitor usage in patients with chronic subdural hematoma: associations with initial presentation and clinical outcome. J Clin Neurosci. 2016;28:82–6.

50. Oh HJ, Lee KS, Shim JJ, Yoon SM, Yun IG, Bae HG. Postoperative course and recurrence of chronic subdural hematoma. J Korean Neurosurg Soc. 2010;48(6):518–23.
51. Oikonomou E, Siasos G, Zaromitidou M, et al. Atorvastatin treatment improves endothelial function through endothelial progenitor cells mobilization in ischemic heart failure patients. Atherosclerosis. 2015;238:159–64.
52. Oprea AD, Popescu WM. Perioperative management of antiplatelet therapy. Br J Anaesth. 2013;111(Suppl 1):i3–i17.
53. Oshida S, Akamatsu Y, Matsumoto Y, et al. A case of chronic subdural hematoma demonstrating the epileptic focus at the area with sulcal hyperintensity on fluid-attenuated inversion recovery image. Radiol Case Rep. 2019;14(9):1109–12.
54. Park M, Kim JM, Kim HJ. Effects of oral streptokinase-streptodornase on remnant chronic subdural hematomas. Korean J Neurotrauma. 2015;11:131–4.
55. Phan K, Abi-Hanna D, Kerferd J, et al. Resumption of antithrombotic agents in chronic subdural hematoma: a systematic review and meta-analysis. World Neurosurg. 2018;109:e792–9.
56. Pickett AM, Taylor DA, Ackman ML. Prolonged infusion of eptifibatide as bridge therapy between bare-metal stent insertion and cardiovascular surgery: case report and review of the literature. Pharmacotherapy. 2010;30(4):127e–33e.
57. Pinggera D, Unterhofer C, Görtz P, Thomé C, Ortler M. Postoperative thromboembolic prophylaxis with low-molecular-weight heparin and risk of rebleeding in patients with chronic subdural hematomas: a comparative retrospective cohort study. World Neurosurg. 2017;104:284–90.
58. Poulsen FR, Munthe S, Soe M, Halle B. Perindopril and residual chronic subdural hematoma volumes six weeks after burr hole surgery: a randomized trial. Clin Neurol Neurosurg. 2014;123:4–8.
59. Pradhanang AB, Sedain G, Shilpakar SK, Sharma MR. Prophylactic use of antiepileptic drug (Phenytoin) in preventing early postoperative seizure in patients with chronic subdural hematoma: a randomized control trial. Indian J Neurosurg. 2019;08(03):168–78.
60. Prud'homme M, Mathieu F, Marcotte N, Cottin S. A pilot placebo controlled randomized controlled trial of Dexamethasone for Chronic Subdural Haematoma. Can J Neurol Sci. 2016;43(2):284–90.
61. Qiu S, Zhuo W, Sun C, Su Z, Yan A, Shen L. Effects of atorvastatin on chronic subdural hematoma: a systematic review. Medicine (Baltimore). 2017;96(26):e7290.
62. Rassi AN, Blackstone E, Militello MA, et al. Safety of "bridging" with eptifibatide for patients with coronary stents before cardiac and non-cardiac surgery. Am J Cardiol. 2012;110(4):485–90.
63. Samokhvalov AV, Irving H, Mohapatra S, Rehm J. Alcohol consumption, unprovoked seizures, and epilepsy: a systematic review and meta-analysis. Epilepsia. 2010;51:1177–84.
64. Savonitto S, Caracciolo M, Cattaneo M, DE Servi S. Management of patients with recently implanted coronary stents on dual antiplatelet therapy who need to undergo major surgery. J Thromb Haemost. 2011;9(11):2133–42.
65. Shapey J, Glancz LJ, Brennan PM. Chronic subdural haematoma in the elderly: is it time for a new paradigm in management? Curr Geriatr Rep. 2016;5:71–7.
66. Shimogawa T, Morioka T, Sayama T, et al. Impact of low coagulation factor XIII activity in patients with chronic subdural hematoma associated with cerebrospinal fluid hypovolemia: a retrospective study. Surg Neurol Int. 2017;8:192.
67. Son S, Yoo CJ, Lee SG, Kim EY, Park CW, Kim WK. Natural course of initially non-operated cases of acute subdural hematoma: the risk factors of hematoma progression. J Korean Neurosurg Soc. 2013;54:211–9.
68. Tahsim-Oglou Y, Beseoglu K, Hänggi D, Stummer W, Steiger H-J. Factors predicting recurrence of chronic subdural hematoma: the influence of intraoperative irrigation and low-molecular-weight heparin thromboprophylaxis. Acta Neurochir. 2012;154(6):1063–8.
69. Tanweer O, Frisoli FA, Bravate C, et al. Tranexamic acid for treatment of residual subdural hematoma after bedside twist-drill evacuation. World Neurosurg. 2016;91:29–33.
70. Thotakura AK, Marabathina NR. Non-surgical treatment of chronic subdural hematoma with steroids. World Neurosurg. 2015;84:1968–72.

71. Todeschi J, Ferracci FX, Metayer T, et al. Impact of discontinuation of antithrombotic therapy after surgery for chronic subdural hematoma. Neurochirurgie. 2020;66(4):195–202.
72. Volovár Š, Tancošová R, Rokyta R. Bridging anticoagulation therapy. Cor Vasa. 2018;60(4):e400–6.
73. Wagner J, Lock JF, Kastner C, et al. Perioperative management of anticoagulant therapy. Innov Surg Sci. 2019;4(4):144–51.
74. Wang D, Li T, Tian Y, et al. Effects of atorvastatin on chronic subdural hematoma: a preliminary report from three medical centers. J Neurol Sci. 2013;336:237–42.
75. Wang W, Feng L, Bai F, Zhang Z, Zhao Y, Ren C. The safety and efficacy of dexmedetomidine vs. sufentanil in monitored anesthesia care during burr-hole surgery for chronic subdural hematoma: a retrospective clinical trial. Front Pharmacol. 2016;7:410.
76. Wang Y, Zhou J, Fan C, et al. Influence of antithrombotic agents on the recurrence of chronic subdural hematomas and the quest about the recommencement of antithrombotic agents: a meta-analysis. J Clin Neurosci. 2017;38:79–83.
77. Weigel R, Hohenstein A, Schlickum L, Weiss C, Schilling L. Angiotensin converting enzyme inhibition for arterial hypertension reduces the risk of recurrence in patients with chronic subdural hematoma possibly by an antiangiogenic mechanism. Neurosurgery. 2007;61:788–92.
78. Won SY, Dubinski D, Sautter L, et al. Seizure and status epilepticus in chronic subdural hematoma. Acta Neurol Scand. 2019;140(3):194–203.
79. Xu M, Chen P, Zhu X, Wang C, Shi X, Yu B. Effects of atorvastatin on conservative and surgical treatments of chronic subdural hematoma in patients. World Neurosurg. 2016;91:23–8.
80. Zanaty M, Park BJ, Seaman SC. Predicting chronic subdural hematoma recurrence and stroke outcomes while withholding antiplatelet and anticoagulant agents. Front Neurol. 2020;10:1401.
81. Zeng J, Yu P, Cui W, Wang X, Ma J, Zeng C. Comparison of HAS-BLED with other risk models for predicting the bleeding risk in anticoagulated patients with atrial fibrillation: a PRISMA-compliant article. Medicine (Baltimore). 2020;99(25):e20782.

Chapter 33
Postoperative Complications of Cranial Chronic Subdural Hematoma

Ali Akhaddar

33.1 Introduction

Although surgical evacuation of intracranial chronic subdural hematoma (CSDH) is thought to be a relatively simple and safe procedure with a low complication rate, reported incidences of postoperative complications vary in literature between 5 and 38% of patients [5, 6, 10, 14, 17, 32, 34, 41, 48, 49, 57]. Complications include those directly related to surgery or surgical technique, while others are nonsurgical (common medical) complications. All complications can adversely impact morbidity and mortality as well as contribute substantially to the costs of treatments and the hospital stay [6, 55]. Postoperative problems occur more often with less experienced surgeons [3]. However, rates of complications are also dependent on patient's factors (e.g., advanced age, general and neurologic conditions, and associated illnesses) as well as types of hematomas, their underlying etiologies, and the surgical procedures used [10, 37].

This chapter provides a comprehensive overview of the main difficulties that are likely to occur after surgical evacuation for intracranial CSDH (Table 33.1) with the aim of helping the responsible medical team to avoid complications.

33.2 Recurrence/Subdural Fluid Reaccumulation

Residual hematoma into the subdural space was not assigned as recurrence because it is a common CT scan finding after surgical drainage and, unless it is associated with neurological symptoms, most patients in this condition can be managed

A. Akhaddar (✉)
Avicenne Military Hospital of Marrakech, Department of Neurosurgery,
Mohammed V University in Rabat, Rabat, Morocco

M. Turgut et al. (eds.), *Subdural Hematoma*,
https://doi.org/10.1007/978-3-030-79371-5_33

Table 33.1 Main postoperative complications after chronic subdural hematoma evacuation

–	**Recurrence and subdural fluid reaccumulation**
–	**Surgical site infections:** Subdural empyema Wound infections Meningitis Brain abscess
–	**New acute intracranial bleeding:** Epidural hematoma Subdural hematoma Intracerebral hematoma Subarachnoid hemorrhage Iatrogenic bleeding/injury
–	**Seizure and status epilepticus**
–	**Tension pneumocephalus**
–	**Other rare complications:** Brain herniation into the subdural space Spinal subdural hematoma Hyperperfusion syndrome Ischemic stroke
–	**Medical (nonsurgical) complications:** Pulmonary Urinary Cardiovascular Thromboembolic Gastrointestinal Renal Septicemia Disseminated intravascular coagulation Neuropsychological

conservatively (Fig. 33.1). Symptomatic recurrence has been seen in 4.9–28% of cases in the 3-month postoperative period [1, 17, 21, 35, 36, 39, 41, 42, 48, 53, 55, 60]. However, in some populations, this complication can reach one in three cases [58]. Symptomatic reaccumulation of the subdural fluid (e.g., recurrence) represents a problematic situation because many patients will need further reoperation(s) and therefore an increased morbid-mortality rate (Fig. 33.2).

Many factors seem to be involved in the occurrence of this complication. Among them, some aspects are still debated like anticoagulant/antiplatelet therapies [42, 64], patients' comorbidities [37, 39], types of hematomas [11, 40, 44], and surgical techniques involved [36, 37]. Treatment of postoperative symptomatic recurrence is frequently surgical, but persistent fluid collection on control computed tomography scan (CT scan) should not be systematically treated unless it increases in size or patient worsening or if there is no clinical recovery. In other words, management should be adapted on a case-by-case basis.

In the series of Nayil and coworkers, 57 of 1181 patients (4.82%) had one recurrence: 43 patients had recurrence on the same side (3.6%) and 14 cases on the

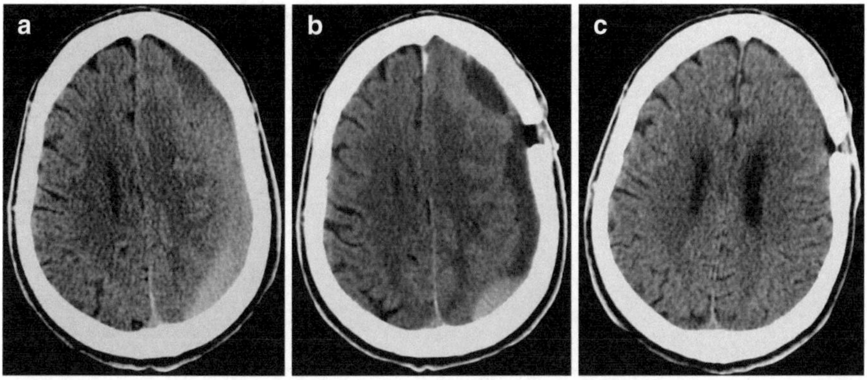

Fig. 33.1 Initial preoperative CT scan (**a**), at 1 week postoperatively (**b**), and 3 months later (**c**) showing a residual collection into the subdural space (**b**) in an asymptomatic patient treated conservatively. Complete disappearance of the SDH at the third month control

contralateral side (1.2%). All these 57 patients were reoperated with hematoma evacuation and postoperative drainage. In addition, 9 patients had two recurrences (0.76%) and were reoperated with craniotomy, evacuation of new hematoma, and neomembranes excision [46]. Parameters such as age, sex, hematoma thickness, midline shift, and hematoma position did not correlate with the recurrence. However, Nayil's team found that the internal architecture of the hematoma and presence of bleeding diathesis influence the recurrence rates [46].

Rauhala et al. treated surgically 1048 patients with CSDH. 278 patients (28%) were reoperated for recurrence. The recurrent hematoma was clinically symptomatic in 229 of the cases, and 49 patients were operated because the follow-up CT scan revealed a voluminous CSDH [55]. According to the study of Motoie, CSDH recurrence was seen in 96 patients (12.2%) among 787. Eleven cases required more than 2 reoperations, 9 cases required 3 reoperations, and 2 cases required 4 reoperations [43].

In Shen's study, a midline shift of more than 10 mm, severe brain atrophy, severe post-surgical pneumocephalus, and a volume of drainage superior to 100 mL were independent risk factors for the recurrence [60]. However, for Huang et al., the volume of the subdural hematoma is not related to recurrence [21]. Concerning the type of CSDH, laminar or layering of the hematoma, thick subdural membranes, high and mixed density lesions, and multiloculated collections are associated with an increased recurrence [11, 21, 40, 44, 46]. For Mori et al., the existence of thin subdural hematoma or effusion contralateral to the site of the first operation result to a high risk of recurrence [41].

Postoperative drainage reduces the recurrence rate. However, the inserted drain type (subdural or subperiosteal) does not seem to influence the time to recurrence [36]. Use of gravity can help the brain to reexpand. Based on Abouzari's results, upright posture soon after the evacuation of CSDH is associated with an increased incidence of recurrence [1].

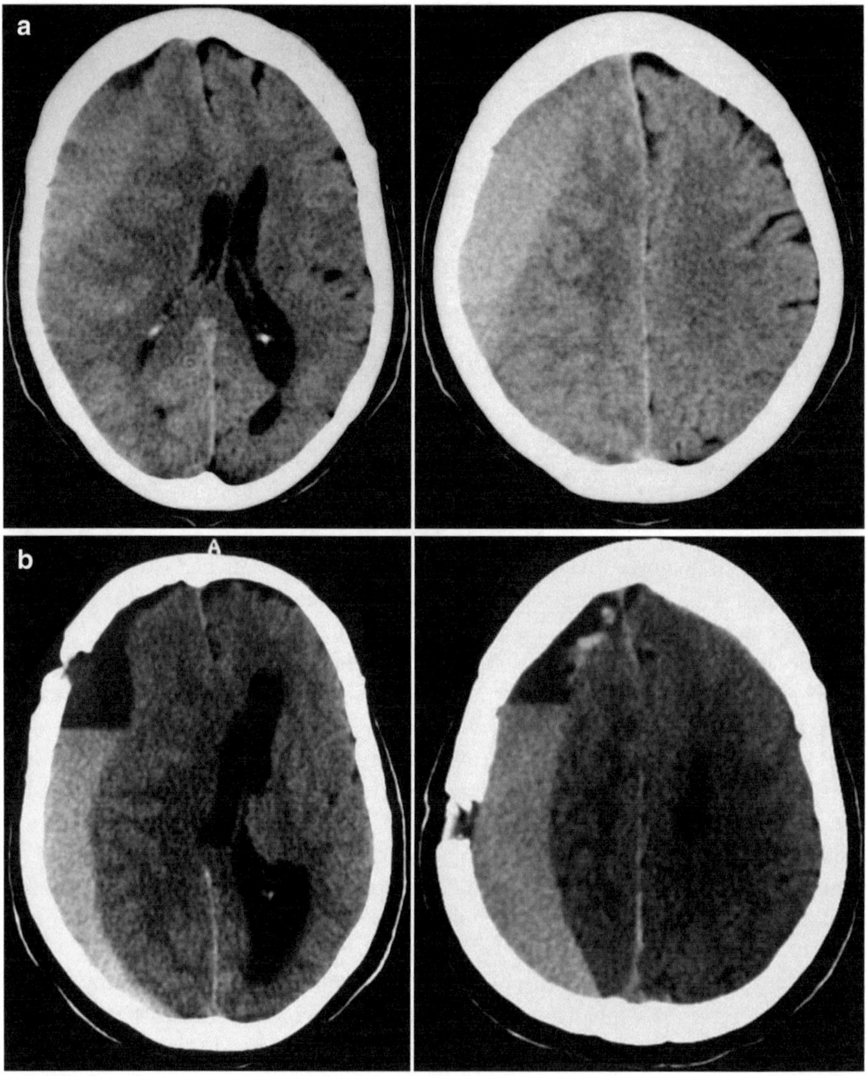

Fig. 33.2 Recurrence of a right chronic subdural hematoma treated 6 weeks previously via two burr holes with subdural closed-system drainage (reappearance of neurological disorders). Initial (**a**) and postoperative control CT scan performed 6 weeks later (**b**)

Although many studies have shown that antiplatelet/anticoagulant agents might facilitate the recurrence of CSDH [42, 64], for Motoie, these drugs were not independent predictors for CSDH recurrence after managing their 96 patients who were reoperated for CSDH recurrence [43].

In literature, almost all of the recurrences were treated successfully with craniostomies and closed-system drainage within 2 months following the first surgical procedure [36, 41, 46, 55]. Therefore, patients with CSDH should be followed up for a minimum of 10 weeks postoperatively to check for recurrence. From our personal experience, corticosteroids can be used as monotherapy or as an adjunct to surgery for some pauci-symptomatic patients. Refractory CSDH may be treated with a variety of surgical techniques, including craniotomy, subdural-peritoneal shunt placement, interventional middle meningeal artery embolization, or subdural catheter injection of tissue plasminogen activator [25, 30].

Reappearance of subdural fluid following surgical drainage of CSDH is not completely understood and it still needs more studies [37].

33.3 Subdural Empyema

Subdural empyemas are by far the most severe surgical site infections following CSDH evacuation. Other infectious complications are less common in particular deep wound infections (Fig. 33.3), meningitis, and brain abscesses [2, 57].

Although rare (less than 2.5% of all surgical complications), subdural empyemas represent serious causes of morbidity and mortality [29, 35, 46, 55, 56, 59, 66]. Most cases occur 1–2 weeks postoperatively. Clinical symptoms vary greatly. Apart from fever and purulent drainage, most cases tend to manifest by the development of new focal neurological deficits or worsening of pre-existing ones, normal or elevated temperature, and progressively impaired level of consciousness. Some cases can be insidious and can cause few or no symptoms (e.g., only an intermittent low-grade fever or general malaise). So, neurosurgeons should consider the possibility

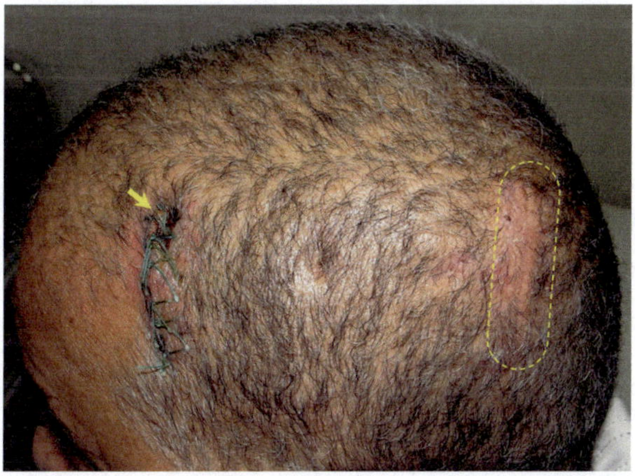

Fig. 33.3 This diabetic patient was operated on 2 weeks ago for chronic subdural hematoma. The posterior incision healed correctly (dotted line); however, the anterior wound presents local signs of inflammation and infection near the incision, superficial wound dehiscence with delayed healing (arrow). (Reproduced from Akhaddar A (editor) Atlas of Infections in Neurosurgery and Spinal surgery (2017). Springer International Publishing; with permission)

of subdural infection in these patients and institute an appropriate diagnostic assessment.

On CT scan, the infected subdural collections have a low or isodensity with surrounding post-contrast enhancement (Figs. 33.4 and 33.5). It is more difficult to differentiate between recurrent CSDH and postsurgical-related subdural empyema without a magnetic resonance imaging (MRI). In that case, post-gadolinium

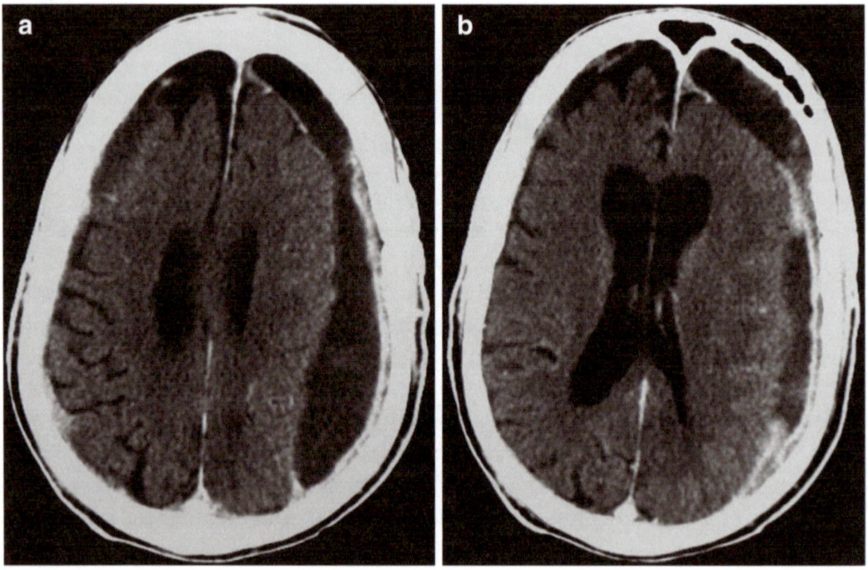

Fig. 33.4 Postoperative subdural empyema in an 80-year-old man operated 4 weeks before for a chronic subdural hematoma. Axial cranial CT scan with contrast injection (**a**, **b**). (Reproduced from Akhaddar A (editor) Atlas of Infections in Neurosurgery and Spinal surgery (2017). Springer International Publishing; with permission)

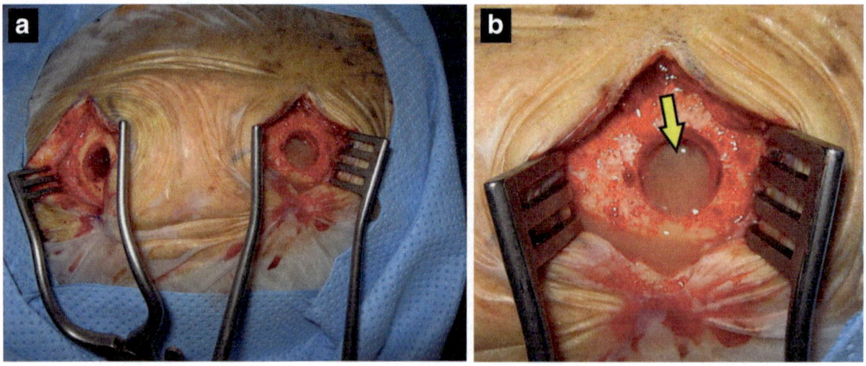

Fig. 33.5 Operative views in the same patient showing the suppurative content of the intracranial subdural collection (arrow) (**a**, **b**). (Reproduced from Akhaddar A (editor) Atlas of Infections in Neurosurgery and Spinal surgery (2017). Springer International Publishing; with permission)

T1-weighted images and diffusion-weighted imaging evaluations may be useful [45] [See Chap. 26 about neuroimaging differential diagnosis of cranial chronic subdural hematoma]. The expression of inflammatory biomarkers is highly variable postoperatively. C-reactive protein (CRP) and Procalcitonin levels are helpful in these conditions. The causative pathogens responsible for the iatrogenic subdural empyema are inconstantly reported and dominated by *Staphylococcus aureus*, *Streptococcus species,* and gram-negative bacteria [13, 35].

Subdural empyema often requires reoperation with cleaning, evacuation of purulent collections, debridement, drainage, and careful wound closure. Medical treatment may start with a broad spectrum of antibiotics, and then a targeted treatment should be initiated according to the antimicrobial susceptibility testing [2, 46].

In his study in 2012, Nayil and his colleagues described nine patients who developed subdural empyema (0.76%) among 1181 who were treated surgically. Six had been operated one time previously for CSDH and three patients had been operated two times. These nine cases had hemiparesis. Two patients had new-onset seizures and four cases developed altered level of consciousness. For most patients, the infected subdural collection was diagnosed within 2 or 3 weeks after the last surgery. For these nine cases, the new surgical procedure had consisted of craniotomy, evacuation of the empyema, and excision of the neomembranes. Unfortunately two patients died [46].

If managed quickly and vigorously, subdural empyemas may resolve without sequelae. However, many neurologic complications and even death may occur. Sequels consist of persistent seizures, residual focal neurologic deficits, and permanent alteration in mental status [29].

33.4 New Acute Intracranial Bleeding

Although uncommon (less than 4% of all complications) [32, 41, 55, 57], acute intracranial bleeding is one of the most serious complications after CSDH surgery. It may increase both morbidity and/or mortality. This postoperative complication can happen either following craniotomy or burr hole procedure for CSDH. Acute subdural hematoma (Figs. 33.6 and 33.7), epidural hematoma (Fig. 33.8) and subarachnoid hemorrhage are the most types of hemorrhage that occur at the surgical site. However, remote intracerebral bleeding from the original site may be seen at different locations, for example, in the ipsilateral side (Fig. 33.9), contralateral side, intraventricular, or in the posterior fossa [4, 22, 50, 62]. Patibandla reported a fatal case with simultaneous multiple intraparenchymal hemorrhages in various intracranial locations (brainstem, cerebral and cerebellar peduncles, right cerebellar hemisphere, right thalamus, and both cerebral hemispheres) after a surgical drainage of a CSDH [51].

The exact pathogenesis of remote intraparenchymal bleeding remains indefinite, but this phenomenon was suspected to be a consequence of various intricate factors like high blood pressure, intracranial hypotension, changes in intracranial pressure,

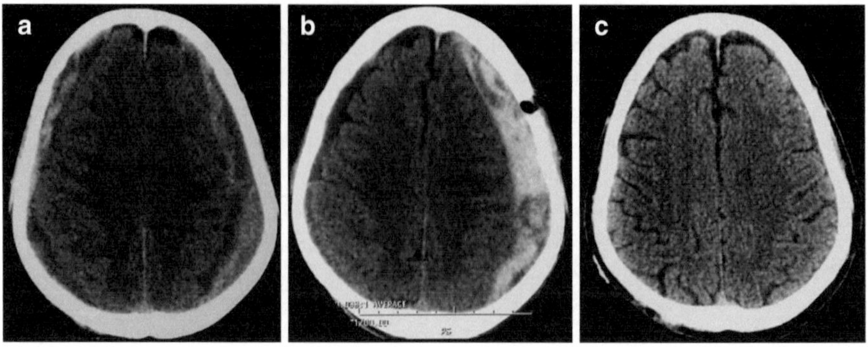

Fig. 33.6 Third day postoperative acute subdural hematoma. The patient was reoperated (Bone flap craniotomy) with a good outcome. Initial axial cranial CT scan (**a**), on the third postoperative day (**b**), and 3 months later (**c**)

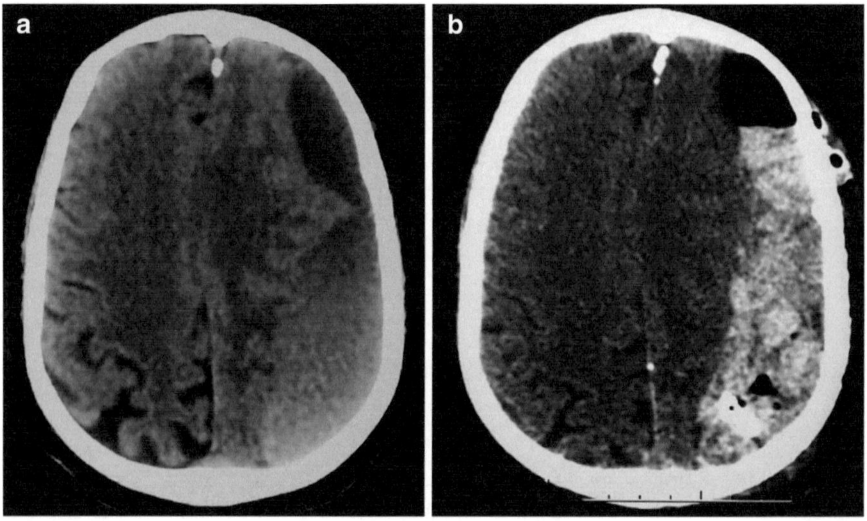

Fig. 33.7 Immediate postoperative subdural bleeding following burr holes evacuation of a chronic SDH. Preoperative (**a**) and urgent postoperative CT scan (**b**)

suction drainage, CSF overdrainage, hemorrhage into previously undetected areas of contusion, and thrombocytopenia [4, 12]. Therefore, many authors recommend slow and gradual brain decompression to prevent rapid changes in blood flow. Kaneshiro and coworkers consider performing an early postoperative CT scan in all suspected patients with postoperative intracranial bleeding [27]. Faced with these variable forms of postoperative bleeding, the indications for a surgical management may not be clear; for that reason, the neurosurgeon's decision must be given on a case-by-case basis.

According to Lee's experience, 14 patients (3.54%) from 395 developed a new acute intracranial bleeding following CSDH surgery. The most common complication was acute epidural hematoma which was adjacent to the burr hole site in seven

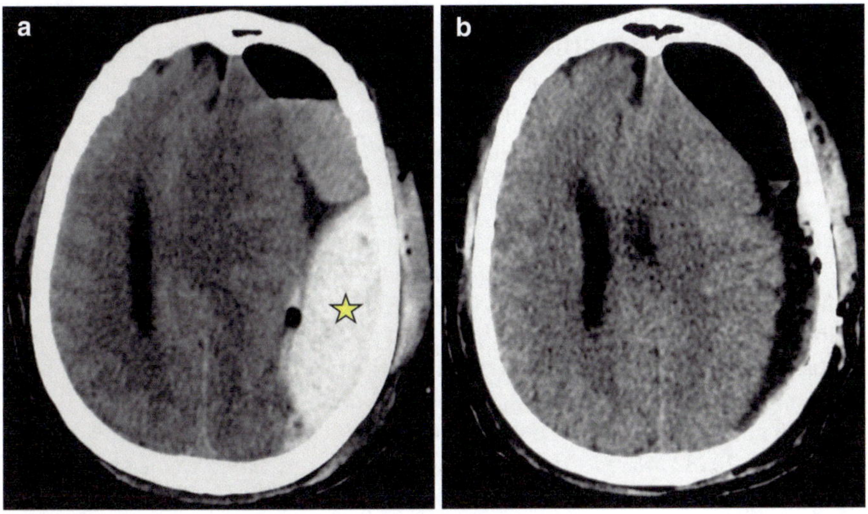

Fig. 33.8 Immediate postoperative acute extradural hematoma (star) following burr holes evacuation of a chronic subdural hematoma. The patient was reoperated urgently through a bone flap craniotomy with a good outcome. Immediate postoperative CT scan (**a**) and following the second surgery (**b**)

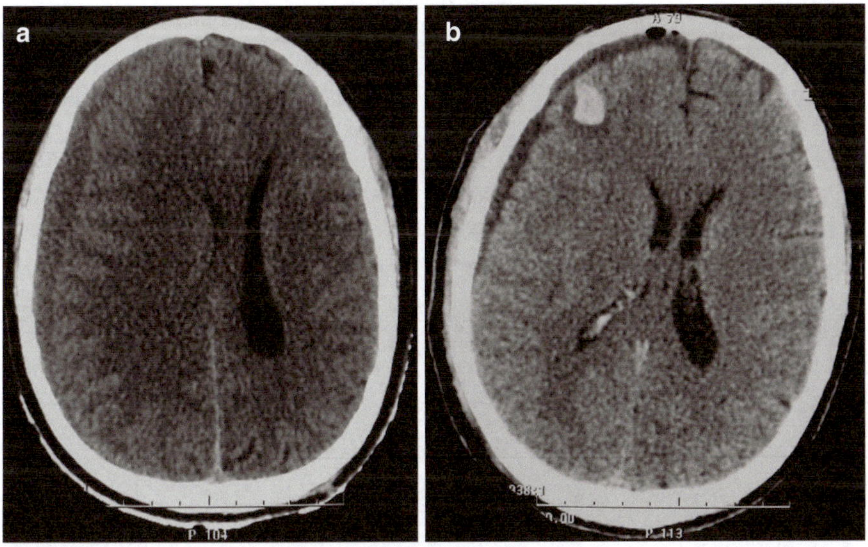

Fig. 33.9 Postoperative remote brain hematoma in the right frontal lobe following surgical evacuation of a chronic SDH. Initial axial cranial CT scan (**a**) and on the third postoperative day (**b**)

patients. Two of these cases underwent craniotomy and hematoma evacuation with a good outcome. Acute subdural hematoma occurred in six patients. Among them, four patients underwent craniectomy and subdural hematoma evacuation. Unfortunately, one nonoperated patient died. In another case, a small intraparenchymal hematoma was seen near the burr hole site [32]. Among the 376 patients operated on for CSDH by Rohde et al., new acute intracranial hemorrhage occurred in 13 patients (3.45%), of which eight cases were intracerebral bleeding (2.12%) and five were acute epidural hematomas (1.33%) [57].

In another work by Nayil et al., five patients (0.42%) from 1181 developed acute subdural hematomas, but two of them were under anticoagulant therapy preoperatively. All these five patients were operated on with evacuation of subdural hematoma but two patients died. Acute extradural hematoma was seen in one patient who recovered well from reoperation. One patient developed a large thalamic hematoma in the immediate postoperative period and died [46].

In addition, iatrogenic bleeding subsequent to surgical evacuation of CSDHshould not be neglected. False move of the skull perforator (Fig. 33.10), wrong drainage insertion (Fig. 33.11), malposition of subdural drain placement (Fig. 33.12), and brain injury irrigation should be mentioned because a few cases have already been reported [9, 26, 32, 46, 52, 65]. In our personal practice, when we need to drain a subdural hematoma we use only a subgaleal soft drain (instead of subdural drains) which reduces the chance of brain injury. In all cases, proper care and vigilance must be taken at the time of inserting and removing the drains.

33.5 Seizure and Status Epilepticus

Global incidence of postoperative seizures is reported between 0.67 and 23% of patients after CSDH evacuation [7, 20, 32, 35, 46, 48, 55, 57, 67] and it may be fatal [33]. This incidence is especially high in those undergoing craniotomy [15]. Hirakawa et al. found that patients who had craniotomy with the opening of the membranes had an increased incidence of epileptic seizures compared to patients

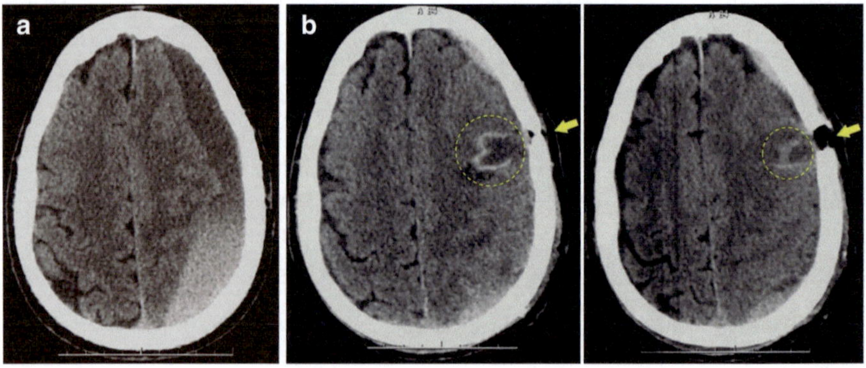

Fig. 33.10 Postoperative frontal cortical brain contusion (dotted circle) following burr hole evacuation (arrow) of a chronic SDH (**a**, **b**). The surgeon had not reported any particular incident during the surgical procedure but it is most likely a false move of the skull perforator

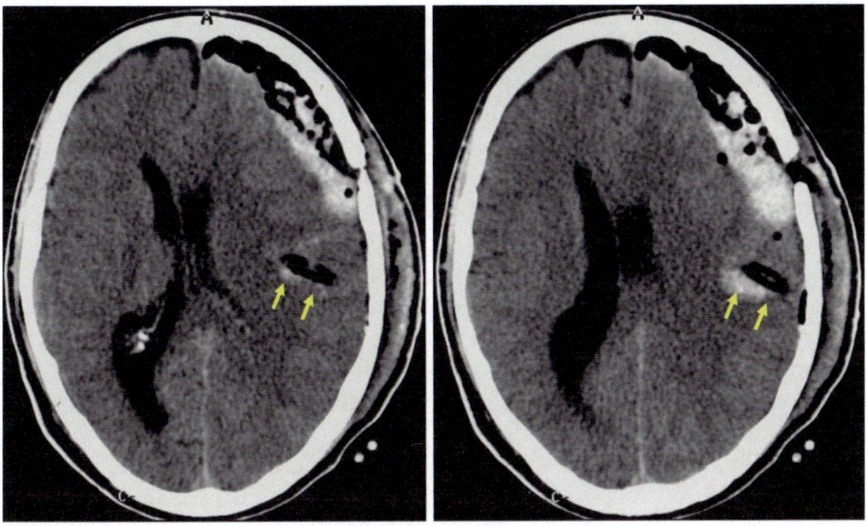

Fig. 33.11 Postoperative axial CT scan showing intraparenchymal deep brain contusions (arrows) following wrong drainage insertion of a chronic SDH

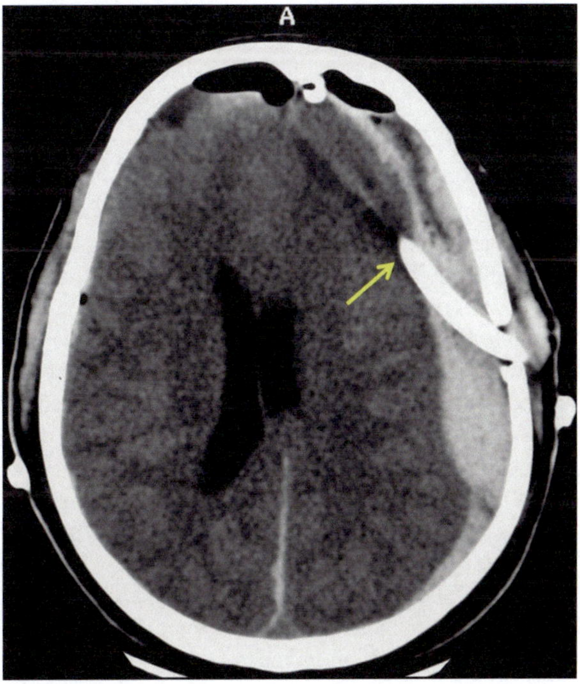

Fig. 33.12 Postoperative axial CT scan showing acute subdural bleeding and frontal cortical brain injury due to malposition of subdural drain placement (arrow) following burr holes chronic SDH evacuation

who underwent burr hole evacuation alone [19]. However, not only the surgical evacuation but also the initial head injury and the compressing hematoma itself can be the source of seizures. On the other hand, patients with a past history of epilepsy are at particular risk to develop postoperative seizures [57]. Cameron et al. recommended that prophylactic anticonvulsants should be started preoperatively and continued for 6 months [7]. However, the effect of the prophylactic antiepileptic drug in reducing the development of new seizure after surgery is still unclear [7, 18].

In the study reported by Lee et al., eight patients (2%) developed new seizures following a burr hole craniostomy. Among them, five patients had aggravated seizures due to new intracranial lesions. Therefore, a timely CT scan evaluation should be performed in patients with newly developed seizures [32]. New onset-seizures were observed in eight patients (0.67%) in the acute postoperative period by Nayil et al. A control CT scan revealed a simple pneumocephalus in all these patients and acute subdural hematoma in another case [46]. However, in regard of the very low incidences of seizures in both Nayil's and Rohde's studies, they do not recommend a routine use of antiepileptic prophylaxis in patients with CSDH [46, 57]. Furthermore, in a Cochrane Register-based search performed by Ratilal et al. in 2013, they concluded that no accepted recommendations were advised about the use of prophylactic anticonvulsants in patients operated on for CSDHs [54].

It is important to add that history of seizure is a well-recognized risk factor for postoperative recurrence of CSDH [11, 68]. For further details, refer to Chap. 10 of the present book about epilepsy and cranial CSDH.

33.6 Tension Pneumocephalus

Pneumocephalus is defined as the existence of air intracranially. This is a common finding seen in the early control CT scan following surgical evacuation of CSDH. Nearly half of the patients can have pneumocephalus postoperatively [23]. However, most pneumocephalus are simple, asymptomatic, and require no treatment. On the contrary, tension pneumocephalus is rare (less than 10% of pneumocephalus) and a most serious condition where the air collection forces the brain parenchyma under pressure leading to neurological deterioration (Fig. 33.13) [41, 53, 56, 57]. Previous fatal cases were also reported due to final brain herniation [61].

The universally proposed hypothesis for the development of tension pneumocephalus is the ball-valve mechanism. For many authors, air influx into the subdural space during surgery is associated with high rates of hematoma recurrence and even subdural empyema [41]. For Ihab, pneumocephalus was found in seven patients among nine with CSDH recurrence [23]. In Shen's study, there was no correlation between brain atrophy and postoperative pneumocephalus following CSDH surgery [60].

Clinical presentation includes headaches, nausea/vomiting, seizures, hemiparesis, vertigo, and progressive neurological deterioration. Tension pneumocephalus usually requires an emergent management [23, 41]. Diagnosis is based on the previous described symptoms associated with unilateral (Fig. 33.13) or bilateral tension pneumocephalus on CT scan. "Mount Fuji sign" is a characteristic aspect of

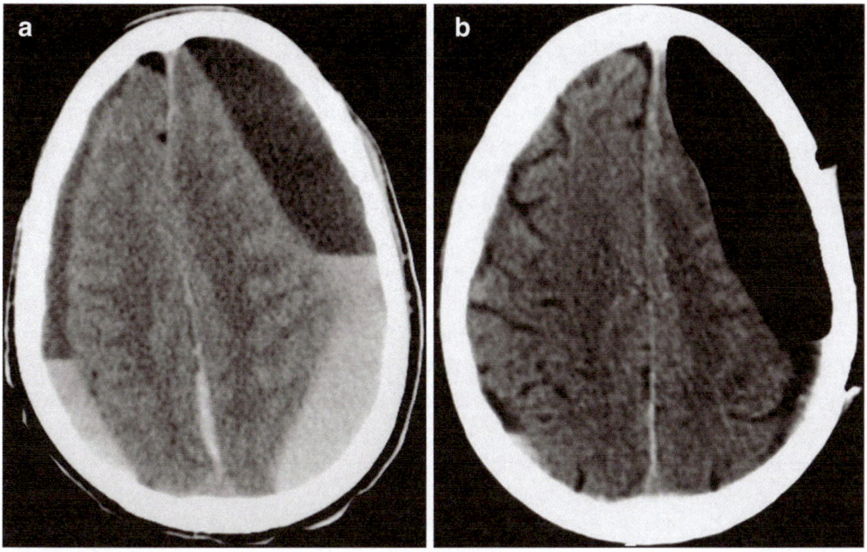

Fig. 33.13 Unilateral postoperative tension pneumocephalus following burr holes surgery for chronic SDH. Initial cranial axial CT scan (**a**) and on the third postoperative day (**b**)

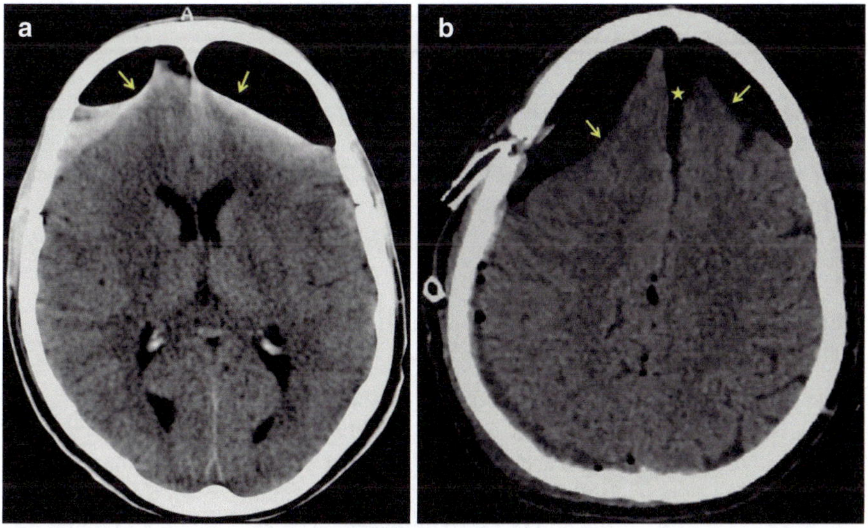

Fig. 33.14 Postoperative cranial axial CT scan in two different patients (**a**, **b**) with bilateral compressive pneumocephalus (arrows) following burr holes surgery for bilateral chronic SDH. Note the frontal interhemispheric pneumocephalus (star) and the "Mount Fuji sign"

bilateral frontal tension pneumocephalus seen on the CT scan: the subdural air separates and compresses the frontal lobes, creating a widened interhemispheric space between the tips of the frontal lobes that mimics the shadow of Japan's Mount Fuji (Fig. 33.14).

Several techniques have been published to prevent the development of tension pneumocephalus after surgery. The best known consist of lumbar intrathecal injection of isotonic saline, ringer's solution, or air during surgery, hyperhydratation of the patient, Trendelenburg positioning of the patient with bed rest for a few days, Valsalva maneuver, intraoperative saline flushing, the replacement of the hematoma with carbon dioxide gas or oxygen, or placement of a subcutaneous reservoir with a catheter introduced into the subdural space [8, 23, 31]. For some authors, the subdural or subcutaneous drain can reduce the occurrence of pneumocephalus as well as fast skin closure. Other simple methods had been demonstrated to be helpful as the supplemental inhalation of 100% oxygen and the decompression of the subdural air by a needle aspiration using a syringe [23, 53]. This last technique was used effectively by Ramachandran et al. for three of their patients with tension pneumocephalus with good results [53]. Furthermore, all the four patients reported by Mori and colleagues were immediately treated by reopening the scalp wound to evacuate the compressing subdural air. Interestingly, Mori's team routinely performs cranial radiography at the end of the surgical procedure to verify the presence of potential pneumocephalus [41]. In the recent studies published by Kawabata, Shen, and You, respectively, severe postoperative pneumocephalus is an independent risk factor for the recurrence of CSDH following surgical drainage [28, 60, 69].

33.7 Other Rare Complications

Some other rare complications have been reported in literature such as brain herniation into the subdural space, spinal subdural hematoma, postoperative hyperperfusion syndrome, and ischemic stroke [16, 24, 38, 47, 70]. All these should at least be mentioned.

33.8 Nonsurgical (Medical) Complications

Like all neurosurgical procedures, surgical evacuations for CSDH are also associated with various nonsurgical "medical" complications. A large number of these postoperative complications is related to the patient's age, general conditions, and comorbidities [46, 53, 55]. Between 0.8 and 22.3% of patients suffer from nonsurgical complications [32, 41, 46, 57, 63]. Pulmonary (especially pneumonia) and urinary problems were among the most common medical complications [32, 57, 63]. Additional common problems are less frequent: gastrointestinal signs, thromboembolic complications, cardiologic problems, renal problems, septicemia, disseminated intravascular coagulation, neuropsychological complications, and cognitive impairments.

For Lee HS and coworkers, two deaths among 39 patients were associated with nonsurgical complications during hospitalization. Pneumonia and sudden cardiac arrest were the causes of death in these two cases who had associated comorbidities. According to multivariate analysis of risk factors performed by Lee's team, pulmonary complications were associated with long hospital stays and patients confined to bed. In addition, old age was a risk factor for cognitive impairment following burr hole drainage; however, the type of anesthesia was not correlated with any nonsurgical complications [32]. On the contrary, Rauhala et al. hypothesized that the frequency of medical complications could be reduced by minimizing the invasiveness of surgical hematoma removal and the anesthesiological management [55]. However, during local anesthesia, emotional stress itself could be the source of cardiac complications in some anxious patients.

Pneumonia was the most frequent medical complication in the series of Rohde (29 cases, 7.7%). Medical complications were fatal in 24 among 376 operated patients. In spite of adequate antibiotic therapy, ten patients died of pneumonia. Cardiac arrhythmia was observed in nine patients and was fatal for five of them. Thromboembolic complications occurred in seven patients, and other septic complications in six [57]. For Rauhala et al. nearly half of the patients operated on for a CSDH and who experienced a medical complication died [55].

33.9 Conclusion

Overall incidence of complications after surgical evacuation of CSDH seems underestimated. In addition, a comparison between different studies remains difficult since methods of data collection and criteria of reporting complications vary greatly. Main surgical risks and complications should be known and clearly explained to the patient or their family before surgery. Many options exist for the management of these complications, but none of them can be considered standard of care. When surgery is considered again, it should be achieved in selected patients, based on the benefit-risk balance. Finally, great caution must be taken perioperatively and during the surgical procedure to reduce postoperative problems that contribute largely to the increase of morbid-mortality rate.

References

1. Abouzari M, Rashidi A, Rezaii J, Esfandiari K, Asadollahi M, Aleali H, et al. The role of postoperative patient posture in the recurrence of traumatic chronic subdural hematoma after burr-hole surgery. Neurosurgery. 2007;61:794–7. https://doi.org/10.1227/01.NEU.0000298908.94129.67.
2. Akhaddar A. Surgical site infections in cranial surgery. In: Akhaddar A, editor. Atlas of infections in neurosurgery and spinal surgery. Cham: Springer International Publishing; 2017. p. 191–215. https://doi.org/10.1007/978-3-319-60086-4_21.
3. Akhaddar A. Letter to the editor: talking about our own complications: is it still a taboo subject in neurosurgery? World Neurosurg. 2020;142:579. https://doi.org/10.1016/j.wneu.2020.07.191.

4. Akhaddar A, Ajja A, Boucetta M. Combined epidural and intracerebral hematomas after evacuation of bilateral chronic subdural hematoma. Neurochirurgie. 2008;54:728–30. https://doi.org/10.1016/j.neuchi.2008.09.001.
5. Borger V, Vatter H, Oszvald Á, Marquardt G, Seifert V, Güresir E. Chronic subdural haematoma in elderly patients: a retrospective analysis of 322 patients between the ages of 65-94 years. Acta Neurochir (Wien). 2012;154:1549–54. https://doi.org/10.1007/s00701-012-1434-x.
6. Bucher B, Maldaner N, Regli L, Sarnthein J, Serra C. Standardized assessment of outcome and complications in chronic subdural hematoma: results from a large case series. Acta Neurochir (Wien). 2019;161:1297–304. https://doi.org/10.1007/s00701-019-03884-7.
7. Cameron MM. Chronic subdural haematoma: a review of 114 cases. J Neurol Neurosurg Psychiatry. 1978;41:834–9. https://doi.org/10.1136/jnnp.41.9.834.
8. Caron JL, Worthington C, Bertrand G. Tension pneumocephalus after evacuation of chronic subdural hematoma and subsequent treatment with continuous lumbar subarachnoid infusion and craniostomy drainage. Neurosurgery. 1985;16:107–10. https://doi.org/10.1227/00006123-198501000-00025.
9. Chan KW, Datta NN. Iatrogenic acute subdural hematoma due to drainage catheter. Surg Neurol. 2000;54:444–6. https://doi.org/10.1016/s0090-3019(00)00323-2.
10. Chari A, Hocking KC, Edlmann E, Turner C, Santarius T, Hutchinson PJ, et al. Core outcomes and common data elements in chronic subdural hematoma: a systematic review of the literature focusing on baseline and peri-operative care data elements. J Neurotrauma. 2016;33:1569–75. https://doi.org/10.1089/neu.2015.4248.
11. Chon KH, Lee JM, Koh EJ, Choi HY. Independent predictors for recurrence of chronic subdural hematoma. Acta Neurochir (Wien). 2012;154:1541–8. https://doi.org/10.1007/s00701-012-1399-9.
12. Cohen-Gadol AA. Remote contralateral intraparenchymal hemorrhage after overdrainage of a chronic subdural hematoma. Int J Surg Case Rep. 2013;4:834–6. https://doi.org/10.1016/j.ijscr.2013.06.014.
13. Dabdoub CB, Adorno JO, Urbano J, Silveira EN, Orlandi BM. Review of the management of infected subdural hematoma. World Neurosurg. 2016;87:663.e1–8. https://doi.org/10.1016/j.wneu.2015.11.015.
14. Farhat Neto J, Araujo JL, Ferraz VR, Haddad L, Veiga JC. Chronic subdural hematoma: epidemiological and prognostic analysis of 176 cases. Rev Col Bras Cir. 2015;42:283–7. https://doi.org/10.1590/0100-69912015005003.
15. Fugate JE. Complications of neurosurgery. Continuum (Minneap Minn). 2015;21(5 Neurocritical Care):1425–44. https://doi.org/10.1212/CON.0000000000000227.
16. Fujita T, Iwamoto Y, Takeuchi H, Tsujino H, Hashimoto N. Lumbar subdural hematoma detected after surgical treatment of chronic intracranial subdural hematoma. World Neurosurg. 2020;134:472–6. https://doi.org/10.1016/j.wneu.2019.11.053.
17. Gelabert-González M, Iglesias-Pais M, García-Allut A, Martínez-Rumbo R. Chronic subdural haematoma: surgical treatment and outcome in 1000 cases. Clin Neurol Neurosurg. 2005;107:223–9. https://doi.org/10.1016/j.clineuro.2004.09.015.
18. Goertz L, Speier J, Schulte AP, Stavrinou P, Krischek B, Goldbrunner R, et al. Independent risk factors for postoperative seizures in chronic subdural hematoma identified by multiple logistic regression analysis. World Neurosurg. 2019;132:e716–21. https://doi.org/10.1016/j.wneu.2019.08.032.
19. Hirakawa K, Hashizume K, Fuchinoue T, Takahashi H, Nomura K. Statistical analysis of chronic subdural hematoma in 309 adult cases. Neurol Med Chir (Tokyo). 1972;12:71–83. https://doi.org/10.2176/nmc.12.71.
20. Huang YH, Yang TM, Lin YJ, Tsai NW, Lin WC, Wang HC, et al. Risk factors and outcome of seizures after chronic subdural hematoma. Neurocrit Care. 2011;14:253–9. https://doi.org/10.1007/s12028-011-9509-8.
21. Huang YH, Lin WC, Lu CH, Chen WF. Volume of chronic subdural haematoma: is it one of the radiographic factors related to recurrence? Injury. 2014;45:1327–31. https://doi.org/10.1016/j.injury.2014.02.023.

22. Hyam JA, Turner J, Peterson D. Cerebellar haemorrhage after repeated burr hole evacuation for chronic subdural haematoma. J Clin Neurosci. 2007;14:83–6. https://doi.org/10.1016/j.jocn.2005.12.048.
23. Ihab Z. Pneumocephalus after surgical evacuation of chronic subdural hematoma: is it a serious complication? Asian J Neurosurg. 2012;7:66–74. https://doi.org/10.4103/1793-5482.98647.
24. Ito S, Miyazaki H, Iino N, Shiokawa Y, Saito I. Acute carotid arterial occlusion after burr hole surgery for chronic subdural haematoma in moyamoya disease. J Clin Neurosci. 2004;11(7):778–80. https://doi.org/10.1016/j.jocn.2003.10.028.
25. Joyce E, Bounajem MT, Scoville J, Thomas AJ, Ogilvy CS, Riina HA, et al. Middle meningeal artery embolization treatment of nonacute subdural hematomas in the elderly: a multiinstitutional experience of 151 cases. Neurosurg Focus. 2020;49:E5. https://doi.org/10.3171/2020.7.FOCUS20518.
26. Kamenova M, Wanderer S, Lipps P, Marbacher S, Mariani L, Soleman J. When the drain hits the brain. World Neurosurg. 2020;138:e426–36. https://doi.org/10.1016/j.wneu.2020.02.166.
27. Kaneshiro Y, Yamauchi S, Urano Y, Murata K. Remote hemorrhage after burr-hole surgery for chronic subdural hematoma: a report of two cases. Surg Neurol Int. 2019;10:18. https://doi.org/10.4103/sni.sni_108_18.
28. Kawabata S, Tani S, Imamura H, Adachi H, Sakai N. Postoperative subdural air collection is a risk factor for chronic subdural hematoma after surgical clipping of cerebral aneurysms. Neurol Med Chir (Tokyo). 2018;58:247–53. https://doi.org/10.2176/nmc.oa.2018-0019.
29. Kim YS, Joo SP, Song DJ, Kim SH, Kim TS. Delayed intracranial subdural empyema following burr hole drainage: case series and literature review. Medicine (Baltimore). 2018;97:e0664. https://doi.org/10.1097/MD.0000000000010664.
30. Lam J, Lee DJ, Oladunjoye A. Subdural catheter injection of tissue plasminogen activator for residual hematoma post drainage of acute-on-chronic subdural hematoma: novel case report of 2 patients. World Neurosurg. 2020;133:266–70. https://doi.org/10.1016/j.wneu.2019.10.007.
31. Lavano A, Benvenuti D, Volpentesta G, Donato G, Marotta R, Zappia M, et al. Symptomatic tension pneumocephalus after evacuation of chronic subdural haematoma: report of seven cases. Clin Neurol Neurosurg. 1990;92:35–41. https://doi.org/10.1016/0303-8467(90)90005-p.
32. Lee HS, Song SW, Chun YI, Choe WJ, Cho J, Moon CT, et al. Complications following burr hole craniostomy and closed-system drainage for subdural lesions. Korean J Neurotrauma. 2018;14:68–75. https://doi.org/10.13004/kjnt.2018.14.2.68.
33. Lee KJ, Eom KS, Park JT, Kim TY. Fatal post-operative epilepticus after burr-hole drainage for chronic subdural hematoma. Korean J Neurotrauma. 2015;11:144–6. https://doi.org/10.13004/kjnt.2015.11.2.144.
34. Lee L, Ker J, Ng HY, Munusamy T, King NK, Kumar D, et al. Outcomes of chronic subdural hematoma drainage in nonagenarians and centenarians: a multicenter study. J Neurosurg. 2016;124:546–51. https://doi.org/10.3171/2014.12.JNS142053.
35. Leung GK, Fan JK, Tam MC, Fan YW. Surgical complications of chronic subdural haematoma: a 5-year audit. Ann Coll Surg Hong Kong. 2001;5:99–103. https://doi.org/10.1046/j.1442-2034.2001.00111.x.
36. Lutz K, Kamenova M, Schaedelin S, Guzman R, Mariani L, Fandino J, et al. Time to and possible risk factors for recurrence after burr-hole drainage of chronic subdural hematoma: a subanalysis of the cSDH-drain randomized controlled trial. World Neurosurg. 2019;132:e283–9. https://doi.org/10.1016/j.wneu.2019.08.175.
37. Maher Hulou M, McLouth CJ, Hayden CS, Sheldrake AK, Parekh M, Dillen WL, et al. Predictors of re-operation in the setting of non-acute subdural hematomas: a 12-year single center retrospective study. J Clin Neurosci. 2020;81:334–9. https://doi.org/10.1016/j.jocn.2020.09.052.
38. Marini A, Spennato P, Aliberti F, Imperato A, Cascone D, Nastro A, et al. Brain herniation into the subdural space: rare iatrogenic complication of treatment of a giant calcified subdural hematoma. World Neurosurg. 2020;140:65–70. https://doi.org/10.1016/j.wneu.2020.05.057.
39. Martinez-Perez R, Tsimpas A, Rayo N, Cepeda S, Lagares A. Role of the patient comorbidity in the recurrence of chronic subdural hematomas. Neurosurg Rev. 2021;44(2):971–6. https://doi.org/10.1007/s10143-020-01274-7.

40. Miki K, Abe H, Morishita T, Hayashi S, Yagi K, Arima H, Inoue T. Double-crescent sign as a predictor of chronic subdural hematoma recurrence following burr-hole surgery. J Neurosurg. 2019;131:1905–11. https://doi.org/10.3171/2018.8.JNS18805.
41. Mori K, Maeda M. Surgical treatment of chronic subdural hematoma in 500 consecutive cases: clinical characteristics, surgical outcome, complications, and recurrence rate. Neurol Med Chir (Tokyo). 2001;41:371–81. https://doi.org/10.2176/nmc.41.371.
42. Motiei-Langroudi R, Stippler M, Shi S, Adeeb N, Gupta R, Griessenauer CJ, et al. Factors predicting reoperation of chronic subdural hematoma following primary surgical evacuation. J Neurosurg. 2018;129:1143–50. https://doi.org/10.3171/2017.6.JNS17130.
43. Motoie R, Karashima S, Otsuji R, Ren N, Nagaoka S, Maeda K, et al. Recurrence in 787 patients with chronic subdural hematoma: retrospective cohort investigation of associated factors including direct oral anticoagulant use. World Neurosurg. 2018;118:e87–91. https://doi.org/10.1016/j.wneu.2018.06.124.
44. Nagatani K, Takeuchi S, Sakakibara F, Otani N, Nawashiro H. Radiological factors related to recurrence of chronic subdural hematoma. Acta Neurochir (Wien). 2011;153:1713. https://doi.org/10.1007/s00701-011-0971-z.
45. Narita E, Maruya J, Nishimaki K, Heianna J, Miyauchi T, Nakahata J, et al. Case of infected subdural hematoma diagnosed by diffusion-weighted imaging. Brain Nerve. 2009;61:319–23.
46. Nayil K, Ramzan A, Sajad A, Zahoor S, Wani A, Nizami F, et al. Subdural hematomas: an analysis of 1181 Kashmiri patients. World Neurosurg. 2012;77:103–10. https://doi.org/10.1016/j.wneu.2011.06.012.
47. Ogasawara K, Ogawa A, Okuguchi T, Kobayashi M, Suzuki M, Yoshimoto T. Postoperative hyperperfusion syndrome in elderly patients with chronic subdural hematoma. Surg Neurol. 2000;54:155–9. https://doi.org/10.1016/s0090-3019(00)00281-0.
48. Ohno K, Maehara T, Ichimura K, Suzuki R, Hirakawa K, Monma S. Low incidence of seizures in patients with chronic subdural haematoma. J Neurol Neurosurg Psychiatry. 1993;56:1231–3. https://doi.org/10.1136/jnnp.56.11.1231.
49. Pang CH, Lee SE, Kim CH, Kim JE, Kang HS, Park CK, et al. Acute intracranial bleeding and recurrence after bur hole craniostomy for chronic subdural hematoma. J Neurosurg. 2015;123:65–74. https://doi.org/10.3171/2014.12.JNS141189.
50. Park KJ, Kang SH, Lee HK, Chung YG. Brain stem hemorrhage following burr hole drainage for chronic subdural hematoma-case report. Neurol Med Chir (Tokyo). 2009;49:594–7. https://doi.org/10.2176/nmc.49.594.
51. Patibandla MR, Thotakura AK, Shukla D, Purohit AK, Addagada GC, Nukavarapu M. Postoperative hematoma involving brainstem, peduncles, cerebellum, deep subcortical white matter, cerebral hemispheres following chronic subdural hematoma evacuation. Asian J Neurosurg. 2017;12:259–62. https://doi.org/10.4103/1793-5482.144163.
52. Pavlov V, Bernard G, Chibbaro S. Chronic subdural haematoma management: an iatrogenic complication. Case report and literature review. BMJ Case Rep. 2012;2012:bcr1220115397. https://doi.org/10.1136/bcr.12.2011.5397.
53. Ramachandran R, Hegde T. Chronic subdural hematomas—causes of morbidity and mortality. Surg Neurol. 2007;67:367–72. https://doi.org/10.1016/j.surneu.2006.07.022.
54. Ratilal BO, Pappamikail L, Costa J, Sampaio C. Anticonvulsants for preventing seizures in patients with chronic subdural haematoma. Cochrane Database Syst Rev. 2013;2013(6):CD004893. https://doi.org/10.1002/14651858.CD004893.pub3.
55. Rauhala M, Helén P, Huhtala H, Heikkilä P, Iverson GL, Niskakangas T, et al. Chronic subdural hematoma-incidence, complications, and financial impact. Acta Neurochir (Wien). 2020;162:2033–43. https://doi.org/10.1007/s00701-020-04398-3.
56. Reinges MH, Hasselberg I, Rohde V, Küker W, Gilsbach JM. Prospective analysis of bedside percutaneous subdural tapping for the treatment of chronic subdural haematoma in adults. J Neurol Neurosurg Psychiatry. 2000;69:40–7. https://doi.org/10.1136/jnnp.69.1.40.

57. Rohde V, Graf G, Hassler W. Complications of burr-hole craniostomy and closed-system drainage for chronic subdural hematomas: a retrospective analysis of 376 patients. Neurosurg Rev. 2002;25:89–94. https://doi.org/10.1007/s101430100182.
58. Schaumann A, Klene W, Rosenstengel C, Ringel F, Tüttenberg J, Vajkoczy P. COXIBRAIN: results of the prospective, randomised, phase II/III study for the selective COX-2 inhibition in chronic subdural haematoma patients. Acta Neurochir (Wien). 2016;158:2039–44. https://doi.org/10.1007/s00701-016-2949-3.
59. Schulz W, Saballus R, Flügel R, Harms L. Das chronische Subduralhämatom. Ein Vergleich zwischen Bohrlochtrepanation und Kraniotomie [Chronic subdural hematoma. A comparison of bore hole trepanation and craniotomy]. Zentralbl Neurochir. 1988;49:280–9.
60. Shen J, Yuan L, Ge R, Wang Q, Zhou W, Jiang XC, et al. Clinical and radiological factors predicting recurrence of chronic subdural hematoma: a retrospective cohort study. Injury. 2019;50:1634–40. https://doi.org/10.1016/j.injury.2019.08.019.
61. Shin HS, Lee SH, Ko HC, Koh JS. Extended pneumocephalus after drainage of chronic subdural hematoma associated with intracranial hypotension: case report with pathophysiologic consideration. J Korean Neurosurg Soc. 2016;59:69–74. https://doi.org/10.3340/jkns.2016.59.1.69.
62. Sun HL, Chang CJ, Hsieh CT. Contralateral acute subdural hematoma occurring after evacuation of subdural hematoma with coexistent contralateral subdural hygroma. Neurosciences (Riyadh). 2014;19:229–32.
63. Thomas PAW, Mitchell PS, Marshman LAG. Early postoperative morbidity after chronic subdural hematoma: predictive usefulness of the physiological and operative severity score for enumeration of mortality and morbidity, American College of Surgeons National Surgical Quality Improvement Program, and American Society of Anesthesiologists Grade in a Prospective Cohort. World Neurosurg. 2019;S1878-8750(18)32942–5. https://doi.org/10.1016/j.wneu.2018.12.119.
64. Torihashi K, Sadamasa N, Yoshida K, Narumi O, Chin M, Yamagata S. Independent predictors for recurrence of chronic subdural hematoma: a review of 343 consecutive surgical cases. Neurosurgery. 2008;63:1125–9. https://doi.org/10.1227/01.NEU.0000335782.60059.17.
65. Vogel TW, Dlouhy BJ, Howard MA 3rd. Don't take the plunge: avoiding adverse events with cranial perforators. J Neurosurg. 2011;115:570–5. https://doi.org/10.3171/2011.3.JNS101310.
66. Weir B. Oncotic pressure of subdural fluids. J Neurosurg. 1980;53:512–5. https://doi.org/10.3171/jns.1980.53.4.0512.
67. Won SY, Konczalla J, Dubinski D, Cattani A, Cuca C, Seifert V, et al. A systematic review of epileptic seizures in adults with subdural haematomas. Seizure. 2017;45:28–35. https://doi.org/10.1016/j.seizure.2016.11.017.
68. Yamamoto H, Hirashima Y, Hamada H, Hayashi N, Origasa H, Endo S. Independent predictors of recurrence of chronic subdural hematoma: results of multivariate analysis performed using a logistic regression model. J Neurosurg. 2003;98:1217–21. https://doi.org/10.3171/jns.2003.98.6.1217.
69. You CG, Zheng XS. Postoperative pneumocephalus increases the recurrence rate of chronic subdural hematoma. Clin Neurol Neurosurg. 2018;166:56–60. https://doi.org/10.1016/j.clineuro.2018.01.029.
70. Zavatto L, Marrone F, Allevi M, Ricci A, Taddei G. Bilateral oculomotor palsy after surgical evacuation of chronic subdural hematoma. World Neurosurg. 2019;127:241–4. https://doi.org/10.1016/j.wneu.2019.04.043.

Chapter 34
Postoperative Management and Follow-Up Strategies for Chronic Subdural Hematoma

Meryem Himmiche, Mohammed Benzagmout, and Faycal Lakhdar

34.1 Introduction

Chronic subdural hematoma (CSDH) is a frequent neurosurgical condition, commonly seen in elderly people. With the frequent use of anticoagulant and antiplatelet agents and the extended life expectancy in the older population, the incidence of this illness continues to increase [58].

The management of CSDH varies according to the patient profile and the best strategy for appropriate treatment is still debated [55]. Indeed, surgical evacuation and drainage of the hematoma in symptomatic patients should lead to a better clinical outcome. However, the postoperative management of CSDH still remains highly empirical resulting in some gaps in our current knowledge. These gaps raise many unanswered questions regarding postoperative care such as the potential value of adjuvant medications to improve outcome. To date, there isn't any uniform care protocol for the optimal management and follow-up of CSDH [7].

The postoperative stage requires developing standard care protocols which is a fundamental requirement that would allow for minimizing complications, preventing recurrences, promoting recovery, and improving the patient outcome [8]. Several factors are important to consider such as the method of anticoagulation correction, commencement/resumption of prophylactic or therapeutic anticoagulation/antiplatelet therapy, early patient mobilization versus bed rest, duration of drain

M. Himmiche
Department of Neurosurgery, Regional Hospital of Laayoune, Laayoune, Morocco

M. Benzagmout (✉) · F. Lakhdar
Department of Neurosurgery, University Hospital of Fez, Fez, Morocco

Clinical Neurosciences Laboratory, Sidi Mohammed Benabdellah University Fez, Fez, Morocco

M. Turgut et al. (eds.), *Subdural Hematoma*,
https://doi.org/10.1007/978-3-030-79371-5_34

placement, perioperative antibiotic application, and the use of adjunctive medications (e.g., antiepileptics or steroids).

In the following sections, we will summarize the postoperative management provided to CSDH neurosurgical patients as well as the clinical and radiological follow-up strategies.

34.2 Postoperative Management

Regardless of the neurosurgical procedure selected to treat the hematoma and the patient's clinical condition, several details should be considered in the postoperative management of CSDH. This management starts in the operating room and includes monitoring the head position as well as the hemodynamic and respiratory parameters. The main goal is to ensure optimal medical treatment in order to stabilize the clinical state of the patient, prevent early complications, and avoid any potential neurological deficits [7].

34.2.1 Patient Care and Monitoring

After the hematoma evacuation, the recovery process will take time and the patient should progressively return to their usual level of energy [7]. The patient should expect to stay in hospital for 2–5 days postoperatively [52], in a standard medical care ward or neurosurgical critical care unit depending on their level of consciousness before surgery and the perioperative patient's clinical status [56].

In a few cases, general anesthesia might be indicated and the postoperative extubation of the patient can take place soon after surgery or may be delayed [7, 50]. Careful postoperative neurologic monitoring is indicated for all patients for a minimum of 6 h after surgery [7].

After surgery, CSDH patients that have a worsening neurological status require crucial medical attention in an intensive care unit (ICU) [13]. An intracranial pressure (ICP) monitor should be instituted promptly in order to manage cranial perfusion pressure in patients with presumed elevation of ICP and who have radiological brain herniation [12]. Consequently, several key elements have to be managed [7]:

- Control of blood pressure, heart rate, and respiratory parameters
- Emergence from anesthesia
- Vigilance and early detection of surgical complications: seizures, stroke, anisocoria, neurological deficit, CSF leak, infection
- Maintaining euthermia and a normal blood glucose level
- Drain monitoring

In general, aged or vulnerable patients require 12–24 h of postoperative hospitalization with ICU-level monitoring; afterwards, they can be discharged to the general neurosurgical floor especially when their preoperative functional level was satisfactory [23]. Early mobilization after day 2 will help to prevent postoperative complications without increasing the risk of recurrence [3, 31].

34.2.2 *Patient Mobilization*

After surgical treatment, the timing of patient mobilization remains controversial and practice patterns are highly variable with regard to early mobilization versus prolonged bed rest [28, 65]. Early mobilization is thought to decrease position-related complications after surgery [31]. However, bed rest can also be planned to promote brain re-expansion, hence decreasing the risk of recurrence after CSDH evacuation [35].

Regarding this aspect, the attitudes of surgeons are quite varied. Some recommend early mobilization during the first 24 h, while others prefer delaying mobilization until after drain removal to promote brain re-expansion and fluid drainage [48]. In fact, it is well known that bed rest in a horizontal position following surgery will positively influence the clinical course by facilitating gravitational drainage of any residual subdural fluid, reducing recurrence rates, and promoting brain re-expansion [35, 65].

In addition, studies have reported no difference in terms of recurrence rates between early mobilization on the first postoperative day compared to delayed mobilization after 3 days or even later. However, they emphasized the value of early postoperative patient mobilization to decrease the risk of complications (urinary tract infection, pneumonia, deep vein thrombosis, and decubitus ulcer formation) [17, 28, 31, 35, 42].

34.2.3 *Head Position*

The role of postoperative head position in the recurrence of CSDH had not been studied sufficiently [27]. A flat head position versus an upright head location soon after surgery seems to not be associated with a significantly increased incidence of postoperative complications [4].

Assuming a 30° head up position in cases of CSDH does not affect the outcome, especially regarding the frequency of symptomatic recurrences, reoperations, or medical complications [27, 62]. Nevertheless, increased recurrence was observed when the headboard level was over-raised by more than 30–40° without other position-related complications [2].

In some studies, an upright posture soon after burr-hole surgery was associated with an increased incidence of CSDH recurrence but not with a significant change in other position-related postsurgical complications [29]. According to this result, an upright position soon after surgery especially in elderly patients is not recommended [2].

It is wise to conclude that patient/head positioning in the postoperative period should be determined based on the patient profile. Nevertheless, special emphasis should be given to all methods of preventing bed rest complications, particularly in elderly fragile patients.

34.2.4 Drain Monitoring and Removal

Burr-hole craniostomy with a closed system drainage is the most common surgical technique used to treat CSDH [16, 53, 64, 74]. Indeed, multiple studies have shown that the use of drainage reduces recurrence significantly and mortality at 6 months [20, 57].

Drainage with a flexible bulb such as a Jackson-Pratt drain has to be managed properly. Fluid inside the bulb should be removed several times per day and the resulting vacuum creates suction which gradually draws hematoma fluid from the subdural space into the bulb. It is important when manipulating the drain to observe the surrounding skin in order to detect any possible signs of wound infection or cranial cerebrospinal fluid leakage.

The effect of a long drainage duration on the functional results and recurrence rates of CSDH has not been studied sufficiently [20]. However, some studies have presumed that it takes at least 3 days of drainage for the CSDH outer membrane to restore the normal balance between coagulation and fibrinolysis after surgery [74].

To date, there is no consensus regarding the necessary duration of the drainage after CSDH surgery. Some authors have systematically removed the draining system 48 h postoperatively [35, 63]. However, others prefer to keep the system draining for longer than 48 h [34, 40, 41, 63, 74]. Commonly, 2–4 days of closed system drainage after a burr-hole craniotomy is an effective choice for treating CSDH, but increasing the drainage duration to 5–7 days can provide better results by decreasing the postoperative residual hematoma thickness and thereby minimizing the recurrence risk without increasing the risk of other complications [29].

34.2.5 Medical Treatment

34.2.5.1 Adjuvant Corticotherapy

There has been increasing evidence that inflammatory mediators play a major role in the pathogenesis of CSDH. In fact, steroids are often used as an adjuvant treatment to surgery [26, 54, 65]. Methylprednisolone and dexamethasone are the two medications widely used in neurosurgical practice. They both improve postoperative outcome and have a beneficial effect on survival [37, 67].

Steroids are used for 21 days to 1 month with a dose of 1 mg/kg/day for methylprednisolone and 4 mg/8 h/day for dexamethasone with a slow taper [36, 49]. The mean total duration of the treatment is approximately 2 months [65, 75]. Steroid treatment is not recommended for all CSDH operated patients [24]. They are indicated for patients with a high recurrence rate risk, i.e., aged people, CSDH with significant midline displacement or a mixed-density hematoma on the CT scan [5]. Clinical and biological follow-up is necessary to limit the adverse effects of corticosteroid use [49].

34.2.5.2 Antiepileptic Prophylaxis

Although the real effectiveness of antiepileptic prophylaxis to reduce the occurrence of postoperative seizures remains controversial, many authors recommend their use in CSDH, particularly when they are associated with other brain injuries that are well known as risk factors for future crises.

Overall, the incidence of postoperative seizures in CSDH patients is low, but their risk is much higher in the presence of a large amount of postoperative pneumocephalus because of the cortical irritation caused by the air bubbles. In addition, it appears that early postoperative seizures have a high incidence of occurring in chronic alcohol consumers [10, 51] and in patients with a mixed-density hematoma on the preoperative CT scan [11].

The identification of high-risk patients and predictors for acute symptomatic seizure/status epilepticus (ASZ/SE) is important because they are associated with a worse functional outcome at discharge as well as at follow-up [69]. A remote stroke, GCS $\leq$ 13 on admission, and recurrent hematoma are all predictors for experiencing ASZ/SE which is unlike drainage insertion [69].

Like Flores et al., we believe that antiepileptic prophylaxis should not be routinely administered if any of the aforementioned seizure risk factors exist [18]. However, pre- and postoperative monitoring by CT scan and EEG before starting a prophylactic antiepileptic treatment is highly recommended. The final prognosis for this kind of postoperative epilepsy remains good.

34.2.5.3 Antibiotic Therapy

Following standard practice patterns, most patients receive prophylactic antibiotics usually as a single-shot dose intraoperatively or also for one postoperative day [65]. However, there is no scientific data supporting long-term prophylactic antibiotic therapy, while the use of a postoperative subdural space drain is widely accepted. Indeed, the absence of direct contact of foreign material with the brain parenchyma potentially minimizes the risk of a postoperative empyema.

34.2.5.4 Venous Thromboembolism (VTE) Prophylaxis

Although patients undergoing neurosurgical procedures are at a high risk for venous thromboembolism, the question of VTE prophylaxis in CSDH patients is still a matter of controversy in the literature. Due to their impaired mobility and various vascular comorbidities, such as coronary artery disease and atrial fibrillation in many elderly patients with CSDH, thromboembolism prophylaxis is often necessary after surgical evacuation and clinicians are challenged to clearly balance the risks and benefits of such treatment.

In many institutions, chemical VTE prophylaxis is routinely started after drain removal [50]. Others consider it reasonable and safe to use early chemical VTE prophylaxis 24 h after surgical intervention in stable patients without an impact on CSDH recurrence [1, 50].

On the other hand, this controversy concerning the use of anticoagulant drugs is sustained by the higher CSDH recurrence rate and VTE-associated complications [1, 50]. The application of postoperative thromboembolism prophylaxis always plays a role in the surgeon's decision-making which obviously causes a selection bias. More studies are needed to compare the risks and benefits of early postoperative chemical VTE prophylaxis and also to determine when is the ideal time to begin treatment [1].

34.2.5.5 Resumption of Anticoagulant/Antiplatelet Drugs

The perioperative management of anticoagulant and antiplatelet drugs is complex and the timing of their resumption is still debated [60]. Although these medications might be given for important indications, the surgical management of CSDH often requires their temporary suspension which could expose the patient to thromboembolic or cardiological complications [19]. Both antiplatelet drugs and anticoagulant therapy are used as curative treatment and for primary and secondary prevention measures in cases of thromboembolic events or coronary arterial diseases. Those drugs have been implicated in both the development and recurrence of CSDH [68], managing these medications postoperatively is complicated without adding the risks of hemorrhage or thromboembolic events [47].

In the literature, multiple variables remain unclear and controversial, including the indication for anticoagulation and antithrombotic treatment, the most appropriate time for postoperative resumption, drug of choice for resumption, risk for future falls and head trauma, and dose and time at which the anticoagulation reaches therapeutic levels postoperatively [10, 43].

In patients undergoing a burr-hole trepanation for CSDH, the early resumption of low-dose ASA (acetylsalicylic acid) therapy is not associated with a high risk of hemorrhage [30]. However, patients with a history of preoperative antithrombotic therapy experienced a high risk of thromboembolic complications; then, resuming antithrombotic therapy earlier by the third day after surgery is reasonable with a low risk of postoperative hemorrhage [22].

For vitamin K antagonists, the European Society of Cardiologists and the European Stroke Initiative recommend suspending all oral anticoagulation therapy for 7–14 days after oral anticoagulation-related intracranial hemorrhage, even in high-risk patients with mechanical heart valves [43].

To date, there is no consensus regarding how to manage these medications postoperatively [47], so it is a highly individualized process, generally left to the neurosurgical team and the investigators to balance the pros and cons of treatment and to establish an adequate protocol with a thorough consideration of the patient age, comorbidities, and respective risk of bleeding and thromboembolism [10, 43, 47].

34.2.5.6 Other Treatments

Several drugs have been suggested and investigated as potential adjunctive therapies for CSDH including angiotensin converting enzyme (ACE) inhibitors, statins, tranexamic acid, celecoxib, Goreisan, and atorvastatin but none of these agents have sufficient evidence to support their routine use [17].

These medications might reduce the risk of CSDH recurrence by exerting different anti-inflammatory and anti-angiogenic actions. Indeed, ACE inhibitors act by reducing the formation of immature vessels in the hematoma wall [17] while statins are known to exhibit anti-inflammatory effects and to facilitate blood vessel repair by recruiting endothelial progenitor cells [17].

Tranexamic acid has been used as an antifibrinolytic drug for bleeding control in pediatric patients and can effectively resolve the CSDH by inhibiting fibrinolysis and the kinin-kallikrein inflammatory system [17, 66]. Celecoxib is a non-steroidal anti-inflammatory drug that acts by inhibiting cyclooxygenase-2 which is significantly higher in CSDH fluid; hence, it was thought to shrink the hematoma volume [17]. Recently, atorvastatin has been reported to be effective in preventing CSDH recurrence [32, 71] and evidence showed that atorvastatin is safe and effective in reducing hematoma volume and improving neurological function of the patients [25].

Finally, Goreisan, a traditional Japanese Kampo medicine, is widely used as adjunctive treatment to prevent CSDH recurrence after surgery [72]. This drug has been used as a diuretic to increase urine output and reduce cerebral edema in a mouse model of ischemic stroke, and also as an adjuvant for patients after surgery to cure CSDH [17].

34.2.6 Patient Discharge

All surgically treated CSDH patients leave the hospital soon after drain removal and recovery. However, some patients are discharged home, some to nursing homes, and others need medical rehabilitation therapy and are transferred to appropriate health care institutions [13, 39].

The median length of hospital stay for surgically treated patients is 3 days without early complications; some elderly patients need more time before discharge. After CSDH surgery, the length of hospital stay has deceased over the years due to the improvement achieved in surgical technique especially with burr-hole craniostomy with drainage performed under local or locoregional anesthesia [6].

34.3 Follow-Up

34.3.1 Clinical Follow-Up

Planned follow-up after surgery and patient discharge is necessary to decrease complication occurrence and allow for selecting patients who will undergo reoperation at an early stage.

One-month, 2–3-month, and 6-month follow-up intervals seem to be sufficient to monitor the evolution of the patient recovery, while several studies showed that recovery occurred within 60 days after surgery [45, 55].

Indeed, the clinical profile of CSDH patients has indicated that a 3-month follow-up period after burr-hole surgery is likely sufficient for most asymptomatic patients because the risk of recurrence thereafter seems to be very low [33].

Clinical follow-up requires special attention to:

- Residual neurological problems including seizures, wound infection, cerebrospinal fluid leak, fever, headache, speech, or motor disturbances.
- Behavioral and cognitive disorders that are mostly assessed using mental tests including the Modified Rankin Scale.
- Any potential adverse effect caused by steroids or antithrombotic drugs.

Finally, the clinical improvement of both motor and cognitive profiles of CSDH patients in the postoperative stage would lead and promote good and rapid recovery.

34.3.2 Radiological Follow-Up

The utility of postoperative imaging remains controversial especially in asymptomatic patients. In common practice, various approaches are used. Some authors are performing routinely a postoperative CT scan for control [70] while others are proceeding in the event of clinical deterioration [59].

A routinely scheduled CT scan after surgery has no convincing effect on the final outcome [46]. However, a CT scan should be performed in patients with neurological deterioration or persisting neurological deficits [61].

It seems reasonable to obtain an imaging control CT scan in the case of clinical symptoms related to raised intracranial pressure and/or cortical irritation. In addition, an early postoperative CT scan might be justified to better appreciate any potential residual subdural collection that could influence brain re-expansion, and to investigate any other risk factors of recurrence [38] or potential predictive signs of seizures such as midline shift and postoperative trapped air [69].

Residual subdural collection is a common feature usually occurring after CSDH evacuation [15], and could be medically treated when necessary [66]. According to Ng et al. [44], residual postoperative hematoma volume can be anticipated from the preoperative hematoma volume. Hence, the postoperative CT scan may not be necessary since it is possible to assess the degree of brain re-expansion based on the suspected residual volume calculated from the preoperative hematoma volume [44].

Based on the earlier discussion, we believe that the decision to perform a postoperative CT scan for control should be tailored according to each patient profile in order to reduce the risks of radiation exposure.

34.4 Rehabilitation Therapy Program

Elderly people with CSDH might show a large spectrum of neurological deficits, including motor, speech, cognitive, and behavioral disorders [21]. After surgery, ambulatory and functional status might remain limited despite successful surgical evacuation [73]. Hence, an adequate rehabilitation program could help to rapidly discharge elderly patients before their full recovery [9]. Physiotherapy has a major role to better improve gait balance and motor weakness. Speech therapy should help speech and communication problems while psychological support allows for promoting rapid social reintegration [14].

34.5 Conclusion

CSDH is the most common clinical entity encountered in daily neurosurgical practice. However, its management remains highly empirical due to some gaps in our current knowledge and raises a number of unanswered questions regarding the appropriate surgical technique and any postoperative processes. To date, there is no standardized postoperative protocol and routine follow-up schedules to manage this well-known disease entity. Improving neurosurgical team knowledge and developing standardized postoperative approaches and follow-up protocols could further optimize patient care and clinical outcomes. Therefore, supporting more basic research and building CSDH multidisciplinary care capacities are a major necessity (Figs. 34.1, 34.2, 34.3, 34.4, and 34.5).

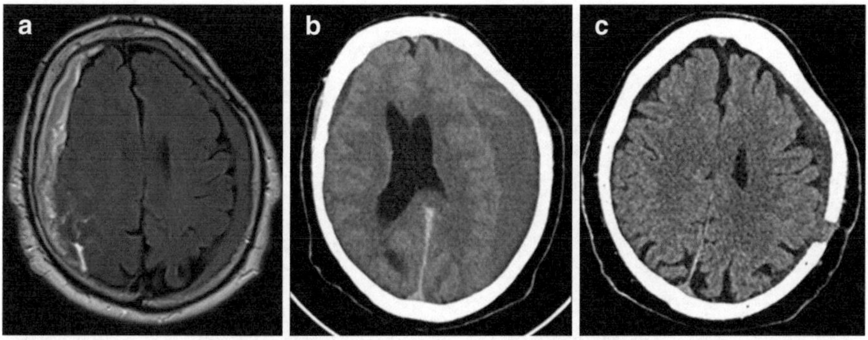

Fig. 34.1 (**a**) Preoperative brain MRI demonstrating bilateral paucisymptomatic frontoparietal CSDH treated conservatively. (**b**) One-month follow-up CT scan demonstrating obvious volume increase of the left CSDH and significant reduction of the right CSDH. (**c**) Postoperative CT scan showing residual left subdural collection

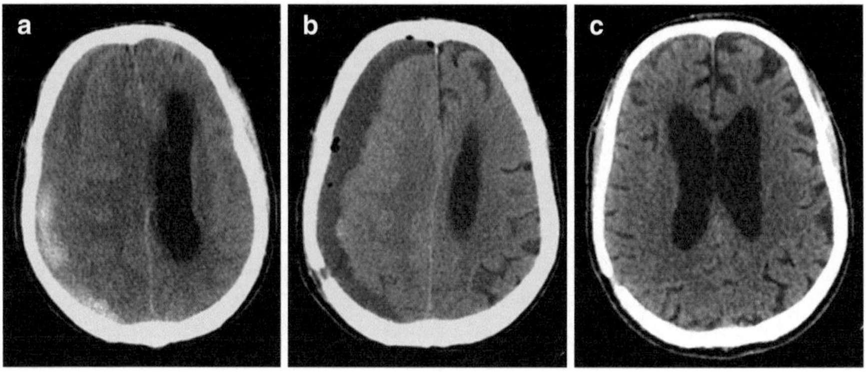

Fig. 34.2 (**a**) Initial CT scan demonstrating large right frontoparietal CSDH. (**b**) Three-week follow-up CT scan demonstrating CSDH recurrence. (**c**) Four-month follow-up CT scan demonstrating total disappearance of the right hematoma

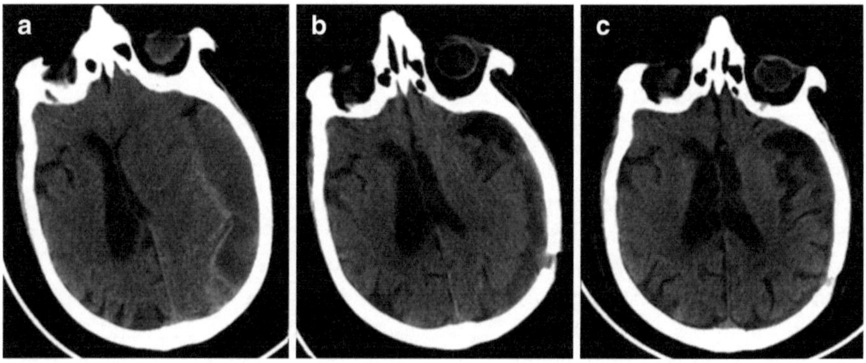

Fig. 34.3 (**a**) Initial brain CT scan demonstrating left compressive CSDH in elderly patient. (**b**) One-month follow-up CT scan demonstrating significant reduction of the CSDH and the related mass effect on the midline structures. (**c**) Four-month follow-up CT scan demonstrating total absence of the CSDH

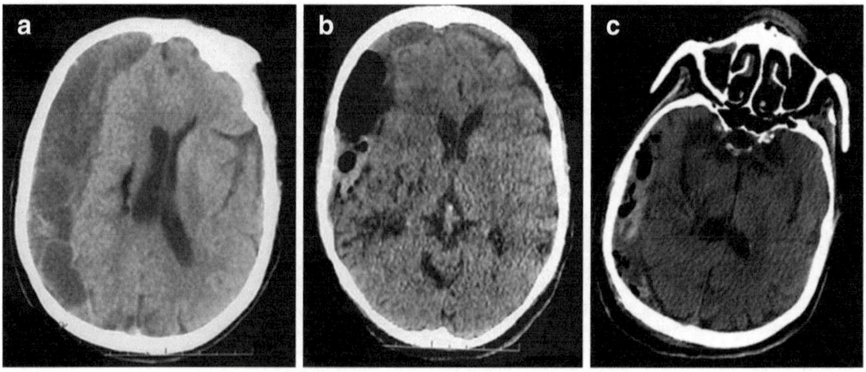

Fig. 34.4 (**a**) Initial brain CT scan demonstrating right compressive frontoparietal CSDH. (**b**, **c**) Immediate postoperative CT scan revealing postoperative pneumocephalus inside the hematoma cavity

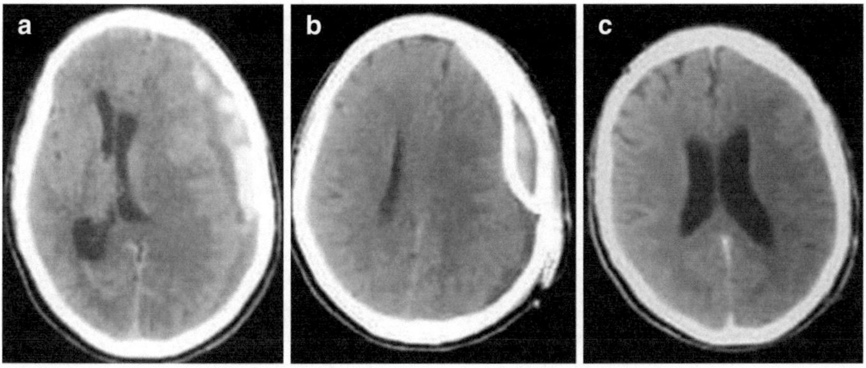

Fig. 34.5 (**a**) Initial brain CT scan demonstrating left CSDH with acute rebleeding. (**b**) Immediate postoperative CT scan showing the drain position. (**c**) Late CT scan demonstrating total resolution of the CSDH

References

1. Abboud T, Dührsen L, Gibbert C, Westphal M, Martens T. Influence of antithrombotic agents on recurrence rate and clinical outcome in patients operated for chronic subdural hematoma. Neurocirugia (Astur). 2018;29(2):86–92.
2. Abouzari M, Rashidi A, Rezaii J, et al. The role of postoperative patient posture in the recurrence of traumatic chronic subdural hematoma after burr-hole surgery. Neurosurgery. 2007;61(4):794–7.
3. Adeolu AA, Rabiu TB, Adeleye AO. Post-operative day two versus day seven mobilization after burr-hole drainage of subacute and chronic subdural haematoma in Nigerians. Br J Neurosurg. 2012;26(5):743–6.
4. Alcalá-Cerra G, Moscote-Salazar LR, Paternina-Caicedo Á, Gutiérrez-Paternina JJ, Niño-Hernández LM, Sabogal-Barrios R. Postoperative bed header position after burr-hole drainage of chronic subdural haematoma: systematic review and meta-analysis of randomised controlled trials. Neurocirugia (Astur). 2014;25(3):99–107.
5. Altaf I, Shams S, Vohra AH. Radiological predictors of recurrence of chronic subdural hematoma. Pak J Med Sci. 2018;34(1):194–7.
6. Balser D, Rodgers SD, Johnson B, Shi C, Tabak E, Samadani U. Evolving management of symptomatic chronic subdural hematoma: experience of a single institution and review of the literature. Neurol Res. 2013;35(3):233–42.
7. Bose G, Luoma AMV. Postoperative care of neurosurgical patients: general principles. Anaesth Intensive Care Med. 2017;18(6):296–303.
8. Brennan PM, Kolias AG, Joannides AJ, et al. The management and outcome for patients with chronic subdural hematoma: a prospective, multicenter, observational cohort study in the United Kingdom. J Neurosurg. 2017;17:1–8.
9. Carlisi E, Feltroni L, Tinelli C, Verlotta M, Gaetani P, Dalla Toffola E. Postoperative rehabilitation for chronic subdural hematoma in the elderly. An observational study focusing on balance, ambulation and discharge destination. Eur J Phys Rehabil Med. 2017;53(1):91–7.
10. Chari A, Clemente Morgado T, Rigamonti D. Recommencement of anticoagulation in chronic subdural haematoma: a systematic review and meta-analysis. Br J Neurosurg. 2014;28(1):2–7.
11. Chen CW, Kuo JR, Lin HJ, et al. Early post-operative seizures after burr-hole drainage for chronic subdural hematoma: correlation with brain CT findings. J Clin Neurosci. 2004;11(7):706–9.

12. China Neurosurgical Critical Care Specialist Council (CNCCSC), Zhao JZ, Zhou DB, et al. The experts consensus for patient management of neurosurgical critical care unit in China. Chin Med J (Engl). 2015;128(9):1252–67.
13. Christopher E, Poon MTC, Glancz LJ, et al. Outcomes following surgery in subgroups of comatose and very elderly patients with chronic subdural hematoma. Neurosurg Rev. 2019;42(2):427–31.
14. Dang B, Chen W, He W, Chen G. Rehabilitation treatment and progress of Traumatic Brain Injury Dysfunction. Neural Plast. 2017;2017:1582182.
15. Dudoit T, Labeyrie PE, Deryckere S, Emery E, Gaberel T. Is systematic post-operative CT scan indicated after chronic subdural hematoma surgery? A case-control study. Acta Neurochir (Wien). 2016;158:1241–6.
16. Farhat Neto J, Araujo JL, Ferraz VR, Haddad L, Veiga JC. Chronic subdural hematoma: epidemiological and prognostic analysis of 176 cases. Rev Col Bras Cir. 2015;42(5):283–7.
17. Feghali J, Yang W, Huang J. Updates in chronic subdural hematoma: epidemiology, etiology, pathogenesis, treatment, and outcome. World Neurosurg. 2020;141:339–45.
18. Flores G, Vicenty JC, Pastrana EA. Post-operative seizures after burr hole evacuation of chronic subdural hematomas: is prophylactic anti-epileptic medication needed? Acta Neurochir (Wien). 2017;159(11):2033–6.
19. Fornebo I, Sjåvik K, Alibeck M, et al. Role of antithrombotic therapy in the risk of hematoma recurrence and thromboembolism after chronic subdural hematoma evacuation: a population-based consecutive cohort study. Acta Neurochir (Wien). 2017;159(11):2045–52.
20. Glancz LJ, Poon MTC, Coulter IC, et al. Does drain position and duration influence outcomes in patients undergoing Burr-Hole evacuation of chronic subdural hematoma? Lessons from a UK multicenter prospective cohort study. Neurosurgery. 2019;85(4):486–93.
21. Gill M, Maheshwari V, Narang A, Lingaraju TS. Impact on cognitive improvement following Burr-Hole evacuation of chronic subdural hematoma: a prospective observational study. J Neurosci Rural Pract. 2018;9(4):457–60.
22. Guha D, Coyne S, Macdonald RL. Timing of the resumption of antithrombotic agents following surgical evacuation of chronic subdural hematomas: a retrospective cohort study. J Neurosurg. 2016;124(3):750–9.
23. Hanak BW, Walcott BP, Nahed BV, et al. Postoperative intensive care unit requirements after elective craniotomy. World Neurosurg. 2014;81(1):165–72.
24. Henaux PL, Le Reste PJ, Laviolle B, Morandi X. Steroids in chronic subdural hematomas (SUCRE trial): study protocol for a randomized controlled trial. Trials. 2017;18(1):252.
25. Huang J, Gao C, Dong J, Zhang J, Jiang R. Drug treatment of chronic subdural hematoma. Expert Opin Pharmacother. 2020;21(4):435–44.
26. Iliescu IA. Current diagnosis and treatment of chronic subdural hematomas. J Med Life. 2015;8(3):278–84.
27. Ishfaq A, Ahmed I, Bhatti SH. Effect of head positioning on outcome after burr hole craniostomy for chronic subdural haematoma. J Coll Physicians Surg Pak. 2009;19(8):492–5.
28. Janowski M, Kunert P. Intravenous fluid administration may improve post-operative course of patients with chronic subdural hematoma: a retrospective study. PLoS One. 2012;7(4):e35634.
29. Kale A, Öz İİ, Gün EG, Kalaycı M, Gül Ş. Is the recurrence rate of chronic subdural hematomas dependent on the duration of drainage? Neurol Res. 2017;39(5):399–402.
30. Kamenova M, Lutz K, Schaedelin S, Fandino J, Mariani L, Soleman J. Does early resumption of low-dose aspirin after evacuation of chronic subdural hematoma with burr-hole drainage Lead to higher recurrence rates? Neurosurgery. 2016;79(5):715–21.
31. Kurabe S, Ozawa T, Watanabe T, Aiba T. Efficacy and safety of postoperative early mobilization for chronic subdural hematoma in elderly patients. Acta Neurochir. 2010;152:1171–4.
32. Liu H, Luo Z, Liu Z, Yang J, Kan S. Atorvastatin may attenuate recurrence of chronic subdural hematoma. Front Neurosci. 2016;10:303.
33. Lutz K, Kamenova M, Schaedelin S, et al. Time to and possible risk factors for recurrence after burr-hole drainage of chronic subdural hematoma: a subanalysis of the cSDH-drain randomized controlled trial. World Neurosurg. 2019;132:e283–9.

34. Matsumoto K, Akagi K, Abekura M, et al. Recurrence factors for chronic subdural hematomas after burr-hole craniostomy and closed system drainage. Neurol Res. 1999;21(3):277–80.
35. Mehta V, Harward SC, Sankey EW, Nayar G, Codd PJ. Evidence based diagnosis and management of chronic subdural hematoma: a review of the literature. J Clin Neurosci. 2018;50:7–15.
36. Merrill SA, Khan D, Richards AE, Kalani MA, Patel NP, Neal MT. Functional recovery following surgery for chronic subdural hematoma. Surg Neurol Int. 2020;11:450.
37. Miah IP, Herklots M, Roks G, et al. Dexamethasone therapy in symptomatic chronic subdural hematoma (DECSA-R): a retrospective evaluation of initial corticosteroid therapy versus primary surgery. J Neurotrauma. 2020;37(2):366–72.
38. Montano N, Stifano V, Skrap B, Mazzucchi E. Management of residual subdural hematoma after burr-hole evacuation. The role of fluid therapy and review of the literature. J Clin Neurosci. 2017;46:26–9.
39. Mulligan P, Raore B, Liu S, Olson JJ. Neurological and functional outcomes of subdural hematoma evacuation in patients over 70 years of age. J Neurosci Rural Pract. 2013;4(3):250–6.
40. Nakaguchi H, Tanishima T, Yoshimasu N. Relationship between drainage catheter location and postoperative recurrence of chronic subdural hematoma after burr-hole irrigation and closed-system drainage. J Neurosurg. 2000;93(5):791–5.
41. Nakaguchi H, Tanishima T, Yoshimasu N. Factors in the natural history of chronic subdural hematomas that influence their postoperative recurrence. J Neurosurg. 2001;95(2):256–62.
42. Nakajima H, Yasui T, Nishikawa M, Kishi H, Kan M. The role of postoperative patient posture in the recurrence of chronic subdural hematoma: a prospective randomized trial. Surg Neurol. 2002;58:385.
43. Nassiri F, Hachem LD, Wang JZ. Reinitiation of anticoagulation after surgical evacuation of subdural hematomas. World Neurosurg. 2020;135:e616–22.
44. Ng HY, Ng WH, King NK. Value of routine early post-operative computed tomography in determining short-term functional outcome after drainage of chronic subdural hematoma: an evaluation of residual volume. Surg Neurol Int. 2014;5:136.
45. Oh HJ, Lee KS, Shim JJ, Yoon SM, Yun IG, Bae HG. Postoperative course and recurrence of chronic subdural hematoma. J Korean Neurosurg Soc. 2010;48(6):518–23.
46. Pedersen CB, Sundbye F, Poulsen FR. No value of routine Brain Computed Tomography 6 weeks after evacuation of chronic subdural hematoma. Surg J (N Y). 2017;3(4):e174–6.
47. Phan K, Abi-Hanna D, Kerferd J, et al. Resumption of antithrombotic agents in chronic subdural hematoma: a systematic review and meta-analysis. World Neurosurg. 2018;109:e792–9.
48. Prud'homme M, Mathieu F, Marcotte N, Cottin S. A pilot placebo controlled randomized controlled trial of Dexamethasone for Chronic Subdural Haematoma. Can J Neurol Sci. 2016;43(2):284–90.
49. Qian Z, Yang D, Sun F, Sun Z. Risk factors for recurrence of chronic subdural hematoma after burr-hole surgery: potential protective role of dexamethasone. Br J Neurosurg. 2017;31(1):84–8.
50. Ragland JT, Lee K. Chronic subdural hematoma ICU management. Neurosurg Clin N Am. 2017;28(2):239–46.
51. Ratilal BO, Pappamikail L, Costa J, Sampaio C. Anticonvulsants for preventing seizures in patients with chronic subdural haematoma. Cochrane Database Syst Rev. 2013;2013(6):CD004893.
52. Rauhala M, Helén P, Huhtala H, et al. Chronic subdural hematoma-incidence, complications, and financial impact. Acta Neurochir (Wien). 2020;162(9):2033–43.
53. Ro HW, Park SK, Jang DK, Yoon WS, Jang KS, Han YM. Preoperative predictive factors for surgical and functional outcomes in chronic subdural hematoma. Acta Neurochir (Wien). 2016;158(1):135–9.
54. Roh D, Reznik M, Claassen J. Chronic subdural medical management. Neurosurg Clin N Am. 2017;28(2):211–7.
55. Sakakibara F, Tsuzuki N, Uozumi Y, Nawashiro H, Shima K. Chronic subdural hematoma—recurrence and prevention. Brain Nerve. 2011;63(1):69–74.

56. Santafé Colomina M, Arikan Abelló F, Sánchez Corral A, Ferrer Roca R. Optimization of the neurosurgical patient in Intensive Care. Med Intensiva. 2019;43(8):489–96.
57. Santarius T, Kirkpatrick PJ, Ganesan D, et al. Use of drains versus no drains after burr-hole evacuation of chronic subdural haematoma: a randomised controlled trial. Lancet. 2009;374(9695):1067–73.
58. Santarius T, Kirkpatrick PJ, Kolias AG, Hutchinson PJ. Working toward rational and evidence-based treatment of chronic subdural hematoma. Clin Neurosurg. 2010;57:112–22.
59. Santarius T, Lawton R, Kirkpatrick PJ, Hutchinson PJ. The management of primary chronic subdural hematoma: a questionnaire survey of practice in the United Kingdom and the Republic of Ireland. Br J Neurosurg. 2008;22:529–234.
60. Scerrati A, Germanò A, Trevisi G, et al. Timing of low-dose aspirin discontinuation and the influence on clinical outcome of patients undergoing surgery for chronic subdural hematoma. World Neurosurg. 2019;129:e695–9.
61. Schucht P, Fischer U, Fung C, et al. Follow-up computed tomography after evacuation of chronic subdural hematoma. N Engl J Med. 2019;380(12):1186–7.
62. Sholapurkar TU, Mahantashetti SS, Shenoy RY, Ghorpade RS, Maste PS. Chronic subdural hematoma: influence of head position (head low/supine) postoperatively on recurrence rate after burr hole craniotomy. J Sci Soc. 2014;41(3):173.
63. Sindou M, Ibrahim I, Maarrawi J. Chronic subdural hematomas: twist drill craniostomy with a closed system of drainage, for 48 hours only, is a valuable surgical treatment. Acta Neurochir. 2010;152(3):545–6.
64. Singh AK, Suryanarayanan B, Choudhary A, Prasad A, Singh S, Gupta LN. A prospective randomized study of use of drain versus no drain after burr-hole evacuation of chronic subdural hematoma. Neurol India. 2014;62(2):169–74.
65. Soleman J, Kamenov M, Lutz K, Guzman R, Fandino J, Mariani L. Drain insertion in chronic subdural hematoma: an international survey of practice. World Neurosurg. 2017;104:528–36.
66. Tanweer O, Frisoli FA, Bravate C, et al. Tranexamic acid for treatment of residual subdural hematoma after bedside twist-drill evacuation. World Neurosurg. 2016;91:29–33.
67. Thotakura AK, Marabathina NR. The role of medical treatment in chronic subdural hematoma. Asian J Neurosurg. 2018;13(4):976–83.
68. Wang H, Zhang M, Zheng H, et al. The effects of antithrombotic drugs on the recurrence and mortality in patients with chronic subdural hematoma: a meta-analysis. Medicine (Baltimore). 2019;98(1):e13972.
69. Won SY, Dubinski D, Sautter L, et al. Seizure and status epilepticus in chronic subdural hematoma. Acta Neurol Scand. 2019;140(3):194–203.
70. Wu L, Ou Y, Liu W. Benefit of postoperative computed tomography in chronic subdural hematoma. J Neurosurg. 2019;131(6):1992–3.
71. Xu M, Chen P, Zhu X, Wang C, Shi X, Yu B. Effects of atorvastatin on conservative and surgical treatments of chronic subdural hematoma in patients. World Neurosurg. 2016;91:23–8.
72. Yasunaga H. Effect of Japanese herbal Kampo medicine Goreisan on reoperation rates after burr-hole surgery for chronic subdural hematoma: analysis of a National Inpatient Database. Evid Based Complement Alternat Med. 2015;2015:817616.
73. Ye HH, Kim JH, Kim YS, Cho CW, Kim DJ. Cognitive impairment in the elderly with chronic subdural hematoma. J Korean Neurotraumatol Soc. 2008;4(2):66–9.
74. Yu GJ, Han CZ, Zhang M, Zhuang HT, Jiang YG. Prolonged drainage reduces the recurrence of chronic subdural hematoma. Br J Neurosurg. 2009;23(6):606–11.
75. Zhang Y, Chen S, Xiao Y, Tang W. Effects of Dexamethasone in the treatment of Recurrent Chronic Subdural Hematoma. World Neurosurg. 2017;105:115–21.

Chapter 35
Corticosteroid Therapy for Chronic Subdural Hematomas

Timothy Beutler and Satish Krishnamurthy

35.1 Introduction

Chronic subdural hematoma (CSDH) is one of the most common neurosurgical conditions, yet the pathophysiology and optimal treatment for the disease remains controversial. Surgical treatment includes a variety of options ranging from traditional open craniotomy to minimally invasive bedside twist drill craniostomy. Despite best surgical management, the recurrence rate of CSDH has been reported as high as 26% [10]. In addition to the risk of recurrence, surgery has the inherent risk of complications including the risks of acute hemorrhage, infection, pneumocephalus, and stroke. For older patients with multiple medical comorbidities, the high rates of recurrence and need for additional procedures can increase the risk for complications.

The theoretical framework for medical management of CSDH is founded in the suspected pathophysiology of the disease. A variety of mechanisms have been implicated including pathways of trauma, angiogenesis, inflammation, recurrent microhemorrhage, exudates, and local coagulopathy [4, 9]. There has been clinical interest in corticosteroids for CSDH because of their known anti-inflammatory and anti-angiogenic effects. Corticosteroids have been investigated not only as monotherapy for treatment of CSDH but also as an adjunct to surgical intervention. The effectiveness of corticosteroids for treating CSDH has been controversial because the majority of the clinical data is derived primarily from retrospective reviews with small sample sizes. Their use has also been associated with side effects including hyperglycemia, infection, and mental status disturbances such as psychosis.

T. Beutler (✉) · S. Krishnamurthy
Department of Neurosurgery, SUNY Upstate Medical University, Syracuse, NY, USA
e-mail: beutlert@upstate.edu; krishnsa@upstate.edu

M. Turgut et al. (eds.), *Subdural Hematoma*,
https://doi.org/10.1007/978-3-030-79371-5_35

In this chapter, the relevant pathophysiology regarding CSDH and corticosteroids is reviewed as well as the evidence regarding the effectiveness of corticosteroids as both monotherapy and adjunctive therapy for CSDH.

35.2 Pathophysiology

CSDH is an encapsulated layered collection of blood, blood degradation products, and fluid between the arachnoid and the dura mater. One of the earliest theories concerning the formation of CSDH is that they are caused by the tearing of bridging veins from the brain as they drain into the dural-venous sinuses. This theory has been disputed because of the long-time course after a trauma that it takes for a CSDH to develop and become symptomatic. CSDH typically become symptomatic on average 4–8 weeks after a trauma; however even a slow venous hemorrhage would accumulate significant mass to become symptomatic within a few hours to days [4]. The slow enlargement of CSDH over time has suggested that hemorrhage is not the only mechanism involved in the expansion of these collections.

Inflammation has long been suspected to play a role in the development of CSDH. The earliest report of inflammation and its role in the pathogenesis of CSDH was described by Virchow in 1857. He referred to the condition as "pachymeningitis haemorrhagica interna" and thought that infection was driving a chronic inflammatory response resulting in fibrin exudation and neovascularization [22]. Our understanding of inflammation has changed much since that time. Now we understand that inflammation occurs not just in response to infection but in response to any cellular or traumatic injury.

Subsequent support for the role of inflammation in the pathogenesis of CSDH has evolved from the work of Inglis in 1946 who identified a specialized layer of modified connective tissue cells in the dura [12]. These cells, which are now called dural border cells, are involved in both phagocytosis of blood products and the development of membranes [6, 17]. It is thought that sustained inflammation results in cellular proliferation forming new membranes and in the release of pro-angiogenic factors contributing to neovascularization [4, 9]. These new blood vessels are considered to be "leaky" and contribute to microhemorrhage and fluid exudation into the newly formed membrane bound spaces.

Corticosteroids have been implicated in many of the mechanisms involved in the formation of CSDH (Fig. 35.1). They are known to mediate anti-inflammatory effects by altering gene expression and the transcription of cytokines and inflammatory proteins [16]. They have been implicated in mediating the cellular differentiation of the immune cells which have been associated with membrane formation [4]. Finally, corticosteroids are suspected of effecting the vascular endothelium and "leaky" blood vessels that are associated with CSDH. The "leaky" endothelium is known to release tissue plasminogen activator and corticosteroids have been shown to mediate the effect by increasing plasminogen

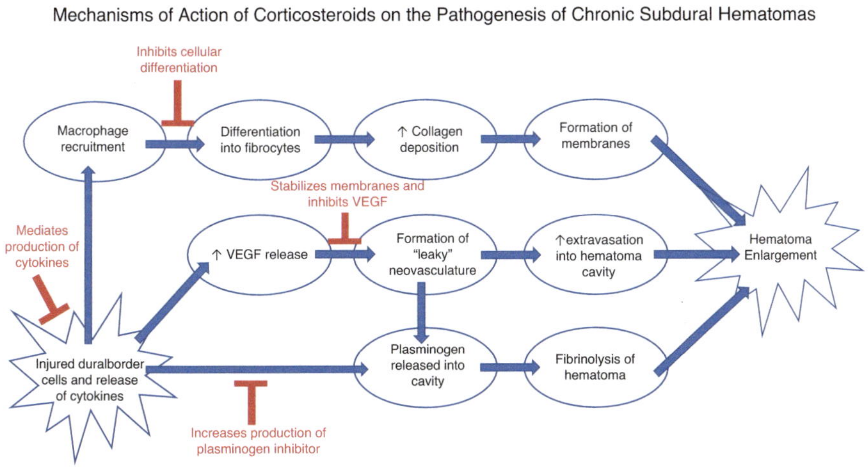

Fig. 35.1 The pathophysiology of CSDH is suspected to involve several pathways of inflammation and neovascularization. Corticosteroids effect the pathogenesis of CSDH through several mechanisms including mediating the production of cytokines, inhibiting cellular differentiation, promoting membrane stabilization, and preventing clot lysis

inhibitor [4]. Corticosteroids also reduce the permeability of the "leaky" blood vessels by mitigating the effects of vascular endothelial growth factor (VEGF). It is thought that corticosteroids can both inhibit the production on VEGF and mitigating the effect of VEGF directly on the vascular endothelium, reducing permeability and fluid accumulation [18].

Corticosteroids have long been used as potential treatment options for CSDH. An early observation by Glover and Labadie in 1976 reported that patients treated with corticosteroids developed significantly smaller and lighter appearing collections that lacked formed membranes [8]. These observations are important because they support the suspected mechanisms of action of corticosteroids in CSDH pathogenesis.

35.3 Corticosteroid Dosing

Corticosteroids have been used as both monotherapy and adjunctive therapy to surgery in the treatment of CSDH. The most common corticosteroid that has been used is dexamethasone; however a few studies have used methylprednisolone. The typical starting daily dose ranges from 12 to 24 mg and is given in divided doses every 6–8 h. The typical tapering course ranges from 2 to 4 weeks. When used as an adjunctive therapy, corticosteroids have been started both preoperatively and postoperatively. There is some weak evidence to suggest a correlation between length of preoperative corticosteroids and decreased risk of CSDH recurrence [1].

35.4 Corticosteroids as Monotherapy

Corticosteroids have been studied as monotherapy for management of patients with CSDH. This option is attractive to some patients and providers because it is a potential nonoperative management option. While there have been no class 1 randomized trials completed that compare corticosteroid treatment to either surgery or placebo, there have been a number of retrospective reviews completed that attempt to address the role of corticosteroids as monotherapy. Because of the retrospective nature of these studies, there is the risk of being confounded by selection bias. Many patients treated with corticosteroid monotherapy have often either refused or were thought to be too high risk for surgical intervention.

One of the first studies to present a significant number of patients treated with corticosteroid monotherapy for CSDH was completed by Sun et al. [19]. They presented a cohort of 26 patients who had been treated with corticosteroid monotherapy and compared their outcomes to patients who were treated with observation, surgery alone and surgery and adjunctive steroids. They found that patients with older age, significant medical comorbidities, and those who refused surgical intervention were often treated with monotherapy. The cohort treated with corticosteroids alone had similar results to those patients treated with surgery and adjunctive corticosteroids. There was also a trend towards improved outcomes in the corticosteroid monotherapy cohort compared to patients treated with either observation or surgery alone.

In 2009, Delgado-López et al. reported a large retrospective series where they stratified patient's neurologic exam at the time of admission [3]. Patients with mild symptoms were started initially on steroids while those with severe symptoms underwent initial surgical management. Asymptomatic patients were not treated. Patients initially assigned to steroid treatment were evaluated after 48–72 h, and if no improvement in their symptoms was noted, then they were offered surgical intervention. They treated nearly 100 patients with corticosteroid monotherapy and reported comparable outcomes to their surgically treated patients even among those with midline shift on imaging.

While there are reports of effective use of corticosteroids as monotherapy for CSDH, there are also reports of worse outcomes. Fountas et al. reported a series of CSDH patients in which patients treated with corticosteroid monotherapy had a significantly higher rate of recurrence (30%) compared to patients treated with burr hole craniostomy alone (7.3%) or combined surgical and corticosteroid treatment (4%) [5]. Although the literature shows varying degrees of efficacy for corticosteroid monotherapy, nonetheless it remains a good treatment option for patients who are either opposed or have contraindications to surgical intervention.

35.5 Corticosteroids as Adjunctive Therapy to Surgery

In addition to monotherapy, corticosteroids have also been studied as a potential adjunctive therapy to surgery. The goal of corticosteroids when used as an adjunctive therapy is to lower the recurrence of CSDH in order to avoid additional procedures without significantly increasing the risk for morbidity or mortality. In addition to several case series, there have been two randomized trials completed looking at corticosteroids as an adjunctive therapy.

Berghauser Pont et al. examined the use of corticosteroids in the preoperative setting [1]. They reviewed nearly 500 patients treated for CSDH. They found that patients treated with preoperative corticosteroids had lower likelihood for recurrence and found a positive correlation between the length of preoperative treatment and risk of recurrence.

Postoperative use of corticosteroids was examined by Qian et al. [15]. They identified advanced age, midline shift, and mixed density hematomas as significant risk factors for CSDH recurrence. They found that high-risk patients treated with a postoperative course of corticosteroids had a lower risk of recurrence than those patients treated with surgery alone. The retrospective study by Fountas et al. also found that patients treated with adjunctive corticosteroids had a lower rate of recurrence compared to those treated with surgery alone [5].

But, the literature regarding the effectiveness of corticosteroids even as an adjunctive treatment is mixed. In one of the few randomized prospective studies that has been completed, Chan et al. found no significant difference in the rates of recurrence and reoperation in patients treated with adjunctive corticosteroids compared to surgery alone [2].

Recently, Hutchinson et al. published the results of a multicenter randomized trial of 680 patients with symptomatic CSDH comparing dexamethasone use to placebo [11]. The design of the trial allowed for surgical intervention if clinically indicated and 94% of the patients underwent surgery. Because of the high rates of surgical intervention and small number of patients receiving corticosteroids as monotherapy, the study primarily examines the use of corticosteroids as adjunctive therapy. While they found lower rates of recurrence and reoperation in the dexamethasone group, they found that corticosteroids were also associated with higher rates of adverse outcomes including infection, hyperglycemia, and altered mental status.

Overall, the data from all of these studies suggest that the outcomes of adjunctive corticosteroid may lower the risk of recurrence and reoperation but may be associated with higher risk of complications. The optimal timing of starting steroids, whether preoperative or postoperative, is unclear, but both have been reported with favorable outcomes.

35.6 Ongoing and Future Studies

Unfortunately, there have been few randomized controlled trials looking at efficacy of corticosteroids and CSDH. Most of the available clinical evidence comes from retrospective observational studies. While these studies provide some valuable information, they are subject to potential bias from non-random allocation. More well-designed randomized trials are needed to compare corticosteroids to placebo, corticosteroids to surgery, and surgery monotherapy to surgery with adjunctive corticosteroids. Given the potential increased risk of complications from corticosteroids, additional research is also needed in order to determine which patients are more likely to have adverse outcomes.

35.7 Positive Prognostic Factors for Corticosteroid Use

Research into the effectiveness of corticosteroids for CSDH has yielded some results on the types of patients who are most likely to benefit from medical management. Some of the variables that have been identified include age, sex, neurologic exam, size of the hematoma, and the density of the collection (Table 35.1) [21].

Age is an independent risk factor for CSDH because age-associated brain atrophy allows for greater accumulation of blood and fluid without the development of symptoms. Patients who are older than 70 and have evidence of brain atrophy and lack symptoms associated with elevated intracranial pressure are thought to be good candidates for potential conservative management [13].

Sex has also been implicated as an important prognostic factor. The overall incidence and prevalence of CSDH is less in women compared to men. Thotakurta and Marabathina have reported better outcomes in women treated with corticosteroid compared to men [20]. This observation is thought to be related to hormonal factors. Histologic studies of CSDH membranes have revealed a higher incidence of estrogen and progesterone receptors in men [7]. It is thought that the local effect of estrogen on the neovascularized membrane results in increased tissue plasminogen activator and increased local fibrinolysis.

Patients with CSDH collections without midline shift and lower density on CT imaging have also been associated with better response to corticosteroid treatment [21]. These findings may also correlate with decreased clinical symptoms as smaller collections tend to present with fewer symptoms.

In regard to corticosteroid monotherapy, the most important factor is the patient's clinical exam. Because initial response to steroids can take from 3 days to a week, patients with worse clinical exams are often taken urgently to surgery. Patients with altered mental status and significant neurology deficits are not good candidates for monotherapy with corticosteroids. Patients with mild symptoms such as headaches have been found to respond well to conservative medical management.

Table 35.1 Favorable factors for corticosteroid use

Age > 70
Female sex
No altered mental status
No significant neurologic deficits
Mild symptoms (such as headaches)
CT imaging with low density collections
CT imaging without midline shift

35.8 Associated Complications

Corticosteroid use has been associated with a number of complications including hyperglycemia, infection, and mental status disturbances. Hyperglycemia is the most frequently reported complication occurring in 6.7–14.8% of patients [10]. Infections have been reported in 1.5–12.5% of patients [10]. The most commonly reported infections are superficial wound infections; however severe infections such as subdural empyema have been reported [2]. Patients with significant comorbidities such as diabetes mellitus are at higher risk for complications. Gastrointestinal hemorrhage is not a common complication because most patients are treated with a proton pump inhibitor, such as omeprazole or pantoprazole, as prophylaxis. The most common mental status disturbance is steroid-induced psychosis. Given the risks associated with corticosteroids, relative contraindications include patients with history of diabetes, gastrointestinal bleeding, and immunocompromise.

Mortality has been reported in 0–4% of patients [14]. When compared to surgery alone, the data regarding mortality is mixed. A recent meta-analysis showed decreased risks of mortality associated with corticosteroid use [10]; however a randomized trial published after the meta-analysis showed an increased risk of mortality [11].

35.9 Conclusion

There is evidence to suggest that chronic inflammation and neovascularization play an important role in the pathogenesis of CSDH. Because of the inflammatory pathways that have been implicated in CSDH formation, corticosteroids have long been employed as a medical treatment option for CSDH. They have been studied as both a monotherapy alternative to surgery and an adjunctive therapy.

The most common corticosteroid that has been used is dexamethasone. The typical starting daily dose ranges from 12 to 24 mg and is given in divided doses every 6–8 h. The typical tapering course ranges from 2 to 4 weeks. The use of corticosteroids in CSDH is generally well tolerated. Common complications include infection, hyperglycemia, and mental status disturbances.

A recent meta-analysis looking at corticosteroid treatment as both monotherapy and adjunctive therapy found no significant difference between treatment modalities and neurologic outcomes compared to standard surgical management [10]. Favorable outcomes with a GOS of 4–5 were reported in up to 90% of patients regardless of primary treatment modality. However, patients treated with surgery and adjunctive corticosteroids were found to have significantly fewer re-interventions and lower mortality.

There is some evidence to suggest the use of corticosteroids in the management of CSDH is safe and can be used as either monotherapy or in combination with surgery as adjunctive therapy. Depending on the clinical presentation the use of

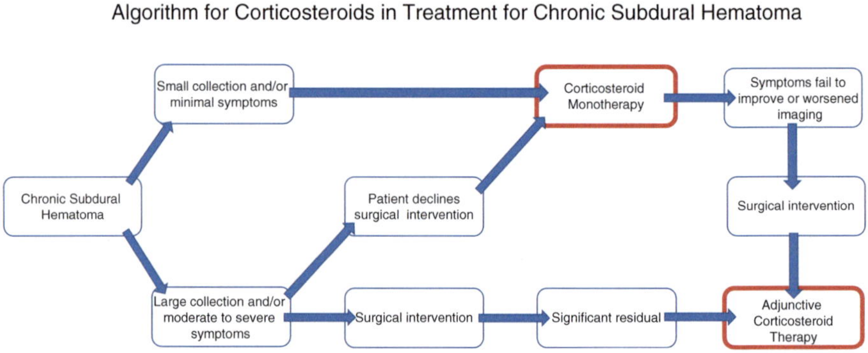

Fig. 35.2 Treatment algorithm for corticosteroids both as monotherapy and as adjunctive therapy to surgery

corticosteroids can be integrated into a treatment protocol for CSDH (Fig. 35.2). Caution should be used when using considering corticosteroids for patients with history of diabetes, gastrointestinal bleeding, or immunocompromise. Corticosteroids are a reasonable monotherapy option for patients with mild symptoms or small collections as well as for patients who either do not want surgery or have contraindications for surgery. For patients with severe symptoms or large collections, corticosteroids can be used as an adjunctive therapy to surgery and may reduce rates of recurrence and reoperation.

References

1. Berghauser Pont LM, Dammers R, Schouten JW, Lingsma HF, Dirven CM. Clinical factors associated with outcome in chronic subdural hematoma: a retrospective cohort study of patients on preoperative corticosteroid therapy. Neurosurgery. 2012;70(4):873–80.
2. Chan DYC, Sun TFD, Poon WS. Steroid for chronic subdural hematoma? A prospective phase IIB pilot randomized controlled trial on the use of dexamethasone with surgical drainage for the reduction of recurrence with reoperation. Chin Neurosurg J. 2015;1(1):2.
3. Delgado-López P, Martín-Velasco V, Castilla-Díez J, Rodríguez-Salazar A, Galacho-Harriero A, Fernández-Arconada O. Dexamethasone treatment in chronic subdural haematoma. Neurocirugia. 2009;20(4):346–59.
4. Edlmann E, Giorgi-Coll S, Whitfield PC, Carpenter KL, Hutchinson PJ. Pathophysiology of chronic subdural haematoma: inflammation, angiogenesis and implications for pharmacotherapy. J Neuroinflammation. 2017;14(1):1–13.
5. Fountas K, Kotlia P, Panagiotopoulos V, Fotakopoulos G. The outcome after surgical vs nonsurgical treatment of chronic subdural hematoma with dexamethasone. Interdiscip Neurosurg. 2019;16:70–4.
6. Friede R, Schachenmayr W. The origin of subdural neomembranes. II. Fine structural of neomembranes. Am J Pathol. 1978;92(1):69.
7. Giuffrè R, Palma E, Liccardo G, Sciarra F, Pastore F, Concolino G. Sex steroid-hormones in the pathogenesis of chronic subdural-hematoma. Neurochirurgia. 1992;35(04):103–7.

8. Glover D, Labadie EL. Physiopathogenesis of subdural hematomas: part 2: inhibition of growth of experimental hematomas with dexamethasone. J Neurosurg. 1976;45(4):393–7.
9. Holl DC, Volovici V, Dirven CM, Peul WC, van Kooten F, Jellema K, et al. Pathophysiology and nonsurgical treatment of chronic subdural hematoma: from past to present to future. World Neurosurg. 2018;116:402–11.e2.
10. Holl DC, Volovici V, Dirven CM, van Kooten F, Miah IP, Jellema K, et al. Corticosteroid treatment compared with surgery in chronic subdural hematoma: a systematic review and meta-analysis. Acta Neurochir. 2019;161(6):1231–42.
11. Hutchinson PJ, Edlmann E, Bulters D, Zolnourian A, Holton P, Suttner N, et al. Trial of dexamethasone for chronic subdural hematoma. N Engl J Med. 2020;383(27):2616–27.
12. Inglis K. Subdural haemorrhage, cysts and false membranes: illustrating the influence of intrinsic factors in disease when development of the body is normal. Brain. 1946;69(3):157–94.
13. Parlato C, Guarracino A, Moraci A. Spontaneous resolution of chronic subdural hematoma. Surg Neurol. 2000;53(4):312–7.
14. Pont BL, Dirven C, Dippel D, Verweij B, Dammers R. The role of corticosteroids in the management of chronic subdural hematoma: a systematic review (vol 19, pg 1397, 2012). Eur J Neurol. 2015;22(12):1575.
15. Qian Z, Yang D, Sun F, Sun Z. Risk factors for recurrence of chronic subdural hematoma after burr hole surgery: potential protective role of dexamethasone. Br J Neurosurg. 2017;31(1):84–8.
16. Rhen T, Cidlowski JA. Antiinflammatory action of glucocorticoids—new mechanisms for old drugs. N Engl J Med. 2005;353(16):1711–23.
17. Schachenmayr W, Friede R. The origin of subdural neomembranes. I. Fine structure of the dura-arachnoid interface in man. Am J Pathol. 1978;92(1):53.
18. Stummer W. Mechanisms of tumor-related brain edema. Neurosurg Focus. 2007;22(5):1–7.
19. Sun T, Boet R, Poon W. Non-surgical primary treatment of chronic subdural haematoma: preliminary results of using dexamethasone. Br J Neurosurg. 2005;19(4):327–33.
20. Thotakura AK, Marabathina NR. Nonsurgical treatment of chronic subdural hematoma with steroids. World Neurosurg. 2015;84(6):1968–72.
21. Thotakura AK, Marabathina NR. The role of medical treatment in chronic subdural hematoma. Asian J Neurosurg. 2018;13(4):976.
22. Virchow R. Haematoma durae matris. Verhandl Phys-Med Gesellsch Wurzburg. 1857;7:134–42.

Chapter 36
Management of Recurrence of Chronic Subdural Hematoma

Mohammed Benzagmout

36.1 Introduction

Drainage of chronic subdural hematoma (CSDH) is a routine procedure usually assigned to residents or the most junior neurosurgeon of the team. Burr hole drainage is the most commonly used surgical technique [2, 28, 50]. The prognosis is usually favorable. However, recurrence of CSDH remains a serious complication accounting for 5–33% of cases [43, 96]. Recurrence can occur early within 3 months after surgery [45], or later [58].

CSDH recurrence is generally defined as an ipsilateral hematoma discovered on follow-up computed tomography (CT) scan that causes neurological symptoms within 3 months after the initial procedure. When the hematoma recurs twice or more, it is called a refractory CSDH [47]. Reoperation is indicated if the original neurologic deficit increases, recurs, does not improve, or if new neurologic symptoms develop.

Several studies have focused on CSDH recurrence to determine its predictors. For such, many risk factors were studied including patient-related factors (age, sex, comorbidities, clinical symptoms, brain atrophy), hematoma characteristics (laterality, thickness, volume, density, mass effect), and surgery-related factors (technique, burr hole number, type of drainage). Although many risk factors have been reported, some are inconsistent, and even controversial or contradictory [13, 18, 22, 53, 55, 77, 80, 84, 85].

It is important to note that CSDH recurrence is not associated with just one risk factor but rather a combination of them. For example, hematoma thickness is closely related to age, brain atrophy, and midline shift, because as the brain atrophies with

M. Benzagmout (✉)
Department of Neurosurgery, University Hospital Hassan II of Fez, Fez, Morocco

Clinical Neurosciences Laboratory, Faculty of Medicine of Fez, Fez, Morocco

M. Turgut et al. (eds.), *Subdural Hematoma*,
https://doi.org/10.1007/978-3-030-79371-5_36

age, older patients are more likely to have a larger preoperative hematoma volume causing significant midline shift. Additionally, older CSDH patients have more comorbidities that can affect their clinical outcome, i.e., the development of postoperative complications.

In this chapter, we will summarize the different risk factors associated with CSDH recurrence, before detailing the available therapeutic options and preventive measures.

36.2 Risk Factors

36.2.1 Patient's Background Factors

36.2.1.1 Age

Age is an important risk factor for CSDH recurrence [59, 84]. Some authors found that older patients experienced a significantly higher recurrence rate and a longer hospital stay [68, 84]. However, others did not find a statistical difference in recurrence rate between different age groups [39, 59].

36.2.1.2 Gender

Some studies have reported that male sex is an independent risk factor for CSDH recurrence, and that males experience more trauma and more complications than females [59]. Other studies did not find a relationship between gender and CSDH recurrence [11, 75].

36.2.1.3 Arterial Hypertension

Arterial hypertension is commonly associated with vascular arteriosclerotic changes, a predisposing factor for ischemic and hemorrhagic complications. Numerous studies demonstrated a higher risk of bleeding in patients with pre-, intra-, and postoperative hypertension [6].

In addition, high blood pressure may also influence postoperative hemostasis. The fragile vessels of the membranes within the CSDH and the vulnerable surgery-injured scalp vessels could explain the higher recurrence risk associated with arterial hypertension. Thus, maintaining a normal blood pressure during the perioperative period is a fundamental rule in the management of CSDH.

36.2.1.4 Intracranial Hypotension

It is well known that intracranial hypotension could lead to CSDH formation. This cause is systematically suspected in young to middle-aged patients who develop CSDH with no past history of cranial trauma or hematological disorders [99].Also, intracranial hypotension could promote CSDH recurrence [34]. Therefore, it is mandatory to consider this possibility and to treat it to avoid recurrences.

36.2.1.5 Diabetes Mellitus

Results regarding this risk factor are also inconsistent in the literature. Pang et al. demonstrated that diabetes mellitus is a significant risk factor for recurrence of CSDH [60]. On the contrary, Yamamoto et al. found that diabetes mellitus may play a role in decreasing the recurrence rate for CSDH [100]. They stated that hyperglycemia raises the blood osmotic pressure and the activation of platelet aggregation which all may help lower the rebleeding tendency of CSDH [100].

36.2.1.6 History of Seizures

In their study, Yamamoto et al. demonstrated that a history of seizures was an independent predictor of CSDH recurrence [100]. Coagulopathy and/or liver dysfunction induced by some anticonvulsant drugs may contribute to the recurrence of CSDH [74].

36.2.1.7 Chronic Alcoholism

Chronic alcoholism is a recognized risk factor for the occurrence and recurrence of CSDH [32]. This increased incidence is explained by brain atrophy and coagulation dysfunction induced by persistent alcohol intake [10]. Besides, chronic alcoholism also exposes the patient to inadvertent and frequent head trauma.

36.2.1.8 Coagulopathy and Underlying Diseases

Patients with hemorrhagic diathesis due to coagulopathy, liver diseases, chronic renal failure, or malignant neoplasms are well known to have a high tendency for CSDH recurrence [32, 33, 92].

Schwarz et al. [69] suspected coagulopathy as a cause of recurrence, especially when no other risk factors were clearly identified. Coagulopathy was not identified with standardized preoperative blood tests (INR, PTT, thrombocytes, anti-thrombin, and fibrinogen) [69]. The intake of vitamin K antagonists seems to be protective against surgical complications [69].

36.2.1.9 Anticoagulant/Antiplatelet Therapy

Anticoagulants and antiplatelet agents have an important role in the pathogenesis of CSDH with a reported incidence rate ranging from 0.6 to 22.5% [10, 42]. These medications inhibit normal hemostatic mechanisms by inhibiting platelet aggregation, decreasing the production of natural platelet aggregates, or interfering with vitamin K metabolism by the liver which significantly increases the risk of developing a recurrent subdural hematoma [64]. In their cohort, Kamenova et al. found that 84.2% of CSDH recurrences occurred before postoperative day 42 [29]. They estimated that there was a continuous increase in the risk of CSDH recurrence (1% per week) if acetylsalicylic acid (ASA) therapy was resumed earlier. However, after day 42, the risk of recurrence decreased. Therefore, they advocated that ASA treatment should be reinstated by week 6 postoperatively. In patients treated for secondary coronary artery disease, early resumption of ASA treatment after 7–10 days may be warranted to prevent the risk of cardiovascular events [29].

As for some former risk factors, several recent studies have reported no relationship between the use of antiplatelet or anticoagulant medications and CSDH recurrence [29, 42, 60].

36.2.2 Radiological Factors

36.2.2.1 Midline Shift

On CT scan, the presence of preoperative midline shift is recognized as a significant risk factor for recurrence of CSDH. The risk increases by a factor of 1.18 per millimeter of deviation from the midline, and up to a factor of 26.93 for a difference of more than 10 mm for surgical complications [69].

Fukuhara and coworkers showed that advanced age, brain atrophy, large hematoma volume, and prolonged compressed parenchyma influenced brain elasticity [19]. It is noteworthy that most often the brain in these conditions poorly re-expands leading to the persistence of postoperative midline displacement [19], hence the higher postoperative recurrence rate [54].

On the other hand, the sudden decrease in intracranial pressure after evacuating a huge CSDH can result in a rapid expansion of the brain parenchyma with subsequent stress on the surrounding vessels which increases the risk of acute rebleeding [6].

36.2.2.2 Cerebral Atrophy

A greater amount of parenchymal brain atrophy was found, on multivariate analysis, to be a predictor of increased postoperative hematoma volume. Brain atrophy is well recognized as a distinct risk factor for both occurrence and recurrence of CSDH [100]. This has been explained by the higher brain elastance associated with advanced age, brain atrophy, and persistence of a notable subdural space [19, 50].

Brain atrophy causes an enlarged subdural space. Therefore, the surgical treatment of CSDH in patients with greater cerebral atrophy and larger extra-axial spaces would be less effective as the pressure gradient driving CSDH efflux is less than that in patients with no atrophy [56]. Secondly, the gap between the dura and the pia mater increases in severe brain atrophy which promotes significant postoperative pneumocephalus. In both conditions, the CSF will accumulate and can be difficult to absorb for an extended period, which may increase the risk of CSDH recurrence.

36.2.2.3 Bilateral CSDH

The bilateral location of CSDH appears to be a risk factor for recurrence in many studies [104]. Schwarz et al. [69] found that patients with bilateral hematomas had roughly a fourfold greater risk for reoperation than patients with a unilateral hematoma. Similarly, Tsai et al. [86] compared unilateral with bilateral hematomas and noted that patients with bilateral hematomas were older and more often on anticoagulants, which may explain the higher risk of complications in those patients.

Tugcu et al. [87] suggested that bilateral hematomas occurred more commonly in patients with brain atrophy, which led to poor postoperative brain re-expansion, and subsequently a higher recurrence rate. Compared with unilateral CSDH, the poor brain re-expansion observed in the bilateral type may result in brain parenchymal shift, blood vessel tearing, significant postoperative pneumocephalus, and cerebrospinal fluid accumulation in the hematoma cavity, hence the higher recurrence rate [35].

Another explanation for the increased complication rate in bilateral CSDH may simply be mathematical in terms that a patient with one hematoma will have a lower risk of reoperation than a patient with two hematomas [69].

Finally, some studies have shown that simultaneous bilateral decompression of bilateral CSDH reduces the potential for complications and the rate of CSDH recurrence; however, others have not corroborated this result [11, 51].

36.2.2.4 Density of the Hematoma

Numerous studies have suggested that preoperative hematoma density is associated with CSDH recurrence, and a hyperdense hematoma is an independent risk factor for recurrence [11, 40]. In hyperdense CSDH, repeated microhemorrhages from the immature capillaries in the outer membrane may explain the high propensity for this CSDH type to recur [40].

Nakaguchi et al. have classified CSDH into four types according to their density and inner structure: **homogenous** (homogenous density), **laminar** (thin high-density layer along the inner membrane), **separated** (two components of different densities), and **trabecular** (non-homogeneous contents with a high-density septum running between the inner and outer membranes in a low-density to isodense background) [55].

Using the Nakaguchi classification, many authors have showed a higher rate of recurrence in separated and laminar hematoma types. The fibrinolytic activity might be higher than the coagulation in these hematoma subtypes, resulting in recurrent hematoma formation [55]. As for Frati et al. [18], they showed a correlation between the concentration of inflammatory cytokines and the recurrence rate, especially in the laminar type.

36.2.2.5 Septations

The presence of septations within the CSDH was previously found to be associated with a high risk of recurrence [75, 81, 100]. Jack et al. [27] demonstrated that the presence of septations was statistically significant for higher residual hematoma volume and CSDH recurrence requiring re-drainage. Tanikawa and colleagues [81] also demonstrated a high rate of recurrence in CSDH harboring a large number of intrahematomal membranes.

Septated hematomas are more difficult to drain because each compartment must be disrupted in order to achieve complete drainage. Interrupting the intrahematomal membranes and connecting all of the hematoma compartments together in order to drain the hematoma fluid may prompt subdural fluid reabsorption and, consequently, prevent fibrinolysis and result in rebleeding [81].

36.2.2.6 Preoperative Hematoma Volume

The hematoma volume is generally calculated on the CT scan using the ABC/2 method [76]. Increased preoperative hematoma volume represents a significant predictor of higher postoperative residual hematoma volume. Obviously, larger hematomas are more difficult to completely drain (particularly through a burr hole). In addition, larger CSDHs have a lower surface-to-volume ratio leading to decreased absorption of the hematoma fluid [17]. Altogether, incomplete drainage and poor thrombosis and re-absorption will likely result in recurrent CSDH.

36.2.2.7 Postoperative Hematoma Volume

The postoperative hematoma volume is strongly indicated as one of the most important radiological predictors for recurrence [62]. Indeed, Ridwan et al. have demonstrated that the risk of recurrence increased significantly when the volume of residual hematoma exceeded 40 mL and/or 40% of the preoperative CSDH volume ("40/40 rule") [62].

It is well known that there is a micro-environment of hyperfibrinolysis and hypercoagulation within the CSDH [100], and that the hematoma resolution is determined by the difference between re-absorption and microvascular leakage [25]. As such, increased postoperative hematoma volume is significantly associated with re-accumulation of CSDH requiring a second surgery.

36.2.2.8 Postoperative Pneumocephalus

Pneumocephalus is a common surgical complication of CSDH drainage [72]. This complication results from misplacement of the cranial burr holes, improper head position, and inadequate filling of the hematoma cavity with saline before the scalp closure is final.

Pneumocephalus increases the recurrence rate of CSDH [102]. Pneumocephalus prompts more postoperative blood accumulation in the hematoma cavity due to the repetitive abrading of the bridging veins by the floating air bubbles generated by patient's head movements [102].

36.2.3 Surgical Factors

36.2.3.1 Surgical Technique

The optimal surgical treatment for CSDH is still a matter of debate. Multiple techniques have been developed over the last few decades. However, to date there is no consensus or guidelines regarding a "standard" surgical technique. The number of burr holes, the size of a burr hole, the usefulness of irrigation, and the location of the drain, whether subdural or subperiosteal, all remain questionable.

Many studies showed that the usage of postoperative drains after burr hole evacuation of primary CSDH is associated with a lower recurrence rate [36, 41, 50]. This finding was supported by the results of a recently published randomized controlled trial [66]. Two meta-analyses concluded that postoperative drainage can reduce the complications and recurrence rate of CSDH, and recommended using drainage routinely [2, 43].

Some authors recommended a closed non-suction drainage system since it was associated with a significantly lower rate of hematoma recurrence without increasing the complication rate [16]. In addition, Smith et al. reviewed four different studies that compared the number of trephinations per subdural hematoma. The authors concluded that two burr holes gave better outcomes than one burr hole in terms of a shorter hospital stay and a lower infection rate [73].

Twist drill craniostomy was proven to be as effective as burr hole craniostomy (BHC) and seemed to be associated with fewer recurrences than the latter with subdural irrigation [52]. Almenawer et al. stated that bedside twist drill drainage showed a slight advantage in terms of complication rates compared with "classic" burr hole trephination [2]. However, in another prospective randomized trial, Gokmen et al. did not detect any significant differences between the two surgical techniques [20].

Today, BHC remains the preferred treatment for CSDH patients [56]. Nonetheless, we believe that the surgical management of CSDH must be tailored to each patient and the challenge is to identify which of those patients should initially be treated with more invasive techniques.

36.2.3.2 Drainage Location

The main cause of hematoma recurrence is believed to be the poor postoperative re-expansion of the brain [50, 55]. Reasons for the latter might be the presence of membranes within the hematoma, decreased blood flow, insufficient drainage, and decreased compliance of the brain parenchyma [50]. Some studies evaluated the correlation between brain compliance and its re-expansion after surgery. They reported that compliance was lower when the postoperative subdural space was more pronounced [19]. Mori and Maeda [50] demonstrated less brain re-expansion in older patients, patients with a past history of an ischemic insult, patients with a significant postoperative subdural air collection, and those receiving anticoagulant treatment.

Regarding the draining catheter location, substantial evidence shows that the frontal location was advantageous with regard to recurrence [55].

36.2.3.3 Volume Drainage

Shen et al. [70] have reported that a drainage volume exceeding 100 mL was an independent risk factor of the recurrence of CSDH. This result might be due to the loss of hemostasis or pia mater rupture during surgery resulting in cerebrospinal fluid (CSF) accumulation in the hematoma cavity, i.e., CSDH recurrence if the CSF is not absorbed.

36.2.3.4 Water Volume and Temperature

Bartley et al. [5] found a significant reduction in recurrence rates of CSDH upon using perioperative irrigation fluid at body temperature (37°) versus irrigation fluid at room temperature (22°). This finding might be explained by the improvement of the coagulation process inside the hematoma [94] and the increase of the solubility and evacuation of the CSDH when performing irrigation at body temperature, thereby facilitating evacuation [8].

Moreover, it was suggested that the quantity of irrigation fluid used intraoperatively has an impact on the risk of recurrence. Roughly speaking, copious irrigation of the subdural space with more than 1400 mL was clearly associated with a reduction of the recurrence risk [78].

36.3 Treatment of Recurrence

36.3.1 Medical Treatment

Several authors discussed the efficacy of corticosteroids in the management of selected cases of recurrent CSDH [53, 83]. Zhang et al. revealed that recurrent CSDH can be successfully treated with dexamethasone without reoperation [103].

Drapkin [15] recommended the use of corticosteroids in the postoperative management of patients with persistent or recurrent symptoms as a measure before reoperation.

It is important to note that some authors have advocated combined therapy (Atorvastatin plus Dexamethasone) for recurrent CSDH. The advantage of this association is to combine anti-inflammatory and angiogenic effects and to simultaneously reduce the risk of complications associated with both drugs [23].

Other authors have advocated the use of tranexamic acid as an adjunctive treatment to surgery when dealing with recurrent CSDH, especially in patients requiring continuous anticoagulant therapy due to a high thromboembolic risk [24]. Tranexamic acid can increase the resolution rate of CSDH, possibly by stabilizing the small bleeds on the membranes surrounding the hematoma, inhibiting the fibrinolytic kinin-kallikrein system, and potentially disrupting the inflammatory process [24].

36.3.2 Surgical Management

36.3.2.1 Burr Hole Evacuation

For the management of the first recurrence, the same surgical technique, usually burr hole craniostomy, irrigation, and drainage, is recommended because it is safe and associated with lower perioperative risks [47]. The same burr hole(s) is/are usually used for the treatment of the recurrence. If the position of the preexisting burr hole(s) does not allow optimal rinsing of the subdural cavity, a new burr hole can be drilled. No special effort is made to disrupt subdural membrane loculations apart from those easily accessible via the burr holes.

Different therapeutic options can be added to burr hole craniostomy to improve the efficacy of the technique, particularly the adjustment of the drainage tube direction [54], irrigation with artificial CSF [1], and fibrin glue injection into the hematoma cavity [93].

In the review of Weigel et al., burr hole drainage was the treatment of choice for recurrent CSDH in 85% of reported cases [95], otherwise craniotomy was used. In case there was considerable disparity between the volume of the brain and the cranial cavity or, on the contrary, intractable high intracranial pressure develops due to brain swelling, craniectomy or mini-craniectomy was indicated [90].

36.3.2.2 Craniotomy

In patients with organized or refractory CSDH, craniotomy could be the ideal surgical option where hematoma evacuation and membranectomy become necessary [63, 90]. Several technical variations of craniotomy have been described in the literature, including large craniotomy or mini-craniotomy (usually defined as a bone flap diameter up to 4 cm), and either partial or total membranectomy [65].

Although mini-craniotomy is a safe, quick, and less invasive surgical technique than a large craniotomy, the removed hematoma volume and the performed membranectomy might be insufficient [47]. Kim et al. reported that the recurrence rate was higher with mini-craniotomy than with a large craniotomy [30].

Many authors agreed that a large craniotomy should be chosen for an organized CSDH since it allows enough room to adequately address the recurrent hematoma, its membrane, and any occasional troublesome bleeding [30, 63, 65].

Regarding membranectomy, it is still controversial whether both outer and inner membranes should be partially or totally removed [88]. On the one hand, resection of the outer and inner membranes may facilitate the release and reabsorption of CSDH contents by cortical glymphatic and dural lymphatic pathways [65]. On the other hand, it prevents rebleeding from macrocapillaries of the outer membrane and helps to re-expand the brain [65]. However, aggressive membranectomy, especially of the inner membrane, can cause cortical venous injury.

36.3.2.3 Endoscopic Surgery

Endoscopic surgery has recently been suggested for the treatment of organized or septated CSDH [46, 79]. Under local anesthesia and enhanced visual control, a flexible endoscope is threaded through a burr hole or mini-craniotomy in order to: divide different septa inside the hematoma cavity, fenestrate the internal membrane, remove solid clot, correctly position the drainage catheter, and coagulate the potential recurrence-causing neovessels [49, 79].

Although endoscopic surgery is a minimally invasive alternative for treating CSDH, residual firm hematoma and persistent membranes are more likely to remain as compared with a large craniotomy, which in turn may give rise to recurrences [63, 79].

36.3.2.4 Ommaya Reservoir Placement

Sato et al. [67] suggested treating recurrent or refractory CSDH using an Ommaya reservoir. Interestingly, Laumer et al. [38] primarily implanted this device in patients in whom the brain did not sufficiently expand after the first burr hole surgery, and additionally in those patients harboring recurrent CSDH. The intervention is performed under general or local anesthesia and consists in threading, through a burr hole, a catheter into the subdural hematoma cavity. Afterwards, the catheter is connected to an Ommaya CSF reservoir placed between the scalp and the bone. The reservoir is then intermittently punctured and drained depending on the amount of accumulated fluid.

This technique represents an interesting surgical alternative for treating recurrent CSDH, especially in patients with severe underlying diseases or a fragile neurological status who could not tolerate a prolonged period of bedrest if they were subjected to multiple operations [37, 67]. The main advantage of this intervention is the shorter immobility period, albeit some minor complications (infection, obstruction of the reservoir, bleeding) could occur [67].

36.3.2.5 Subdural Peritoneal Shunt

Peritoneal drainage of CSDH using a low-pressure valve was successfully performed first in children [4]. The procedure was advocated as a treatment modality for recurrent CSDH, even in the elderly [61]. The employed drainage systems are usually valveless. Low-pressure valves have also been successfully used, particularly in younger patients [9].

The technique appears simple, safe, and effective in treating recurrent CSDH [48]. However, inserting a subdural peritoneal shunt requires general anesthesia and is associated with a longer operative time and a relatively higher risk of postoperative infection and abdominal complications than some other treatment methods.

Drainage for about 6 weeks is usually sufficient in most cases [48] and the shunt can be removed afterwards. On occasion, the subdural catheter becomes strongly adherent to the underlying brain cortex within 3 months of placement, and in this case its removal is inadvisable because of the risk of complications, primarily that of hemorrhage.

36.3.3 Endovascular Treatment

Embolization of the middle meningeal artery (MMA) has recently been considered as the most reasonable and effective treatment for recurrent CSDH, with minimal surgical invasiveness [12, 82]. Histological studies revealed that the MMA feeds the outer membrane and perhaps enhances the expansion of the CSDH [80]. Embolization of the MMA may disrupt the blood supply to the outer membrane and thereby prevent hematoma enlargement [12, 82]. By targeting the origin of the bleeding, this method appears reasonable and is effective.

Altogether, the treatment outcomes have been generally good despite some recurrent cases [12]. In the latter cases, inadequate embolization or recanalization of the MMA was deemed responsible for the CSDH recurrence; a second embolization or using burr hole irrigation and drainage achieved a complete cure [12]. To avoid treatment failure, liquid embolic materials such as *N*-butyl 2-cyanoacrylate or polyvinyl alcohol with coil embolization should be utilized [12].

Finally, embolization of the MMA might be contraindicated or unsuitable, e.g., in patients with severe renal failure or when the MMA is not accessible [47].

36.4 Prevention of Recurrence

36.4.1 Surgical Tips

Burr hole irrigation and drainage has been widely performed as the gold-standard treatment for CSDH [66, 99]. One of the best ways to prevent recurrence is to ensure good surgical evacuation of the hematoma by fully respecting the well-known key steps of the surgical procedure.

A meta-analysis of five randomized trials indicated a significant reduction in the recurrence rate when drains were inserted following hematoma evacuation [2, 66]. Several surgical tips and technical nuances have been described to reduce the risk of CSDH recurrence. Placing closed-system drainage or irrigating with artificial CSF were associated with reduced recurrence in a randomized controlled trial [1, 99]. Irrigation with a large amount of fluid, during the procedure, and intravenous fluid administration of at least 2000 mL for 3 days postoperatively were also associated with a reduced recurrence rate [78].

Similar reduction in recurrence was also obtained upon irrigating the hematoma cavity with a thrombin solution [71], or adding tissue plasminogen activator (tPA) to the irrigation fluid [57]. This practice increases the amount of drained fluid after hematoma evacuation, especially in the presence of residual solid clot.

To prevent recurrence of hematoma, Aoki et al. [3] filled the hematoma cavity with oxygen via percutaneous subdural tapping. Similarly, Kitakami et al. used CO_2 gas to fill the hematoma cavity, and observed a rapid disappearance of the hematoma cavity and re-expansion of the brain within 24 h of CO_2 injection [31]. In addition, Xu et al. [97] suggested locally applying methylprednisolone sodium succinate into the hematoma cavity combined with surgery to prevent recurrence.

36.4.2 Adjunctive Treatment

Adjunctive therapies such as corticosteroids, angiotensin-converting enzyme inhibitors, tranexamic acid, atorvastatin, and Kampo medicine have often been used for preventing recurrence of CSDH.

Regarding adjunctive corticosteroid therapy, preoperative dexamethasone administration might be effective in preventing CSDH recurrence, especially in the layered-type of hematoma [53]. Berghauser et al. reported that a longer preoperative administration period of dexamethasone is associated with a lower CSDH recurrence rate [7]. This beneficial effect could be explained by the corticosteroid suppression of vascular endothelial growth factor (VEGF) [53]. However, some authors do not share the same opinion regarding the risk of recurrence [77].

It has also reported that the use of angiotensin-converting enzyme (ACE) inhibitors decreases the risk of CSDH recurrence [96]. This might be related to the anti-angiogenic properties of this medication class [96]. ACE inhibitors were found to inhibit the development of immature and new blood vessels in the neomembrane of the hematoma [26].

Recently, atorvastatin has been reported to be effective in preventing CSDH recurrence [44, 98]. Wang et al. [91] have reported a rat model of subdural hematoma treated with atorvastatin, and concluded that atorvastatin at a low dose is effective in inducing angiogenesis and vascular maturation, leading to significant reduction in subdural hematoma formation and the associated neurological consequences.

In Japan, Kampo medicines, such as Goreisan, are widely used as an adjunctive therapy for preventing recurrence of CSDH because of the low incidence of side effects [101]. Goto et al. confirmed that Goreisan is effective in preventing CSDH recurrence after surgery [21]. The authors believe that Goreisan reduces the hematoma volume by inhibiting apoquaporin-4 expressed in the outer membrane of the CSDH, thus decreasing its permeability [89, 101].

36.5 Conclusion

CSDH is a common neurosurgical condition. After surgical evacuation, recurrence of CSDH represents a significant issue in neurosurgical practice with an incidence that ranges from 5 to 33% and its treatment is widely debated [43, 95]. Therefore, a comprehensive understanding of the underlying risk factors will offer an opportunity to improve the surgical results and clinical outcome.

The treatment modalities for recurrent CSDH are still debatable. Although newer surgical techniques seem to provide reasonable alternatives to burr hole evacuation, none has been proven to be highly effective in the treatment of recurrent CSDH. Most recurrent subdural hematomas can be managed successfully via burr hole craniostomy and postoperative closed-system drainage. Refractory hematomas may require craniotomy with membranectomy, subdural-peritoneal shunt drainage, placement of a subdural catheter connected to an Ommaya reservoir with serial tapping, endoscopic removal, continuous postoperative irrigation and drainage, or injection of isotonic fluid into the ventricular space to promote brain re-expansion [14].

CSDH surgeries are expected to increase, hence the need to optimize treatment strategies with evidence-based treatments [2]. More investigations are needed to clarify the indications of currently available surgical techniques in the management of recurrent CSDH. In our opinion, the appropriate surgical technique must be selected depending on the patient background, clinical status, and radiological records.

Since most of the available data are extracted from retrospective studies conducted on a limited number of patients with heterogeneous clinical and/or radiological characteristics, different selection biases are suspected. Therefore, large multicenter prospective randomized controlled trials on a large number of patients are warranted to determine the most effective perioperative strategies to use in CSDH management.

References

1. Adachi A, Higuchi Y, Fujikawa A, Machida T, Sueyoshi S, Harigaya K, et al. Risk factors in chronic subdural hematoma: comparison of irrigation with artificial cerebrospinal fluid and normal saline in a cohort analysis. PLoS One. 2014;9:e103703.
2. Almenawer SA, Farrokhyar F, Hong C, Alhazzani W, Manoranjan B, Yaras-cavitch B, et al. Chronic subdural hematoma management: a systematic review and meta-analysis of 34,829 patients. Ann Surg. 2014;259(3):449–57.
3. Aoki N. A new therapeutic method for chronic subdural hematoma in adults: replacement of the hematoma with oxygen via percutaneous subdural tapping. Surg Neurol. 1992;38:253–6.
4. Aoki N, Mizutani H, Masuzawa H. Unilateral subdural peritoneal shunting for bilateral hematoma in infancy: report of three cases. J Neurosurg. 1985;63:134–7.
5. Bartley A, Jakola AS, Tisell M. The influence of irrigation fluid temperature on recurrence in the evacuation of chronic subdural hematoma. Acta Neurochir. 2020;162(3):485–8.
6. Basali A, Mascha EJ, Kalfas I, Schubert A. Relation between perioperative hypertension and intracranial hemorrhage after craniotomy. Anesthesiology. 2000;93:48–54.
7. Berghauser Pont LM, Dammers R, Schouten JW, Lingsma HF, Dirven CM. Clinical factors associated with outcome in chronic subdural hematoma: a retrospective cohort study of patients on pre-operative corticosteroid therapy. Neurosurgery. 2012;70(4):873–80.
8. Black S, Muller F. On the effect of temperature on aqueous solubility of organic solids. Org Process Res Dev. 2010;14(3):661–5.
9. Cameron MM. Chronic subdural hematoma: a review of 114 cases. J Neurol Neurosurg Psychiatry. 1978;41:834–9.
10. Chen JC, Levy ML. Causes, epidemiology, and risk factors of chronic subdural hematoma. Neurosurg Clin N Am. 2000;11:399–406.
11. Chen FM, Wang K, Xu KL, Wang L, Zhan TX, Cheng F, et al. Predictors of acute intracranial hemorrhage and recurrence of chronic subdural hematoma following burr hole drainage. BMC Neurol. 2020;20(1):92.
12. Chihara H, Imamura H, Ogura T, Adachi H, Imai Y, Sakai N. Recurrence of a refractory chronic subdural hematoma after middle meningeal artery embolization that required craniotomy. NMC Case Rep J. 2014;1:1–5.
13. Chon KH, Lee JM, Koh EJ, Choi HY. Independent predictors for recurrence of chronic subdural hematoma. Acta Neurochir. 2012;154(9):1541–8.
14. Desai VR, Scranton RA, Britz GW. Management of recurrent subdural hematomas. Neurosurg Clin N Am. 2017;28(2):279–86.
15. Drapkin AJ. Chronic subdural hematoma: pathophysiological basis for treatment. Br J Neurosurg. 1991;5:467–73.
16. Ducruet AF, Grobelny BT, Zacharia BE, Hickman ZL, DeRosa PL, Anderson K, et al. The surgical management of chronic subdural hematoma. Neurosurg Rev. 2012;35:155–69.
17. El-Kadi H, Miele VJ, Kaufman HH. Prognosis of chronic subdural hematomas. Neurosurg Clin N Am. 2000;11:553–5567.
18. Frati A, Salvati M, Mainiero F, Ippoliti F, Rocchi G, Raco A, et al. Inflammation markers and risk factors for recurrence in 35 patients with a posttraumatic chronic subdural hematoma: a prospective study. J Neurosurg. 2004;100(1):24–32.
19. Fukuhara T, Gotoh M, Asari S, Ohmoto T, Akioka T. The relationship between brain surface elastance and brain reexpansion after evacuation of chronic subdural hematoma. Surg Neurol. 1996;45:570–4.
20. Gokmen M, Sucu HK, Ergin A, Gokmen A, Bezircio Lu H. Randomized comparative study of burr-hole craniostomy versus twist drill craniostomy: surgical management of unilateral hemispheric chronic subdural hematomas. Zentralbl Neurochir. 2008;69:129–33.
21. Goto S, Kato K, Yamamoto T, Shimato S, Ohshima T, Nishizawa T. Effectiveness of Goreisan in preventing recurrence of chronic subdural hematoma. Asian J Neurosurg. 2018;13:370–4.

22. Han MH, Ryu JI, Kim CH, Kim JM, Cheong JH, Yi HJ. Predictive factors for recurrence and clinical outcomes in patients with chronic subdural hematoma. J Neurosurg. 2017;127(5):1117–25.
23. Huang J, Li L, Zhang J, Gao C, Quan W, Tian Y, et al. Treatment of relapsed chronic subdural hematoma in four young children with atorvastatin and low-dose dexamethasone. Pharmacotherapy. 2019;39(7):783–9.
24. Iorio-Morin C, Blanchard J, Richer M, Mathieu D. Tranexamic Acid in Chronic Subdural Hematomas (TRACS): study protocol for a randomized controlled trial. Trials. 2016;17(1):235.
25. Ito H, Komai T, Yamamoto S. Fibrinolytic enzyme in the lining walls of chronic subdural hematoma. J Neurosurg. 1978;48:197–200.
26. Ivamoto HS, Lemos HP Jr, Atallah AN. Surgical treatments for chronic subdural hematomas: a comprehensive systematic review. World Neurosurg. 2016;86:399–418.
27. Jack A, O'Kelly C, McDougall C, Findlay JM. Predicting recurrence after chronic subdural hematoma drainage. Can J Neurol Sci. 2015;42(1):34–9.
28. Jang KM, Kwon JT, Hwang SN, Park YS, Nam TK. Comparison of the outcomes and recurrence with three surgical techniques for chronic subdural hematoma: single, double burr hole, and double burr hole drainage with irrigation. Korean J Neurotrauma. 2015;11(2):75–80.
29. Kamenova M, Lutz K, Schaedelin S, Fandino J, Mariani L, Soleman J. Does early resumption of low-dose Aspirin after evacuation of chronic subdural hematoma with burr-hole drainage lead to higher recurrence rates? Neurosurgery. 2016;79(5):715–21.
30. Kim JH, Kang DS, Kim JH, Kong MH, Song KY. Chronic subdural hematoma treated by small or large craniotomy with membranectomy as the initial treatment. J Korean Neurosurg Soc. 2011;50:103–8.
31. Kitakami A, Ogawa A, Hakozaki S, Kidoguchi J, Obonai C, Kubo N. Carbon dioxide gas replacement of chronic subdural hematoma using single burr-hole irrigation. Surg Neurol. 1995;43:574–7.
32. Ko BS, Lee JK, Seo BR, Moon SJ, Kim JH, Kim SH. Clinical analysis of risk factors related to recurrent chronic subdural hematoma. J Korean Neurosurg Soc. 2008;43:11–5.
33. Konig SA, Schick U, Dohnert J, Goldammer A, Vitzthum HE. Coagulopathy and outcome in patients with chronic subdural hematoma. Acta Neurol Scand. 2003;107:110–6.
34. Kristof RA, Grimm JM, Stoffel-Wagner B. Cerebrospinal fluid leakage into the subdural space: possible influence on the pathogenesis and recurrence frequency of chronic subdural hematoma and subdural hygroma. J Neurosurg. 2008;108:275–80.
35. Kung WM, Hung KS, Chiu WT, Tsai SH, Lin JW, Wang YC, et al. Quantitative assessment of impaired post evacuation brain re-expansion in bilateral chronic subdural hematoma: possible mechanism of the higher recurrence rate. Injury. 2012;43(5):598–602.
36. Kutty SA, Johny M. Chronic subdural hematoma: a comparison of recurrence rates following burr-hole craniostomy with and without drains. Turk Neurosurg. 2014;24(4):494–7.
37. Laumer R. Implantation of a reservoir for refractory chronic subdural hematoma. Neurosurgery. 2002;50(3):672.
38. Laumer R, Schramm J, Leykauf K. Implantation of a reservoir for recurrent subdural hematoma drainage. Neurosurgery. 1989;25(6):991–6.
39. Liliang PC, Tsai YD, Liang CL, Lee TC, Chen HJ. Chronic subdural hematoma in young and extremely aged adults: a comparative study of two age groups. Injury. 2002;33:345–8.
40. Lin CC, Lu YM, Chen TH, Wang SP, Hsiao SH, Lin MS. Quantitative assessment of post-operative recurrence of chronic subdural hematoma using mean hematoma density. Brain Inj. 2014;28(8):1082–6.
41. Lind CR, Lind CJ, Mee EW. Reduction in the number of repeated operations for the treatment of subacute and chronic subdural hematomas by placement of subdural drains. J Neurosurg. 2003;99:44–6.
42. Lindvall P, Koskinen LO. Anticoagulants and antiplatelet agents and the risk of development and recurrence of chronic subdural hematomas. J Clin Neurosci. 2009;16:1287–90.

43. Liu W, Bakker NA, Groen RJ. Chronic subdural hematoma: a systematic review and meta-analysis of surgical procedures. J Neurosurg. 2014;121:665–73.
44. Liu H, Luo Z, Liu Z, Yang J, Kan S. Atorvastatin may attenuate recurrence of chronic subdural hematoma. Front Neurosci. 2016;10:303.
45. Lutz K, Kamenova M, Schaedelin S, Guzman R, Mariani L, Fandino J, Soleman J. Time to and possible risk factors for recurrence after Burr-hole drainage of chronic subdural hematoma: a subanalysis of the cSDH-drain randomized controlled trial. World Neurosurg. 2019;132:e283–9.
46. Majovsky M, Masopust V, Netuka D, Benes V. Flexible endoscope-assisted evacuation of chronic subdural hematomas. Acta Neurochir. 2016;158:1987–92.
47. Matsumoto H, Hanayama H, Okada T, Sakurai Y, Minami H, Masuda A, et al. Which surgical procedure is effective for refractory chronic subdural hematoma? Analysis of our surgical procedures and literature review. J Clin Neurosci. 2018;49:40–7.
48. Misra M, Salazar JL, Bloom DM. Subdural-peritoneal shunt: treatment for bilateral chronic subdural hematoma. Surg Neurol. 1996;46(4):378–83.
49. Mobbs R, Khong P. Endoscopic-assisted evacuation of subdural collections. J Clin Neurosci. 2009;16:701–4.
50. Mori K, Maeda M. Surgical treatment of chronic subdural hematoma in 500 consecutive cases: clinical characteristics, surgical outcome, complications, and recurrence rate. Neurol Med Chir. 2001;41(8):371–81.
51. Motiei-Langroudi R, Thomas AJ, Ascanio L, Alturki A, Papavassiliou E, Kasper EM, et al. Factors predicting the need for surgery of the opposite side after unilateral evacuation of bilateral chronic subdural hematomas. Neurosurgery. 2018;85(5):648–55.
52. Muzii VF, Bistazzoni S, Zalaffi A, Carangelo B, Mariottini A, Palma L. Chronic subdural hematoma: comparison of two surgical techniques. Preliminary results of a prospective randomized study. J Neurosurg Sci. 2005;49:41–6.
53. Nagatani K, Wada K, Takeuchi S, Nawashiro H. Corticosteroid suppression of vascular endothelial growth factor and recurrence of chronic subdural hematoma. Neurosurgery. 2012;70:E1334.
54. Nakaguchi H, Tanishima T, Yoshimasu N. Relationship between drainage catheter location and postoperative recurrence of chronic subdural hematoma after burr-hole irrigation and closed-system drainage. J Neurosurg. 2000;93(5):791–5.
55. Nakaguchi H, Tanishima T, Yoshimasu N. Factors in the natural history of chronic subdural hematomas that influence their postoperative recurrence. J Neurosurg. 2001;95(2):256–62.
56. Neal MT, Hsu W, Urban JE, Angelo NM, Sweasey TA, Branch CL Jr. The subdural evacuation port system: outcomes from a single institution experience and predictors of success. Clin Neurol Neurosurg. 2013;115(6):658–64.
57. Neils DM, Singanallur PS, Wang H, Tracy P, Klopfenstein J, Dinh D, et al. Recurrence-free chronic subdural hematomas: a retrospective analysis of the instillation of tissue plasminogen activator in addition to twist drill or burr-hole drainage in the treatment of chronic subdural hematomas. World Neurosurg. 2012;78:145–9.
58. Oh HJ, Lee KS, Shim JJ, Yoon SM, Yun IG, Bae HG. Postoperative course and recurrence of chronic subdural hematoma. J Korean Neurosurg Soc. 2010;48:518–23.
59. Ou Y, Dong J, Wu L, Xu L, Wang L, Liu B, et al. A comparative study of chronic subdural hematoma in three age ranges: below 40 years, 41-79 years, and 80 years and older. Clin Neurol Neurosurg. 2019;178:63–9.
60. Pang CH, Lee SE, Kim CH, Kim JE, Kang HS, Park CK, et al. Acute intracranial bleeding and recurrence after bur hole craniostomy for chronic subdural hematoma. J Neurosurg. 2015;123(1):65–74.
61. Probst C. Peritoneal drainage of chronic subdural hematomas in older patients. J Neurosurg. 1988;68(6):908–11.
62. Ridwan S, Bohrer AM, Grote A, Simon M. Surgical treatment of chronic subdural hematoma: predicting recurrence and cure. World Neurosurg. 2019;128:e1010–23.

63. Rocchi G, Caroli E, Salvati M, Delfini R. Membranectomy in organized chronic subdural hematomas: indications and technical notes. Surg Neurol. 2007;67:374–80.
64. Rust T, Kiemer N, Erasmus A. Chronic subdural hematomas and anticoagulation or antithrombotic therapy. J Clin Neurosci. 2006;13(8):823–7.
65. Sahyouni R, Mahboubi H, Tran P, Roufail JS, Chen JW. Membranectomy in chronic subdural hematoma: meta-analysis. World Neurosurg. 2017;104:418–29.
66. Santarius T, Kirkpatrick PJ, Ganesan D, Chia HL, Jalloh I, Smielewski P, et al. Use of drains versus no drains after burr-hole evacuation of chronic subdural hematoma: a randomized controlled trial. Lancet. 2009;374:1067–73.
67. Sato M, Iwatsuki K, Akiyama C, Kumura E, Yoshimine T. Implantation of a reservoir for refractory chronic subdural hematoma. Neurosurgery. 2001;48:1297–301.
68. Schoedel P, Bruendl E, Hochreiter A, Scheitzach J, Bele S, Brawanski A, Schebesch KM. Restoration of functional integrity after evacuation of chronic subdural hematoma-an age-adjusted analysis of 697 patients. World Neurosurg. 2016;94:465–70.
69. Schwarz F, Loos F, Dünisch P, Sakr Y, Safatli DA, Kalff R, Ewald C. Risk factors for reoperation after initial burr hole trephination in chronic subdural hematomas. Clin Neurol Neurosurg. 2015;138:66–71.
70. Shen J, Yuan L, Ge R, Wang Q, Zhou W, Jiang XC, Shao X. Clinical and radiological factors predicting recurrence of chronic subdural hematoma: a retrospective cohort study. Injury. 2019;50(10):1634–40.
71. Shimamura N, Ogasawara Y, Naraoka M, Ohnkuma H. Irrigation with thrombin solution reduces recurrence of chronic subdural hematoma in high-risk patients: preliminary report. J Neurotrauma. 2009;26:1929–33.
72. Shin HS, Lee SH, Ko HC, Koh JS. Extended pneumocephalus after drainage of chronic subdural hematoma associated with intracranial hypotension: case report with pathophysiologic consideration. J Korean Neurosurg Soc. 2016;59(1):69–74.
73. Smith MD, Kishikova L, Norris JM. Surgical management of chronic subdural hematoma: one hole or two? Int J Surg. 2012;10:450–2.
74. So CC, Wong KF. Valproate-associated dysmyelopoiesis in elderly patients. Am J Clin Pathol. 2002;118:225–8.
75. Stanisic M, Lund-Johansen M, Mahesparan R. Treatment of chronic subdural hematoma by burr-hole craniostomy in adults: influence of some factors on postoperative recurrence. Acta Neurochir. 2005;147:1249–57.
76. Sucu HK, Gokmen M, Gelal F. The value of XYZ/2 technique compared with computer-assisted volumetric analysis to estimate the volume of chronic subdural hematoma. Stroke. 2005;36:998–1000.
77. Sun TF, Boet R, Poon WS. Non-surgical primary treatment of chronic subdural haematoma: preliminary results of using dexamethasone. Br J Neurosurg. 2005;19:327–33.
78. Tahsim-Oglou Y, Beseoglu K, Hänggi D, Stummer W, Steiger H-J. Factors predicting recurrence of chronic subdural hematoma: the influence of intraoperative irrigation and low-molecular-weight heparin thromboprophylaxis. Acta Neurochir. 2012;154(6):1063–8.
79. Takahashi S, Yazaki T, Nitori N, Kano T, Yoshida K, Kawase T. Neuroendoscope assisted removal of an organized chronic subdural hematoma in a patient on bevacizumab therapy–case report. Neurol Med Chir. 2011;51:515–8.
80. Tanaka T, Kaimori M. Histological study of vascular structure between the dura mater and the outer membrane in chronic subdural hematoma in an adult. No Shinkei Geka. 1999;27:431–6.
81. Tanikawa M, Mase M, Yamada K, Yamashita N, Matsumoto T, Banno T, Miyati T. Surgical treatment of chronic subdural hematoma based on intrahematomal membrane structure on MRI. Acta Neurochir. 2001;143(6):613–9.
82. Tempaku A, Yamauchi S, Ikeda H, Tsubota N, Furukawa H, Maeda D, et al. Usefulness of interventional embolization of the middle meningeal artery for recurrent chronic subdural hematoma: five cases and a review of the literature. Interv Neuroradiol. 2015;21:366–71.

83. Thotakura AK, Marabathina NR. Nonsurgical treatment of chronic subdural hematoma with steroids. World Neurosurg. 2015;84(6):1968–72.
84. Toi H, Kinoshita K, Hirai S, Takai H, Hara K, Matsushita N, et al. Present epidemiology of chronic subdural hematoma in Japan: analysis of 63,358 cases recorded in a national administrative database. J Neurosurg. 2018;128:222–8.
85. Torihashi K, Sadamasa N, Yoshida K, Narumi O, Chin M, Yamagata S. Independent predictors for recurrence of chronic subdural hematoma: a review of 343 consecutive surgical cases. Neurosurgery. 2008;63(6):1125–9.
86. Tsai TH, Lieu AS, Hwang SL, Huang TY, Hwang YF. A comparative study of the patients with bilateral or unilateral chronic subdural hematoma: precipitating factors and postoperative outcomes. J Trauma. 2010;68:571–5.
87. Tugcu B, Tanriverdi O, Baydin S, Hergunsel B, Gunaldi O, Ofluoglu E, et al. Can recurrence of chronic subdural hematoma be predicted? A retrospective analysis of 292 cases. J Neurol Surg A Cent Eur Neurosurg. 2014;75(1):37–41.
88. Unterhofer C, Freyschlag CF, Thome C, Ortler M. Opening the internal hematoma membrane does not alter the recurrence rate of chronic subdural hematomas: a prospective randomized trial. World Neurosurg. 2016;92:31–6.
89. Utsuki S, Oka H, Kijima C, Inukai M, Abe K, Fujii K. Role of saireito in postoperative chronic subdural hematoma recurrence prevention. J Tradit Med. 2012;29:137–42.
90. Voelker JL, Sambasivan M. The role of craniotomy and trephination in the treatment of chronic subdural hematoma. Neurosurg Clin N Am. 2000;11:535–40.
91. Wang D, Li T, Wei H, Wang Y, Yang G, Tian Y, et al. Atorvastatin enhances angiogenesis to reduce subdural hematoma in a rat model. J Neurol Sci. 2016a;362:91–9.
92. Wang Y, Zhou J, Fan C, Wang D, Jiao F, Liu B, Zhang Q. Influence of antithrombotic agents on the recurrence of chronic subdural hematomas and the quest about the recommencement of antithrombotic agents: a meta-analysis. J Clin Neurosci. 2016b;38:79–83.
93. Watanabe S, Amagasaki K, Shono N, Nakaguchi H. Fibrin glue injection into the hematoma cavity for refractory chronic subdural hematoma: a case report. Surg Neurol Int. 2016;7(Suppl 37):S876–9.
94. Watts DD, Trask A, Soeken K, Perdue P, Dols S, Kaufmann C. Hypothermic coagulopathy in trauma: effect on varying levels of enzyme speed, platelet function and fibrinolytic activity. J Trauma. 1998;44(5):846–54.
95. Weigel R, Schmiedek P, Krauss JK. Outcome of contemporary surgery for chronic subdural hematoma: evidence based review. J Neurol Neurosurg Psychiatry. 2003;74:937–43.
96. Weigel R, Hohenstein A, Schlickum L, Weiss C, Schilling L. Angiotensin converting enzyme inhibition for arterial hypertension reduces the risk of recurrence in patients with chronic subdural hematoma possibly by an antiangiogenic mechanism. Neurosurgery. 2007;61:788–92.
97. Xu XP, Liu C, Liu J, Pang YG, Lu O XD, Fu J, et al. Local application of corticosteroids combined with surgery for the treatment of chronic subdural hematoma. Turk Neurosurg. 2015;25(2):252–5.
98. Xu M, Chen P, Zhu X, Wang C, Shi X, Yu B. Effects of atorvastatin on conservative and surgical treatments of chronic subdural hematoma in patients. World Neurosurg. 2016;91:23–8.
99. Yadav YR, Parihar V, Namdev H, Bajaj J. Chronic subdural hematoma. Asian J Neurosurg. 2016;11(4):330–42.
100. Yamamoto H, Hirashima Y, Hamada H, Hayashi N, Origasa H, Endo S. Independent predictors of recurrence of chronic subdural hematoma: results of multivariate analysis performed using a logistic regression model. J Neurosurg. 2003;98(6):1217–21.
101. Yasunaga H. Effect of japanese herbal Kampo medicine Goreisan on reoperation rates after burr-hole surgery for chronic subdural hematoma: analysis of a National Inpatient Database. Evid Based Complement Alternat Med. 2015;2015:817616.
102. You CG, Zheng XS. Postoperative pneumocephalus increases the recurrence rate of chronic subdural hematoma. Clin Neurol Neurosurg. 2018;166:56–60.
103. Zhang Y, Chen S, Xiao Y, Tang W. Effects of dexamethasone in the treatment of recurrent chronic subdural hematoma. World Neurosurg. 2017;105:115–21.
104. Zumofen D, Regli L, Levivier M, Krayenbuhl N. Chronic subdural hematomas treated by burr hole trepanation and a subperiostal drainage system. Neurosurgery. 2009;64:1116–21.

Chapter 37
Rehabilitation for Chronic Subdural Hematoma in the Elderly

Engin Taştaban and Mehmet Turgut

37.1 Introduction

Chronic subdural hematoma (CSDH) is a frequent disease in neurosurgical practice, particularly in elderly patients [12, 18]. This disorder often occurs in the elderly after a minor injury [5]. Other risk factors for CSDH include male gender, history of chronic alcoholism, presence of hematological coagulopathies, and use of anticoagulant drugs [28, 37]. The incidence of CSDH in the population ranges from 8.2 to 14.0 per 100,000 people per years.

CSDH is characterized by a collection of blood and blood breakdown products in the subdural space with a relatively slow but progressive course of disease, over an extended period [16, 20]. On the other hand, it is possible to diagnose CSDH quickly using computed tomography or magnetic resonance imaging, demonstrating a characteristic crescent-shaped space occupying lesion [9]. Unfortunately, however, recurrence was reported to be 6.1–22%, although surgical treatment is effective in the management of patients with CSDH [13].

Clinical presentation of CSDH is variable with both onset of symptoms and their progression extending from days to weeks in duration [22, 32]. Symptoms and signs develop if the mass effect caused by the hematoma within the subdural space results in an intolerable compression of the cerebral cortex. In clinical practice, patients with CSDH have multiple symptoms, including weakness, headache, mental status

E. Taştaban (✉)
Department of Physical Medicine and Rehabilitation, Adnan Menderes University Faculty of Medicine, Aydın, Turkey

M. Turgut
Department of Neurosurgery, Aydın Adnan Menderes University Faculty of Medicine, Efeler, Aydın, Turkey

Department of Histology and Embryology, Aydın Adnan Menderes University Health Sciences Institute, Efeler, Aydın, Turkey

M. Turgut et al. (eds.), *Subdural Hematoma*,
https://doi.org/10.1007/978-3-030-79371-5_37

changes, aphasia, apraxia, incoordination, visuospatial dysfunction, gait changes, falls, and seizures [18].

Clinically, hemiparesis was found in most patients of CSDH [2]. Hemiparesis can initially be transitory and then persistent. As a rule, weakness of the extremities is generally mild, but there is a disproportionate drowsiness associated with neurological deficit. Neurologically, the deficit is usually contralateral, although there are case reports with ipsilateral clinical symptoms and signs. Gait disturbance and falls are a common presenting symptom in patients with CSDH [31]. It is important to know that recurrent falls are considered a major risk for development of CSDH. Although, development of a CSDH may cause recurrent falls possibly due to altered mental status of these patients or their neurological deficits.

37.2 Inpatient Rehabilitation Management

Despite recent developments in surgical and pharmacologic treatment, CSDH is still a debilitating condition [3]. Rehabilitation interventions allow for reduced physical limitations, reduced joint pain, improved quality of life, and decreased complications, but the ideal mobilization period following surgical treatment of CSDH is not known [19, 29]. However, it is generally accepted that early postoperative bed rest in patients with CSDH reduces recurrence rates due to providing expansion of the cerebral cortex [21]. On the other hand, it is well known that early mobilization is useful to decrease various complications of immobility, in particular venous thromboembolism and hospital-acquired infections [8]. In a recent systematic review, Cunningham et al. found that regular physical activity is associated with decreased rates of mortality, recurrent falls, cognitive decline, and depression in CSDH patients aged 60 years and older [11].

Patients with CSDH are candidates for rehabilitation programs in both the hospital and outpatient settings. Using rehabilitation programs that start in the intensive care unit and then continue into outpatient clinics, it is possible to provide significant clinical improvement in patients with CSDH [25]. An exercise program which consists of individual physical therapy and then an independent home program is applied by a rehabilitation team that are trained in mobility, self-care skills, and other activities of daily living of patients with CSDH [8]. There is no doubt that providing a maximal functional range of motion is the major aim of the exercise program for patients with CSDH. Technically, an increased range of motion is obtained using the process of exercise where the main purpose of flexibility stretching is to increase the range of motion and physical function and must be performed in a period of 5–7 days per week [27]. The stretching will be more effective if the muscles have been warmed with active exercise or with an external heating modality.

The production of full joint range of motion and the strength which is necessary to complete these skills is obtained with motion and resistance exercises and the use of various orthoses [6]. Soft tissue and joint mobilization as well as the prevention of contractures are obtained with early mobility [15]. Passive range of motion and active range of motion with maximal stretching should be performed daily in all motions. Strength training should be targeted towards the key muscle groups responsible for improved function to optimize the translation to functional gain [34]. Regular therapeutic exercise provides full strength, complete range of motion, and coordination, thereby reducing the risks of cardiovascular complications and osteoporosis [4]. Recently, Carlisi et al. suggested that an assisted rehabilitation program may help improve short-term postoperative balance and ambulatory status [8].

Weakness and reduced endurance are frequently observed after hospitalization of the patient in the intensive care unit due to prolonged bed rest. The presence of weakness may lead to various abnormalities in the gait and trials for ambulation have to start with standing at the bedside. In a previous study, Weiss et al. demonstrated that early physical therapy intervention improves recovery of muscle strength after stroke [33]. Activities for enhancement of the range of motion are vital for success of the rehabilitation used for the resolution of soft tissue contractures. The aim of active and passive stretching is completely empiric, but there is evidence that stretching may reduce development of contractures in such patients [1]. It is important to know that flexibility activities should be used for the affected muscle groups. There is no doubt that analgesic drugs may be necessary during the passive and active motions when the intensity of pain is severe.

37.3 Physical Therapeutic Modalities

Increasingly, some physical therapeutic modalities like electrical therapy, thermotherapy, and application of heat/cold are commonly used in the rehabilitation of patients with CSDH to relieve pain and increase the flexibility of muscles and joints [24]. It is well known that heat therapy relieves stiffness of joints and muscles, thus providing the therapeutic effect of stretching. Electrical therapy (i.e., transcutaneous electrical nerve stimulation) is used for pain control and muscle stimulation. These modalities may relieve the pain of joints and muscle and may therefore reduce the need for analgesic drugs [10].

37.4 Frailty

Frailty is widely accepted as a multifactorial syndrome characterized by presence of chronic illness, increased body fat mass, and older age where there is an increased risk for falls in these patients, resulting in increased morbidity and mortality rates [14]. In a previous systematic review of the treatment of frailty, it was concluded that therapeutic exercises are very effective for the prevention of serious adverse events [14].

37.5 Falls

It has been reported that falls are frequent among the patients with CSDH and are a major cause of morbidity in these patients [2]. Therefore, patients with CSDH should be investigated carefully for the diagnosis of balance impairment and/or muscle strength asymmetry as a risk factor for falling. Impairments in physical function affecting balance and mobility include reduced muscle strength, power and endurance, changes in soft tissues restricting joint range, reduced coordination, and disordered sensory and perceptual processes and cognitive dysfunction that are responsible for an increased incidence of falls. The rehabilitation team must be careful in the presence of risk factors. As expected, age-related changes and neurologic dysfunctions regarding gait are also important risk factors for falling [35].

37.6 Assistive Devices

It is well known that the use of assistive devices, which are external devices that assist a patient to perform a particular task, may be necessary for ambulation of some patients with CSDH [23]. In particular, quad and three-point canes provide adequate stability for these patients, by increasing the diameter of the cane base [23]. In such patients, use of a walker allows the patient to transport items from place to place, thus providing increased stability [23]. Therefore, the benefits of assistive devices have been recognized in particular for older people with CSDH in recent years.

37.7 Osteoporosis

Today, some authors believe that corticosteroids are useful in the management of patients with CSDH [19]. It has been suggested that the use of preoperative and postoperative corticosteroids prevent the development of recurrent CSDH [26]. In addition to exercise program, various drugs including calcium and vitamin D supplementation, use of oral antiresorptive agents, such as alendronate sodium or risedronate are routinely used in the medical treatment of patients with osteoporosis [7]. Regular weight-bearing or resistance training exercises can improve bone mass and minimize falls. An exercise program including walking, weight training, balance exercises, posture, and flexibility may be used in patients with CSDH [17]. It has been suggested that spinal extension exercises and progressive resistive back-strengthening exercises are useful to reduce the development of lumbar lordosis [30]. Furthermore, use of rigid thoracolumbar orthoses is recommended to provide extension of the spine in the presence of compression fractures in these patients [30].

37.8 Contractures

The term "contracture," limiting motion of the joint in certain directions and thus restricting its function, means a fixed stiffness of a soft tissue such as muscle, as a potential cause of pain and skin breakdown [36]. Wong et al. suggested that prolonged joint immobilization results in development of the contracture [36]. It is well known that some precautions such as proper positioning, passive range of motion, and stretching exercises are useful for prevention of contractures of the joints [36]. Positioning strategies are necessary for maintaining soft tissue length and some protective devices like static and dynamic splints are usually used for this purpose [35].

37.9 Outpatient Rehabilitation Management

Outpatient rehabilitation management is important in maintaining exercise capacity and lifelong function of the patient with CSDH. Modifying the environment prevents further injury and a positive impact on quality of life for these patients [35]. Use of nonslip rugs, improved lighting, and decreased bed height may be useful for the prevention of fall-related injuries in patients with CSDH [35].

37.10 Conclusion

After surgical and medical treatments of patients with CSDH, restricted ambulatory and functional status may influence the activities of daily living. An adequate education regarding the importance of exercise should be provided in outpatient rehabilitation programs for lifelong function. Today, it is well known that physical rehabilitation enables the patient to be more functional and to increase their quality of life.

References

1. Ada L, Dorsch S, Canning CG. Strengthening interventions increase strength and improve activity after stroke: a systematic review. Aust J Physiother. 2006;52:241–8.
2. Adhiyaman V, Asghar M, Ganeshram KN, Bhowmick BK. Chronic subdural haematoma in the elderly. Postgrad Med J. 2002;78:71–5.
3. Almenawer SA, Farrokhyar F, Hong C, Alhazzani W, Manoranjan B, Yarascavitch B, Arjmand P, Baronia B, Reddy K, Murty N, Singh S. Chronic subdural hematoma management: a systematic review and meta-analysis of 34,829 patients. Ann Surg. 2014;259:449–57.

4. American College of Sports Medicine, Chodzko-Zajko WJ, Proctor DN, Fiatarone Singh MA, Minson CT, Nigg CR, Salem GJ, Skinner JS. American College of Sports Medicine position stand. Exercise and physical activity for older adults. Med Sci Sports Exerc. 2009;41:1510–30.
5. Borger V, Vatter H, Oszvald A, Marquardt G, Seifert V, Guresir E. Chronic subdural haematoma in elderly patients: a retrospective analysis of 322 patients between the ages of 65-94 years. Acta Neurochir. 2012;154:1549–54.
6. Cadore EL, Pinto RS, Bottaro M, Izquierdo M. Strength and endurance training prescription in healthy and frail elderly. Aging Dis. 2014;5:183–95.
7. Camacho PM, Petak SM, Binkley N, Diab DL, Eldeiry LS, Farooki A, Harris ST, Hurley DL, Kelly J, Lewiecki EM, Pessah-Pollack R, McClung M, Wimalawansa SJ, Watts NB. American Association of Clinical Endocrinologists/American College of Endocrinology Clinical Practice Guidelines for the diagnosis and treatment of postmenopausal osteoporosis-2020 Update. Endocr Pract. 2020;26:1–46.
8. Carlisi E, Feltroni L, Tinelli C, Verlotta M, Gaetani P, Dalla Toffola E. Postoperative rehabilitation for chronic subdural hematoma in the elderly. An observational study focusing on balance, ambulation and discharge destination. Eur J Phys Rehabil Med. 2017;53:91–7.
9. Carroll JJ, Lavine SD, Meyers PM. Imaging of subdural hematomas. Neurosurg Clin N Am. 2017;28:179–203.
10. Chen N, Wang J, Mucelli A, Zhang X, Wang C. Electro-acupuncture is beneficial for knee osteoarthritis: the evidence from meta-analysis of randomized controlled trials. Am J Chin Med. 2017;45:965–85.
11. Cunningham C, O'Sullivan R, Caserotti P, Tully MA. Consequences of physical inactivity in older adults: a systematic review of reviews and meta-analyses. Scand J Med Sci Sports. 2020;30:816–27.
12. Dumont TM, Rughani AI, Goeckes T, Tranmer BI. Chronic subdural hematoma: a sentinel health event. World Neurosurg. 2013;80:889–92.
13. Edlmann E, Giorgi-Coll S, Whitfield PC, Carpenter KLH, Hutchinson PJ. Pathophysiology of chronic subdural haematoma: inflammation, angiogenesis and implications for pharmacotherapy. J Neuroinflammation. 2017;14:108.
14. Fried LP, Tangen CM, Walston J, Newman AB, Hirsch C, Gottdiener J, Seeman T, Tracy R, Kop WJ, Burke G, McBurnie MA. Frailty in older adults: evidence for a phenotype. J Gerontol A Biol Sci Med Sci. 2001;56:M146–56.
15. Han P, Zhang W, Kang L, Ma Y, Fu L, Jia L, Yu H, Chen X, Hou L, Wang L, Yu X, Kohzuki M, Guo Q. Clinical evidence of exercise benefits for stroke. Adv Exp Med Biol. 2017;1000:131–51.
16. Holl DC, Volovici V, Dirven CMF, Peul WC, van Kooten F, Jellema K, van der Gaag NA, Miah IP, Kho KH, den Hertog HM, Lingsma HF, Dammers R. Pathophysiology and nonsurgical treatment of chronic subdural hematoma: from past to present to future. World Neurosurg. 2018;116:402–11.
17. Kirazli Y, Atamaz Calis F, El O, Gokce Kutsal Y, Peker O, Sindel D, Tuzun S, Gogas Yavuz D, Durmaz B, Akarirmak U, Bodur H, Hamuryudan V, Inceboz U, Oncel S. Updated approach for the management of osteoporosis in Turkey: a consensus report. Arch Osteoporos. 2020;15:137.
18. Kolias AG, Chari A, Santarius T, Hutchinson PJ. Chronic subdural haematoma: modern management and emerging therapies. Nat Rev Neurol. 2014;10:570–8.
19. Kurabe S, Ozawa T, Watanabe T, Aiba T. Efficacy and safety of postoperative early mobilization for chronic subdural hematoma in elderly patients. Acta Neurochir. 2010;152:1171–4.
20. Kwon CS, Al-Awar O, Richards O, Izu A, Lengvenis G. Predicting prognosis of patients with chronic subdural hematoma: a new scoring system. World Neurosurg. 2018;109:e707–14.
21. Mehta V, Harward SC, Sankey EW, Nayar G, Codd PJ. Evidence based diagnosis and management of chronic subdural hematoma: a review of the literature. J Clin Neurosci. 2018;50:7–15.
22. Merrill SA, Khan D, Richards AE, Kalani MA, Patel NP, Neal MT. Functional recovery following surgery for chronic subdural hematoma. Surg Neurol Int. 2020;11:450.
23. Panel on Prevention of Falls in Older Persons, American Geriatrics Society and British Geriatrics Society. Summary of the Updated American Geriatrics Society/British Geriatrics

Society clinical practice guideline for prevention of falls in older persons. J Am Geriatr Soc. 2011;59:148–57.
24. Paolillo FR, Paolillo AR, Joao JP, Frasca D, Duchene M, Joao HA, Bagnato VS. Ultrasound plus low-level laser therapy for knee osteoarthritis rehabilitation: a randomized, placebo-controlled trial. Rheumatol Int. 2018;38:785–93.
25. Ragland JT, Lee K. Chronic subdural hematoma ICU management. Neurosurg Clin N Am. 2017;28:239–46.
26. Roh D, Reznik M, Claassen J. Chronic subdural medical management. Neurosurg Clin N Am. 2017;28:211–7.
27. Sady SP, Wortman M, Blanke D. Flexibility training: ballistic, static or proprioceptive neuromuscular facilitation? Arch Phys Med Rehabil. 1982;63:261–3.
28. Sahyouni R, Goshtasbi K, Mahmoodi A, Tran DK, Chen JW. Chronic subdural hematoma: a historical and clinical perspective. World Neurosurg. 2017;108:948–53.
29. Shapey J, Glancz LJ, Brennan PM. Chronic subdural haematoma in the elderly: is it time for a new paradigm in management? Curr Geriatr Rep. 2016;5:71–7.
30. Sinaki M. Critical appraisal of physical rehabilitation measures after osteoporotic vertebral fracture. Osteoporos Int. 2003;14:773–9.
31. Tabuchi S, Kadowaki M. Chronic subdural hematoma in patients over 90 years old in a super-aged society. J Clin Med Res. 2014;6:379–83.
32. Uno M, Toi H, Hirai S. Chronic subdural hematoma in elderly patients: is this disease benign? Neurol Med Chir. 2017;57:402–9.
33. Weiss A, Suzuki T, Bean J, Fielding RA. High intensity strength training improves strength and functional performance after stroke. Am J Phys Med Rehabil. 2000;79:369–76; quiz 391–64.
34. Williams G, Kahn M, Randall A. Strength training for walking in neurologic rehabilitation is not task specific: a focused review. Am J Phys Med Rehabil. 2014;93:511–22.
35. Winstein CJ, Stein J, Arena R, Bates B, Cherney LR, Cramer SC, Deruyter F, Eng JJ, Fisher B, Harvey RL, Lang CE, MacKay-Lyons M, Ottenbacher KJ, Pugh S, Reeves MJ, Richards LG, Stiers W, Zorowitz RD. Guidelines for adult stroke rehabilitation and recovery: a guideline for healthcare professionals from the American Heart Association/American Stroke Association. Stroke. 2016;47:e98–e169.
36. Wong K, Trudel G, Laneuville O. Noninflammatory joint contractures arising from immobility: animal models to future treatments. Biomed Res Int. 2015;2015:848290.
37. Yang W, Huang J. Chronic subdural hematoma: epidemiology and natural history. Neurosurg Clin N Am. 2017;28:205–10.

Chapter 38
Outcome and Prognosis of Chronic Subdural Hematoma

Serdar Ercan, Zeki Serdar Ataizi, and Kemal Yücesoy

38.1 Introduction

Chronic subdural hematoma (CSDH) is a hemorrhagic collection of at least 21 days located between the dura and arachnoid membrane. This collection is a more common pathology in adults, especially in elderly patients. Thickening of the outer layer of the dura occurs due to the synthesis of dural collagen and the clustering of fibroblasts on the inner surface of the dura after subdural hemorrhage develops. As time passes, the subdural hematoma (SDH) liquefies and takes the form of a hygroma. During this period, calcifications in the inner wall of the dura and septa in the hemorrhage may form. Hygromas are thought to passively cause brain atrophy, trauma to neural tissue, dehydration, and an increase in intracranial pressure.

Surgical evacuation is among the options available to reduce the mass effect of bleeding. Evacuation can be accomplished with many different techniques. Unilateral or bilateral hematoma drainage is recommended in patients with liquefied blood, without membranes or a calcified hematoma [8, 42]. The prognosis for CSDH is generally considered to be good. However, there have been many studies showing that CSDH can lead to patient morbidity and mortality [6, 9].

S. Ercan (✉)
Department of Neurosurgery, Eskisehir City Hospital, Eskisehir, Turkey

Z. S. Ataizi
Department of Neurosurgery, Yunus Emre State Hospital, Eskisehir, Turkey

K. Yücesoy
Department of Neurosurgery, Bahcesehir University, Faculty of Medicine, Istanbul, Turkey

M. Turgut et al. (eds.), *Subdural Hematoma*,
https://doi.org/10.1007/978-3-030-79371-5_38

38.2 Age and Prognosis

As the proportion of the elderly in the population increases, the number of patients presenting with subdural hematoma will continue to increase. Age is directly related to prognosis [9, 10, 26, 32, 43]. Gonzales-Vargas et al. reported that the prognosis was significantly worse in patients over 80 years of age [17]. This view is supported by similar studies [16, 43]. However, although advanced age is one of the reasons for poor prognosis, this should be ignored when deciding on surgical intervention. Despite their advanced age, there are many elderly patients who recover after surgical intervention [15, 38, 56].

Although advanced age is a criterion for poor prognosis, no significant difference was observed between age groups [42]. Gelabert-Gonzales et al. in their series of 1000 patients emphasized that cognitive changes were more common in patients over 70 years of age (33.8%) compared to younger patients (21.7%) with increased intracranial pressure [16]. Asghar reported that the most common clinical symptoms in patients over 65 years of age were mental disorders [2].

38.3 Surgical Technique and Prognosis

Some techniques for surgical treatment of CSDH such as twist drill craniostomy (TDC), burr-hole craniostomy (BHC), craniotomy/minicraniotomy have been described over the years [11, 49]. The aim of surgery is to evacuate the hematoma and to reduce the intracranial pressure. Tabaddor and Shulman showed in their closed system drainage twist drill craniostomy study that the intracranial pressure decreased to zero after 20% of the subdural fluid accumulation was evacuated [47]. They suggested that this 20% volume decrease is usually sufficient to cause significant clinical improvement [47]. Markwalder et al. reported that in burr-hole craniotomy studies with closed system drainage, 78% of patients could still have a subdural collection that did not affect healing up to the tenth postoperative day. It is known that the subdural collection is completely resorbed on CT in 85% of patients by 40 days after surgery. For this reason, they suggest that there is no need to intervene with the collection as long as the patient does not improve or clinically deteriorate [31].

Weigel et al. found no significant difference in recovery and mortality between these three surgical techniques [53]. However, they reported that TDC had a significantly higher recurrence rate compared to BHC and craniotomy, and they concluded that BHC provided the best treatment-to-complication ratio. In contrast, Ducruet stated that BHC resulted in a higher rate of complications compared to TDC and craniotomy [16]. Additionally, they recommended TDC as the first-line intervention because BHC resulted in less recurrence than TDC and craniotomy, and recommended that the craniotomy technique should be used for patients with extensive

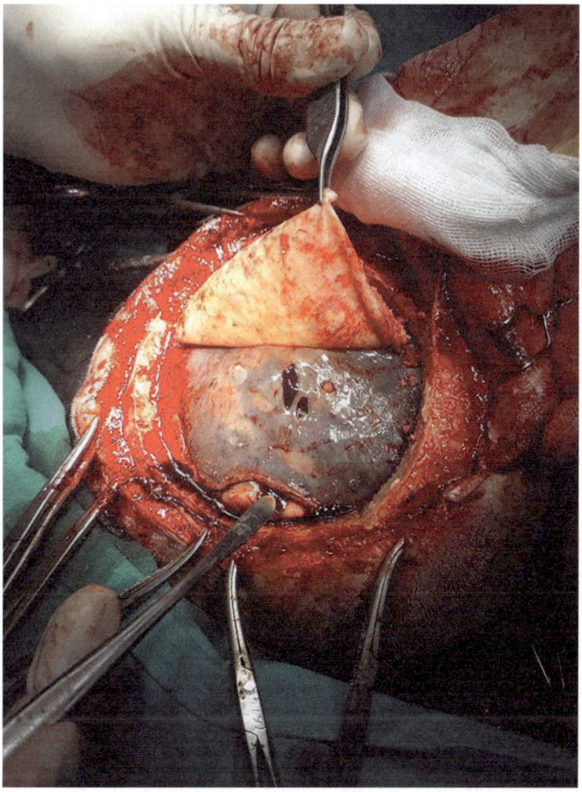

Fig. 38.1 The craniotomy technique used for the patient due to the extensive membrane formation

membrane formation (Fig. 38.1) [11]. Almenawer reported that there was no significant difference in recovery, recurrence, morbidity, or mortality rates between TDC and BHC, and craniotomy caused a higher complication rate [1].

38.4 Rebleeding

CSDH recurrence is an important problem observed in approximately 5–30% of patients. Risk factors that cause recurrent bleeding include advanced age, male gender, brain atrophy, and use of anticoagulants or antiplatelet drugs [39]. Septated CSDH is a special type of hematoma that contains individual spaces divided into different sections by fibrin. These septations constitute a completely independent risk factor for recurrence [7]. Since only the liquid form of CSDH can be evacuated with burr-hole drainage, the septa remain inside the hematoma. Although the complication rate is high in the presence of thick septa, the craniectomy technique should be used [55]. Twist drill craniostomy technique was found to have a higher recurrence rate compared to other burr-hole craniostomy and classical craniotomy techniques. In addition, the use of a closed system drainage after burr-hole craniostomy reduces the risk. It has been stated that the rate of recurrence increased significantly in patients who did not have a drainage system and who only underwent burr-hole craniostomy compared to patients who underwent drainage [34]. Some of the factors that increase the risk of rebleeding are the patient being older than 70 years of age, a history of pre-existing cerebral infarction, and taking anticoagulant or antiplatelet therapy. In addition to advanced age, thick subdural membrane bleeding and bilateral bleeding further increase the risk.

38.5 Brain Expansion

Factors that reduce re-expansion of the brain after surgery are similar to those that cause recurrence. A history of pre-existing cerebral infarction, tension pneumocephalus due to the presence of air in the subdural space, and intracranial hypotension affect brain compliance and prevent postoperative expansion. It has been reported that diseases such as arterial hypertension and diabetes mellitus do not affect the re-expansion of the cortex [5]. Radiological findings can show significant hematomas with or without shifting of the midline brain structures. Hematoma width and a shift of the midline are indicative of poor prognosis. Septa have been associated with higher recurrence rates [24, 33, 36, 43, 52, 54]. Postoperative bed rest, intravenous volume replacement, or fluid intake after evacuation of CSDH facilitate the re-expansion of the brain. In addition, there are clinical studies showing that the application of CO_2 or O_2 to the surgical area helps the brain to re-expand after craniotomy, before closing the dura or replacing the bone flap [16].

38.6 Mortality and Morbidity

One of the most important factors affecting mortality and morbidity in patients with CSDH is the patient's preoperative Glasgow Coma Score (GCS). Having a GCS between 3 and 12 and an ASA of 3 or more increases mortality and morbidity. Rohde et al. stated that the overall mortality rate was 13.3% [42]. In addition, the presence of additional systemic and/or central nervous system pathologies such as the presence of infection and venous thromboembolism worsen the clinical picture. The complication rate varies between 6 and 32% [41, 46].

In their study on mortality rates, Weigel and colleagues compared the mortality rates for twist drill craniostomy technique (2.7%), burr-hole craniostomy technique (2.9%), and craniotomy (4.6%) and showed that there was no significant difference between them [21]. In similar cohort studies comparing surgical techniques, it was stated that there was no significant difference between those surgical techniques when they compared recurrence rates, reoperation, length of hospital stay, neurological recovery, and mortality rates [11, 34]. The 4% mortality rate is similar to the previously reported mortality rates [4].

Rebleeding is now considered a complication affecting morbidity [4, 27]. Brodbelt et al. defined morbidity as any complication occurring during or after surgery other than recurrence. They found that craniotomy (12.3%) had higher morbidity rates than twist drill craniostomy (3%) and burr-hole craniostomy (3.8%) [5]. Therefore, reoperation after craniotomy is observed more frequently than for other surgical techniques. However, neurological improvement is best achieved in cases with craniotomy [11]. Post-surgical infection rates are variable and reported by Borger as 3.6%, Gelabert as 1.7%, and Rohde as 2.1% [16, 42]. The relationship between the neurological status of the patient at admission and their poor prognosis has been reported in previous studies [13, 30, 31, 43]. Ramachandran found that GCS at admission and the presence of comorbid diseases are associated with the GOS [40].

38.7 Epilepsy

Central nervous system complications in CSDH can be in the form of seizures, acute subdural and intracerebral hemorrhage, tension pneumocephalus, subdural empyema, and wound infection [32]. In CSDH, the hematoma causes epilepsy by irritating the cortical surface with blood compounds and later causing irritation with degradation products [14]. In particular, the separation of hemoglobin on the cortical surface is highly epileptogenic [18, 20]. It has been reported that seizures are observed in 24% in acute SDH and in 11% in chronic SDH [19, 22, 50]. For patients with CSDH, the risk factors for seizures are different from those for acute SDH. A prospective study reported that alcoholism is a risk factor for seizures in CSDH [12]. Previous studies have shown that the rate of a poor functional outcome increases gradually with age. In contrast, patients under 75 years of age have been reported to recover without an increase in this complication rate compared to older patients [16, 23, 28]. Although 2–19% seizure rates have been reported in patients with CSDH, many studies have different rates or descriptions of seizures. Oshida et al. observed transient hyperemia of the cortex under the CSDH immediately after surgical evacuation in elderly patients [39]. They suggested that this finding may be related to complications such as acute intracranial bleeding and seizures. Similarly, van Havenbergh et al. reported that the capsule left in situ may be responsible for late epilepsy [21]. For these reasons, the role of prophylactic anticonvulsant drugs in CSDH patients was analyzed and it was concluded that patients who received prophylactic phenytoin had a significant decrease in seizure development.

Today, there are controversial suggestions regarding prophylactic anticonvulsant drug therapy for patients with CSDH. A retrospective study focusing on surgically treated patients with CSDH showed that the use of prophylactic phenytoin effectively reduced seizures; however, the outcome benefit was not fully defined [28]. Another study reported that prophylactic antiepileptic drug therapy resulted in a lower incidence of seizures in CSDHs. Conversely, there was no benefit in patients treated prophylactically with AEDs after discharge [39]. Even though the use of a prophylactic anticonvulsant has been recommended for 6 months, due to the variable incidence of epileptic seizures in patients with CSDH, there is currently no consensus recommendation for the use of prophylactic antiepileptic drugs in these patients [37, 44, 45].

38.8 Antiagregan Therapy

CSDH is one of the most important pathologies observed in neurosurgery especially in the elderly population after mild head trauma. To the best of our knowledge, known risk factors for bleeding include old age, previous cranial hemorrhage, intracranial hypotension, and pre-trauma anticoagulant or antiaggregant therapy [3, 25, 29]. It has been reported that 16–76% of patients presenting with CSDH have a history of antiaggregation therapy [35, 48, 51].

Evaluation with brain CT in the early postoperative period will help in making the decision to initiate anticoagulant and antiaggregant treatment. In anticoagulant therapy, the correct timing is one of the important factors that prevents recurrent bleeding or clinical deterioration of the patient. Although it is known that aspirin poses a risk for postoperative intracranial bleeding and CSDH, it is recommended to continue aspirin in patients without radiological bleeding signs on CT [35].

38.9 Conclusion

Age is directly related to prognosis and advanced age is one of the main reasons for poor prognosis. However, this should be ignored when deciding on surgical intervention. Despite the advanced age, there are many elderly patients who recover after surgical intervention. The aim of surgery is to evacuate the hematoma and to reduce the intracranial pressure. Previous studies recommend TDC as a first-line intervention despite BHC resulting in less recurrence than TDC and craniotomy, and recommended that the craniotomy technique should be used for patients with extensive membrane formation. Even though the use of a prophylactic anticonvulsants has been recommended for 6 months from the time of diagnosis, due to the variable incidence of epileptic seizures in patients with CSDH, there is currently no consensus recommendation for the use of prophylactic antiepileptic drugs.

References

1. Almenawer SA, Farrokhyar F, Hong C, Alhazzani W, Manoranjan B, Yarascavitch B, Arjmand P, Baronia B, Reddy K, Murty N. Chronic subdural hematoma management: a systematic review and meta-analysis of 34829 patients. Ann Surg. 2014;259:449–57.
2. Asghar M, Adhiyaman V, Greenway MW, Bhowmick BK, Bates A. Chronic subdural haematoma in the elderly—a North Wales experience. J R Soc Med. 2002;95:290–2.
3. Aspegren OP, Åstrand R, Lundgren MI, Romner B. Anticoagulation therapy a risk factor for the development of chronic subdural hematoma. Clin Neurol Neurosurg. 2013;115:981–4.
4. Borger V, Vatter H, Oszvald A, Marquardt G, Seifert V, Guresir E. Chronic subdural haematoma in elderly patients: a retrospective analysis of 322 patients between the ages of 65-94 years. Acta Neurochir (Wien). 2012;154:1549–54.
5. Brodbelt A, Warnke P, Weigel R, Krauss JK. Outcome of contemporary surgery for chronic subdural haematoma: evidence based review [3] (multiple letters). J Neurol Neurosurg Psychiatry. 2004;75:1209–10.
6. Bucher B, Maldaner N, Regli L, Sarnthein J, Serra C. Standardized assessment of outcome and complications in chronic subdural hematoma: results from a large case series. Acta Neurochir (Wien). 2019;161:1297–304.
7. Cai Q, Guo Q, Zhang F, Sun D, Zhang W, Ji B, Chen Z, Mao S. Evacuation of chronic and subacute subdural hematoma via transcranial neuroendoscopic approach. Neuropsychiatr Dis Treat. 2019;15:385–90.
8. Cenic A, Bhandari M, Reddy K. Management of chronic subdural hematoma: a national survey and literature review. Can J Neurol Sci. 2005;32:501–6.
9. Cofano F, Pesce A, Vercelli G, Mammi M, Massara A, Minardi M, Palmieri M, D'Andrea G, Fronda C, Lanotte MM, Tartara F, Zenga F, Frati A, Garbossa D. Risk of recurrence of chronic subdural hematomas after surgery: a multicenter observational cohort study. Front Neurol. 2020;11:1–10.
10. Delgado PD, Cogolludo FJ, Mateo O, Cancela P, Garcia R, Carrillo R. Early prognosis in chronic subdural hematomas. Multivariate analysis of 137 cases. Rev Neurol. 2000;30:811–7.
11. Ducruet AF, Grobelny BT, Zacharia BE, Hickman ZL, DeRosa PL, Anderson K, Sussman E, Carpenter A, Connolly ES. The surgical management of chronic subdural hematoma. Neurosurg Rev. 2012;35:155–69.
12. Dudek H, Michno T, Michalski J, Kaczmarek M, Drapało L. Late posttraumatic epilepsy in patients with an alcoholic problem treated surgically for posttraumatic chronic subdural hematomas. Rocz Akad Med Bialymst. 1999;44:119–27.
13. El-Kadi H, Miele VJ, Kaufman HH. Prognosis of chronic subdural hematomas. Neurosurg Clin N Am. 2000;11:553–67.
14. Frey LC. Epidemiology of posttraumatic epilepsy: a critical review. Epilepsia. 2003;44:11–7.
15. Fukui S. Evaluation of surgical treatment for chronic subdural hematoma in extremely aged (over 80 years old) patients (in Japanese). No To Shinkei. 1993;45:449–53.
16. Gelabert-González M, Iglesias-Pais M, García-Allut A, Martínez-Rumbo R. Chronic subdural haematoma: surgical treatment and outcome in 1000 cases. Clin Neurol Neurosurg. 2005;107:223–9.
17. González-Vargas PM, Thenier-Villa JL, Calero Félix L, Galárraga Campoverde RA, Martín-Gallego Á, de la Lama Zaragoza A, Conde Alonso CM. Factors that negatively influence the Glasgow Outcome Scale in patients with chronic subdural hematomas. An analytical and retrospective study in a tertiary center. Interdiscip Neurosurg. 2020;20:100606.
18. Haltiner AM, Temkin NR, Dikmen SS. Risk of seizure recurrence after the first late posttraumatic seizure. Arch Phys Med Rehabil. 1997;78:835–40.
19. Hamasaki T, Yamada K, Kuratsu J. Seizures as a presenting symptom in neurosurgical patients: a retrospective single-institution analysis. Clin Neurol Neurosurg. 2013;115:2336–40.
20. Hammond EJ, Ramsay RE, Villarreal HJ, Wilder BJ. Effects of intracortical injection of blood and blood components on the electrocorticogram. Epilepsia. 1980;21:3–14.

21. van Havenbergh T, van Calenbergh F, Goffin J, Plets C. Outcome of chronic subdural haematoma: analysis of prognostic factors. Br J Neurosurg. 1996;10:35–9.
22. Huang KT, Bi WL, Abd-El-Barr M, Yan SC, Tafel IJ, Dunn IF, Gormley WB. The neurocritical and neurosurgical care of subdural hematomas. Neurocrit Care. 2016;24:294–307.
23. Huang Y-H, Lin W-C, Lu C-H, Chen W-F. Volume of chronic subdural haematoma: is it one of the radiographic factors related to recurrence? Injury. 2014;45:1327–31.
24. Juković MF, Stojanović DB. Midline shift threshold value for hemiparesis in chronic subdural hematoma. Srp Arh Celok Lek. 2015;143:386–90.
25. Kamenova M, Lutz K, Schaedelin S, Fandino J, Mariani L, Soleman J. Does early resumption of low-dose aspirin after evacuation of chronic subdural hematoma with burr-hole drainage lead to higher recurrence rates? Neurosurgery. 2016;79:715–21.
26. Krupp WF, Jans PJ. Treatment of chronic subdural haematoma with burr-hole craniostomy and closed drainage. Br J Neurosurg. 1995;9:619–28.
27. Lee L, Ker J, Ng HY, Munusamy T, King NKK, Kumar D, Ng WH. Outcomes of chronic subdural hematoma drainage in nonagenarians and centenarians: a multicenter study. J Neurosurg. 2016;124:546–51.
28. Leroy H-A, Aboukais R, Reyns N, Bourgeois P, Labreuche J, Duhamel A, Lejeune J-P. Predictors of functional outcomes and recurrence of chronic subdural hematomas. J Clin Neurosci. 2015;22:1895–900.
29. Lindvall P, Koskinen L-OD. Anticoagulants and antiplatelet agents and the risk of development and recurrence of chronic subdural haematomas. J Clin Neurosci. 2009;16:1287–90.
30. Markwalder T-M. Chronic subdural hematomas: a review. J Neurosurg. 1981;54:637–45.
31. Markwalder TM, Steinsiepe KF, Rohner M, Reichenbach W, Markwalder H. The course of chronic subdural hematomas after burr-hole craniostomy and closed-system drainage. J Neurosurg. 1981;55:390–6.
32. Mori K, Maeda M. Surgical treatment of chronic subdural hematoma in 500 consecutive cases: clinical characteristics, surgical outcome, complications, and recurrence rate. Neurol Med Chir (Tokyo). 2001;41:371–81.
33. Motiei-Langroudi R, Alterman RL, Stippler M, Phan K, Alturki AY, Papavassiliou E, Kasper EM, Arle J, Ogilvy CS, Thomas AJ. Factors influencing the presence of hemiparesis in chronic subdural hematoma. J Neurosurg. 2019;131:1926–30.
34. Muzii VF, Bistazzoni S, Zalaffi A, Carangelo B, Mariottini A, Palma L. Chronic subdural hematoma: comparison of two surgical techniques. Preliminary results of a prospective randomized study. J Neurosurg Sci. 2005;49:41–7.
35. Nathan S, Goodarzi Z, Jette N, Gallagher C, Holroyd-Leduc J. Anticoagulant and antiplatelet use in seniors with chronic subdural hematoma: systematic review. Neurology. 2017;88:1889–93.
36. Oh H-J, Lee K-S, Shim J-J, Yoon S-M, Yun I-G, Bae H-G. Postoperative course and recurrence of chronic subdural hematoma. J Korean Neurosurg Soc. 2010;48:518–23.
37. Ohno K, Maehara T, Ichimura K, Suzuki R, Hirakawa K, Monma S. Low incidence of seizures in patients with chronic subdural haematoma. J Neurol Neurosurg Psychiatry. 1993;56:1231–3.
38. Ooba S, Shiomi N, Shigemori M. Clinical features and surgical results of chronic subdural hematoma in the extremely aged patients (in Japanese). No Shinkei Geka. 2006;34:273–8.
39. Oshida S, Akamatsu Y, Matsumoto Y, Ishigame S, Ogasawara Y, Aso K, Kashimura H. A case of chronic subdural hematoma demonstrating the epileptic focus at the area with sulcal hyperintensity on fluid-attenuated inversion recovery image. Radiol Case Rep. 2019;14:1109–12.
40. Ramachandran R, Hegde T. Chronic subdural hematomas-causes of morbidity and mortality. Surg Neurol. 2007;67:367–72.
41. Reponen E, Korja M, Niemi T, Silvasti-Lundell M, Hernesniemi J, Tuominen H. Preoperative identification of neurosurgery patients with a high risk of in-hospital complications: a prospective cohort of 418 consecutive elective craniotomy patients. J Neurosurg. 2015;123:594–604.
42. Rohde V, Graf G, Hassler W. Complications of burr-hole craniostomy and closed-system drainage for chronic subdural hematomas: a retrospective analysis of 376 patients. Neurosurg Rev. 2002;25:89–94.

43. Rovlias A, Theodoropoulos S, Papoutsakis D. Chronic subdural hematoma: surgical management and outcome in 986 cases: a classification and regression tree approach. Surg Neurol Int. 2015;6:127.
44. Rubin G, Rappaport ZH. Epilepsy in chronic subdural haematoma. Acta Neurochir (Wien). 1993;123:39–42.
45. Sabo RA, Hanigan WC, Aldag JC. Chronic subdural hematomas and seizures: the role of prophylactic anticonvulsive medication. Surg Neurol. 1995;43:579–82.
46. Sase T, Furuya Y, Tanaka Y. Hospital discharge arrangements for very elderly patients with chronic subdural hematoma (in Japanese). No Shinkei Geka. 2020;48:1115–20.
47. Schmidek HH, Sweet WH. Surgical management of chronic subdural hematoma in adults. In: Operative neurosurgical techniques. 2012. p. 1573–8.
48. Soleman J, Kamenova M, Guzman R, Mariani L. The management of patients with chronic subdural hematoma treated with low-dose acetylsalicylic acid: an international survey of practice. World Neurosurg. 2017;107:778–88.
49. Tabaddor K, Shulman K. Definitive treatment of chronic subdural hematoma by twist-drill craniostomy and closed-system drainage. J Neurosurg. 1977;46:220–6.
50. Temkin NR, Dikmen SS, Wilensky AJ, Keihm J, Chabal S, Winn HR. A randomized, double-blind study of phenytoin for the prevention of post-traumatic seizures. N Engl J Med. 1990;323:497–502.
51. Wada M, Yamakami I, Higuchi Y, Tanaka M, Suda S, Ono J, Saeki N. Influence of antiplatelet therapy on postoperative recurrence of chronic subdural hematoma: a multicenter retrospective study in 719 patients. Clin Neurol Neurosurg. 2014;120:49–54.
52. Wakuta N, Abe H, Nonaka M, Morishita T, Higashi T, Arima H, Inoue T. Analysis of endoscopic findings in the chronic subdural hematoma cavity: bleeding factors in chronic subdural hematoma natural history and as predictors of recurrence. World Neurosurg. 2019;124:e241–51.
53. Weigel R, Schmiedek P, Krauss JK. Outcome of contemporary surgery for chronic subdural haematoma: evidence based review. J Neurol Neurosurg Psychiatry. 2003;74:937–43.
54. Yan K, Gao H, Wang Q, Xu X, Wu W, Zhou X, Xu W, Ye F. Endoscopic surgery to chronic subdural hematoma with neovessel septation: technical notes and literature review. Neurol Res. 2016;38:467–76.
55. Yan K, Gao H, Zhou X, Wu W, Xu W, Xu Y, Gong K, Xue X, Wang Q, Na H. A retrospective analysis of postoperative recurrence of septated chronic subdural haematoma: endoscopic surgery versus burr hole craniotomy. Neurol Res. 2017;39:803–12.
56. Zingale A, Albanese V, Romano A, Distefano G, Chiaramonte J. Traumatic chronic subdural hematoma over 80 years. A preliminary prospective study. J Neurosurg Sci. 1997;41:169–73.

Chapter 39
Medicolegal Aspects of Subdural Hematoma

Mehmet Turgut and Erdal Kalkan

39.1 Introduction

Today, thousands of people suffer from a subdural hematoma (SDH) each year as a result of a head injury caused by motor vehicle accidents, falls, etc. worldwide. The incidence of SDH increases with age and it can be difficult to diagnose a case of SDH because the symptoms can be slow to develop. Unfortunately, further injury can occur due to misdiagnosis or negligent surgery, called medical malpractice, in such cases. It is well known that SDHs are more common in the elderly, athletes experiencing head trauma, bleeding disorders such as hemophilia and sickle cell disease, patients who take anticoagulation, alcoholics, and premature babies [7, 8, 13, 26]. In such cases, a comprehensive physical and neurological examination are a necessary part of the diagnostic evaluation.

Clinically, it is important to know that SDHs that develop more slowly as in the chronic subdural hematoma (CSDH) might be mistaken for other conditions, such as multiple myeloma, brain tumor, stroke, or dementia [6, 10, 23]. Furthermore, an elderly person may not remember or forget hitting their head, and sometimes the traumatic event was very minor and may have occurred weeks or months before the development of symptoms of SDH. Surgically, cases with SDHs are treated by drilling a hole into the skull to relieve the pressure on the brain, in addition to medical treatment. Unfortunately, however, many hospitals and physicians may make

M. Turgut (✉)
Department of Neurosurgery, Aydın Adnan Menderes University Faculty of Medicine, Efeler, Aydın, Turkey

Department of Histology and Embryology, Aydın Adnan Menderes University Health Sciences Institute, Efeler, Aydın, Turkey

E. Kalkan
Department of Neurosurgery, Private Medova Hospital, Konya, Turkey

M. Turgut et al. (eds.), *Subdural Hematoma*,
https://doi.org/10.1007/978-3-030-79371-5_39

clinical errors regarding the diagnosis and treatment of SDH, leading to permanent neurological injuries [6, 10].

In this chapter, various case scenarios of malpractice regarding the management of SDH, including those with missed or delayed diagnosis and treatment, those with a failure in the care of risk factors, neonatal premature babies undergoing vacuum or forceps-assisted deliveries, and those with (SBS). These cases are discussed in detail following a brief general review of SDH that was the cause of malpractice act.

39.2 Subdural Hematoma as a Cause of Malpractice Act

A SDH is characterized by a collection of blood between the dura mater and the arachnoid mater (Fig. 39.1). As a result of tears in bridging veins between the brain and these meningeal layers, a SDH develops that may cause compression of the surrounding brain tissue and signs of life-threatening increased intracranial pressure (IICP).

As discussed in detail in earlier chapters of this book, SDH is subdivided into acute, subacute, and chronic forms, taking into account the time elapsed after the onset of bleeding. SDHs are caused by a head injury causing vascular shear injuries due to various rotational or linear forces as the mechanism for their occurrence [12, 26]. Typically, the vessels extend along the inside of the skull that overlies the convexity of the brain, confined by dural structures such as the tentorium cerebelli and

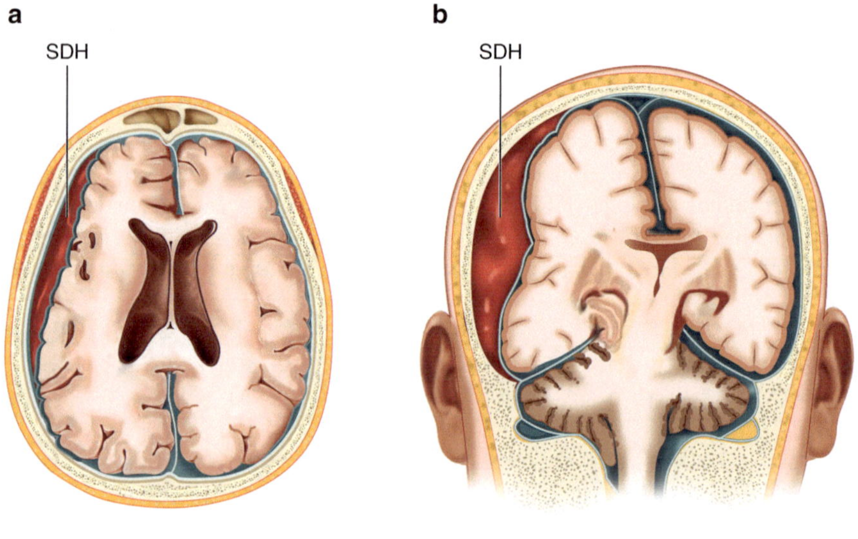

Fig. 39.1 A schematic drawing of axial (**a**) and coronal (**b**) sections showing blood collection between the dura mater and the arachnoid mater, called subdural hematoma (SDH), was produced by medical illustrator Sercan Çelebi

falx cerebri, thus creating a "concave" shape, in contrast to their epidural counterparts, which cannot cross the sutures of the skull, leading to a "biconvex lens" shape [10, 29].

Even following a relatively minor traumatic event, as a rule, SDHs may develop in those infants who have enlarged subdural spaces and elderly alcoholic people who have cortical cerebral atrophy, increasing the length of the bridging veins and thus increasing the likelihood of shear forces causing a vessel to tear. Furthermore, a SDH is frequently encountered in patients receiving antiplatelet or anticoagulant drugs, such as warfarin and aspirin. Moreover, an arachnoid cyst and cerebrospinal fluid (CSF) leaks in the juvenile age group are additional risk factors for the development of SDH, owing to a reduction in CSF pressure and leading to disruption of the bridging veins caused by pulling the arachnoid away from the dura mater [3, 9, 15, 22, 31]. Medicolegally, it is also important to remember that SDH may be seen in cases of SBS [20].

Clinically, it is very important to keep in mind that signs and symptoms of SDHs may develop within minutes in the acute form, but they can be delayed for months or years in the chronic form [13, 16, 18, 26]. In clinical practice, cases with SDH have any combination of the following symptoms including loss of consciousness, headache, nausea or vomiting, confusion, drowsiness, lethargy, dizziness, disorientation, inability to speak, weakness on one side of the body, difficulty walking, loss of balance, memory loss, altered breathing patterns, tinnitus, seizures, personality changes, psychiatric manifestations, blurred vision, irritability and enlarged head in babies, etc. [13, 16, 26, 28].

Radiologically, it is important that a computed tomography (CT) scan and/or magnetic resonance imaging (MRI) scan are obtained following a complete neurological examination in order to diagnose SDHs. SDHs are classically crescent-shaped on a CT scan, but they can have a convex appearance, especially in the early stages of bleeding causing difficulty in diagnosing SDH from its epidural counterpart [5, 10, 27, 29].

Treatment of a SDH depends on its size and rate of enlargement. Asymptomatic or small SDHs may be managed conservatively by careful clinical and radiological monitoring, but symptomatic or large collections should be treated by inserting a catheter for removal of the blood with suction or irrigation through a burr-hole or via craniotomy [13, 25, 26]. In addition, patients should be treated with anticonvulsant drugs for a long period of time. Acute SDHs generally expand at a slower rate than their epidural counterparts with an arterial bleeding source, but they have a high rate of mortality (50–90% of cases) because of the presence of associated serious traumatic injuries. Postoperative complications can include IICP, brain edema, recurrent bleeding, infection, and seizures [13].

Although SDH can also occur with normal, term deliveries, newborn premature babies have the highest risk for development of a SDH. In premature babies, one of the risk factors for development of SDH is use of a vacuum or forceps during the delivery that results in injury of tiny blood vessels in the involved brain. If a baby is diagnosed with a SDH, in addition to blood transfusion, surgical intervention may be needed to prevent brain damage or death. From a medicolegal standpoint of view, it is considered malpractice act for pediatrician to miss the diagnosis of a SDH that any reasonable prudent physician would make without difficulty. Indeed, to obtain a neurosurgical consultation following a cranial ultrasound (USG), CT scan, and/or MRI scan may indicate the need for surgery in some of these cases [5]. In these cases, as suggested by pediatric neurosurgeons, it is possible to perform a proper surgical procedure to improve the prognosis, if the correct diagnosis of SDH is made without delay.

Classically, SBS is a difficult diagnostic challenge with medicolegal implications and should be considered in pediatric cases with a triad of bilateral SDH, retinal hemorrhages, and encephalopathy as an indication of traumatic cranial injury, after excluding other etiologies with radiological studies and laboratory testing, although it has been under-reported in the literature [20, 21, 24, 30]. Recently, Lynøe et al. assessed the diagnostic value of the triad in the identification of traumatic shaking and they found that there was a little supportive scientific evidence (low-quality evidence) [19]. In such cases, however, it is important to realize that the neurosurgeon must report such suspected child abuse cases to the responsible legal authorities, in particular in the presence of a calcified or ossified chronic SDH in a baby associated with any kind of physical injury [1, 14, 21, 24, 30]. From a legal point of view, we believe that keeping the medical documents of patients with calcified or ossified chronic SDHs in our private archives in addition to that of the hospital may be useful.

As described below in detail, the common cases for negligence include a delay in diagnosis and treatment of SDH, a delay in obtaining an USG, CT, or MRI scan as a diagnostic study, or poor management of anticoagulation including monitoring of coagulation parameters such as the International Normalized Ratio (INR) when taking any anticoagulant drug for another health problem.

39.3 Case Scenarios of Malpractice upon Negligent Management of Subdural Hematoma

The examples of the case scenarios of malpractice with negligent management of SDH described below provide some useful guidelines regarding the correct diagnosis and proper management for physicians treating these cases.

39.3.1 Missed or Delayed Diagnosis and Treatment of SDH

Case 1: A claim settled for "delayed diagnosis" of SDH leading to death

A brief case scenario may be as follows: "*The deceased ... year old man who fell down a flight of stairs ... he had ... a reduced Glasgow Coma Scale (GCS) score and ... He was noted to be on warfarin ... for a heart ... he was sent for an urgent*

CT scan ... the radiologist reported that the scan did not show any intracranial bleeding, no attempt was made to reverse the deceased's warfarin and increase his clotting factors. ... later, ... a second radiologist ... identified a ... SDH. ... this information was conveyed to the consultant in charge of the deceased's care ..., there was a failure to contact the on-call neurosurgeons for advice or to stop/reverse the warfarin, which represented a significant bleeding risk for the SDH. ... the deceased was transferred to the ... which was not aware that the deceased had a brain injury while being on warfarin. Later that day, the deceased suffered a catastrophic neurological decline ... A repeat CT scan showed that the SDH had progressed and had caused midline shift of the deceased's brain, with almost total compression of the right ventricle. ... nothing could further be done for the deceased. ... he passed away the next day."

In this case scenario, there was a failure to contact the on-call neurosurgeons for advice or to stop/reverse the warfarin. Thus, it is expected that the expert will confirm negligence in the failure to identify SDH on CT scan, which results in the failure to stop the drug warfarin. Admittedly, the advice if contacted by the on-duty neurosurgeon would be to stop the warfarin and reverse its effects by using the appropriate medications. There is no doubt that if these failures had not existed, the deceased should have survived. Medicolegally, it is obvious that this failure led to the deceased's SDH bleeding again or continuing to bleed, leading to significant neurological impairment and death.

Case 2: A claim settled against a hospital for death of the patient following "delayed diagnosis" of a SDH

A brief case scenario may be as follows: "*The patient, ... was admitted to ... hospital with a headache, blurred vision, ... vomiting, ... and a swollen and droopy left eye. A CT scan took place and was reported to be normal. She was admitted to a medical ward for observation and to await an MRI scan. ... Six days passed by while an MRI scan was awaited. There was no review by the hospital's on-call neurologist. .... Her left pupil was fixed and dilated, ... A CT scan of her head took place but was reported as being normal. ... A repeat CT scan revealed an acute subdural haematoma and the neurosurgical team at another hospital was contacted for advice. ... at another hospital, her pupils were found to be bilaterally fixed and dilated, and ... she had suffered irreversible brain injury. Brain stem tests were performed and her death was confirmed.*"

In this case scenario, there was a failure to consider SDH as an etiology or to refer such patient for neurological opinion for symptoms. Thus, it is expected that the expert report from a consultant radiologist and a consultant physician will confirm negligence regarding the radiological and clinical management of the patient that fall below the appropriate standard. According to the standard management algorithm for SDH, it is crucial to follow an active diagnostic strategy rather than observing the patient because an expanding intracranial lesion causing symptoms and neurological loss can result in a catastrophic outcome. In this case, there was also a radiological failure in the reporting of the study, which should have identified a SDH and prompted a neurosurgical review. Admittedly, the patient could have survived if these failures had not existed. Medicolegally, it is obvious that these errors led to a failure to carry out urgent neurosurgical intervention to prevent further bleeding, resulting in the patient's neurological deterioration and death.

39.3.2 Failure in the Care of Risk Factors

Case 1: A claim settled for failure to monitor platelet count and/or to give fresh frozen plasma for SDH leading to brain damage

A brief case scenario may be as follows: "*A patient presented ... with blood in his urine, a history of recent nose bleeds, petechiae on his legs and arms, ... complete blood count (CBC) showed the patient had an undetectable level of platelets ... hematologists ...were contacted to evaluate ... The patient was diagnosed with... idiopathic thrombocytopenic purpura (ITP) ... The hematologists did not order any platelets ...the patient had no further blood work to check on his platelets. Afterwards, the patient developed a headache ... that increased dramatically, ... leading to vomit, and .. he became lethargic. A CT scan revealed a new SDH... Neurosurgery was called emergently ... for ... evacuation of the blood. ... After he recovered from his operations, he was sent to a rehabilitation hospital ... today he is known to have vision problems and speech and language difficulties.*"

In this case scenario, there was a failure to give platelets for a SDH leading to brain damage. Thus, it is expected that the expert report from a consultant hematologist will confirm negligence regarding treatment of the patient by failing to give fresh frozen plasma and platelet replacement prior to the brain hemorrhage, because of the fact that the platelets of the patient were undetectable upon arrival. It is expected that the hematologist should order fresh frozen plasma and platelets for such a patient with ITP appropriately when the patient is actually having a brain bleed.

39.3.3 Neonatal Premature Babies Undergoing Vacuum Extraction or Forceps-Assisted Deliveries

Case 1: A claim settled for failure to have a CT and electroencephalogram (EEG) for correct diagnosis and proper treatment

A brief case scenario may be as follows: "*A baby with a gestational age of 36 weeks was born vaginally, with vacuum assistance ... A vacuum cup was applied at 500 mmHg and ... Apgar score was 9 at 5 min. At 5 h of age the infant had increasing respiratory distress and ... stopped breathing, endotracheal intubation was applied and the infant was transferred to our tertiary care facility ... On admission haemoglobin and platelets values of the baby had decreased from 15.7 g/dL and to 9.4 g/dL and 69,000, respectively, suggesting consumptive coagulopathy ... Unfortunately, any further investigation was not taken for investigation of coagulopathy. Then, the baby was taken to a tertiary hospital; CT revealed bilateral SDH, an EEG revealed an epileptic focus and the phenobarbitone was continued. ... the infant was extubated on the 12th day of life and was followed with CT..."*

In this case scenario, there was a failure to properly investigate the possibility of SDH using USG, CT, and EEG for treatment of the neonatal baby with a history of use of a vacuum or forceps during the delivery. Thus, it is expected that the expert will confirm negligence for the pediatrician treating the baby in the failure to identify SDH as a cause of coagulopathy, which may cause an epileptic seizure. Medicolegally, it is the duty of the physician to properly investigate the causes of coagulopathy; the failure to promptly diagnose and initiate appropriate management may compromise a baby's outcome. A proper surgical procedure to improve the prognosis is possible if a neurosurgical consultation is obtained in such cases without delay.

39.3.4 "Shaken Baby Syndrome" as a Cause of Bilateral SDH

Case 1: A claim settled against physicians for failure to investigate the possibility of abuse

A brief case scenario may be as follows: "*In January 2019, 2½ month old baby was taken to a community hospital with fever and seizures... The baby was stabilised and sent home, although several cigarette burn marks were noticed on the forearm of the baby. One week later, however, the baby was taken to a tertiary hospital* via *ambulance for further care as he developed progressive hemiparesis and ... In addition to presence of retinal hemorrhages, the CT scan revealed bilateral chronic CSDH, ...resulting in an irreversible brain injury and the report noted that the possibility of SBS was high ... Following further investigation, the baby was removed from his parents care and the child's father was charged with child abuse ...*"

In this case scenario, there was a failure to properly investigate the possibility of abuse during the treatment of the baby. Thus, it is expected that the expert will confirm negligence for the physician seeing the injured baby in their failure to identify SDH on CT scan, which resulted in an irreversible brain injury. There is no doubt that if this failure had not existed, the baby would not have sustained a brain injury. Medicolegally, it is obvious that this failure led to the baby's CSDH, leading to significant neurological impairment. It is the duty of the physician to properly investigate the causes of injuries in such cases in order to prevent such future tragedies, if not to detect the presence of signs of external injuries. Undoubtedly, the failure to promptly diagnose and initiate appropriate management can seriously compromise a baby's outcome, as it did in this baby.

39.4 Comment upon Case Scenarios

As seen in the case scenarios given above, malpractice related to the negligent management of SDH includes missed or delayed diagnosis, mistakes in neurological treatment, delayed treatment, and neurosurgical errors. Unfortunately, the consequences of such cases can be catastrophic and the loss of employment may cause significant financial strain.

World Medical Association (WMA) defines malpractice as "*damage caused by the physician not performing the standard, up-to-date practice during treatment, lack of skills or not giving the treatment to the patient*" [2, 4, 11, 17]. Medicolegally, the attorney (physician) is not responsible for the failure to achieve the result he desired while fulfilling his obligation to treat the subject according to the power of the attorney (physician) contract, but he is responsible for the damages arising from the lack of diligence in his effort, transactions, actions, and behaviors to achieve this result [17]. Importantly, the attorney (physician) has to act with care and is responsible for even the slightest fault [17]. Therefore, all the flaws of the doctor within the profession, even if they are mild, should be considered as an element of responsibility [17]. More importantly, the doctor is obligated to carry out researches to eliminate this hesitation in cases that cause a hesitation, even at a minimum level, and to take protective measures in the meantime [17]. While making a choice between various treatment methods, the characteristics of the patient and their disease should be taken into consideration, avoiding attitudes and behaviors that would put her/his patient at risk, and choosing the safest way [17]. Indeed, the client (the patient) has the right to expect that the attorney (physician), who is a professional doctor, show meticulous care and attention at all stages of the treatment.

In the case scenarios examined under a total of the four headings above, reasons such as delay in diagnosis, inadequacy in radiological and clinical management, failure to take precautions for thrombocytopenia as a result of not being able to evaluate the laboratory results correctly, not being able to predict the development of SDH due to neonatal coagulopathy, and error and delay in diagnosis in SBS have been revealed. The attorney (physician)'s duty is not to act with the guarantee of healing the patient completely. However, the attorney (physician) is obliged to approach her/his patient with care.

39.5 Conclusion

Even today SDH might be mistaken for other clinical conditions because of the high incidence of errors regarding its diagnosis and treatment, leading to potential devastating permanent injuries. Therefore, cases of malpractice regarding the management of SDH, including those with missed or delayed diagnosis and treatment, those with failure in the care for risk factors, neonatal premature babies undergoing vacuum or forceps-assisted deliveries, and those with SBS are frequently encountered. Medicolegally, it is important to know that every physician as an attorney of his/her patient should keep in mind that any negligence, carelessness, and lack of care in any of these stages will cause serious malpractices during the management of cases with SDH.

References

1. Al Wohaibi M, Russell N, Al Ferayan A. A baby with armoured brain. CMAJ. 2003;169:46–7.
2. Arıkan M, Kalkan E, Erdi F, Deniz M, İzci E. The distinction between cases and malpractice-complications in medical law: the perspectives of the senior students of the faculty of medicine and the faculty of law, problems and suggestions for solution (in Turkish). Türk Nöroşir. 2016;26:40–8.
3. Beck J, Gralla J, Fung C, Ulrich CT, Schucht P, Fichtner J, Andereggen L, Gosau M, Hattingen E, Gutbrod K, Z'Graggen WJ, Reinert M, Hüsler J, Ozdoba C, Raabe A. Spinal cerebrospinal fluid leak as the cause of chronic subdural hematomas in nongeriatric patients. J Neurosurg. 2014;121:1380–7.
4. Birtek F. Complication-malpractice distinction in terms of medical interventions (in Turkish). İstanbul Barosu Dergisi. 2007;81:1997–2007.
5. Carroll JJ, Lavine SD, Meyers PM. Imaging of subdural hematomas. Neurosurg Clin N Am. 2017;28:179–203.
6. Catana D, Koziarz A, Cenic A, Nath S, Singh S, Almenawer SA, Kachur E. Subdural hematoma mimickers: a systematic review. World Neurosurg. 2016;93:73–80.
7. Dobran M, Iacoangeli M, Scortichini AR, Mancini F, Benigni R, Nasi D, Gladi M, Scerrati M. Spontaneous chronic subdural hematoma in young adult: the role of missing coagulation facto. G Chir. 2017;38:66–70.
8. Ellis GL. Subdural hematoma in the elderly. Emerg Med Clin North Am. 1990;8:281–94.
9. Gregori F, Colistra D, Mancarella C, Chiarella V, Marotta N, Domenicucci M. Arachnoid cyst in young soccer players complicated by chronic subdural hematoma: personal experience and review of the literature. Acta Neurol Belg. 2020;120:235–46.
10. Grelat M, Madkouri R, Bousquet O. Acute isodense subdural hematoma on computed tomography scan-diagnostic and therapeutic trap: a case report. J Med Case Rep. 2016;10:43.
11. Hakeri H. Distiction between malpractice and complication in medical law (in Turkish). Toraks Cerrahisi Bülteni. 2014;1:23–8.
12. Holl DC, Volovici V, Dirven CMF, Peul WC, van Kooten F, Jellema K, van der Gaag NA, Miah IP, Kho KH, den Hertog HM, Lingsma HF, Dammers R, Dutch Chronic Subdural Hematoma Research Group (DSHR). Pathophysiology and nonsurgical treatment of chronic subdural hematoma: from past to present to future. World Neurosurg. 2018;116:402–411.e2.
13. Iliescu IA. Current diagnosis and treatment of chronic subdural haematomas. J Med Life. 2015;8:278–84.
14. Ingraham FD, Matson DD. Subdural hematoma in infancy. J Pediatr. 1944;25:1–37.
15. Johnson R, Amine A, Farhat H. Spontaneous acute subdural hematoma associated with arachnoid cyst and intra-cystic hemorrhage. Cureus. 2018;10:e3383.
16. Kar SK, Kumar D, Singh P, Upadhyay PK. Psychiatric manifestation of chronic subdural hematoma: the unfolding of mystery in a homeless patient. Indian J Psychol Med. 2015;37:239–42.
17. Kök N. Malpractice and complication distinction. In: Kalkan E, Serel TA, Yılmaz EN, editors. Legal guide for physicians (in Turkish). Ankara: Turkish Neurosurgery Academy Publications No: 1, Sage Publishing; 2018. p. 109–39.
18. Kushner D. Mild traumatic brain injury: toward understanding manifestations and treatment. Arch Intern Med. 1998;158:1617–24.
19. Lynøe N, Elinder G, Hallberg B, Rosén M, Sundgren P, Eriksson A. Insufficient evidence for 'shaken baby syndrome'—a systematic review. Acta Paediatr. 2017;106:1021–7.
20. Martin HA, Woodson A, Christian CW, Helfaer MA, Raghupathi R, Huh JW. Shaken baby syndrome. Crit Care Nurs Clin North Am. 2006;18:279–86.
21. Mian M, Shah J, Dalpiaz A, Schwamb R, Miao Y, Warren K, Khan S. Shaken baby syndrome: a review. Fetal Pediatr Pathol. 2015;34:169–75.
22. Mori K, Yamamoto T, Horinaka N, Maeda M. Arachnoid cyst is a risk factor for chronic subdural hematoma in juveniles: twelve cases of chronic subdural hematoma associated with arachnoid cyst. J Neurotrauma. 2002;19:1017–27.

23. Prajsnar-Borak A, Balak N, Von Pein H, Glaser M, Boor S, Stadie A. Intracranial multiple myeloma may imitate subdural hemorrhage: how to overcome diagnostic limitations and avoid errors in treatment. Neurol Neurochir Pol. 2017;51:252–8.
24. Richards PG, Bertocci GE, Bonshek RE, Giangrande PL, Gregson RM, Jaspan T, Jenny C, Klein N, Lawler W, Peters M, Rorke-Adams LB, Vyas H, Wade A. Shaken baby syndrome. Arch Dis Child. 2006;91:205–6.
25. Santarius T, Kirkpatrick PJ, Ganesan D, Chia HL, Jalloh I, Smielewski P, Richards HK, Marcus H, Parker RA, Price SJ, Kirollos RW, Pickard JD, Hutchinson PJ. Use of drains versus no drains after burr-hole evacuation of chronic subdural haematoma: a randomised controlled trial. Lancet. 2009;374:1067–73.
26. Schmidt L, Gørtz S, Wohlfahrt J, Melbye M, Munch TN. Recurrence of subdural haematoma in a population-based cohort—risks and predictive factors. PLoS One. 2015;10:e0140450.
27. Sieswerda-Hoogendoorn T, Postema FAM, Verbaan D, Majoie CB, van Rijn RR. Age determination of subdural hematomas with CT and MRI: a systematic review. Eur J Radiol. 2014;83:1257–68.
28. Stone JL, Rifai MH, Sugar O, Lang RG, Oldershaw JB, Moody RA. Subdural hematomas. I. Acute subdural hematoma: progress in definition, clinical pathology, and therapy. Surg Neurol. 1983;19:216–31.
29. Tans JT. Computed tomography of extracerebral hematoma. Clin Neurol Neurosurg. 1977;79:296–306.
30. Vinchon M. Shaken baby syndrome: what certainty do we have? Childs Nerv Syst. 2017;33:1727–33.
31. Wu X, Li G, Zhao J, Zhu X, Zhang Y, Hou K. Arachnoid cyst-associated chronic subdural hematoma: report of 14 cases and a systematic literature review. World Neurosurg. 2018;109:e118–30.

Chapter 40
Spinal Subdural Hematomas

Arsal Acarbaş, Alican Tahta, and Mehmet Turgut

40.1 Introduction

Spinal subdural hematoma (SDH) is an infrequent condition where blood clot is located in the spinal subdural space. This entity may cause permanent or temporary neurological deficits by compressing the spinal cord, cauda equina or spinal nerve roots [25]. Therefore, devastating results may occur if spinal SDH is not diagnosed and treated immediately. Spinal SDH was first described by Duverney in 1682 [24] and it constitutes 4.1% of all spinal hematomas. Improvements in imaging methods have increased detection rates of spinal SDHs [25]. Especially in patients with progressive neurological deficits, a rapid diagnosis should be made with appropriate radiological imaging methods and proper treatment should be initiated.

In this chapter, we will review the epidemiology, etiology, pathogenesis, clinical presentation, radiological features, and treatment of spinal SDH in detail.

A. Acarbaş (✉)
Department of Neurosurgery, Mugla Sıtkı Kocman University Faculty of Medicine, Muğla, Turkey

A. Tahta
Department of Neurosurgery, Istanbul Medipol University Faculty of Medicine, Istanbul, Turkey

M. Turgut
Department of Neurosurgery, Aydın Adnan Menderes University Faculty of Medicine, Efeler, Aydın, Turkey

Department of Histology and Embryology, Aydın Adnan Menderes University Health Sciences Institute, Efeler, Aydın, Turkey

M. Turgut et al. (eds.), *Subdural Hematoma*,
https://doi.org/10.1007/978-3-030-79371-5_40

40.2 Epidemiology

Spinal SDH is a rare entity, much more so than spinal epidural hematomas. In a meta-analysis consisting of over 600 spinal hematomas, only 4% of the cases were spinal SDH [13]. Spinal SDH is generally caused by a traumatic event, spinal surgery, or lumbar puncture [4, 8, 23]. Since it is a rare condition and the patients reported in the literature are mostly case reports, its incidence remains unknown.

Notably, there is a small predominance of spontaneous spinal SDH in women (1.25/1) [20]. Spinal SDH has two peaks of incidence throughout life: the first one is between the first and second decades of life and the second one is at 60 years of age [20, 22]. The first peak is related to bleeding caused by hematologic diseases, while the second peak is associated with vascular diseases and anticoagulant therapy [20, 22].

Although there is a substantial affinity for the lower thoracic and lumbar regions for spinal SDHs in the patients between 46–60 years old and 61–75 years old, in children aged less than 15 years, spinal SDH usually occurs in the cervical and cervicothoracic regions of the spine, and in 16- to 30-year-old patients, there is a small predominance of SDHs in the cervical and cervicothoracic regions of the spine [13]. Also, the thoracic region was found to be the most common location for idiopathic spinal SDH (9/21 42.9%) in a review of literature published by Wang et al. [24].

40.3 Etiology

Spinal SDH is generally caused by a traumatic event, spinal surgery, or lumbar puncture, but it may be related to spinal manipulation, called chiropractic therapy [2, 9, 17]. It has been also encountered in patients with various hematologic disorders, spinal cord lesions, neoplasms, or vascular malformations [6, 9, 23]. Spontaneous spinal SDHs are mainly associated with coagulopathies, vascular malformations, and iatrogenic causes [20].

Bleeding abnormalities are frequently the result of impairment of the hemostatic mechanism, such as in classical hemophilia, severe thrombocytopenia, acute leukemia, polycythemia vera, and bleeding diathesis [4, 22]. In addition to pregnancy and eclampsia, many rheumatologic diseases including ankylosing spondylitis, rheumatoid arthritis, and systemic lupus erythematosus and congenital connective tissue and renal diseases such as fibromuscular dysplasia, cystic fibrosis, and polycystic kidneys are reported to be risk factors for spinal SDH in the literature [5, 6, 22]. In the vast majority of cases of spontaneous spinal SDH, an underlying hematologic or iatrogenic cause can be identified [7, 9, 25]. However, most patients have no identifiable cause which is called idiopathic spinal SDH; therefore, further investigation is necessary in these cases to determine the correct diagnosis [7, 9, 25]. Spinal SDH has been reported that is located in the thoracic region of the spine, involving more than one vertebral level [20]. Various hematologic diseases with coagulopathies and the use of anticoagulant therapy were responsible in nearly half of all patients with spinal SDH [22, 25].

40.4 Pathogenesis

Anatomically, the spinal subdural space has no bridging veins, in contrast to its intracranial counterpart [3]. The pathogenesis of spinal SDH is not clear because of the absence of bridging veins, which are usually implicated in the development of intracranial SDH, within the spinal canal [22]. It has been suggested that the hemorrhage in cases of spinal SDH may be related to perforation of vessels within the subarachnoid space following the Valsalva maneuver, which is associated with an increased intra-abdominal and intra-thoracic pressure [8]. Based on their experiences, some authors have noted that the cerebrospinal fluid (CSF) pressure was equal to the pressure in the extradural venous plexus, suggesting the existence of a close association of increased intrathecal pressure with high pressure in the extradural venous plexus [1, 9, 13, 19, 20, 22].

It is important to realize that any hemorrhage from the vessels within the subarachnoid space is diluted by CSF, preventing the development of a solid hematoma in the spinal canal [22]. Interestingly, there are rare case reports with spinal subarachnoid hemorrhage (SAH) coexisting with spinal SDH in the literature [18, 22]. In these cases, it is accepted that any hemorrhage within the subarachnoid space may perforate into the subdural space in the presence of a higher volume of blood [22]. Also, any hemorrhage in cases with spinal SDH may be related to the perforation of fine vessels on the dural surface [11]. Therefore it is not easy to determine the source of the hemorrhage in cases with spinal SDH involving the subarachnoid space or subdural space [22]. Other theories, including intradural migration from the upper intracranial space or clival region to lower areas in the spine, have also been investigated extensively [3, 16]. Moreover, there are case reports with spinal SDH occurring due to a strong back massage and paraspinal muscle needling in the literature [9, 17].

In general, there is a multifactorial etiology in most of the cases of spinal SDH, but the exact cause of the hemorrhage cannot be identified in 29.7% of these cases which are known as idiopathic spinal SDH [13]. Furthermore, spinal SDH may be related to the use of anticoagulant therapy, the presence of any congenital vascular malformation, and epidural spinal anesthetic procedures associated with anticoagulants [4, 13, 15, 23]. It is widely accepted that there should be "locus minoris resistentiae" in combination with an increased pressure in the interior vertebral venous plexus and/or oral anticoagulant therapy for the development of spontaneous spinal SDH [13]. Therefore, indications for the use of spinal anesthetic procedures in cases receiving anticoagulant drugs should be restricted and close follow-up of these patients is necessary [13]. It has been concluded that the following precautions should be considered to prevent the development of spinal SDHs: (a) careful patient selection; (b) non-traumatic lumbar puncture; (c) time interval of at least 1 h between spinal anesthesia and heparinization protocol; and (d) follow-up of hematologic coagulation parameters [13].

40.5 Clinical Presentation

According to a review of the literature, the most frequent initial symptoms in 63% of patients with spinal SDH are back pain and interscapular pain, but headache as an initial symptom is rarely seen in such cases [1, 3, 13]. Patients with spinal SDH presents with intense, stabbing pain at the location of the hemorrhage, called "coup de poignard," which may be short term in duration but then a progressive paralysis below the affected spinal level will develop. Interestingly, meningitis symptoms, loss of consciousness, and epilepsy may also develop, if there is an associated SAH, leading to a misdiagnosis of the intracerebral hematoma [13].

Spinal SDH may present with rapidly progressive neurological symptoms [6]. Clinically, symptoms in patients with spinal SDH may simulate those of spinal cord injury, spinal cord compression, or cauda equina syndrome [22]. Spinal SDH often presents initially with back pain and/or radicular pain [22]. As a rule, neurological symptoms may be different according to the level of the spinal SDH, monosegmental or multisegmental, from one segment to seven segments according to the extent of the hemorrhage [14, 23]. Similarly, the time interval from the initial symptoms to the onset severe neurologic deficits may be different occurring from over a few hours to 3 weeks [14]. On the other hand, the degree of neurological deficit (motor, sensory, or sphincter dysfunction) may vary from a mild monoparesis to quadriplegia [14]. Despite current imaging techniques, it is possible to overlook the correct diagnosis in asymptomatic patients with spinal SDH [18].

40.6 Radiological Findings

Anatomically, spinal epidural hematomas are frequently localized in the posterior aspect of the spinal canal and the vast majority of spinal epidural hematomas occur in the cervicothoracic and thoracolumbar regions of the spine because vulnerable portions of the epidural venous plexus are also located in the same aspect of the spinal canal [16, 21]. Spinal SDHs occur within the dural sac; therefore, unlike epidural hematomas, the epidural fat is preserved and the dura is not displaced inward [21]. It is bounded by the paired lateral denticulate ligaments and the dorsal septum, forming the inverted Mercedes-Benz sign on axial images [12, 21]. As such, the SDH compresses the nerve roots but does not extend into the neural foramina or make direct contact with bone. Smaller collections do not expand the potential subdural space; therefore, they do not cause the inverted Mercedes-Benz sign [16, 21].

40.7 Computed Tomography

Computed tomography (CT) is the workhorse of emergency medicine and is usually utilized before magnetic resonance imaging (MRI) for emergencies. However, spinal SDHs can easily be missed in the acute setting, especially if they are small. After having identified a spinal SDH on MRI, it is good practice to review the CT study and use a narrow window in an attempt to identify the hematoma. Moreover, revisiting the CT study can sometimes help clarify the diagnosis. A crescentic hyperdense collection may be observed as adhering to the inner edge of the dura mater, separated from the hypodense epidural fat [21].

40.8 Magnetic Resonance Imaging

MRI is the best of choice of imaging modality in the diagnosis of spinal cord injuries, including spinal SDH and other spinal cord pathologies. MRI is the standard modality for both identification and characterization of spinal SDHs [10, 19, 21]. Signal characteristics vary depending on the age of the blood and can be identified chronologically: the hyperacute SDH is iso/hypointense on T1-weighted images and hyperintense on T2-weighted images, the acute SDH is mildly hypo-/isointense on T1-weighted images and hypointense on T2-weighted images. The early subacute SDH is hyperintense on T1-weighted images and hypointense on T2-weighted images and the late subacute SDH is hyperintense on T1-weighted and T2-weighted images. The chronic SDH is generally hypointense on T1-weighted and T2-weighted images [16, 25]. The previously described "Y" shaped sign (Inverted Mercedes Benz sign) is a result of the encasement of blood around an arachnoid lined neural structure and is useful in making the diagnosis of an epidural hematoma from a subdural one [16, 21]. After having confirmed the location of the collection as subdural on axial images, sagittal images can be utilized for detecting its extent. As a rule, the hemorrhagic lesion with a liquid nature should be considered if it has the contour of the compressed arachnoid mater similar to two convex discs in apposition to each other in the sagittal projections of the MRI, in particular for those located in a dependent area (L5-S1) [16, 21]. However, intradural lymphomas generally have a fusiform or sausage shape, but they may demonstrate any shape [16, 18, 21].

40.9 Treatment

As a rule, the neurological examination of the patient is important in order to choose a treatment option for these lesions [1]. There are no definite guidelines for management [8, 22, 23]. Some reports have suggested that treatment involves conservative management with serial MRIs, but others have advocated for a decompressive surgical technique, including removal of the lamina, in patients with spinal SDH, although there is no clinical improvement in some cases after the surgical decompression [18, 19, 23, 25].

Proposed treatments for spinal SDH include both operative and nonoperative options, in addition to lumbar puncture [1]. Some authors reported successful results with conservative treatment in patients presenting with a large clival SDH and spinal extension [1, 22, 25]. But overall, many authors have suggested that surgical decompression, consisting of laminectomy and removal of the hematoma, must be performed without delay for patients with compression due to a spinal SDH with progressive neurological deterioration [2, 13, 24]. The neurological status at presentation is the strongest predictor of outcome [13, 23]. According to our practice, surgical intervention is the best option for reversing the neurological deficits in patients with spinal SDHs. The main aim of surgery is to improve the quality of life by relief of pain and the restoration of neurological functions. Decompressive laminectomy with a mid-line dural opening and evacuation of the SDH should be performed [13]. In cases with SDH with posterior localization and without any coagulopathy, percutaneous drainage may be an alternative therapy [14, 22]. Some authors suggest that the timing of the operation should be immediate and some others recommend normalizing or at least improving coagulation values preoperatively [8, 13, 18].

40.10 Illustrative Case

A 29-year-old pregnant woman underwent an emergency C-section operation with spinal anesthesia for preeclampsia. One day later, perimesencephalic SAH was detected on the cranial CT examination, which was performed because of headache, numbness in the left arm, and neck stiffness. Cranial, cervical, and thoracic spinal MRIs were urgently scheduled based upon the complaint of increasing headache and onset of numbness in the legs 20 min after CT examination. The procedure was terminated due to acute paraplegia while the patient was in the MRI scanner. After the cervical and thoracic spinal MRI revealed a massive SDH extending from the clivus to the T10 level, and a subdural nidal appearance (arteriovenous malformation?) anterior to the spinal cord at the C6-C7 level, the patient was taken into the operating room under emergent conditions (Fig. 40.1). A C6 and C7 total laminectomy was performed. When the dura was incised, SDH was identified surrounding the entire cord. A dense hematoma localized anterior to the spinal cord at the C6-C7 level was removed. No vascular nidus was found at this level. On the post-op neurological examination of the patient, no abnormal findings were observed except for the left triceps having 3/5 muscle strength. No deficits were detected in the patient's neurological examination at the 1 month follow-up.

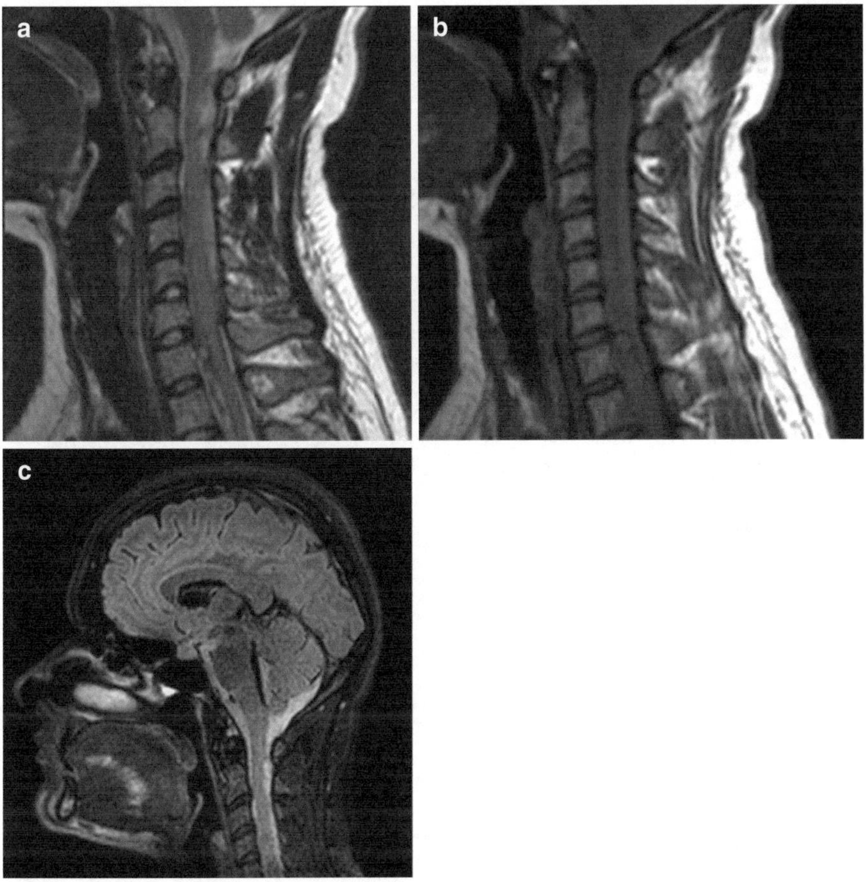

Fig. 40.1 (**a**) On T2W images, a dorsally located hyperintense collection was detected. (**b**) On T1W images, the signal of the entire subdural space (both anterior and posterior to spinal cord) has increased due to subdural hematoma, and the bleeding is observed down to the T10 level. (**c**) On FLAIR images, the signal of the entire subdural space has increased from the clivus and cisterna magna down to the T10 level

40.11 Conclusion

Selection of a proper treatment algorithm for spinal SDH is challenging because it is a rare neurosurgical entity. In particular, spontaneous spinal SDH is an extremely rare condition and is less common in the absence of an identifiable etiology. Even today spinal SDH remain poorly understood. If spinal SDH is suspected, the first choice of radiological imaging method should be MRI. Even if some other treatments are considered, surgical decompression should be the first treatment modality. Especially, if the neurological examination of patient demonstrates progressive worsening, the surgeon must consider decompression.

References

1. Ahn ES, Smith ER. Acute clival and spinal subdural hematoma with spontaneous resolution: clinical and radiographic correlation in support of a proposed pathophysiological mechanism: case report. J Neurosurg. 2005;103:175–9.
2. Benyaich Z, Laghmari M, Lmejjati M, Aniba K, Ghannane H, Benali SA. Acute lumbar spinal subdural hematoma inducing paraplegia after lumbar spinal manipulation: case report and literature review. World Neurosurg. 2019;128:182–5.
3. Bortolotti C, Wang H, Fraser K, Lanzino G. Subacute spinal subdural hematoma after spontaneous resolution of cranial subdural hematoma: causal relationship or coincidence?: case report. J Neurosurg Spine. 2004;100:372–4.
4. Cha Y-H, Chi JH, Barbaro NM. Spontaneous spinal subdural hematoma associated with low-molecular-weight heparin: case report. J Neurosurg Spine. 2005;2:612–3.
5. Esfahani DR, Shah HP, Behbahani M, Arnone GD, Mehta AI. Spinal subdural hematoma and ankylosing spondylitis: case report and review of literature. Spinal Cord Ser Cases. 2018;4:1–5.
6. Gabl M, Kostron H. Acute spinal subdural haematoma. Neurochirurgia. 1988;31:99–100.
7. Hsieh JK, Colby S, Nichols D, Kondylis E, Liu JK. Delayed development of spinal subdural hematoma following cranial trauma: a case report and review of the literature. World Neurosurg. 2020;141:44–51.
8. Hung K-S, Lui C-C, Wang C-H, Wang C-J, Howng S-L. Traumatic spinal subdural hematoma with spontaneous resolution. Spine. 2002;27:E534–8.
9. Ji GY, Oh CH, Choi W-S, Lee J-B. Three cases of hemiplegia after cervical paraspinal muscle needling. Spine J. 2015;15:e9–e13.
10. Johnson P, Hahn F, McConnell J, Graham E, Leibrock L. The importance of MRI findings for the diagnosis of nontraumatic lumbar subacute subdural haematomas. Acta Neurochir (Wien). 1991;113:186–8.
11. Kakitsubata Y, Theodorou SJ, Theodorou DJ, Miyata Y, Ito Y, Yuki Y, Honbu K, Maehara T. Spontaneous spinal subarachnoid hemorrhage associated with subdural hematoma at different spinal levels. Emerg Radiol. 2010;17:69–72.
12. Kasliwal MK, Shannon LR, O'Toole JE, Byrne RW. Inverted Mercedes Benz sign in lumbar spinal subdural hematoma. J Emerg Med. 2014;47:692–3.
13. Kreppel D, Antoniadis G, Seeling W. Spinal hematoma: a literature survey with meta-analysis of 613 patients. Neurosurg Rev. 2003;26:1–49.
14. Kyriakides AE, Lalam RK, El Masry WS. Acute spontaneous spinal subdural hematoma presenting as paraplegia: a rare case. Spine. 2007;32:E619–22.
15. Maddali P, Walker B, Fisahn C, Page J, Diaz V, Zwillman ME, Oskouian RJ, Tubbs RS, Moisi M. Subdural thoracolumbar spine hematoma after spinal anesthesia: a rare occurrence and literature review of spinal hematomas after spinal anesthesia. Cureus. 2017;9:e1032.
16. Manish K, Chandrakant S, Abhay M. Spinal subdural haematoma. J Orthop Case Rep. 2015;5:72–4.
17. Maste P, Paik S-H, Oh J-K, Kim Y-C, Park M-S, Kim T-H, Kwak Y-H, Jung J-K, Lee H-W, Kim SW. Acute spinal subdural hematoma after vigorous back massage: a case report and review of literature. Spine. 2014;39:E1545–8.
18. Mavroudakis N, Levivier M, Rodesch G. Central cord syndrome due to a spontaneously regressive spinal subdural hematoma. Neurology. 1990;40:1306.
19. Park YJ, Kim SW, Ju CI, Wang HS. Spontaneous resolution of non-traumatic cervical spinal subdural hematoma presenting acute hemiparesis: a case report. Korean J Spine. 2012;9:257.
20. Pereira BJA, de Almeida AN, Muio VMF, de Oliveira JG, de Holanda CVM, Fonseca NC. Predictors of outcome in nontraumatic spontaneous acute spinal subdural hematoma: case report and literature review. World Neurosurg. 2016;89:574–7.
21. Pierce JL, Donahue JH, Nacey NC, Quirk CR, Perry MT, Faulconer N, Falkowski GA, Maldonado MD, Shaeffer CA, Shen FH. Spinal hematomas: what a radiologist needs to know. Radiographics. 2018;38:1516–35.

22. Rettenmaier LA, Holland MT, Abel TJ. Acute, nontraumatic spontaneous spinal subdural hematoma: a case report and systematic review of the literature. Case Rep Neurol Med. 2017;2017:2431041.
23. Thiex R, Thron A, Gilsbach JM, Rohde V. Functional outcome after surgical treatment of spontaneous and nonspontaneous spinal subdural hematomas. J Neurosurg Spine. 2005;3:12–6.
24. Wang Y, Zheng H, Ji Y, Lu Q, Li X, Jiang X. Idiopathic spinal subdural hematoma: case report and review of the literature. World Neurosurg. 2018;116:378–82.
25. Yokota K, Kawano O, Kaneyama H, Maeda T, Nakashima Y. Acute spinal subdural hematoma: a case report of spontaneous recovery from paraplegia. Medicine. 2020;99:e20032.

Conclusion

Subdural hematomas (SDHs), with the exception of those located in the spine, are a common neurosurgical disease entity where the management is still a point of discussion due to the evolving medical and surgical therapeutic options that have become available. Because of the increasing life expectancy of elderly patients and the widespread use of anticoagulant therapy, the incidence of SDHs is increasing worldwide. The various forms of intracranial and intraspinal SDHs that are considered acute, subacute, and chronic in nature will influence the clinical presentation and direct the form of therapeutic management that is pursued. The clinical presentation of patients with SDHs will determine which type of diagnostic neuroimaging study is performed, whether it be computed tomography or magnetic resonance imaging, which will help to better delineate the location, extent, and in some cases the etiology of the hemorrhagic collection. The clinical history of the patient can occasionally provide valuable information that can yield an explanation for the SDH development such as in the case of electroconvulsive therapy, lumbar puncture, cerebrospinal fluid diversion, spontaneous intracranial hypotension, anticoagulant therapy, head trauma, or a sports-related injury.

The management of SDHs is still primarily surgical and is intended to relieve the intracranial or intraspinal mass effect and pressure on the brain or spinal cord although less invasive techniques that include endoscopy or meningeal artery embolization have been added to the neurosurgeon's armamentarium. In a similar fashion, medical management of SDHs has advanced through the use of corticosteroid therapy, atorvastatin, and tranexamic acid. Despite the best medical efforts, complications still can occur that lead to hematoma recurrence and repeat drainage.

M. Turgut et al. (eds.), *Subdural Hematoma*,
https://doi.org/10.1007/978-3-030-79371-5

Rehabilitation therapy is an essential part of patient recovery due to the preponderance of elderly patients that develop SDHs. Medicolegal concerns are centered around diagnostic and treatment errors in adults and non-accidental trauma in children.

Aydın, Turkey Mehmet Turgut, MD, PhD
Marrakech, Morocco Ali Akhaddar, MD, IFAANS
Syracuse, NY, USA Walter A. Hall, MD, MBA
Ankara, Turkey Ahmet T. Turgut, MD

Index

M. Turgut et al. (eds.), *Subdural Hematoma*,
https://doi.org/10.1007/978-3-030-79371-5

GPSR Compliance

The European Union's (EU) General Product Safety Regulation (GPSR) is a set of rules that requires consumer products to be safe and our obligations to ensure this.

If you have any concerns about our products, you can contact us on ProductSafety@springernature.com

In case Publisher is established outside the EU, the EU authorized representative is:

Springer Nature Customer Service Center GmbH
Europaplatz 3
69115 Heidelberg, Germany

Batch number: 10777430

Printed by Printforce, the Netherlands